Upper Extremity Injuries in the Athlete

Upper Extremity Injuries in the Athlete

Edited by

Arthur M. Pappas, M.D.

Professor and Chairman
Department of Orthopedics and Physical Rehabilitation
University of Massachusetts Medical School
Worcester, Massachusetts
Medical Director
Boston Red Sox Baseball Team
Boston, Massachusetts

In Association With

Janet Walzer, M.Ed.

Editor
Department of Orthopedics and Physical Rehabilitation
University of Massachusetts Medical School
Worcester, Massachusetts

Churchill Livingstone

New York, Edinburgh, London, Madrid, Melbourne, Milan, Tokyo

Library of Congress Cataloging-in-Publication Data

Upper extremity injuries in the athlete / edited by Arthur M. Pappas,
    in association with Janet Walzer.
        p.   cm.
    Includes bibliographical references and index.
    ISBN 0–443–08836–5
    1.   Arm—Wounds and injuries.   2. Sports injuries.   I. Pappas,
Arthur M.   II. Walzer, Janet.
    [DNLM: 1. Arm Injuries—diagnosis.   2. Arm Injuries—therapy.
3. Athletic   Injuries.   4. Arm—physiologogy.   WE 805 U686 1995]
    RD557.U674 1995
    617.5'7'0088796—dc20
    DNLM/DLC
    for Library of Congress   94–33757
                                                                CIP

© Churchill Livingstone Inc. 1995

Distributed in the United Kingdom by Churchill Livingstone, Robert Stevenson House, 1–3 Baxter's Place, Leith Walk, Edinburgh EH1 3AF, and by associated companies, branches, and representatives throughout the world.

Accurate indications, adverse reactions, and dosage schedules for drugs are provided in this book, but it is possible that they may change. The reader is urged to review the package information data of the manufacturers of the medications mentioned.

The Publishers have made every effort to trace the copyright holders for borrowed material. If they have inadvertently overlooked any, they will be pleased to make the necessary arrangements at the first opportunity.

Acquisitions Editor: *Jennifer Mitchell*
Assistant Editor: *Carol Bader*
Copy Editor: *Bridgett L. Dickinson*
Production Supervisor: *Sharon Tuder*
Cover Design: *Paul Moran*

Production services provided by Bermedica Production, Ltd.

Printed in the United States of America

First published in 1995   7   6   5   4   3   2   1

Contributors

R. Maxwell Alley, M.D.
Capital Region Orthopaedic Associates, Albany, New York

William B. Balcom, M.D.
Norwich Orthopedic Group, Norwich, Connecticut

Thomas F. Breen, M.D.
Assistant Professor, Department of Orthopedics and Physical Rehabilitation, University of Massachusetts Medical School, Worcester, Massachusetts

Brian D. Busconi, M.D.
Sports Medicine Fellow, Department of Orthopedics and Physical Rehabilitation, University of Massachusetts Medical School, Worcester, Massachusetts

James M. Coumas, M.D.
Department of Radiology, Carolinas Medical Center, Charlotte, North Carolina

Nancy M. Cummings, M.D.
Instructor, Department of Orthopedic Surgery, Harvard Medical School; Department of Orthopedic Surgery, Beth Israel Hospital, Boston, Massachusetts

Kathleen A. Curtis, Ph.D., P.T.
Assistant Professor, Division of Physical Therapy, Department of Orthopaedics and Rehabilitation, University of Miami School of Medicine, Coral Gables, Florida

Richard Diana, M.D.
New Haven Orthopedic Group, Hamden, Connecticut

Dudley A. Ferrari, M.D.
Assistant Professor, Department of Orthopedics and Physical Rehabilitation, University of Massachusetts Medical School, Worcester, Massachusetts

Thomas P. Goss, M.D.
Professor, Department of Orthopedics and Physical Rehabilitation, University of Massachusetts Medical School, Worcester, Massachusetts

Randall R. Long, M.D., Ph.D.
Associate Professor, Department of Neurology, University of Massachusetts Medical School, Worcester, Massachusetts

Claire F. McCarthy, P.T., M.S.
Director of Physical and Occupational Therapy, Children's Hospital, Boston, Massachusetts

William J. Morgan, M.D.
Associate Professor, Department of Orthopedics and Physical Rehabilitation, University of Massachusetts Medical School, Worcester, Massachusetts; Hand Surgical Consultant, Boston Red Sox Baseball Team and Boston Celtics Basketball Team, Boston, Massachusetts

Arthur M. Pappas, M.D.
Professor and Chairman, Department of Orthopedics and Physical Rehabilitation, University of Massachusetts Medical School, Worcester, Massachusetts; Medical Director, Boston Red Sox Baseball Team, Boston, Massachusetts

Terry F. Reardon, M.D.
Orthopedic Associates of Middletown, Middletown, Connecticut

Michael J. Rohrer, M.D.
Assistant Professor, Division of Vascular Surgery, Department of Surgery, University of Massachusetts Medical School, Worcester, Massachusetts

Lisa A. Schulz, O.T.R./L., C.H.T.
Department of Orthopedics and Physical Rehabilitation, University of Massachusetts Medical School, Worcester, Massachusetts

Robert S. Skerker, M.D.
Morristown Memorial Hospital, The Rehabilitation Institute, Morristown, New Jersey

John Vitolo, M.D.
Northwest Jersey Orthopedics, Madison, New Jersey

Janet Walzer, M.Ed.
Editor, Department of Orthopedics and Physical Rehabilitation, University of Massachusetts Medical School, Worcester, Massachusetts

Richard M. Zawacki, P.T., M.S.
Boston Red Sox Baseball Team, Boston, Massachusetts

Foreword

In his new book, *Upper Extremity Injuries in the Athlete,* Dr. Arthur Pappas has made an excellent and timely contribution to the literature on the diagnosis and treatment of athletic injuries. This work is a very thoughtful summation of Dr. Pappas' years of experience in treating high performance, recreational, and adolescent athletes, particularly those involved with overhead throwing activities. He not only conveys to the reader his own vast experience, which has come from years of careful physical examination and thoughtful observation, but also succinctly and appropriately addresses the value and limitations of the new technologies available to the health care professional for the diagnosis and treatment of these difficult problems.

The general outline of this book flows in a meaningful way. The sections on anatomy and physical diagnosis are particularly pertinent. Dr. Pappas stresses the importance of understanding the biomechanics of throwing to better appreciate the stresses placed on the neurovascular structures of the upper extremities as well as the capsular and ligamentous supports. His thoughtful approach to diagnosis is supplemented by his clear indications for special diagnostic tests, such as arthrograms, magnetic resonance imaging, computed tomography, and bone scans.

Perhaps one of the most helpful messages in this book is the approach to rehabilitation of these injuries. He emphatically outlines the need to educate the injured athlete about what the patient will need to do to return to a functional level of activity and then stresses the need to involve parents, coaches, and trainers, as well as physical therapists, in the various stages of the rehabilitation process.

Upper Extremity Injuries in the Athlete should be available on the book shelves in all athletic training rooms and will prove to be of great value to all physicians, orthopedic surgeons, trainers, and physical therapists who see and treat both competitive and recreational athletes.

Arthur L. Boland, M.D., P.C.
Head Surgeon
Harvard University Athletic Department
Chief
Department of Orthopedics
Harvard University Health Sciences
Boston, Massachusetts

Worces

C
Di

Preface

Upper Extremity Injuries in the Athlete is directed to all health care professionals who provide advice and care to patients with athletic injuries. The scope and significance of upper extremity injuries in the athlete are reflected in the range of those who seek care. From the weekend tennis player to the professional baseball player, each has individual anatomic and clinical characteristics. The approach and goal is the same for every athlete regardless of the level or skill: a successful return to sport.

The purpose of this text is to provide the health care professional with the anatomic and pathologic basis of specific injuries along with the details of diagnosis and appropriate treatment. This information is conveyed through case studies and by relevant illustrations. Realistic situations are outlined using a wide range of athletic activities and skill levels.

The first section, *Principles of Evaluation and Care of the Upper Extremity,* provides general principles of evaluation in the care of the upper extremity injury with a progression to specific populations. The next four sections follow a regional sequence with the first chapters of each section focusing on anatomy and function, followed by information on acute and chronic injuries.

Although operative treatment is necessary in certain cases, the emphasis is on the importance of conditioning and rehabilitation to prevent injury and re-injury. It is hoped that this particular focus will provide new information for the health care professional and thereby benefit the athlete with an upper extremity injury.

Arthur M. Pappas, M.D.
Janet Walzer, M.Ed.

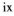

Acknowledgments

The editors gratefully acknowledge and appreciate the following individuals for their contributions and commitment to *Upper Extremity Injuries in the Athlete:* the contributing authors; Joy Marlowe for her artwork; Richard Waite, M.D., for his assistance in interpreting radiologic images; Caroline Kuzia, Karen Lawton, and Linda Olsen for their word processing; and Charlene Baron and Biomedical Media, University of Massachusetts Medical Center for their technical assistance and photography.

Contents

Color plates follow page 214.

1

Diagnostic Imaging

James M. Coumas

The anatomic complexity of the upper extremity mandates strong communication between the athletic patient and the referring physician; the physician must then transfer this information to the radiologist. This line of communication is critical in determining the appropriate imaging technique or sequence of radiographs to be used in the diagnostic examination. This chapter outlines the principal radiologic modalities used in the evaluation of the upper extremity and provides insight into common applications, individual strengths or limitations of specific modalities, and cost-effective utilization.

PLAIN FILM RADIOGRAPHY

Plain film radiographs (conventional roentgenography) are essential in the evaluation of upper extremity sports disability. The plain film radiograph is a survey that provides the physician with valuable information, ranging from the integrity of the articulation by its bony and soft tissue components to the extent of immobilization, characterized by its degree of osteopenia. It is essential to evaluate any musculoskeletal area in at least two tangential planes. Routine views in the evaluation of the shoulder should include an image in the anteroposterior (AP) projection in internal and external rotation and an image in the axillary or Y projection (Fig. 1-1).

Plain film radiographs are particularly helpful in the evaluation of trauma, including fracture or dislocation,

and inflammatory processes such as calcific tendinitis, bursitis, inflammatory arthropathy, and instability. Plain film radiographs are the most cost-effective initial approach to diagnostic imaging. While they may not always provide the total amount of information required, they will often indicate which additional technique(s) will be most helpful and how the examination should be performed for a complete evaluation. The limitations of the plain film radiograph are its static rather than dynamic evaluation, and its inability to accurately assess soft tissue injury. In many cases, plain films alone may not provide sufficient information to guide surgical repair. This is best exemplified in the wrist where evaluation of instability is accomplished dynamically by using fluoroscopy with videotape recording (Fig. 1-2).

A number of special views that augment the routine radiographs are available at each articulation to further investigate various anatomic and/or functional components. Table 1-1 lists those views most helpful in upper extremity imaging.

ARTHROGRAPHY

Through the years, multiple imaging techniques have evolved that, along with plain film radiographs, contribute to the assessment of musculoskeletal disability. For example, shoulder arthrography has existed since 1939 when Lindblom[1] performed single-contrast arthrograms to document ruptures of the rotator cuff.

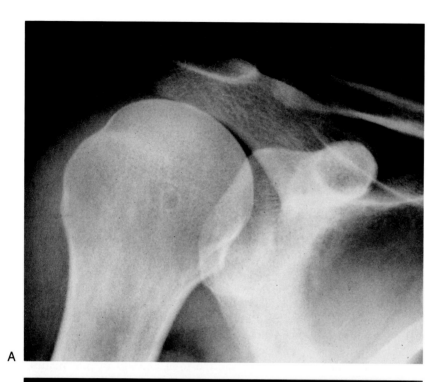

A

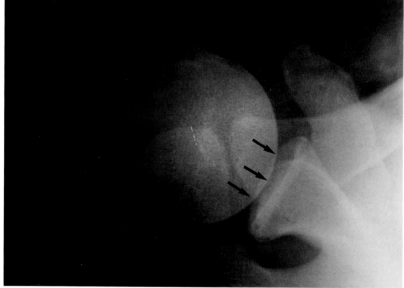

B

Figure 1-1 Plain film radiographs. **(A)** AP view of the shoulder in neutral position allows for evaluation of arthritis, calcific tendinitis/bursitis, chronic rotator cuff disease and neoplastic processes. **(B)** Axial view is extremely helpful in the evaluation of subluxation/dislocation, joint congruence *(arrows),* and degenerative processes about the glenohumeral articulation. Together tangential views complement one another and provide a more effective survey of any articulating joint. *(Figure continues.)*

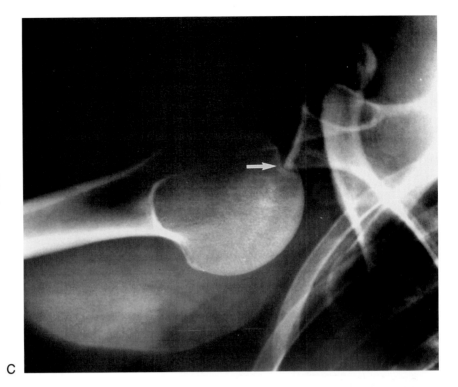

Figure 1-1 *(Continued)* **(C)** Modified axial view of anteriorly and inferiorly dislocated humeral head with associated Hill-Sachs defect *(arrows).*

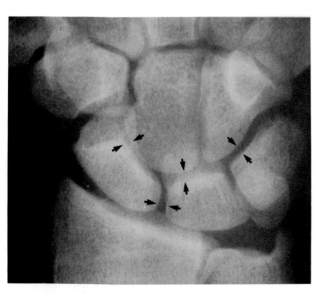

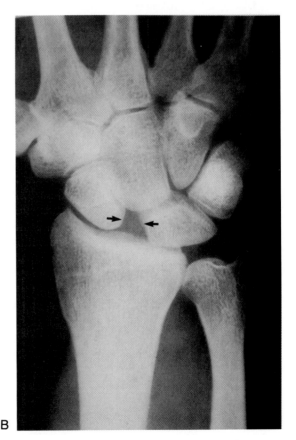

Figure 1-2 Stress radiograph of the wrist. **(A)** Symmetric intercarpal distance and alignment in the normal wrist *(arrows).* **(B)** Stress film in the "clenched fist" position documents widening of the scapholunate intercarpal distance *(arrows)* and ligamentous injury.

Table 1-1   Additional Plain Film Views

Articulation	View/Projection	Anatomy Evaluated
Wrist	AP compression view	Subluxation of carpal bones
	PA oblique with radial flexion	Scaphoid trauma
	PA with ulnar deviation	Scaphoid trauma
	Lateral oblique view	Scaphoid trauma
	Ulnar oblique view (supinated oblique view)	Pisiform and pisitriquetral joint
	Carpal tunnel view	Hook of hamate; trapezium; pisiform
Elbow	Radial head, capitellum view	Radial head; capitellum; coronoid process
	Ulnar sulcus view (ulnar notch view)	Olecranon; epicondyles; ulna notch
Shoulder	West point view	Glenohumeral alignment anterior interior glenoid rim; posterior acromion
	Transthoracic view	Glenohumeral alignment
	AP oblique view	Osteophytes from inferior acromion and distal clavicle
	Didiee view (PA or AP axial)	Hill-Sachs defect
	45° Stryker view	Glenoid and glenoid cavity
	Bicipital groove view	Configuration of bicipital groove
	Scapula AP view	Entire scapula
	Lateral scapula view	Body of scapula; coracoid process; acromium

AP, anteroposterior; PA, posteroanterior.

A single-contrast technique using iodinated contrast material alone, or double-contrast arthrography with the addition of air, may be employed. In either case, evaluation of the intra-articular components is performed by providing a radiopaque coating to the joint's inner structures and subsequent distention of the joint capsule.

At present, most upper extremity arthrography performed is double-contrast, with the exception of single-contrast arthrography of the wrist. In certain cases of adhesive capsulitis of the shoulder, therapeutic distention and lysis of the adhesions is attempted by manipulating the controlled force of fluid hydraulics associated with single-contrast arthrography.

In the shoulder, arthrography can be used in the evaluation of full and partial rotator cuff tears, adhesive capsulitis, cartilage defects, biceps tendon tears, radiolucent loose bodies, and assessment of the rotator cuff after surgical repair (Fig. 1-3). In the past, air-only shoulder arthrography was used for patients with documented iodinated contrast allergic reactions; magnetic resonance imaging now fills that role.

Indications for arthrographic evaluation of the elbow parallel those of the shoulder, with emphasis on the assessment of post-traumatic abnormalities. Abnormalities of the elbow, such as loose bodies, osteochondritis dissecans focusing on the integrity of overlying cartilage, synovial proliferation, and capsular integrity,

are well demonstrated on both single- and double-contrast elbow arthrography[2] (Fig. 1-4).

For the wrist, arthrography is most frequently performed in cases of persistent pain or limited movement following trauma. It is generally coupled with fluoroscopic videotape recording for optimal evaluation of the integrity of the intrinsic carpal ligaments both statically and dynamically. The lack of tendon or muscular attachments to the proximal carpal bones is unique and ensures a strong dependence on intact intrinsic intercarpal ligaments for stability. At present, a three-compartment sequential wrist arthrogram is obtained for complete evaluation of the distal radioulnar joint, midcarpal joint, and radiocarpal joint complexes[3] (Fig. 1-5). Digital subtraction imaging has also been advocated as an enhancement to wrist arthrography.

Limitations of arthrography are well documented in the literature. False-negative studies have been reported in cases of scar formation in full-thickness rotator cuff tears of the shoulder or incomplete tears limited to the bursal aspect of the rotator cuff.[4] Similarly, false-negative studies have been reported in cases of intrinsic carpal ligament injury with subsequent adhesion and scar formation.[3] Another disadvantage of arthrography is the requisite introduction of a needle into the joint space, thus classifying it as an invasive technique.

The improved intra-articular visualization associated with distention of the joint capsule, whether by

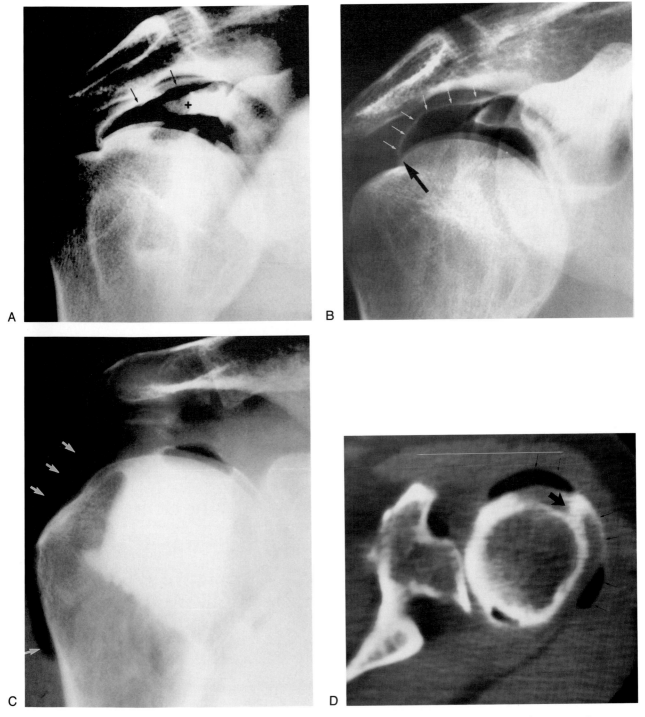

Figure 1-3 Shoulder arthrography. **(A)** Normal shoulder in external rotation shows a sharp continuous coating of contrast material to the undersurface of the rotator cuff *(arrows)*. The longhead of the biceps tendon is also well shown in external rotation (+). **(B)** Normal shoulder in internal rotation shows the posterior component of the rotator cuff in tangent. No imbibition of contrast material into the cuff is noted to suggest a tear *(white arrows)*. Note the normal insertion of the rotator cuff at the greater tuberosity of the humerus adjacent to the articular margin anteriorly and posteriorly *(black arrow)*. **(C)** Abnormal arthrogram of the shoulder shows air and contrast material filling the subacromial and subdeltoid bursa consistent with a full-thickness tear of the rotator cuff *(arrows)*. **(D)** CT arthrogram of the shoulder delineates the full-thickness tear of the rotator cuff filled with contrast material *(large arrow)* and extravasation of air and contrast material into the subdeltoid bursae *(small arrows)*. *(Figure continues.)*

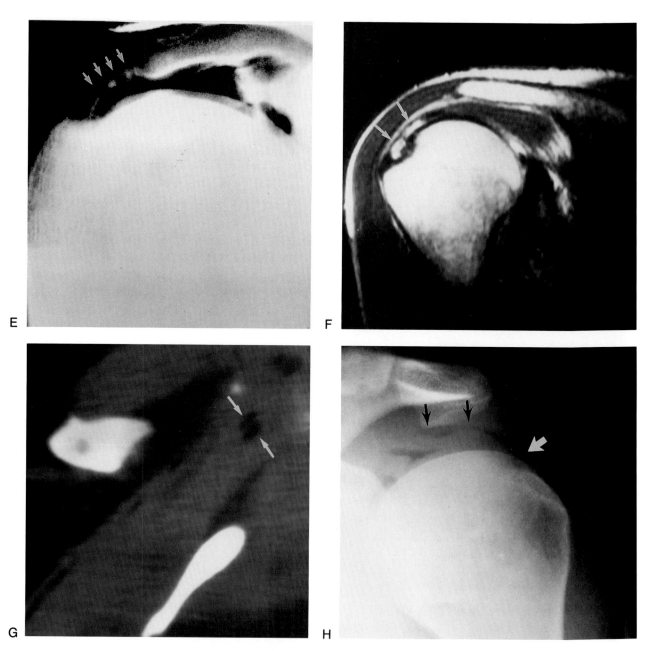

Figure 1-3 *(Continued)* **(E)** Abnormal arthrogram of the shoulder shows imbibition of contrast material into the undersurface of the rotator cuff *(arrows)* near its insertion into the greater tuberosity consistent with an incomplete tear. **(F)** Magnetic resonsance imaging of patient in Fig. E with T_2-weighted spin echo imaging shows increased signal intensity within the rotator cuff *(arrows)* confined to the humeral aspect consistent with an incomplete tear of the rotator cuff. **(G)** Air-only arthrogram of the shoulder in a patient with documented allergy to contrast material. Air introduced into the glenohumeral joint promptly tracks into the subacromial bursae *(arrows)* confirming full thickness tear. **(H)** CT arthrogram of the shoulder of patient in Fig. G shows air tracking into supraspinatus tendon *(white arrow)* and beyond the normal insertion of the rotator cuff into subacromial/deltoid bursae *(black arrows)*.

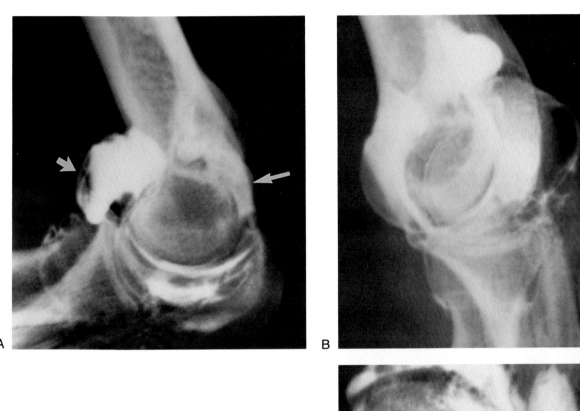

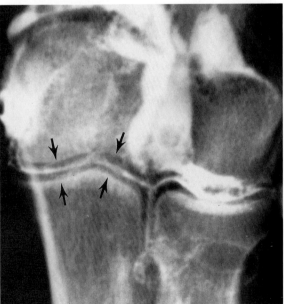

Figure 1-4 Elbow arthrography. **(A)** Lateral view of the elbow shows normal filling of the anterior and posterior recesses with contrast material *(arrows)*. **(B)** Oblique view confirms the absence of intracapsular loose bodies or synovial hypertrophy. **(C)** AP view shows symmetric joint space and cartilage thickness *(arrows)*.

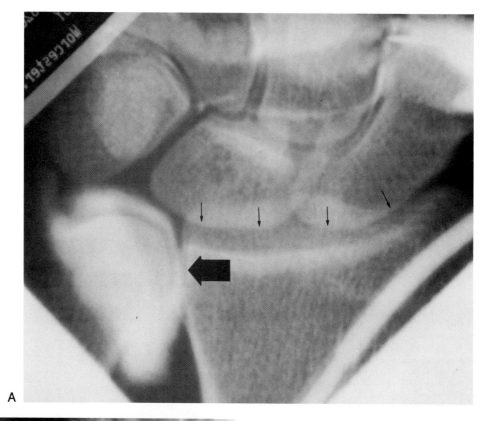

A

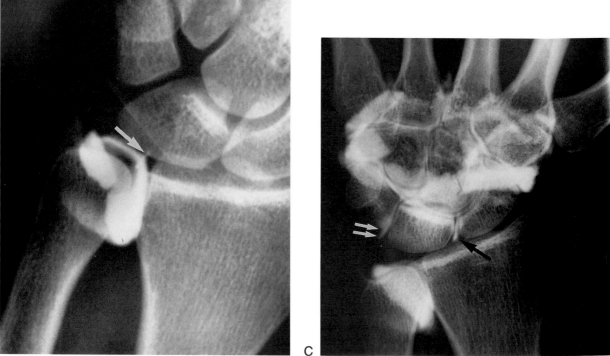

B   C

Figure 1-5 Wrist arthrography. **(A)** PA view shows normal filling of the distal radioulnar joint with contrast material *(wide arrow)* and no extension of contrast material to the radiocarpal joint *(small arrows)*. **(B)** Abnormal intravasation of contrast material introduced into the distal radioulnar joint tracks into the triangular fibrocartilage consistent with a tear *(arrow)*. **(C)** Normal filling of the midcarpal joint with contrast material showing intact scapholunate *(black arrow)* and lunatotriquetral ligaments *(white arrows)*. *(Figure continues.)*

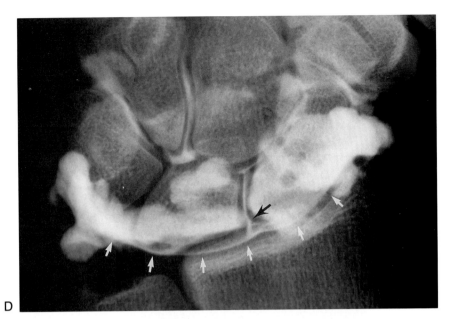

D

Figure 1-5 *(Continued)* **(D)** Abnormal midcarpal joint arthrogram shows tracking of contrast material through torn scapholunate ligament *(black arrow)* and into radiocarpal joint *(white arrows)*. **(E)** Normal arthrogram of the radiocarpal joint. No extension of contrast material into the distal radioulnar joint or midcarpal joint noted. Normal filling of the volar *(large arrow)* and prestyloid *(small arrows)* recesses. **(F)** Abnormal radiocarpal joint arthrogram shows filling of the distal radioulnar joint during radiocarpal joint injection consistent with a tear of the triangular fibrocartilage *(arrow)*.

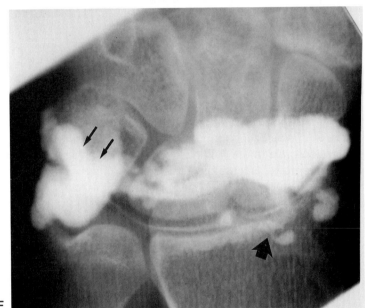

E

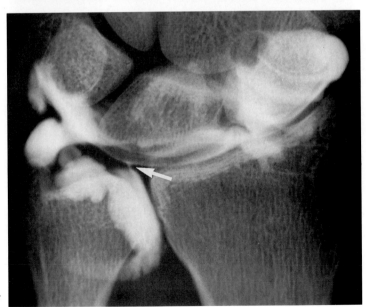

F

air or iodinated contrast agent, has led to a combination of arthrographic techniques with tomography, computed tomography, and, most recently, magnetic resonance imaging.

COMPUTED ARTHROTOMOGRAPHY

Arthrotomography of the shoulder was initially introduced as a technique for the evaluation of labral tears.[5] This has subsequently been replaced by computed arthrotomography, which generates much less radiation exposure while providing exquisite soft tissue detail and superior cross-sectional images (Fig. 1-6). Similarly, arthrotomography of the elbow was initially used as a technique in the assessment of osteocartilaginous fragments and articular cartilage integrity. This technique has also been replaced by computed arthrotomography.[6]

Computed arthrotomography of the shoulder requires computed tomography to be performed as quickly as possible after completion of a double-contrast arthrogram of the shoulder. This time constraint becomes even more stringent in computed arthrotomography of the elbow due to the rapid resorption of contrast material in synovial extensions of this articulation. The addition of epinephrine (0.1 to 0.2 ml of 1:1,000 solution) to the contrast agent is helpful in reducing venous resorption of the intra-articular iodinated contrast material.

In the shoulder, computed arthrotomography allows delineation of the superior, middle, and inferior glenohumeral ligaments, in addition to the capsular insertions, the subscapularis tendon, and the long head of the biceps tendon[7] (Fig. 1-7). Rotator cuff abnormalities involving the humeral surface of the rotator cuff are well shown and classified as partial- or full-thickness tears. Intrasubstance tears or partial tears involving the bursal aspect of the rotator cuff are not visualized.

Double-contrast computed arthrotomography remains the technique of choice for study of the glenoid labrum and can provide a more accurate assessment of subluxation and anatomic instability (Fig. 1-8). Dynamic evaluation can be incorporated into the computed tomography (CT) arthrographic examination of the shoulder for increased sensitivity in the evaluation of capsular shearing and instability.[8] This is also particularly advantageous in the analysis of labral injury. Dynamic evaluation will extend and change the position of the glenohumeral ligaments and capsule, thereby displacing an otherwise nondisplaced labral tear (Fig. 1-9). The most common interpretive difficulties associated with computed arthrotomography of the shoulder include variations in the morphology and size of the anterior labrum and confusion of the middle glenohumeral ligament for a torn labral fragment. Significant normal variation in the origin and size of the middle glenohumeral ligament is to be expected.[9]

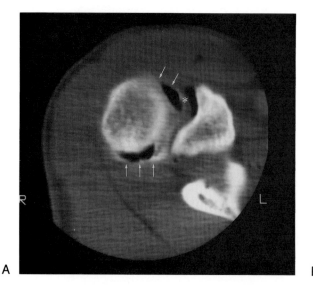 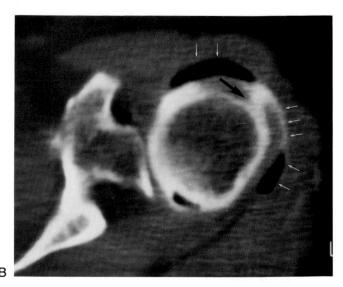

Figure 1-6 CT arthrography of the shoulder. **(A)** Normal axial image of the glenohumeral joint with air distending the anterior and posterior recesses *(arrows)*, normal superior glenohumeral ligament (*) and no extension of air or contrast material into the subdeltoid bursae. **(B)** Abnormal axial section shows extravasation of contrast material through a tear in the rotator cuff *(arrow)* with air and contrast material within the subdeltoid bursae *(arrows)*.

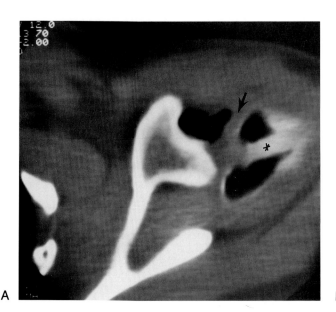

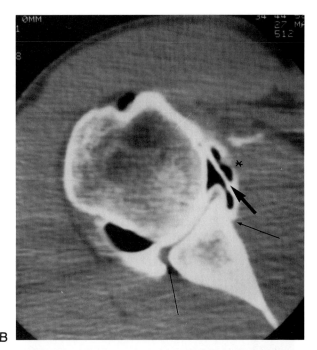

Figure 1-7 CT arthrography of glenohumeral ligaments and capsular insertions. **(A)** Axial section through the superior glenohumeral joint shows the superior glenohumeral ligament *(arrow)* and longhead of the biceps tendon (*). **(B)** Axial section through the midglenohumeral joint shows the middle glenohumeral ligament *(wide arrow)* deep to the subscapularis tendon (*). Note normal anterior and posterior capsular attachments *(long arrows)*. **(C)** Axial section through the inferior glenohumeral joint shows the inferior glenohumeral ligament *(arrow)*. Note longhead of biceps tendon *(arrowhead)*.

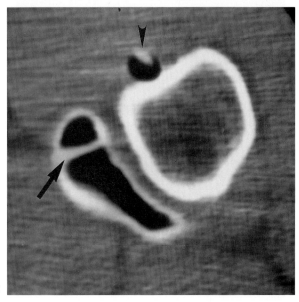

CT arthrography of the elbow has proven effective in the evaluation of the integrity of the articular cartilage, especially in the evaluation of osteochondritis dissecans. In addition, small rents in the capsule or post-traumatic intra-articular abnormalities leading to a restriction in range of motion are well assessed with CT arthrography (Fig. 1-10). The major limitation of CT arthrography of the elbow involves the evaluation of the extra-articular soft tissues, which incur a high rate of injury and subsequent complications in patients with trauma to this joint.

CT arthrography of the wrist has thus far remained limited to cases in which arthrography raises the question of an intra-articular cartilaginous loose body and ligamentous disruption. Computed tomography alone has been especially useful in cases of bony trauma to the wrist or assessment of postoperative bony union of the wrist.[10]

While computed arthrotomography represents an increase in medical costs over either arthrography or CT alone, together they provide a critical evaluation of the intra-articular components of the joint, determine the integrity of the joint capsule, and, with dynamic examination, evaluate joint stability. Early and accurate diagnosis of articular pathology may help to decrease morbidity and cost to the patient overall. The

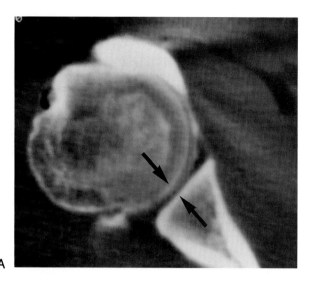
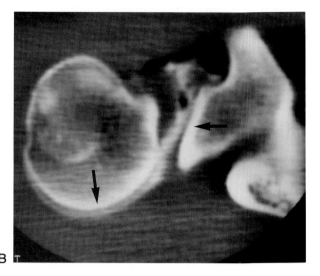

Figure 1-8 Instability: dynamic evaluation of the shoulder. **(A)** Axial section through the midglenohumeral joint in external position shows normal alignment of the humeral head and glenoid fossa *(arrows)*. **(B)** Axial section through the midglenohumeral joint maintained in internal rotation shows posterior subluxation of the humeral head with reference to the glenoid fossa *(arrows)*.

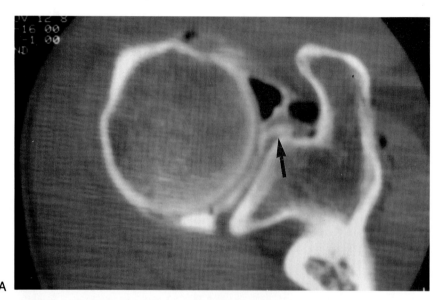

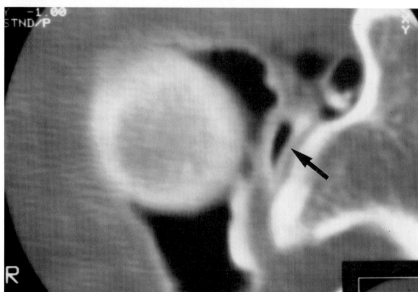

Figure 1-9 Labral tear: dynamic evaluation. **(A)** Axial section through superior glenohumeral joint in neutral position shows linear imbibition of contrast material into anterior superior glenoid labrum *(arrow)*. **(B)** With external rotation, the labral tear is distracted with air and contrast filling the gaping tear *(arrow)*.

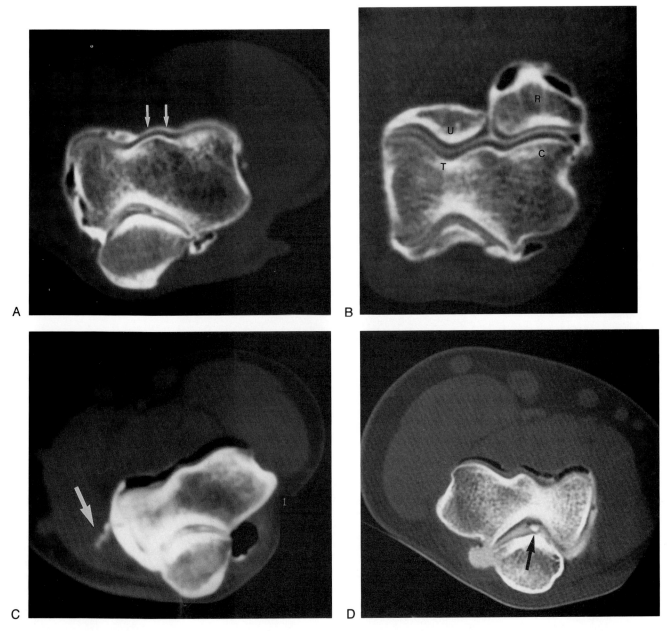

Figure 1-10 Elbow CT arthrography. **(A)** Axial section through the elbow shows contrast material coating normal articular cartilage *(arrows)*. **(B)** Coronal section through the elbow shows normal radial head *(R)*, capitellum *(C)*, ulna *(U)*, and trochlear *(T)* articulations outlined by contrast material. **(C)** Axial CT section through the elbow delineates a focus of contrast material beyond the confines of the normal capsule and medial collateral ligament consistent with a tear *(arrow)*. **(D)** Axial CT section shows intra-articular loose body *(arrow)*. *(Figure continues.)*

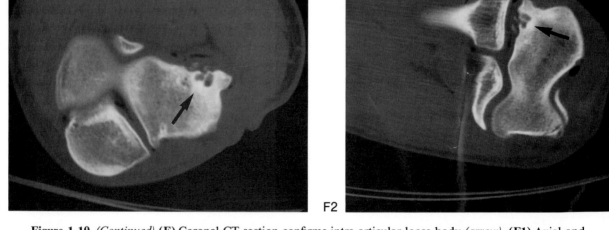

Figure 1-10 *(Continued)* **(E)** Coronal CT section confirms intra-articular loose body *(arrow).* **(F1)** Axial and **(F2)** coronal CT sections show irregularity of the capitellum consistent with osteochondritis dissecans *(arrow).*

major shortcomings of CT or computed arthrotomography lie in the evaluation of the juxta-articular soft tissues.

MAGNETIC RESONANCE IMAGING

Magnetic resonance imaging (MRI) is the newest modality used in imaging of the musculoskeletal system. The elimination of ionizing radiation, its noninvasive nature, and its multiplanar capability make it ideal for the evaluation of the upper extremity. In contrast to CT, MRI provides exquisite soft tissue contrast and multiplanar imaging without need of articular or intravenous contrast material.

In the shoulder, normal anatomy of the rotator cuff, labrum, capsular insertions, bony skeleton, and marrow compartment are well delineated by MRI[11] (Fig. 1-11). There have been numerous reports comparing shoulder MRI to standard CT arthrography.[12-14] At the present time, these techniques complement one another, each with its own particular strengths and applications. MRI is preferable in the evaluation of a soft tissue mass, cases of inflammation, and intrasubstance or incomplete tears of the rotator cuff (Fig. 1-12). CT arthrotomography is helpful in the assessment of bony and capsular integrity, glenohumeral instability, and labral injury (Fig. 1-13). The ability to image the marrow compartment with MRI is useful in cases of contusion/trauma, infection, and neoplastic or metastatic processes.

In the elbow, MRI provides exquisite delineation of muscles and associated tendons and ligaments. Differentiation and delineation of neurovascular structures is excellent.[15] Associated soft tissue inflammation and/or bursitis can be demonstrated. Capsular and ligamentous integrity are well shown and enhanced by the presence of an associated joint effusion (Fig. 1-14).

Magnetic resonance imaging of the wrist is useful in the evaluation of carpal marrow abnormalities, such as bony contusion, nondisplaced fractures, or avascular necrosis (Fig. 1-15). The noninvasive delineation of the intrinsic and extrinsic ligaments of the wrist and superb soft tissue contrast detects tenosynovitis-tendinosis and abnormalities of the carpal tunnel, and allows the differentiation and characterization of soft tissue masses as well (Fig. 1-16). MRI provides postsurgical evaluation with specific emphasis on soft tissue masses and recurrent carpal tunnel symptomatology.

The cost of MRI varies widely throughout the United States, depending on the following factors: necessity of contrast agent, cost of imaging unit, geographic location, and complexity of the examination. CT and MRI complement one another and should not be viewed as mutually exclusive in all cases. In general, CT is less expensive and requires less time per examination. If both techniques can provide the necessary information, CT should be considered the study of choice. However, in many instances (particularly those requiring evaluation of the soft tissues), MRI is superior and should be considered the procedure of choice. This reinforces the need for clear lines of communication between the radiologist and the referring physician, as well as the need for radiologists to understand the information sought and to play a pivotal role in medical efficacy and cost containment. Furthermore, it becomes imperative for referring physicians to understand the strengths and limitations of the imaging facility they use. It may prove more accurate and cost-effective to evaluate shoulder instability by dynamic CT arthrography at one institution, while MRI may be more accurate and specific when performed by experienced personnel with state-of-the-art equipment elsewhere.

Although definitive algorithms for the diagnostic evaluation of upper extremity trauma or injury have not been established, we believe the least expensive approach to obtaining the desired information should be employed. As such, the utility of MRI for the primary evaluation of a loose body is neither more precise nor cost-effective when compared to arthrography.

NUCLEAR SCINTIGRAPHY, BONE SCAN, AND ULTRASOUND

Additional imaging tools used in the study of the upper extremity include nuclear scintigraphy, bone scanning, and ultrasound. In the past, nuclear scintigraphy has been advantageous in the evaluation of metastatic disease, primary bone tumors, infection, and trauma in which the plain film radiographs often appear normal. Magnetic resonance imaging has replaced many of the areas previously requiring scintigraphic examination. Bone scintigraphy can be particularly beneficial in analyzing the extent of a disease or assessing the activity of a specific skeletal lesion. This is often difficult to evaluate radiographically, with conclusions often based more on clinical and secondary findings than on radiologic techniques and/or MRI.

In the injured athlete, bone scintigraphy is especially helpful in demonstrating the location and extent of skeletal injury when plain film radiographs are unremarkable or when determining reactivation or reinjury at a previously traumatized site. An impaction or compression injury to a chondro-osseous area (e.g., articular or subchondral) may not be identified on plain radiographs, yet the athlete may continue to experience

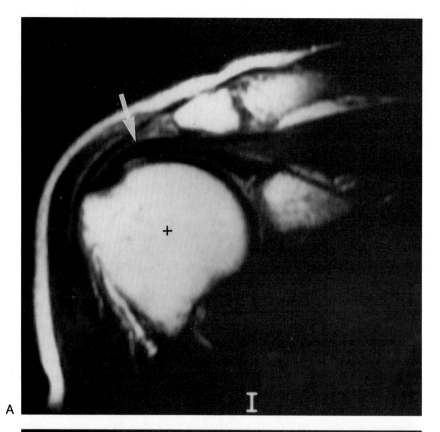

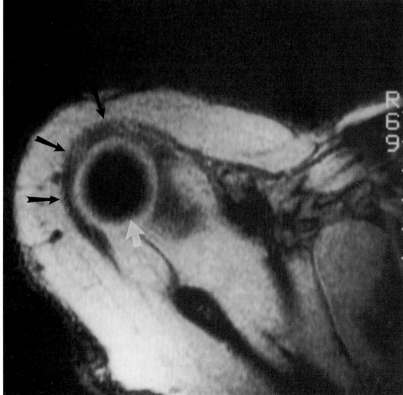

Figure 1-11 MRI of the shoulder. **(A)** Coronal T_1-weighted MR (TR/TE, 400/20) image shows the normal homogeneous low-signal intensity of the rotator cuff *(arrow)*. Note normal homogeneous high-signal intensity of fatty marrow canal (+). **(B)** Gradient echo axial MR (TR/TE/F, 500/13/20) image shows the normal homogeneous low-signal intensity of the rotator cuff *(black arrows)*. Note homogeneous suppression of marrow canal *(white arrow)*.

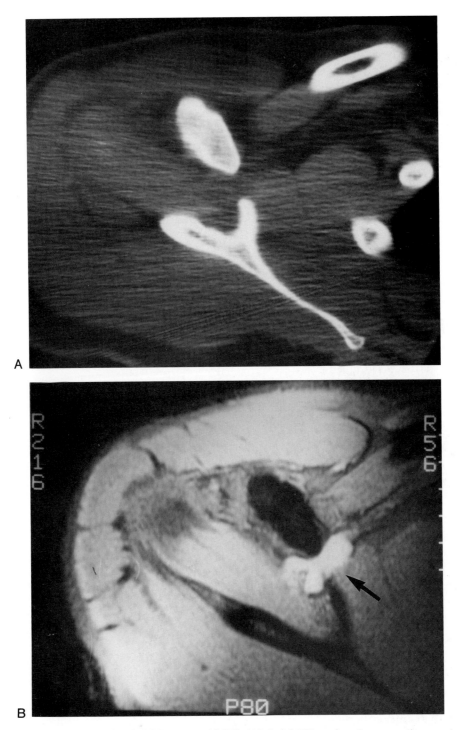

Figure 1-12 Soft tissue evaluation by CT scan and MRI. **(A)** Axial CT section shows no discrete abnormality. **(B)** Gradient echo MR axial image in the same patient clearly delineates a soft tissue mass in the suprascapular notch consistent with a ganglion *(arrow).*

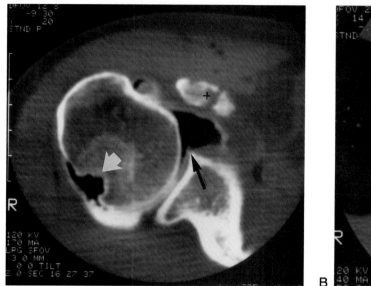
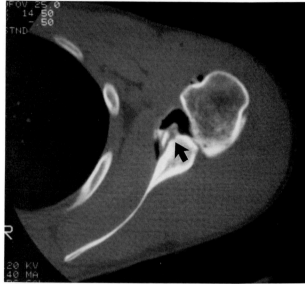
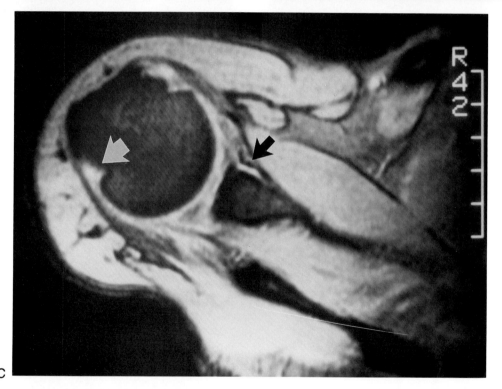

Figure 1-13 Instability of the shoulder, evaluation by CT and MRI. **(A)** Axial CT section shows Hill-Sachs lesion *(white arrow),* torn anterior superior labrum *(black arrow),* and fracture of the coracoid (+) associated with traumatic dislocation and subsequent recurrent instability. **(B)** Axial CT section more inferiorly shows associated Bankart lesion *(arrow).* **(C)** Gradient echo MR axial image in a different patient shows Hill-Sachs lesion *(white arrow)* and Bankart lesion *(black arrow)* associated with recurrent posttraumatic instability.

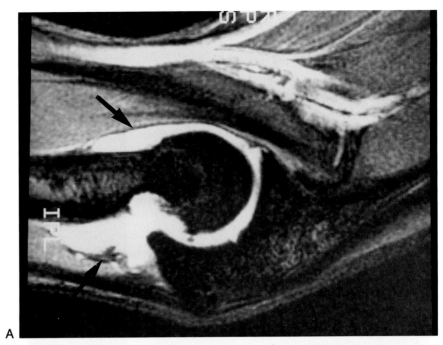

A

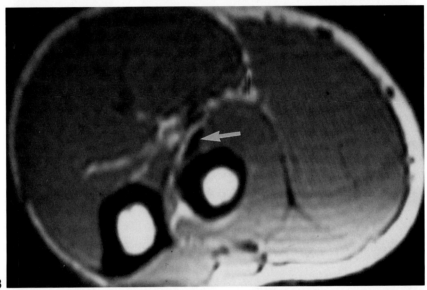

Figure 1-14 MRI of the elbow. (A) Gradient echo MR sagittal image shows prominent joint effusion *(arrows).* (B) Proton spin MR axial image shows normal biceps tendon *(arrow).* (C) T$_2$-weighted MR axial image shows increased signal intensity within the biceps tendon consistent with a tear *(arrow). (Figure continues.)*

B

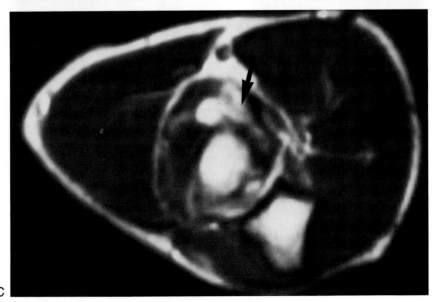

C

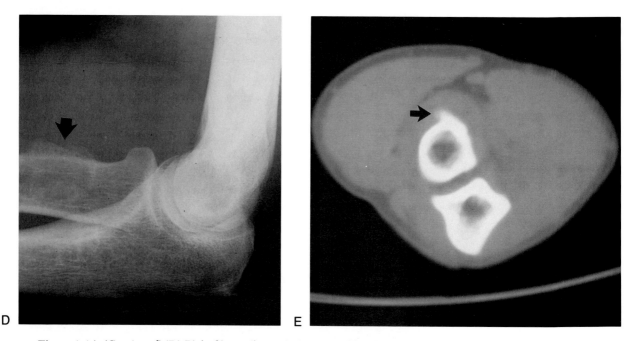

Figure 1-14 *(Continued)* **(D)** Plain film radiograph shows proliferative mineralization at the insertion of biceps tendon consistent with a previous avulsion or tear *(arrow).* **(E)** Axial CT scan confirms proliferative mineralization at the site of previous injury *(arrow).*

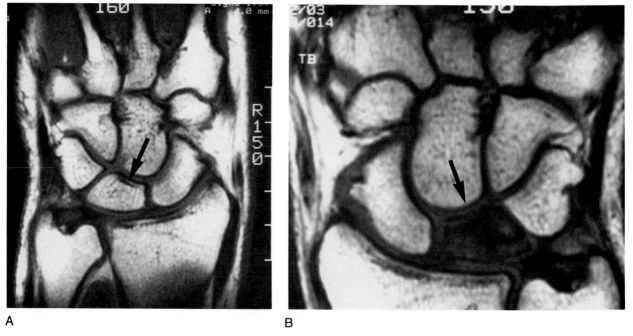

Figure 1-15 MRI of the wrist. **(A)** Coronal T_1-weighted MR image of the wrist shows the normal increase in signal intensity associated with normal marrow *(arrow).* **(B)** Coronal T_1-weighted MR image shows the loss of normal increased marrow signal intensity associated with Kienböck's disease *(arrow).*

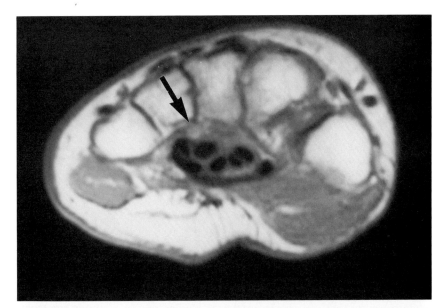

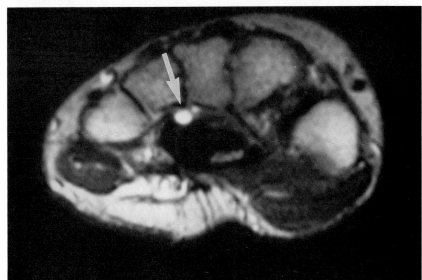

Figure 1-16 MRI of the wrist. **(A)** Intermediate and T_2-weighted images show increased signal intensity of a soft tissue mass within the carpal tunnel consistent with a ganglion *(arrows)*. **(B)** Gradient echo axial image shows increased signal intensity within the extensor carpi ulnaris tendon *(large arrow)* in addition to circumferential fluid within the tendon sheath *(small arrows)* consistent with tenosynovitis/tendinosis.

A

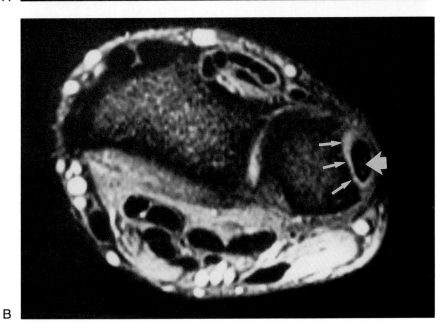

B

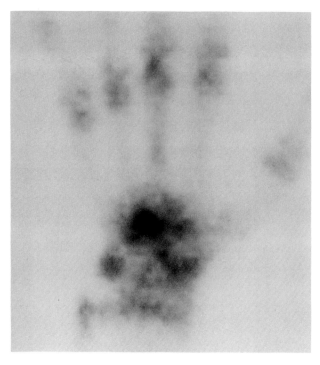

Figure 1-17 Bone scintigraphy consistent with carpal injury.

pain during attempted athletic functions. A bone scintigraphic examination may reveal findings consistent with focal changes that define the location of a performance impairment problem (e.g., carpal injury with negative radiographs) (Fig. 1-17). Nuclear scintigraphy is less costly than MRI, and is closer to the expense of an unenhanced CT examination. However, once a scintigraphic examination has been performed, radiographic assessment can be better tailored to the individual patient. Additional information can be obtained by doing a "spec" scan, particularly when there is an overlap of several structures (e.g., the glenohumeral joint).

Sonographic evaluation of the shoulder has recently gained many advocates as an alternative method of tendinous evaluation.[16] Potential advantages include the use of nonionizing radiation, its noninvasive nature, and ease of performing the examination with dynamic and real-time components. Additionally, sonography is significantly less expensive than scintigraphy, CT, or MRI. The disadvantages, however, include its operator-dependent nature and limitations in the assessment of all integral components at an articulation. In the shoulder, imaging is mainly confined to the rotator cuff and biceps tendon, and no evaluation of labral or capsular abnormalities is possible. Ultrasound of the elbow has been limited to evaluation of the soft tissues. This is true at the level of the wrist as well, where

the anatomy of tendinous structures, especially discontinuity, can be demonstrated. Finally, orthopedic surgeons have been somewhat hesitant to depend solely on the ultrasound image, as the anatomic delineation is much less clear when compared to CT and MRI.

REFERENCES

1. Lindblom K: Arthrography and roentgenology in ruptures of tendons of the shoulder joint. Acta Radiol 20:548, 1939
2. Sauser DD, Thorderson SH, Fahr LM: Imaging of the elbow. Radiol Clin North Am 28:923, 1990
3. Levinsohn ME, Palmer AK, Cohen AB, Zinberg E: Wrist arthrography: the value of the three compartment injection technique. Skelet Radiol 16:539, 1987
4. Killoran PJ, Marcove RC, Freiberger RH: Shoulder arthrography. AJR 103:658, 1968
5. El-Khoury GY, Albright JP, Abu Yousef MM, Montgomery WJ, Tuck SL: Arthrotomography of the glenoid labrum. Radiology 131:333, 1979
6. Singson RD, Feldman F, Rosenberg ZS. Elbow joint: assessment with double contrast CT arthrography. Radiology 160:167, 1986
7. Manaster BJ: Digital wrist arthrography: precision in determining the site of radiocarpal-midcarpal communication. AJR 147:153, 1986
8. Coumas JM, Waite RJ, Goss TP et al: CT and MR evaluation of the labral capsular ligamentous complex of the shoulder. AJR 158:591, 1992
9. McNiesch LM, Callaghan JJ: CT arthrography of the shoulder: variations of the glenoid labrum. AJR 149:963, 1987
10. Howard BA, Rubenstein JD: Computed tomography of the wrist. In Bloem JL, Satoris DJ (eds): MRI & CT of Musculoskeletal System: A Text Atlas. Williams & Wilkins, Baltimore, 1992
11. Rafii M, Minkoft J, DeStefano V: Diagnostic imaging of the shoulder. In Nicholas, JA, Heishman EB (eds): The Upper Extremity in Sports Medicine. CV Mosby, St. Louis, 1990
12. Kieft GJ, Bloem JL, Rozing PM, Obermann WR: MR imaging of the anterior dislocation of the shoulder: comparison with CT arthrography. AJR 150:1083, 1988
13. Seeger LL, Gold RH, Bassett LW: Shoulder instability: evaluation with MR imaging. Radiology 168:695, 1988
14. Habibian A, Staufer A, Resnick D et al: Comparison of conventional and computed arthrotomography with MR of the shoulder. J Comput Assist Tomogr 13:968, 1989
15. Frocrain L, Lucas C, deKorvin B et al: MRI anatomy of the nerves of the upper limb. J Clin Anat 11:141, 1989
16. Middleton WD, Reinus WR, Totty WG et al: Ultrasonography of the rotator cuff and biceps tendon. J Bone Joint Surg [Am] 68:440, 1986

2

Principles of Rehabilitation of the Injured Athlete

Robert S. Skerker
Lisa A. Schulz

This chapter provides a broad overview of the rehabilitation process for the athlete with an upper extremity injury. We discuss the athlete and the rehabilitation team, examine pain and performance along with the important psychological aspects of caring for the injured athlete, outline principles used in rehabilitation, and explain modalities used during the rehabilitative process.

THE ATHLETE AND THE REHABILITATION TEAM

The general principles of rehabilitative care for an acute physical injury apply to both the general and the athletic populations. The primary goal is to facilitate the athlete's return to sport as safely and quickly as possible, and the work of the rehabilitation team members must be compatible with this goal. The treatment team must provide the athlete with the necessary therapeutic resources and education about the injury, rehabilitative process, recovery time, and subsequent performance expectations. The rehabilitation team members must be knowledgeable about the sport, the role of the individual team member, the injury, and the psychological impact of the injury on the athlete. The rehabilitative process represents a continuum between the members of the rehabilitation team, the coaches, and the athlete (often parents as well) until the return to sport is complete.

Differences may exist between a competitive amateur and a professional athlete. At times, there may be a premature expectation for a professional to perform at preinjury level. Rate of progression varies among individual athletes. The same type of injury in two athletes can present different functional expectations and, as such, affects treatment. A dislocated finger (interphalangeal joint) in a quarterback's throwing hand will be managed differently from the hand of a football lineman, and the impact on return to competition will vary as well. Given the demands of each position, the lineman may be able to return to competition shortly following reduction, while the quarterback may remain out of competition for days to weeks due to the need for good digit range of motion and fine dexterity skills.

Although the specific protocols and techniques will vary, depending on the type of injury and the athlete's response to treatment, the following goals should be part of every rehabilitation program: (1) decrease pain and inflammatory response; (2) reduce edema; (3) maximize range of motion; (4) improve muscle control and coordination; and (5) increase strength, endurance, and proprioceptive awareness. Many of the treatment techniques used will address multiple areas simultaneously.

Individual rehabilitation programs are developed to accommodate the availability of resources, personnel, and personal concerns. An athlete who is involved on the collegiate or professional level receives daily attention (i.e., daily training room visits with evaluation and treatment) as opposed to the individual who must independently coordinate care within general guidelines provided by health care professionals. The availability of personnel (e.g., certified athletic trainer, physical therapist, exercise physiologist, registered occupational therapist) and therapeutic equipment becomes significant in relation to rehabilitation and recovery. The specific age group of the athlete (pediatric/adolescent, mature, middle aged, and senior) is another factor that should be considered in the rehabilitation process. A shoulder joint injury illustrates the differences that may exist between age groups. A shoulder injury in a growing child may lead to growth-related problems; a middle-aged athlete with shoulder problems may have an inflammatory condition or microtrauma to the tissues; and the mature/senior athlete may have difficulties secondary to degenerative changes.

As in other areas of medical rehabilitation, a team approach to the management of the injured athlete is beneficial. A physician should serve as the team advisor, organizing the rehabilitation program of the injured athlete. Among the important members of this team are the athletic team trainers, therapists, coaches, exercise physiologists, and sports psychologists. The team physician is the link between the other professional health staff and the coaching staff, continually updating the coach on a player's progress toward recovery and making medical judgments as to a safe level of participation. Furthermore, good communication between the coaches and the medical staff may help identify certain practices or training techniques that predispose a returning player to further injury. The medical personnel assume 100 percent of the care of an injured athlete during the initial phases of the rehabilitation program. During the latter phases of rehabilitation (integrated functions and return to sport), the medical staff role decreases and the role of the coaching staff increases.[1]

The athletic trainers and therapists who perform the daily preventive and rehabilitative work with the athletes are critical members of the rehabilitation team. These professionals generally have a keen understanding of team psychology and the dynamics between players and coaches and therefore are in a unique position to serve as intermediary between an off-site treating physician and the team. In this regard, they must be included in the diagnostic evaluation and treatment program as much as possible. Their duties include designing and implementing the rehabilitation program, recording daily progress and treatment, and reassessing status, along with providing protective equipment, taping joints, providing massage therapy, and assisting with modality usage.

The exercise physiologist has various responsibilities, including the development of a conditioning program during preseason training. Preseason physiologic testing and conditioning programs prepare both the whole team and each individual member for the upcoming competitive season (see Ch. 16). There is evidence that improved aerobic conditioning decreases injury rates even in contact sports such as football[2,3] (R.S. Skerker, W.C. Etchison, B. McCluskey, and J.M. Henderson, unpublished observations, 1991). The development of specific weight-training regimens for strength and body mass increase is generally the concern of the weight-training coach.

Nutrition becomes increasingly important with an injured athlete due to changes in nutritional needs for healing and the caloric impact of decreased physical activity. In addition, with decreased physical activity there may be a slowing of the baseline metabolic rate. This, combined with decreased energy expenditure (due to decreased physical activity), can result in significant weight gain if the athlete does not modify caloric intake. The athlete's understanding of nutrition and performance may influence the response to nutritional guidance and recommended changes. Although coaches, teammates, and lay peers are often the source of nutritional information for the athlete, this information is not always appropriate. In addition, an athlete's perception of "good nutrition" may be influenced by commercialism and potential financial gains as well as cultural aspects of upbringing.

Another consideration is the value that the athlete attaches to a certain food or supplement. Although a scientific correlation between improved performance and faster healing time may not be apparent, denying an athlete a food that is associated with success may have a negative effect on his or her performance.[4] Monitoring the athlete's diet may be a challenge. Food provided by the team can be controlled for fat, calories, and nutritional value. Food eaten at home and while traveling, however, is not as easily supervised. Coaches and trainers should consistently monitor the athlete's diet and provide ongoing nutritional education. In general, a balanced diet provides the most appropriate nutrition for athletes of all ages.

PSYCHOLOGICAL ASPECTS OF CARING FOR THE INJURED ATHLETE

The psychological effect of injury to the athlete is another critical factor influencing the rehabilitation process. In order to facilitate rehabilitation, it is imperative that the athlete's response to the injury is understood with the teaching of coping strategies incorporated into the rehabilitation program. In addition, the expectations for recovery and return to competition by the athlete, as well as by the coaching staff and other team personnel, will have an impact on the rehabilitation process. Education regarding realistic rehabilitation expectations should begin early. Inappropriate expectations for early return to competition, for example, will put additional stress on the athlete and may impede the rehabilitation progress.

Psychologically, the athlete should have an idea of the degree of severity of a temporary disability, as well as the expected length of time for recuperation. As with other patients, it is important for athletes to know they have some control over the rehabilitation process. In this regard, the treating staff should discuss the rationale for pursuing a certain course of rehabilitation and then offer alternatives for implementing the specified program. Although these patients may not have full knowledge of the medical aspects of their recovery and rehabilitation, their feelings and concerns are important, since they must undergo the prescribed course of therapy. The staff should also present realistic expectations for the athlete to keep in mind during the rehabilitation process. An athlete who has insight into the rehabilitation process and participates in goal-setting will be more motivated to follow the prescribed course and ultimately should be in better condition both physically and psychologically.

Research has shown that more seriously injured athletes experience tension, depression, anger, and fatigue. An individual's age and status has an impact on how he or she experiences the injury. It has been suggested by some authors that athletes may progress through a grief cycle similar to that of terminally ill patients.[5] In the loss-of-health models, such as those discussed by Kubler-Ross, these stages are (1) disbelief, denial, and isolation; (2) anger; (3) bargaining; (4) depression; and (5) acceptance.[5a] Although athletes may in fact experience simultaneous elevations in depression, anger, and tension, the cause may be due to serious losses as a consequence of the injury, for example, loss of position on the team, income, scholarship, teammate support, self-esteem, and sports skills. Intervention strategies for coping with these psychological stressors should be geared to the individual athlete. Communication with the coaching staff and team members is often a key component in the management of these issues.[5] Other authors, however, believe that, although these loss-of-health models may be helpful to anticipate responses, athletes may in fact respond somewhat differently to injury.[5]

It has been shown that the potential for injury increases if the athlete has recently experienced significant stress, causing decreased attention to performance and physical and mental fatigue, which may increase risk of injury and potential reinjury.[6]

A comprehensive protocol for assessment and intervention concerning the psychological aspects of athletic injury has been established by Smith and colleagues.[5] The program includes an assessment of the significance of the injury to the athlete and other psychological concerns, followed by referral to the team counselor for additional assessment of coping skills and emotional state. Intervention includes education on coping mechanisms, such as motivational analysis, goal-setting, expectations for success, relaxation exercises, and systematic mental rehearsal and imagery.[7] Additionally, the athlete may need other support and encouragement on a day-to-day basis in order to stay motivated to comply with the rehabilitation program. Goal-setting and documentation of progress can become important factors for motivation.

One additional psychological aspect of an athletic injury concerns the general decrease in exercise that accompanies an injury. Engaging in physical activity and exercise will moderate depression. It follows then that encouraging the athlete to exercise uninjured body parts (i.e., lower extremity and general aerobic conditioning with hand injuries) as soon as possible will help to lessen depression and enhance coping strategies. Fears of reinjury and decreased self-esteem may also be lessened if the athlete is engaged in activities designed to maintain general skills and endurance necessary for high-level performance. Imagery techniques that reduce anxiety are often quite helpful. Sports psychologists help the team and individual player work through feelings of inadequacy secondary to injury, and can be quite beneficial in helping the athlete focus on and attain specific goals. In particular, they may help the athlete's psychological progress through the rehabilitation program and return to competition.

PAIN AND PERFORMANCE

Pain and the athlete's response to it is an important aspect of rehabilitation in the acute phase as well as throughout the rehabilitation program. Pain is a protective mechanism employed by the body to warn of trauma or further injury.[8,9] It is not only an unpleasant physical stimulus but also affects individuals psychologically. An individual's pain threshold is often determined by personal and cultural characteristics as much as by physiology.

Pain can be categorized two ways: *expected* or *unexpected.* Expected pain is the discomfort that occurs postperformance (i.e., the physiological response to lactic acid and metabolic waste products) or discomfort associated with conditioning. Unexpected pain is the pain resulting from an injury. The type of pain experienced depends on the athlete's perception. During rehabilitation, if an athlete confuses or misinterprets the type of pain experienced, it can adversely affect the program.[8,10] For example, if an athlete perceives the "expected" pain from an exercise program as "unexpected," and subsequently reduces the intensity of the rehabilitation program, then the athlete may be at increased risk for reinjury when returning to competition. In addition, the athlete's rehabilitation progress may be slowed and deconditioning prolonged. It should also be remembered that each individual has a unique pain tolerance, and thus two athletes with the same injury may have different recovery times.

Some discomfort is a normal component of the rehabilitation process. Education on pain and appropriate pain responses should be included in the rehabilitation program, beginning in the acute phase. For example, in certain situations, stretching will cause some athletes expected discomfort, while others will perceive it as unexpected pain.

When the athlete first returns to competition, there may be a period of time when some amount of discomfort or pain is felt during competition. The impact of the pain on the athlete's performance will vary depending upon a number factors. A football lineman returning to competition following a finger dislocation may experience some discomfort, but this should not inhibit his ability to block. Yet a gymnast competing for the first time on the uneven parallel bars following a similar injury may risk a fall if the pain is significant and prevents a strong grip on the bar.

With the return to competition, there is also often a fear of reinjury. Playing with pain will often contribute to this fear. Conversely, an athlete's motion may be altered due to the fear of pain. The athlete's complaints of continued, worsening, or new pain that occur with competition must be evaluated in order to rule out reinjury and to reassure the athlete that competition is acceptable.

INFLAMMATION, TISSUE DAMAGE, AND REPAIR

Rehabilitation techniques (e.g., exercises, heat treatments, stretching) are attempts to modify the inflammatory and repair process of the injured tissue. The following is a summary of inflammation and repair and then a discussion on the repair of individual tissue types.

Cornelius Celsus, a Roman writer of the first century, described the four cardinal signs of inflammation: *rubor* (redness); *tumor* (swelling); *calor* (heat); and *dolor* (pain). Later, a fifth clinical sign, loss of function, was added by Virchow. These classical clinical signs are the result of a complex series of events that are still not completely understood today. In the realm of sports medicine, inflammation is usually a response to tissue damage (i.e., contusion of muscle, tendon or ligament disruption, laceration of skin, fracture of bone), with induction of changes in vascular flow, vascular permeability, and leukocyte exudation.

Very early after injury, vascular flow is diminished due to vasoconstriction, which is usually fleeting and followed by vasodilation. As this occurs, increased amounts of blood enter the injured area, resulting in local warmth and redness. Some degree of transudation may occur, but the majority of fluid transudating from the intravascular compartment to the extravascular space occurs from increased vascular permeability, and thus the clinical sign of swelling is revealed. As these processes occur, leukocytes (primarily neutrophils and monocytes) invade the injured area. Leukocytes escape from the vascular space by literally squeezing through the junctions between the endothelial cells lining the blood vessel (endothelial cells) and then migrating toward the injury via a process known as *chemotaxis,* that is, locomotion oriented along a chemical gradient. Leukocytes enter the damaged area and begin to release enzymes that degrade cellular material and debris. Blood plasma entering the area brings other chemical mediators of inflammation.

Table 2-1 summarizes some of the most likely mediators of inflammation and their actions. The biochemistry is complex and in some cases not well understood. However, they serve to mediate the common clinical signs of inflammation, including vasodilation, increased vascular permeability, chemotaxis, warmth, pain, and tissue damage.

There are three phases in the wound healing process: inflammation, fibroplasia, and remodeling. Inflammation is the earliest phase of healing damaged tissues or organs and results in cleaning the damaged areas such that the next phases of healing can occur. Repair usu-

Table 2-1   Likely Mediators in Inflammation

Vasodilation
   Prostaglandins
Increased vascular permeability
   Vasoactive amines
   C3a and C5a (through liberating amines)
   Bradykinin
   Leukotriene C, D, E
Chemotaxis
   C5a
   Leukotriene B$_4$
   Other chemotactic lipids
   Neutrophil cationic proteins
Fever
   Endogenous pyrogen
   Prostaglandins
Pain
   Prostaglandins
   Bradykinin
Tissue damage
   Neutrophil and macrophage lysosomal enzymes
   Oxygen metabolites

ally involves two processes: (1) the replacement of injured tissue by parenchymal cells of the same type (known as regeneration), sometimes leaving little or no residue of injury; and (2) replacement by connective tissue or scar formation.

The mechanisms of repair and wound healing are quite complex, involving regeneration of parenchymal cells, migration and proliferation of both parenchymal and connective tissue cells, synthesis of extracellular matrix proteins, remodeling of connective tissue, and collagenization and acquisition of wound strength. The development of wound strength is thought to be related to fibroblast proliferation and the deposition of collagen, which ultimately provides tensile strength to healing wounds. However, fibroblasts also synthesize elastic fibers and secrete the various glycosamingoglycans. The healing wound is a dynamic and changing environment, involving a variety of events and dependent on interactions between cells and local factors (e.g., PO$_2$, pH, immune reactions), which turn on or turn off the synthesis or degradation of extracellular matrix proteins, as well as proliferation and migration of cells.

Using skin as a model organ for a discussion of wound strength, it is believed that a sutured incision (healing by primary intention) has approximately 70 percent of the strength of unwounded skin largely due to the tensile strength of the sutures. Systemic influences such as poor nutrition, diabetes, and systemic glucocorticoids may lead to problems with wound healing. Local factors such as inadequate blood supply (seen in patients with peripheral vascular disease), local

infection, foreign bodies, pressure, and shear forces may result in delayed and/or poor quality healing.

The specific tissue injured should also be considered in the treatment of sports injuries for two reasons: (1) some tissues do not heal with replacement of parenchymal cells, thus scar must form (such as articular cartilage); (2) some tissues heal better when immobilized for a period of time (i.e., bone) but then need to be mobilized for stronger wound healing and improved function (i.e., tendon). The next section gives specific information on damage and repair of muscle, ligament, tendon, and bone.

Muscle Fiber

Throughout life, skeletal muscle fibers are repeatedly damaged and undergo repair. Injury can be caused by abnormalities within the fiber such as ischemia (lack of oxygen supply), disease, metabolic deficiencies, or denervation. In sports medicine, however, we typically think of external and functional events causing skeletal muscle fiber damage, such as compression, contusion, excessive stretch,[11] and excessive exercise.[12] As with other tissues, muscle has the capacity to heal by regeneration.[12] Initially, damaged cells leak endogenous proteases that autodigest damaged cells. Inflammatory mediator chemicals soon attract or induce macrophages, which infiltrate the area of damage and clean up cellular debris. Satellite cells then begin to proliferate at the damaged areas to align themselves along the basal lamina and fuse into myotubes. The myotubes then mature and differentiate into muscle cells, generating myofibrillar proteins. The proteins then assemble into disorganized myofibers, which begin to align in the direction of mature muscle. Maturity brings further organization, recovery of contractile abilities, and increasing tensile strength.

It is well documented that lengthening muscle contractions (i.e., eccentric contractions) are damaging to muscle fibers and may in part explain why eccentric contractions produce more postexercise muscle soreness than concentric contractions.[12] The extent of damage can vary from an imperceptible change in molecules of actin and myosin filaments to a gross change in the whole muscle visible to the eye.[13]

More extreme damage, such as that which occurs from increased loads, greater stretching, or longer periods of eccentric work, may cause muscle fibers to disrupt. The weakest zone in a mechanically stretched muscle is at the myotendinous junction, with a tear most commonly occurring during a forceful eccentric contraction. For example, biceps brachii muscle ruptures commonly occur at the myotendinous junction. These injuries often occur during sudden placement of a load greater than the biceps can resist. Therefore, the muscle rapidly stretches while the fibers are vigorously contracting in an eccentric manner to control the rate of stretch. The forces, however, are too great, and the muscle fails at the weakest point, the myotendinous junction.

Clinically, muscle injuries are called strains and Table 2-2 outlines relevant information regarding classification of these injuries.

Coaches and trainers have advocated the benefits of stretching muscles before and after athletic participation. Recent research suggests several reasons why stretching had been experimentally noted to be helpful.[11] Stretching results in increased length of the muscle-tendon unit and therefore should contribute toward greater flexibility. Repetitive stretching results in a reduction in the peak load or tensile stress placed on a muscle-tendon unit, which may lessen the chances of injury.

Ligament

Clinically, injuries to ligaments are called sprains and can be categorized based on degree of severity, as shown in Table 2-2 and Figure 2-1. After ligament sprains were produced in experimental animals, Miltner and colleagues[14] examined them histologically to study the healing process. One week after mild injury, edema and fibroblastic proliferation occur. The surrounding synovium is also inflamed, and the inflammatory process continues into the second and third weeks. During this period, subcutaneous hemorrhage begins to resolve and fibroblastic proliferation continues. By 6 weeks, the cellular response has subsided, and the healing process with fibrous tissue has begun. More severe sprains follow the same healing

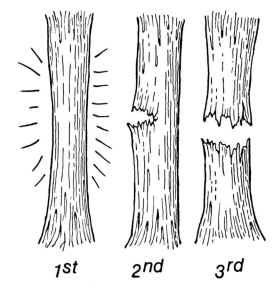

Figure 2-1 Grades of severity of strains and sprains.

progression, but the repair process may take 8 to 10 weeks, depending on the maturity and strength of the tissue. Generally, by 6 to 8 weeks individuals can return to athletic activities.

Many investigators believe that joint range of motion exercises ultimately result in stronger ligament healing, although it is agreed that early immobilization to protect the area during the initial stage of healing may be important.[15-17] Considerable clinical evidence suggests that chronic joint instability resulting from ligamentous laxity will lead to late degenerative changes within the joint. For example, untreated ulnar collateral ligament tears of the thumb metacarpophalangeal joint commonly lead to post-traumatic arthritis.[18,19] These injuries often do not heal well through secondary intention due to interposition of soft tissues such as the adductor pollicis aponeurosis between the

Table 2-2 Guidelines for Sprains and Strains

	Grade		
	I	II	III
Description	Mild stretch	Moderate stretch; partial tear	Severe stretch; complete tear
Observation	Minimal swelling	Moderate swelling	Moderate to major swelling
Palpation	Mild point tenderness; no palpable defect	Localized pain; palpable abnormality or defect	Pain on limited exam; palpable defect
Stability	Stable	Instability with stress	Instability demonstrable during exam
Active motion	Full with mild discomfort	Incomplete motion with pain	Pain with minimal motion
Functional activity	Limited with discomfort	Pain with attempt	Not able to perform
Associated injury	Unlikely	Probable at mild to moderate degree	Probable severe injury of multiple structures

ends of the ruptured ligament (Stenner lesion). An incomplete tear (i.e., partial tear or sprain) of the thumb metacarpophalangeal joint ulnar collateral ligament is treated with immobilization in a thumb spica cast or splint. A distinction is made between complete tear and partial tear, noting that surgical repair is not necessarily better at conferring stability than healing by secondary intention in cases of partial tear.[20]

Tendon

Tendon healing incorporates a combination of both intrinsic and extrinsic mechanisms. For many years it was thought that tendons healed by the proliferation of cells from surrounding damaged tissues.[21] In 1970, Potenza[21] stated that "flexor tendons are not healed by any intrinsic tenoblastic response of their own." This concept has since been challenged and modified. Gelberman and Manske[22] have reported that tendons do in fact demonstrate intrinsic healing. Their work, both in vivo and in vitro, demonstrated that lacerated tendons placed in a tissue culture media demonstrated a tenoblastic response, in isolation from other injured structures, supporting the theory of intrinsic tendon healing. Tendon healing occurs through a combination of intrinsic and extrinsic mechanisms.

The tendon healing process proceeds, as with other tissues, through an initial inflammatory phase followed by a fibroblastic phase and finally to scar remodeling. Inflammation occurs 1 to 3 days after injury/surgery and is marked by the appearance of cells originating from the extrinsic peritenon and intrinsic epitenon and endotenon. Collagen synthesis begins within the first week following repair, with the fibroblasts becoming the predominant cells.[23] The change in tensile strength as healing progresses is a cause for concern. Healing tendons have their lowest tensile strength at 5 to 15 days postrepair. During the first 5 days after tendon repair, the tendon strength is provided by the suture used for the repair. After 5 days, the strength of the tendon decreases secondary to the repaired area being bridged primarily by fibrin from the clot. The suture material is also becoming weaker during this period. At this point (days 5 to 15), the athlete is at increased risk for tendon rerupture and additional injury due to the decreased tendon tensile strength. Tendon strength begins to increase after 15 days, as the network of collagen fibrils becomes more organized. Providing controlled stress to the healing tendon will further increase the tensile strength of the tendon.[24] In most cases, the tendon will be strong enough so that the athlete can begin resistive exercise at 8 weeks, and return to athletic activities 12 weeks after tendon repair (Table 2-3).

Bone

A fractured bone initiates a sequence of inflammation, repair, and remodeling that is conceptually similar to that of other tissue.[25] Initial trauma injures the bone and surrounding soft tissues, including periosteum and muscle. Hematoma develops within the medullary canal between fracture fragments and beneath elevated periosteum. Primary damage to bone blood vessels and elevated local pressures clot capil-

Table 2-3   Tendon Wound Healing

Time from Operation	Paratenon Reaction	Gap	Stumps	Union
3 days	Cellular (leukocytes, histiocytes, lymphocytes, fibroblasts), vascular	Cellular and vascular from sheath	Anuclear necrosis at ends	Silk
1 wk	Cellular and vascular	Cellular and vascular from sheath	Tenoblasts (mitoses), vascular	Cellular and vascular from sheath
2 wk	Cellular, fibrosis, vascular	Tenoblasts from stumps invade gap	Tenoblasts with active mitoses, vascular	Granulation tissue from sheath
3 wk	Fibrosis and vascular	Tenoblasts from stumps fill entire gap	Tenoblasts more mature	Tenoblasts, vascular
4 wk	Fibrous tissue sheath separates from tendon	Tenoblasts with wavy fibers (collagen), vascular	Tenoblasts with wavy fibers (collagen), vascular	Tenoblasts with wavy fibers (collagen), vascular
5 wk	Mature fibrous sheath	Tenoblasts more mature, with stress lines	Tenoblasts more mature, more collagen	Tenoblasts more collagen stress lines
7 wk	Synovia, mature fibrous sheath	Young adult tendon cells	Young adult tendon cells	Young adult tendon cells
8 wk		Mature tendon cells	Mature tendon cells	Mature tendon cells

laries and thus prevents nutrients from reaching osteocytes. Other tissues including marrow, periosteum, and muscle also die and contribute necrotic debris to the fracture site. As these cells die, inflammatory mediators are released, which bring polymorphonuclear leukocytes, macrophages, lymphocytes, and osteoclasts into the area where they clean up the cellular and acellular debris, readying the region for repair.

As the inflammatory phase wanes, the reparative process begins with angiogenesis, bringing in new capillary buds and a new blood suppy to the region. With the new blood supply comes pluripotential mesenchymal cells that form fibrous tissue, cartilage, and eventually new bone which slowly mineralizes. Clinically, fracture union occurs with the fracture becoming stabilized by callus. Physical exam reveals that the fracture site becomes pain-free and radiographs show bone crossing the fracture site. At this stage (8 to 12 weeks), the fracture site is still weaker than surrounding normal bone.

During the final stages of healing, the fracture site continues to gain strength. Remodeling of bone occurs with the replacement of woven bone (or callus) with lamellar bone and absorption of unneeded callus. Radioisotope scanning demonstrates that this metabolic stage continues for years after clinical fracture union. Remodeling is directly related to stresses and strains placed across the healing bone such that changes in bone architecture provide more or less strength as needed.

The observation that changes in bone architecture are associated with changes in loading is referred to as *Wolff's law*. Electrical fields influence fracture healing such that electropositivity occurs on the convex surface and electronegativity on the concave surface of a bone subject to stress. Evidence suggests that osteoclastic activity (cells that digest bone cells and matrix) predominates in regions of electropositivity and osteoblastic activity (cells that create new bone) prevails in areas of electronegativity. Thus, alterations in electric fields that affect cellular behavior and bone structure may reflect Wolff's law. Eventually, remodeling is complete when the mechanical properties of the original tissues are restored. However, bone is a complex organ system and its structure continues to change (albeit imperceptibly) throughout one's life.

THE FIVE PHASES OF SPORTS REHABILITATION

The rehabilitation process following any type of soft tissue or bony injury can be divided into a series of progressive phases. These phases have overlapping elements and should be viewed as a continuum rather than as discrete entities. Different aspects of rehabilitation are emphasized in each phase (Table 2-4). As the athlete progresses through the phases of rehabilitation, the injured structures are simultaneously moving through the repair process. The five phases of sport injury rehabilitation[1] as outlined in Table 2-4 are acute injury, initial rehabilitation, progressive rehabilitation, integrated functions, and return to sport.

Phase I: Acute Injury

The functional goals for the first phase of rehabilitation are (1) to prepare the area for healing, (2) to avoid additional injury, (3) to reduce swelling resulting from the inflammatory process, and (4) to decrease pain.

The body begins to respond to the injury during the acute injury phase. The wound healing process is the body's response to an injury and follows a predictable series of events, as already reviewed under specific tissue injuries. Time frames and the response will vary with the type of tissue injured. The inflammatory period predominates during the acute injury phase of rehabilitation. This phase has usually run its course by the fourth day postinjury or -surgery.

Problems can occur if rehabilitation of the injured athlete does not begin at the moment of injury. After an acute injury, an athlete may go to the local emergency room where he or she is often told that no fractures have been sustained. With this diagnosis, the athlete believes there is no injury and, despite pain and swelling, continues with full activity, leading to further injury of the already damaged structures. It should be stressed to the athlete that a negative radiograph does not preclude the presence of an injury. Rather, the athlete should be informed of the likelihood of soft tissue injury, and appropriate treatment should be initiated.

This phase is characterized by increased vascularity to the area (as indicated by swelling, warmth, and erythema), specific chemical changes that mediate cellular activities, and wound decontamination. Pain, edema, and inflammation often can be managed by a combination of rehabilitation treatments, including *p*rotection, *r*est, *i*ce or cold, *c*ompression, and *e*levation (PRICE). Depending upon the type of injury and patient compliance, immobilization (protection and rest) can be accomplished through casts, splints, or simple positioning (pillows, slings, etc.). Rest to the injured area should be complete. The athlete's use of the injured extremity is limited, not only for sports-related activities, but all activities of daily living (ADL). Local anesthetics should not be injected into the acutely

Table 2-4 Guidelines for Athletic Injury Rehabilitation

Phase	Pathologic Process	Functional Goals	Rehabilitation Treatment

I. Acute injury	Tissue injury
	  Hematoma
	  Edema
	  Inflammation
	  Necrosis
		Protection
		  Limit injury
		  Limit swelling
		  Limit pain
			Price
			  Protection
			  Rest
			  Ice
			  Compression
			  Elevation

II. Initial rehabilitation	Fibroblastic stage
	  Decreasing inflammation
	  Edema beginning to wane
	  Minimal tensile strength
	    (0–15%)
		Progressive
		  Pain-free range of motion
			Active/active assisted range of motion
			Limited short-arc resistance
			Cold
			Gentle isometrics
			Early aerobics

III. Progressive rehabilitation	Early tissue repair
	  Primitive collagen & early
	    tissue maturation
	  Moderate tensile strength
	    (15–50%)
		Improve range of motion
		Increase strength
		Limited activity skills
		Ongoing protection prn
			Passive/active range of motion
			  stretching
			Progressive resistive exercise
			  with isotonic and/or isokin-
			  etic exercises
			Increased aerobic activities

IV. Integrated functions	Mature collagen
	Tissue characteristics now
	  evident
	Tensile strength better
	  (50–90%)
		Increase skills
		Increase strength
		Enhance flexibility
			Advanced progressive resistive
			  exercise
			Flexibility exercises
			Coordination training
			Proprioceptive training

V. Return to sport	Tissue remodeling
	Tissue characteristics ma-
	  turing
	Tensile strength increased
	  (90–99%)
		Maximize skills
		Simulated participation
		Prevent reinjury
			Maintain strength and flexibil-
			  ity
			Advanced coordination activi-
			  ties
			Protect previously injured area
			  from reinjury

painful area because pain offers a component of protection that helps the athlete avoid further injury. Instead, appropriate oral analgesics and anti-inflammatory medication should be used as indicated by the examiner's assessment of the extent of injury. Some health professionals believe that anti-inflammatory medications are contraindicated because they modify the inflammatory response and therefore delay healing. Cold, compression, and elevation all serve to control edema and inflammation and thus limit the extent of secondary tissue injury (see the section on *cryotherapy*). Depending on the location and extent of injury, the acute injury phase will last from 24 to 96 hours. During this phase, the athlete should avoid activities that will exacerbate the injury.

Phase II: Initial Rehabilitation

Progressive pain-free recovery of maximum range of motion is the functional goal of the second phase of rehabilitation.[1] Movement is encouraged within a pain-free arc by using active-assisted range of motion.

Exercises such as active and active-assisted motion may be used to enhance collagen extensibility and alignment, which in turn permits easier motion. In some cases, specific techniques such as continuous passive motion, (see the section, *Range of Motion*) may be needed. Following motion treatment, the injured area may then benefit from cryotherapy to prevent rebound swelling. Toward the end of this phase, gentle isometric strengthening may be initiated to begin strengthening and to retrain neuromuscular coordination that has been lost as a result of the injury. In addition, aerobic activities should be incorporated into the athlete's program to maintain general conditioning. Consideration must be given to the types of activities incorporated into the conditioning program so as not to jeopardize the injured upper extremity. For example, treadmill work and lower extremity weight training can often begin early without exacerbating upper extremity problems.

During the second phase of rehabilitation, the inflammatory process is still present but waning, and, as a consequence, edema gradually decreases though its management remains an important goal. It is important to monitor treatment activities and progress during this phase so the inflammatory response is not exacerbated, and a negative pain-inflammation cycle is not initiated. The earliest fibroblastic stage of healing has now begun: proliferative activity leads to an abundance of fibroblasts within the damaged tissues, which contribute to collagen formation. Scar formation begins with early collagen bundle organization. This histologic process of early healing is associated with significant loss of tensile strength within the damaged tissues, which continue to require protection.

Phase III: Progressive Rehabilitation

Once the patient has reached the point of nearly full, relatively pain-free, passive and active range of motion, more aggressive rehabilitation components for increasing strength and endurance can begin. Conditioning should continue in the third phase of rehabilitation, with increasing aerobic activities as tolerated by the athlete.

Toward the end of the progressive rehabilitation phase, isotonic and/or isokinetic strengthening exercises may be safely incorporated into the rehabilitation program. These activities permit a greater range of physiologic response to the exercise program. Graded therapy putty and hand grippers and free weights are often used for a progressive resistive exercise program (PRE). In addition, equipment such as the Baltimore Therapeutic Equipment work simulator (BTE) can be used to provide very specific, graded exercise programs for upper extremity rehabilitation. Using various attachments with the BTE, PREs for all structures of the upper extremity can be designed (Fig. 2-2). An upper extremity ergometer such as the UBE can provide graded upper extremity resistance as well as an aerobic workout. The Cybex System can also be used for graded upper extremity resistive exercise.

Concurrently with the strengthening program, the athlete's coordination should be assessed and any deficits addressed. Changes in sensibility, and even minimal limitations in range of motion can adversely affect the athlete's coordination and skill performance. Relearning of skills is often necessary following an injury. The specifics of any coordination program will be determined by the amount of deficit the athlete demonstrates and the specific skills required for the sport. Once again, activity simulation can be used as a treatment technique, such as in the improving of coordination.

At this point in the healing process (early tissue repair), there is sufficient muscle strength, as compared to the normal side, for progression to limited activity

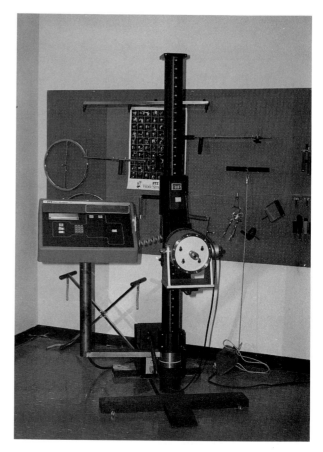

Figure 2-2 BTE work simulator.

skills. For example, a pitcher with rotator cuff tendonitis in this phase of recovery may be able to start light tossing exercises with a football to regain confidence and coordination in the involved muscle groups. A tennis player (statuspost lateral epicondyle release) may begin some gentle swinging with a tennis racquet, and a quarterback with a volar plate injury can begin grasping a football to regain proximal interphalangeal joint extension. This is also the time to determine whether protection will be necessary for the athlete to advance safely to the next phase of rehabilitation. If needed, external protection can be provided by taping or functional bracing (see Ch. 8).

In this third phase of rehabilitation, the fibroblastic stage of wound healing begins to overlap with the early tissue specific repair stage of wound healing. This is a lengthy process in which remodeling and realignment of collagen fibers occur according to the tensile forces to which the scar is exposed. As tensile strength improves in tissues such as tendon and ligament, it is appropriate to increase range of motion to the normal full arc. Clinical factors such as a decrease in pain, swelling, and increased tolerance of motion serve to guide the clinician during this phase.

Phase IV: Integrated Functions

The functional goals (Table 2-4) of the fourth phase are several: (1) to enhance flexibility to preinjury conditions (and possibly superior to preinjury standards if relative inflexibility was the cause of the injury); (2) to increase strength; (3) to increase specific athletic skills; and (4) to improve exercise tolerance. Additionally, protective equipment needs, activity modification, and proprioception should be assessed further during this phase.

Proprioception is the sense of where one's limbs are in three-dimensional space, the speed of movement of individual limb segments, and how these movements affect the body and athletic activity undertaken. Proprioceptive awareness takes place on a subconscious level during the heat of competition, but training can improve it. Maneuvers that simulate the actual skill needed to play the specific sport must be practiced repeatedly. For example, a basketball player recuperating from an olecranon injury will need to practice his free throw motion to regain necessary neuromuscular coordination. Pitchers recuperating from an injury may now start practicing the pitching motion with light, short tosses, advancing to longer, faster throwing as tolerated (see Ch. 16). As mentioned above, the BTE can be adapted to simulate many useful activities as well as serve as a component in the athlete's strengthening program.

During the integrated functions phase of rehabilitation, the maturation stage of healing continues to progress. The injured tissues are gradually assuming more normal architecture and function. This process can be augmented with the use of modalities such as scar compression, splinting, and heat. Although scar tissue is not as strong as uninjured tissue, it is appropriate to begin integrated functions, since the healing tissues are ready to withstand the stress that will be placed on them.

During phase IV, care begins to transfer from health professionals to the coaching staff such that the coach becomes an important contributor to the athlete's rehabilitation. Strong communication between the coaching staff and the rehabilitation team is imperative for successful rehabilitation.

Phase V: Return to Sport

During the fifth phase, the rehabilitation team progressively transfers responsibilities for the athlete's performance to the coaching staff. At this point, the rehabilitation team's role is to ensure that the athlete has achieved a return to normal strength as determined by physical examination or by objective isokinetic testing.

The rehabilitation team must also evaluate the need to continue maintenance exercises and external protection to aid maximal recovery and minimize the possibility of reinjury.

Using their knowledge of sports, healing, and rehabilitation, the coaching staff's major functional goal, in conjunction with the experience of the athlete, physician, and trainer, is to determine clinical readiness for return to full competition. It is at this point that the athlete progresses from simulation to competition. While the athlete is returning to a highly competitive level, he or she has to be reminded of the importance of continuing a progressive rehabilitation and conditioning program to maximize abilities and to limit the chance of reinjury. Tissue remodeling occurs to the point where mature tissue characteristics and integrity are present.

THERAPEUTIC MODALITIES IN SPORTS REHABILITATION

The therapeutic modalities of cold, compression, motion, progressive resistive exercise, heat, and electricity are used by rehabilitation professionals throughout the five phases of rehabilitation to facilitate treatment goals. Each modality is incorporated into the program for a specific purpose, based upon the athlete's stage of rehabilitation and response to treatment. The following discussion of therapeutic modalities should not be considered exhaustive; readers interested in further details, including technique of application, should seek other sources.[26-28]

Cryotherapy

Cryotherapy, the therapeutic application of local cold, is restricted to superficial structures. It is used to decrease edema and serves as both an analgesic and anesthetic. It limits local tissue damage by minimizing hypoxic tissue necrosis, edema, and inflammation.[29-31] Common acute inflammatory conditions seen in sports medicine clinics respond well to cryotherapy. Acute epicondylitis, bursitis, and tenosynovitis may be managed with cold during the acute injury phase. In general, agents that are primitive but effective such as ice, cold water, skin refrigerants, refrigeration units, and chemical packs are used.

Cooling a local area results in an initial period of vasoconstriction due to regional reflexes and increased sympathetic constrictor tone.[32-35] It is believed that vasoconstriction continues until subcutaneous temperatures fall to about 15°C (59°F). Below 15°C (59°F), blood vessels dilate as a result of paralysis of contractile mechanisms or blockage of sympathetic constrictor signals. If skin cooling continues to a temperature of 0°C (32°F), an increase in cutaneous blood flow may actually be noted.[33] As skin cooling progresses, an equilibrium temperature of about 12 to 13°C (53 to 55°F) is reached in a 10-minute time span. Subcutaneous tissue temperatures decline by 3 to 5°C (37 to 41°F) and deep muscle temperature decreases the least. In 10 minutes, deep muscle temperature may be lessened by only 1°C (34°F).[36] The slowness of the drop in deep muscle temperature is primarily due to the insulating quality of fat. It has been shown that the muscle of a thin person is cooled in approximately 10 minutes, while the cooling would take approximately a half hour in an overweight person.[36]

The most common technique of application is the melting of ice together with cold water, thereby creating a slush at 0°C (32°F). The affected area is then treated with submersion or topical application. This technique is often carried out for 20 to 30 minutes, and may be combined with local compression to inhibit interstitial fluid collection, which arises as a consequence of an acute inflammatory process from tissue trauma. Several devices are commercially available that work to cool an injured structure while providing some compression. For example, the Aircast Company makes sleeves for shoulders and elbows that are filled with ice water such that the joint is subject to cooling and compression at the same time.

Other application techniques include the use of iced whirlpools, which employ heat or cold transfer across a temperature gradient via convection currents. An iced whirlpool treatment may employ a slurry of ice and water (about 0°C [32°F]) rapidly churning while the treated limb is immersed for 10 to 20 minutes per session.

Ice is an extremely safe modality, although it should be remembered that too vigorous or too prolonged an application can cause tissue damage from ischemia and/or cellular death from freezing; in susceptible persons, exacerbations of Raynaud's disease should be prevented. Cold-induced hypersensitivity reactions and urticaria must also be considered. Topical applications of ice to insensate skin are safer than heat but not without risk. Finally, neural tissue is very sensitive to temperature changes. Our experience and the sports medicine literature document cold-induced peripheral nerve injuries,[37] thus we caution against prolonged cold directly over superficial nerves.

On the field, use of chemical refrigerants (e.g., ethyl chloride, fluoromethane) as a temporary method to cool the skin has some merit, since the effect is as a topical anesthetic. Chemical packs that employ endothermic reactions may be applied, but their cooling properties are inferior to those of ice and carry the risk of leaking and causing chemical burns to the skin.

Edema Management

One of the primary goals in the acute injury phase of the rehabilitation process is edema management. Those methods used to decrease pain and inflammation will also help to reduce edema. Elevation is also vitally important in the management of edema. Splint or cast immobilization should be in the functional position as dictated by the specific type of injury. Improper positioning, in conjunction with edema, can impede the athlete's ability to regain full range of motion. (Fig. 2-3) (e.g., a radius fracture immobilized with cast distal to the proximal palmar crease may result in limited metacarpophalangeal joint range; a Boxer's fracture immobilized with metacarpophalangeal joint extension and/or proximal interphalangeal joint flexion may result in permanent contracture at these joints).

In addition to positioning, there are a number of techniques that can be used to decrease edema. If there are no contraindications secondary to vascular compromise, infection, or unstable fracture, compression (via gloves, coban wrapping, elastic bandage wrapping, or pneumatic pumps) is an effective method for treating edema. Coban wrapping provides constant gentle compression. Coban wrap is a self-adhering, elasticized wrap most commonly used for smaller areas such as digits (1-in. coban) or hands (2-in. coban). If compression is needed for larger areas (e.g., hand and forearm), an elasticized stockinette or elastic bandage can be used to provide the compression. Wrapping should always be done distal to proximal (Fig. 2-4). Distal aspects of digits should be visible and tips should be checked regularly for color, temperature, and sensation. Instruction on wrap application as well as a list of warning signals, (throbbing, numbness or tingling of the digits, decreased temperature of digit tips, and color change of digit tip, i.e., cyanosis, to dark blue or purple) should be

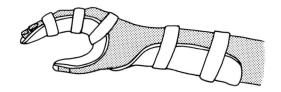

Figure 2-3 Volar resting splint.

given to the patient. In the acute injury phase, compression will be most effective for decreasing edema. There are a number of machines available (e.g., Jobst pump) to provide pneumatic compression. Intermittent periods of compression are generally followed by compression wrapping or gloving to maintain the edema control.

Limiting or decreasing edema will facilitate the achievement of other rehabilitation goals, such as increased range of motion. Maximal range of motion is critical to regaining full functional use of the upper extremity. Range of motion should be addressed in the rehabilitation program as early as possible. The type of injury and its initial management, open versus closed (i.e., surgical fixation or repair vs conservative treatment) will determine the time frame for introducing a range of motion program (time frames will be discussed specifically for each diagnosis in specific chapters).

Early motion is often used for edema management. The patient should be instructed to perform active or active-assisted motion to all (stable) upper extremity joints three to five times per day. The time frame for initiation of range of motion is dictated by the specific injury (e.g., digit range of motion with radius fracture can be initiated immediately, while active-assisted motion with flexor tendon injuries is not initiated until $3\frac{1}{2}$ weeks). Continuous passive motion can be useful for reducing edema as well as for managing pain.[38] It is the "pumping" effect of the motion that facilitates the reduction of the swelling. Finally, retrograde massage has also proven successful in the reduction of edema. Patients should be taught to perform this procedure three to five times per day, followed by compression wrapping.

Range of Motion

Throughout the initial phases of rehabilitation, treatment is geared toward minimizing any "pain cycle" response (Fig. 2-5). The "pain cycle" consists of an initial injury and inflammation that causes pain. This pain leads to decreased use or disuse of the injured extremity, which then leads to atrophy and fibrosis. This in turn facilitates a decrease in flexibility and development of contractures, followed by altered function, weakness, and, ultimately, decreased performance. Early initiation of range of motion and education on pain will help the athlete caught in this cycle.

A motion program consists of active, active-assistive, and passive range of motion exercises. The active range of motion arc is the amount of motion the athlete is able to obtain without external assistance. Active-assisted motion combines the athlete's power with external assistance, while passive motion is achieved solely through external forces. Patients must be active participants in the program and should be instructed on a self-range program to be completed at least five times per day (Fig. 2-6), ideally every 1 to 2 waking hours. Written instructions and diagrams on the technique, along with advising patients of any precautions or contraindications, will ensure that exercises are performed correctly. The frequency of the treatment provided by the therapist will vary depending upon the nature of the injury, the athlete's status (weekend athlete, competitive amateur, or professional) and motivation level. For individuals with more involved injuries or with decreased comprehension of the home program, more directly supervised, daily treatment may be necessary, while less involved, compliant athletes may require

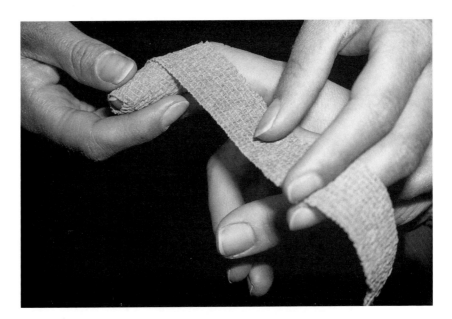

Figure 2-4 Coban wrapping of digit.

only weekly monitoring by the health care provider to assess progress and update the home program. Use of any pain or anti-inflammatory medications should be monitored by the physician.

The progress of a range of motion program will be unique for each athlete. As healing progresses, the injured structures will be able to tolerate increased stress without risk of reinjury, and the athlete will be able to tolerate increased stress without an adverse pain response. The arc of motion provided should be increased as tolerated by the athlete. If an increase in pain or edema occurs following an exercise session, it is an indication that the exercise was too aggressive and should be moderated. The adage "no pain, no gain" should not be used as a criterion for the progression of the treatment program. Icing can be used following a range of motion treatment session to limit any localized inflammatory response that may be present secondary to the stress applied to the healing tissues.

Plyometrics are exercises or patterns of function that are performed to integrate muscle function and speed of movement. The goal of plyometrics is to maximize the muscle activity from complete concentric contraction to complete eccentric contraction. Plyometrics should not be used until late in phase III or in phase IV

of rehabilitation. If used too soon, reinjury or additional injury can result. Plyometrics should not be used if there is pain, instability, or weak muscles.

Joint Mobilization and Splinting

Joint mobilization techniques can be used by a therapist to facilitate increased range of motion. Serial static and dynamic splinting are other useful methods for improving range of motion. With serial splinting, a prolonged (6 to 8 hours), gentle, passive stretch is applied to the tissues. The tissues respond by accommodating to the stretch and lengthening. The duration of the stretch must be long enough to alter new tissue synthesis.[39] Dynamic splinting is used to provide a more aggressive stretch to the tissues for a shorter duration of time (45 minutes to 1 hour). Once again, the tissues accommodate to the stress provided by the splint. The type of splint used is best determined by the type of injury, precautions, patient compliance, and physiologic response to the splint.

The initiation of these modalities will generally occur at the end of the initial rehabilitation phase and can continue through the progressive rehabilitation

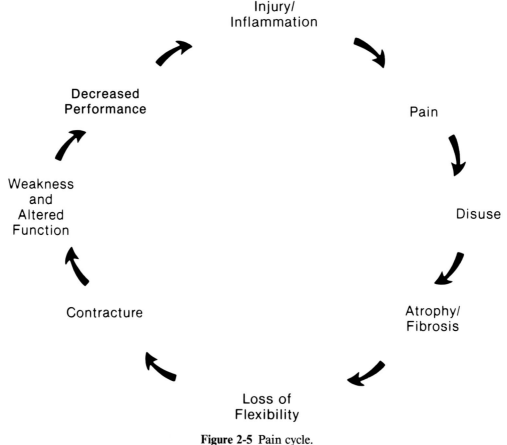

Figure 2-5 Pain cycle.

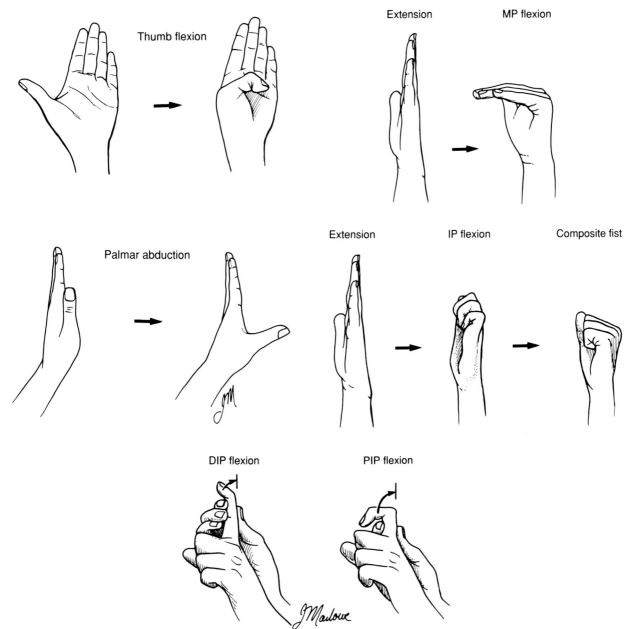

Thumb flexion

Extension · MP flexion

Palmar abduction

Extension · IP flexion · Composite fist

DIP flexion · PIP flexion

Figure 2-6 Self-range program.

phase. By the time the patient has progressed to the integrated functions phase, use of this type of splinting modality generally will no longer be necessary. Caution must be exercised with all range of motion and splinting programs to minimize microtrauma to the healing structures. Pain may be used as a guide for treatment intensity.

Continuous Passive Motion

Continuous passive motion (CPM), a modality utilized to promote increased motion, uses machines de-signed to move body parts through specified arcs of motion. CPM works most effectively to maintain range of motion gains obtained through mobilization, splinting, and other exercises. It is not effective for moving a stiff joint through an arc of motion. The full application and benefit gained by the use of CPM has been increasingly explored over the past 20 years. The detrimental effects of immobilization are well-documented in the literature. Significant numbers of animal model studies have shown the beneficial effects of CPM on the healing of various tissues, including articular cartilage, ligament, and tendon.[38,40] Use of CPM immediately following injury contributes to improved nourishment and indirect healing of articular cartilage, increased tensile strength and intrinsic healing of tendons with decreased adhesion formation, and maintenance of joint nutrition and integrity. Gelberman and Manske[22] reported in a prospective, randomized study that statistically significant improvements in outcome following zone II flexor tendon injuries are obtained with use of CPM as compared to standard flexor tendon management protocols.

In addition, we have successfully treated intra-articular proximal interphalangeal joint and metacarpophalangeal joint fractures with CPM immediately postoperatively and have seen full range of motion without evidence of early degenerative joint changes.

Scar Management

As the healing process proceeds, scar tissue is formed. Scar tissue can be remodeled so that it performs similarly to the tissue it is replacing; however, if scar management does not occur, the scar tissue will remain thick, adherent, minimally extensible, and often hypersensitive. Scar management modalities include massage, compression, and ultrasound. Silicone-based products, such as elastomer, otoform, and silicone gel sheets, can be used to provide constant, uniform pressure to scars. They can be secured with elastic wraps or incorporated into splints. As with other treatment modalities, the time frame for the initiation of scar management will be based upon the type of injury and the healing process along with the patient's response to treatment (Fig. 2-7).

Therapeutic Heat

Therapeutic heat increases collagen extensibility, decreases joint stiffness, produces pain relief, relieves muscle spasm, and increases local blood flow. Thera-

peutic heat should not be used in the acute injury or the initial rehabilitation phases of sports rehabilitation because it tends to exacerbate edema. Heat, however, becomes very important in the progressive and latter phases of rehabilitation due to its analgesic effect and positive influence on tissue extensibility which ultimately enhance joint range of motion.

Therapeutic heating modalities are commonly classified by those providing superficial tissue temperature increases (e.g., hot packs, paraffin baths, hydrotherapy or whirlpool treatments, and infrared or luminous heat lamps) and those producing temperature increases in deep tissues such as muscles, ligaments, tendons, periosteum, and joint capsules. The deep heating modalities are called diathermy (e.g., microwave diathermy, shortwave diathermy, and ultrasound diathermy).

The therapeutically effective temperature range for heating biologic tissues is 40 to 45.5°C (104 to 113.9°F) (Fig. 2-8). Higher temperatures cannot be maintained for as long as lower temperatures, since tissue damage occurs at an increasing rate with increasing temperature. Thus the skin can tolerate a drop of water at 45°C (113°F) for 1 hour but can only tolerate a drop of water at 65°C (149°F) for approximately 1 second before damage occurs (Fig. 2-9). Within the therapeutic temperature range, the approximate therapeutic duration is 3 to 30 minutes. Other determinants of the physiologic action to heat include the rate of tissue temperature rise and the size of the treatment area. It should be remembered that for every 1°C (34°F) rise in body temperature, the metabolic demand for O_2 increases by 10 percent.

Shortwave and microwave diathermy produce heating of tissues as a result of resistance to the passage of high-frequency electromagnetic currents that are created. Heating of deep tissues occurs by causing rapid motion of molecules within tissues. Neither modality is recommended as a form of deep heating, as each has been replaced by ultrasound diathermy.

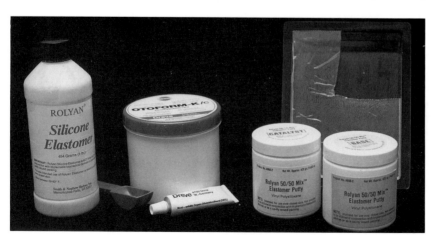

Figure 2-7 Commercially available silicon-based products used for scar compression.

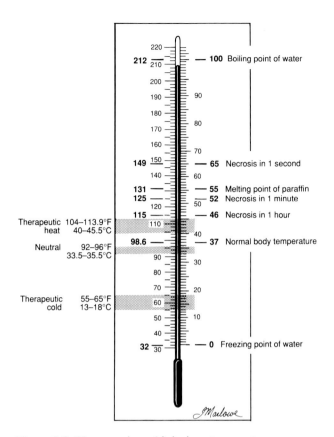

Figure 2-8 Therapeutic and injurious temperature ranges.

Ultrasound

Unlike microwave and shortwave diathermy, ultrasound does not use electromagnetic energy to heat tissues. Ultrasound equipment works by transforming electrical energy into acoustical vibrations (sound) (Fig. 2-10). Ultrasound heats deep tissues by sending

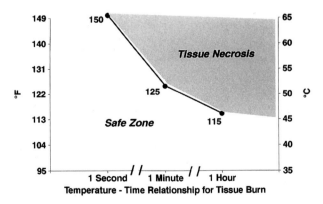

Figure 2-9 Temperature-time relationship for tissue burn.

acoustical vibrations through them, causing vibration of molecules which in turn produces heat. Tissue interfaces (such as the muscle-periosteum interface) are selectively heated because of reflection and formation of shear waves as the acoustical vibrations travel through tissues of varying acoustic impedance.[27,36] Ultrasound is relatively ineffective at heating surfaces but is the most effective modality for heating deep tissues and may penetrate to depths of 4 to 6 cm. Therefore, ultrasound is the method of choice for heating deep tissues and joints and is the most common form of diathermy currently used in sports rehabilitation.

Ultrasound has reported benefits (e.g., treatment of joint contractures, inflammation, tendon repairs) and precautions (e.g., prohibited with ischemic tissue, limited exposure to superficial nerves) when applied to sport injury rehabilitation. It may be used for treating joint contractures and scar formation, to reduce pain and muscle spasm, and is commonly used in the management of bursitis, tendonitis, and periarticular calcium deposits. It can be used in individuals who have metallic implants, and in fact, is the only safe form of deep heating which allows this.[21] It may also be used as an adjunct in wound healing whereby clinicians employ ultrasound to repaired tendons to aid healing and to prevent adhesions to the tendon sheath. The literature, however, is inconclusive as to its benefits and potential complications when used after tendon repairs.[41,42]

In summary, therapeutic ultrasound is recommended as a deep heating modality in sports rehabilitation, provided that appropriate indications and precautions are followed.

Phonophoresis

Phonophoresis utilizes therapeutic ultrasound in conjunction with a medication-laden ultrasound coupling media to drive the medication across the skin and into subcutaneous tissues.[43,44] There is clinical evidence that the use of hydrocortisone enhances the therapeutic benefit of ultrasound. The exact way ultrasound aids permeation of drug into subcutaneous tissues is not known.[45]

A common clinical practice is to mix hydrocortisone powder in an ointment or cream to form a 10 percent-by-weight compound and then use this as the coupling medium. The clinician should be aware that some of these preparations have relatively low ultrasound transmissivity because microscopic amounts of air introduced during the mixing process block sound wave transmission.[46] Many pharmacists will mix a 10 percent hydrocortisone medium or commercial preparations of 10 percent hydrocortisone can be purchased

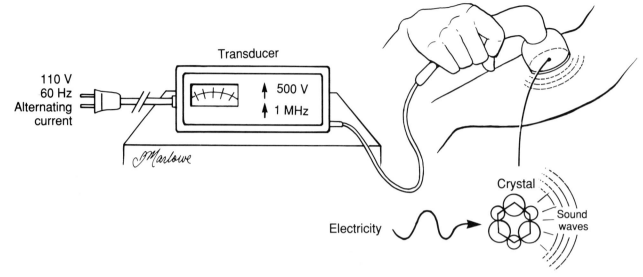

Figure 2-10 Household current to high voltage ultrasound.

from suppliers.* Patients may experience beneficial effects from the use of phonophoresis for rehabilitating sports injuries such as epicondylitis, tendonitis, and bursitis. Generally, the individual is given a daily treatment of 5 to 10 minutes for a total of 10 to 14 treatments. We recommend a trial of this modality on a case by-weight compound and then use this as the coupling medium. The clinician should be aware that some of these preparations have relatively low ultrasound

Electrical Stimulation

Neuromuscular electrical stimulation (NMES) has been clinically used to activate electrically excitable tissues (muscle and nerve), and is reported to modulate pain, control edema, improve strength, aid tissue repair, and help drive ions across living tissues.

Transcutaneous electrical nerve stimulation (TENS) utilizes short duration, high-frequency, low-intensity galvanic pulses delivered above the sensory nerve threshold and below the motor nerve threshold. It is thought that pain fiber transmission is blocked peripherally or there is an activation of central inhibiting fibers (similar to the original gate control theory of pain proposed by Melzack and Wall[47]) that modulates pain. Its clinical utility has been shown[48-50] and it is also well accepted for the management of postoperative pain. We recommend its usage for pain control when other standard approaches fail (e.g., analgesics, ice, compression).

Electrically elicited rhythmic muscle contractions may be used for edema control by aiding lymphatic and venous drainage.[51,52] Galvanic (direct) current has also been shown to aid wound healing at rates 1.5 to 2.5 faster than control groups.[53,55] We believe that research studies are still lacking in these areas, and thus at this time cannot recommend electrical stimulation as an accepted modality for edema control or wound healing.

One of the most promising applications of neuromuscular electrical stimulation is that of facilitating strength gain in weakened muscles. We believe that neuromuscular electrical stimulation may be beneficial in those with nonneurologic muscle weakness, and recommend using this procedure as a facilitator of strength gain in selected individuals with nonneurologic weakness, along with other standard approaches to building strength. One example of this benefit has been demonstrated using neuromuscular electrical stimulation after anterior cruciate ligament reconstruction. Patients who had neuromuscular electrical stimulation applied to the quadriceps muscle demonstrated significantly greater quadriceps strength gains when compared to controls. These strength gains could be correlated with functional improvements in gait kinematics and mechanics versus the control group.[55]

Iontophoresis

Iontophoresis, the application of electricity to drive ions across living tissues, has been in use for more than a half-century.[26] The electricity employed for ion transfer is continuous low-voltage galvanic (direct) current provided by a low-voltage generator or a battery-powered unit. The basis for ion transfer is that

---

* Ultracort (10 percent hydrocortisone in an aqueous ultrasound transmission gel). Lyne Laboratories, Inc. 260 Toscal Drive, Stoughton, MA 02072-9990. 617-344-4676.

like charges repel each other. Therefore, a positively charged ion will travel away from the positively charged electrode (anode) and toward the negatively charged electrode (cathode). While doing so, a therapeutically active ion will enter the dermis and ideally the subcutaneous tissues. Certain researchers, however, believe that ion penetration is generally less than 1 cm, which is less than ideal.[45] The majority of active ions are deposited directly beneath the active electrode with further penetration depending on local blood flow for transport to deeper tissues.[26]

Iontophoresis has become a common treatment regimen in sports rehabilitation. Typically, medications such as dexamethasone disodium phosphate (Decadron), salicylic acid, or lidocaine (Xylocaine)[56] are delivered to the skin to relieve inflammation and pain. Several commercial units for patient use are presently marketed.* Chemical burns, heat burns, and cutaneous sensitivity to the applied ions are complications to be avoided. Further clinical research is needed before we can recommend this as standard practice.[57,58]

For athletes who have trouble with injections, the application of pain relief and anti-inflammatory medications without injection via phonophoresis or iontophoresis may be useful. In general, we do not believe there is enough clinical validity to recommend them as a first line of treatment.

REFERENCES

1. Pappas AM: Rehabilitation. In Dyment PG (ed): Sports Medicine: Health Care for Young Athletes. 2nd Ed. American Academy of Pediatrics, 1991 Elk Grove Village, IL
2. Cahill BR, Grifith EH: Effect of preseason conditioning on the incidence and severity of high school football knee injuries. Am J Sports Med 6:180, 1978
3. Gliem GW, Witman PA, Nicholas JA: Indirect assessment of cardiovascular "demands" using telemetry on professional football players. Am J Sports Med 9:178, 1981
4. Wilmore JH, Freund BJ: Nutritional enhancement of athletic performance. p. 67. In: Sensible Fitness. Leisure Press, Champaign, IL, 1986
5. Smith AM, Scott SG, Wiese DM: The psychological effects of sports injuries. Sports Med 9:352, 1990
5a. Kubler-Ross E: On Death and Dying. pp. 86–111. MacMillan, New York, 1969
6. Kerr G, Fowler B: The relationship between psychological factors and sports injuries. Sports Med 6:127, 1988
7. Smith AM, Scott DO, O'fallon WM et al: Emotional responses of athletes to injury. Mayo Clin Proc 65:38, 1990
8. Kelley MJ Jr: Psychological risk factors and sports injuries. J Sports Med Phys Fitn 30:202, 1990
9. Prentice W: Therapeutic Modalities in Sports Medicine. pp. 1–15. CV Mosby, St. Louis, MO, 1986
10. Reynolds G, Higdon H: Positive Pain. Superfit. (Spring), 90:65, 1986
11. Taylor DC, Dalton JD, Seaber AV, Garrett WE: Viscoelastic properties of muscle-tendon units, the biomechanical effects of stretching. Am J Sports Med 18:300, 1990
12. Lieber, RL: Skeletal Muscle Structure and Function: Implications for Rehabilitation and Sports Medicine. Williams & Wilkins, Baltimore, 1992
13. Russell B, Dix DJ, Haller DL, Jacobs-El J: Repair of injured skeletal muscle: a molecular approach. Med Sci Sports Exerc 24:189, 1992
14. Miltner LJ, Hu CH, Fang HC: Experimental joint sprain. Arch Surg 35:234, 1934
15. Goldstein WM, Barmada R: Early mobilization of rabbit medial collateral ligament repairs: biomechanic and histologic study. Arch Phys Med Rehabil 65:239, 1984
16. O'Donoghue DH, Frank GR, Jeter GL et al: Repair and reconstruction of the anterior cruciate ligament in dogs. J Bone Joint Surg [Am] 53:710, 1971
17. Vailas AC, Tipton CM, Matthes RD, Gart M: Physical activity and its influence on the repair process of medial collateral ligaments. Connect Tissue Res 9:25, 1981
18. Green DP, Rowland SA: Fractures and dislocations in the hand. Ch. 7. In Rockwood CA, Green DP, Bucholz RW (eds): Fractures in Adults. 3rd Ed. JB Lippincott, Philadelphia, 1991
19. Neviaser RJ, Wilson JN, Lievano A: Rupture of the ulnar collateral ligament of the thumb. J Bone Joint Surg [Am] 53:1357, 1971
20. Daniels K, Dee R: Ligaments: structure, function, and repair. p. 48. In: Dee R, Mango E, Hurst LC (eds): Principles of Orthopaedic Practice. McGraw-Hill, New York, 1989
21. Potenza AD: Flexor tendon injuries. Orthop Clin North Am 1:2, 1970
22. Gelberman RH, Nunley II JA et al: Influences of the protected passive mobilization interval on flexor tendon healing. Clin Orthop 264:189–199, 1991
23. Gelberman R, Goldberg V, Kai-Wan A, Banes A: Tendon. p. 9. In Woo SL-Y, Buckwalter JA (eds): Injury and Repair of the Musculoskeletal Soft Tissues. American Academy of Orthopedic Surgeons, 1988, Park Ridge, IL
24. Strickland JW: Biological rationale, clinical application, and results of early motion following flexor tendon repair. J Hand Therapy 71, 1989
25. Buckwalter JA, Cruess RL: Healing of musculoskeletal tissues. Ch. 2. pp. 181–222. In Rockwood CA, Green DP, Bucholz RW (eds): Fractures in Adults. 3rd Ed. JB Lippincott, Philadelphia, 1991
26. Kahn J: Iontophoresis. p. 119. In: Principles and Practice of Electrotherapy, 2nd Ed. Churchill Livingstone, New York, 1991

---

* Phoresor electronic transdermal drug delivery system. IOMED, Inc. 1290 West 2320 South Salt Lake City, UT 84119. (800) 621-3347.

27. Michlovitz SL: Thermal Agents in Rehabilitation. FA Davis, Philadelphia, 1986

28. Snyder-Mackler L, Robinson AJ: Clinical Electrophysiology, Electrotherapy and Electrophysiologic Testing. Williams & Wilkins, Baltimore, 1989

29. Basur RL, Shepherd E, Monzas GL: A cooling method in the treatment of ankle sprains. Practitioner 216:708, 1976

30. Knight KL: Ice, compression and elevation in the immediate care of traumatic injuries. p. 15. In Knight KL (ed): Cryotherapy: Theory, Technique and Physiology. 1st Ed. Chattanooga Corporation, Chattanooga, TN, 1985

31. Schaubel HJ: The local use of ice after orthopedic procedures. Am J Surg 72:711, 1946

32. Franchiment P, Juchmes J, Lecomite J: Hydrotherapy: mechanisms and indications. Pharmacol Ther 20:79, 1983

33. Guyton AC: Muscle blood flow during exercise: cerebral, splanchnic, and skin blood flows. p. 336. In Textbook of Medical Physiology. 7th Ed. WB Saunders, Philadelphia, 1986

34. Perkins JF, Li MC, Hoffman F et al: Sudden vasoconstriction in denervated or sympathectomized paws exposed to cold. Am J Physiol 155:165, 1948

35. Schmidt KL, Oh VR, Rocher G et al: Heat, cold, and inflammation. Rheumatology 38:391, 1979

36. Lehmann JF, deLateur BJ: Therapeutic heat. In Lehmann JF (ed): Therapeutic Heat and Cold. 4th Ed. Williams & Wilkins, Baltimore, 1990

37. Drez D, DC Faust, JP Evans: Cryotherapy and nerve palsy. Am J Sports Med 9:256, 1981

38. Salter RB: The biological concept of continuous passive motion of synovial joints: the first 18 years of basic research and its clinical application. Clin Orthop 242:12, 1989

39. Colditz JC: Dynamic splinting of the stiff hand. p. 342. In Hunter JM, Schneider LH, Mackin EJ, Callahan AD (eds): Rehabilitation of the Hand: Surgery and Therapy. 3rd Ed. CV Mosby, St. Louis, 1990

40. Namba RS, Kabo JM, Dorey FJ, Meals RA: Continuous passive motion versus immobilization: the effect on posttraumatic joint stiffness. In Section III Basic Science and Pathology. Clin Orthop 267:218, 1991

41. Enwemeka CS: The effects of therapeutic ultrasound on tendon healing a biomechanical study. Am J Phys Med Rehabil 68:283, 1989

42. Roberts M, Rutherford JH, Harris D: The effect of ultrasound on flexor tendon repairs in the rabbit. Hand 14:17, 1982

43. Davick JR, Martin RK, Albright JP: Distribution and deposition of tritiated cortisol using phonophoresis. Phys Ther 68:1672, 1988

44. Griffin JE, Touchstone JC: Ultrasonic movement of corticosteroid into pig tissue. Proc Soc Exp Biol Med 109:461, 1962

45. Tyle P, Agrawala P: Drug delivery by phonophoresis. [Reveiw]. Pharm Res 6:355, 1989

46. Warren CG, Koblanski JN, Sigelman RA: Ultrasound coupling media: their relative transmissivity. Arch Phys Med Rehabil 57:218, 1976

47. Melzack R, Wall PD: Pain mechanisms: a new theory. Science 150:971, 1965

48. Ersek RA: Low back pain: prompt relief with transcutaneous neurostimulation—a report of 35 consecutive patients. Orthop Rev 5:27, 1976

49. Nathan PW, Wall PD: Treatment of post-herpetic neuralgia by prolonged electrical stimulation. Br Med J 3:645, 1974

50. Roberts HJ: TENS in the management of pancreatitis pain. South Med J 71:396, 1978

51. Apperty FL, Cary MK: The control of circulatory stasis by the electrical stimulation of large muscle group. Am J Med Sci 216:403, 1948

52. Doran FSA, White M, Frury M: A clinical trial designed to test the relative value of two simple methods of reducing the risk of venous stasis in the lower limbs during surgical operations, the danger of thrombosis and a subsequent pulmonary embolism, with a survey of the problem. Br J Surg 57:20, 1970

53. Carley P, Wainapel SF: Electrotherapy for acceleration of wound healing: low intensity direct current. Arch Phys Med Rehabil 66:443, 1985

54. Wolcott L, Wheeler P, Hardwicke H et al: Accelerated healing of skin ulcers by electrotherapy. South Med J 62:795, 1969

55. Snyder-Mackler L, Ladin Z, Schepsis A, Young JC: Electrical stimulation of the thigh muscles after reconstruction of the anterior cruciate ligament. J Bone Joint Surg 73A:1025, 1991

56. Novak EJ: Experimental transmission of lidocaine through intact skin by ultrasound. Arch Phys Med Rehabil 5:231, 1964

57. Glick E, Snyder-Mackler L: Iontophoresis. In Snyder-Mackler L, Robinson AJ (eds): Clinical Electrophysiology, Electrotherapy, and Electrophysiologic Testing. Williams & Wilkins, Baltimore, 1989

58. Henley EJ: Transcutaneous drug delivery: iontophoresis, phonophoresis. Crit Rev Phys Rehabil Med 2:139, 1991

3

Nerve Anatomy and Diagnostic Principles

Randall R. Long

Peripheral nerve involvement should always be considered when assessing the upper extremity of an injured athlete. Although peripheral nerve injuries are not a common finding in upper extremity athletic injuries, peripheral nerve dysfunction can disturb the level of musculoskeletal performance required for competitive and even recreational sports, and, in turn, predispose the individual to further injury. More significant nerve pathology will have a major impact on the rate and extent of recovery from injury and can lead to abrupt disruption and, potentially, termination of athletic careers.

Peripheral nerve injuries in athletes fall into two major groups: acute and chronic. Acute nerve injury may be associated with otherwise obvious musculoskeletal trauma, particularly fractures or dislocations in which there is an appreciable displacement of normal structures. Acute nerve injuries are recognizable primarily by virtue of associated motor and sensory deficits. Chronic peripheral mononeuropathies are associated with a repetitive athletic activity in a given sport, and can be compared to repetitive use or entrapment neuropathies in occupational medicine. Chronic mononeuropathies may also present with objective clinical deficits, but the presentation is usually more vague. Recurrent use-related pain may be the only early manifestation. In such cases, there may be pain at the site of injury, but it is more often referred to the

nerve's sensory field or to muscles and joints innervated by the nerve. The following discussion will review relevant peripheral nerve anatomy, the pathogenesis of peripheral nerve injury and general diagnostic principles. The clinical aspects of injury to the individual nerves of the upper limb are discussed in Chapter 4.

ANATOMIC ORGANIZATION

The peripheral nervous system (PNS) consists of parallel axons, myelin sheaths and Schwann cells, both longitudinal (endoneurium and epineurium) and circumferential (perineurium) connective tissue elements, and blood vessels (vasa nervorum). The sensory and motor portions of the peripheral nervous system extend centrally to the dorsal horn or dorsal column nuclei and to the anterior horn cell, respectively.

The functional subunits of the nerve are the axon and the Schwann cell. Pathologic insults affect either axons, Schwann cells, or both. A process that primarily affects axons may impair the ability to conduct electrical impulses or lead to axonal degeneration distal to the site of injury. If Schwann cells are the major target of injury, segmental demyelination occurs, slowing or blocking conduction of electrical impulses. Subsequent remyelination may restore conduction, but remyelinated internodes are shorter and thinner than normal, and conduction across remyelinated segments is slower than normal. Extensive segmental demyelination may in turn cause secondary axonal degeneration. If axons are transected, the distal axon and its myelin degenerate simultaneously—a process known as wallerian degeneration. If motor axons undergo either axonal or Wallerian degeneration, the muscle cells they innervate will undergo denervation atrophy. Segmental demyelination of motor axons does not lead to denervation changes in muscle, even if electrical conduction is blocked. These basic pathologic processes are illustrated in Figure 3-1.

The cell bodies of motor axons lie within the ventral horns of the spinal cord. The cell bodies of sensory axons reside in the dorsal root ganglia, their central axons projecting to the dorsal horns or ascending sensory tracts. Motor axons exit exclusively via the ventral roots, while most sensory axons enter via the dorsal roots. Once the dorsal and ventral roots join to form the spinal nerves, a number of merging and diverging connections serve to group together axons with common peripheral distributions.

At the cervical levels that subserve upper limb function, the spinal nerves reorganize to form the trunks and cords of the brachial plexus and then the major peripheral nerves of the limb. The anatomic organization of the peripheral nervous system relevant to the upper limb can be viewed as composed of the following levels: cervical cord segments, dorsal and ventral spinal roots, plexus trunks, plexus cords, and specific peripheral nerves (Fig. 3-2). The clinical manifestations of

injury at each level are unique and provide the basis for accurate clinical diagnosis.

It is useful to keep in mind not only the site of origin of each nerve from the brachial plexus, but also the contributions to each from the relevant roots, and thus the pathways through the plexus (Table 3-1).

BRACHIAL PLEXUS

Figure 3-3 provides a schematic diagram of the right brachial plexus, viewed from the front. The superior, middle, and inferior trunks and their divisions are key to understanding the organization of the brachial plexus. Each trunk divides into an anterior and posterior division, all three posterior divisions joining to form the posterior cord. The anterior divisions of the superior and middle trunks form the lateral cord; the medial cord is the extension of the remaining anterior division of the inferior trunk.

Long Thoracic Nerve

The long thoracic nerve is the most proximal in its origin, formed by the confluence of posterior branches from the C5, C6, and C7 roots. The C5 and C6 contributions join, pass through the medial scalene muscle, and then join the C7 branch. Thereafter the nerve passes laterally and inferiorly behind the brachial plexus and the major vessels to first reach the anterior

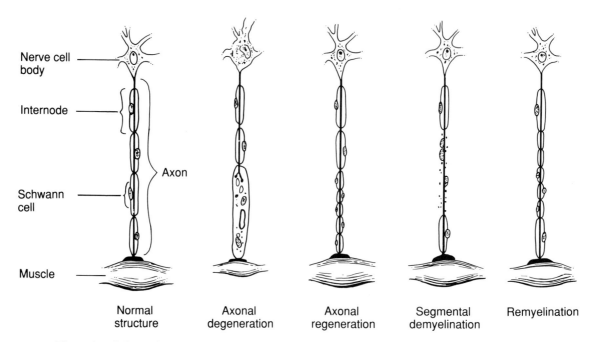

Figure 3-1 Schematic summary of pathologic processes in peripheral nerve injury and recovery.

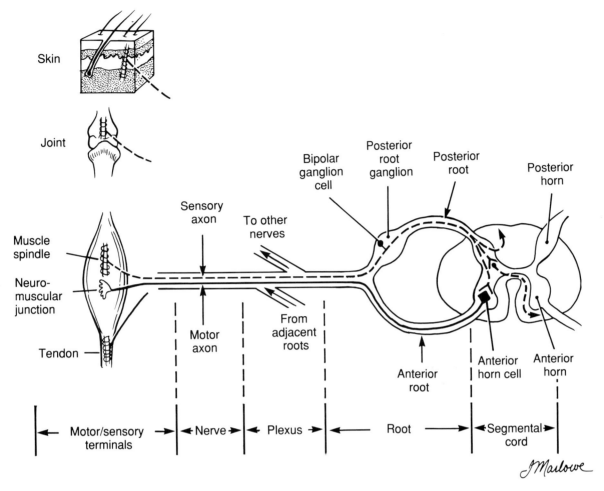

Figure 3-2 Organization of the peripheral nervous system, emphasizing the differentiation between segmental cord, root, plexus, and peripheral nerve levels.

portion of the serratus anterior along the posterolateral chest wall. It innervates only the serratus anterior muscle.

Suprascapular Nerve

The suprascapular nerve arises posteriorly from the superior trunk of the brachial plexus, just proximal to the bifurcation of the trunk into anterior and posterior divisions. The suprascapular nerve therefore carries mostly axons which go to or from the C5 and C6 roots, a few representing C4 in certain individuals. The nerve traverses the posterior cervical triangle lying anterior to the trapezius until it reaches the scapular notch. At this point, the nerve accompanies the suprascapular artery but is separated from it by the overlying transverse scapular ligament. The nerve next crosses the supraspinatus fossa, sending branches to the supraspinatus and articular branches to the glenohumeral and acromio-

clavicular joints before reaching the spinoglenoid notch of the scapula. It then descends through the spinoglenoid notch, sending its terminal branches to the infraspinatus. Beyond muscle afferents, the only sensory axons within the suprascapular nerve are articular, since there is no cutaneous representation. The articular branches may underlie referred pain to the shoulder, an important clinical consideration.

Axillary Nerve

The axillary nerve arises from the posterior cord of the brachial plexus at its terminal bifurcation (i.e., at the radial nerve's point of origin). Its axons, however, are limited to C5 and C6 contributions via the superior trunk. The axillary nerve passes under the coracoid process and laterally between the subscapularis muscle and the axillary artery. At about the point of origin of the posterior humeral circumflex artery, the nerve

Table 3-1   Major Peripheral Nerves of the Upper Limb

Nerve	Roots of Origin	Plexus Origin	Muscles	Function	Sensory
Long thoracic	C5, C6, C7	Branches arising directly from distal roots	Serratus anterior	Scapular stabilization	Muscle only
Suprascapular	C5, C6	Origin from superior trunk	Supraspinatus, infraspinatus	Shoulder abduction and external rotation	Glenohumeral and acromioclavicular joints
Subscapular	C5, C6, C7	Origin from posterior cord, via posterior divisions of superior and middle trunks	Subscapularis, teres major	Shoulder adduction and internal rotation	Muscle only
Musculo-cutaneous	C5, C6, C7	Origin at terminal bifurcation of lateral cord, via anterior divisions of superior and middle trunks	Coracobrachialis, biceps, brachialis	Shoulder and elbow flexion	Radial forearm
Axillary	C5, C6	Origin at terminal bifurcation of posterior cord, via posterior division of superior trunk	Deltoid, teres minor	Shoulder abduction and external rotation	Lateral arm and inferior shoulder capsule
Radial	C5, C6, C7, C8	Origin at terminal bifurcation of posterior cord, via posterior divisions of all trunks	Triceps, anconeus and all forearm extensors	Elbow, wrist, and digit extension; forearm supination	Dorsolateral forearm and hand
Ulnar	C8, T1	Origin at terminal bifurcation of medial cord, via anterior division of inferior trunk	Flexor carpi uln flex dig prof IV hand intrinsics (except abd poll, brev, oppon poll and 1st lumb)	Ulnar wrist and finger flexion; intrinsic hand functions (except thumb)	Ulnar palm; 5th digit and ulnar $\frac{1}{2}$ of 4th digit
Median	C6, C7, C8, T1	Origin at juncture of terminal bifurcations from medial and lateral cords, via anterior divisions of all trunks	Pronator teres, forearm flexors, abd poll brev, and opponens poll	Forearm pronation; wrist & finger flexion thumb abduction & opposition	Non-ulnar palm; ventral digits 1–3 and $\frac{1}{2}$ of 4th digit

turns posteriorly into the quadrilateral or quadrangular space. Within the quadrilateral space, the axillary nerve forms two major and one minor division. The superoanterior branch curves around the surgical neck of the humerus to innervate the anterior portion of the deltoid and some overlying skin (an autonomous cutaneous area of clinical importance) before terminating as the superolateral brachial cutaneous nerve of the arm, while the inferoposterior branch innervates the teres minor and the posterior deltoid. The minor branch is articular, supplying an inferior portion of the shoulder capsule.

Musculocutaneous Nerve

The musculocutaneous nerve arises at the terminal bifurcation of the lateral cord of the brachial plexus, the other major branch of the lateral cord joining with a branch from the medial cord to form the median nerve. Its axons are contributed largely by the C5 and C6 roots, although there may be a variable contribution from C7. The point of musculocutaneous origin is near the inferior margin of the pectoralis minor. The nerve then enters the arm lying lateral to the axillary artery. It penetrates and innervates the coracobrachialis and de-

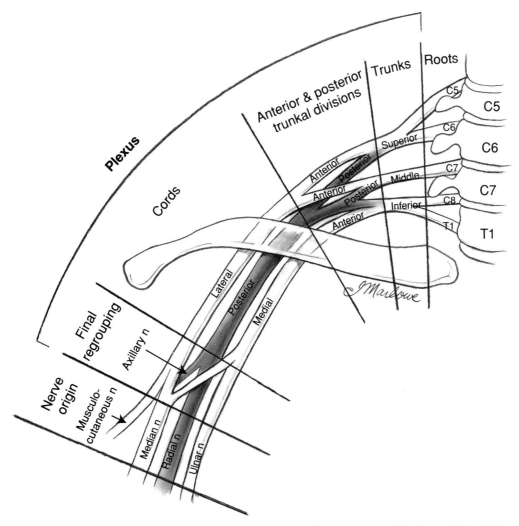

Figure 3-3 Right brachial plexus, viewed from the front. It emphasizes plexus organization and the origins of the major nerves of the upper limb.

scends between the biceps and brachialis muscles, angling in a medial to lateral direction. The branches to biceps and brachialis originate after the nerve exits from the coracobrachialis. The sensory termination of the musculocutaneous nerve, the lateral antebrachial cutaneous nerve of the forearm, penetrates the brachial fascia and becomes superficial a few centimeters above the antecubital crease, lateral to the biceps tendon.

Ulnar Nerve

The ulnar nerve arises at the terminal bifurcation of the medial cord of the brachial plexus, thus consisting of axons to and from the C8 and T1 roots. The nerve initially lies posterior to the axillary artery, and then continues into the arm with the brachial artery lying

just medial to it. In the upper arm, it is within a common neurovascular bundle, which also contains the median nerve and the two medial cutaneous nerves of the arm and forearm. These latter two sensory nerves also arise from the medial cord, just proximal to its terminal bifurcation. The ulnar nerve departs this bundle at the point of coracobrachialis attachment to the humerus, penetrating the medial intermuscular septum and angling posteriorly under cover of the medial head of the triceps.

As it approaches the elbow, and as the medial head of the triceps thins into its tendinous insertion onto the olecranon process of the ulna (the arcade of Struthers), the nerve passes posterior to the medial epicondyle (the ulnar groove) and medial to the ulnar collateral ligament and the olecranon itself. Upon exiting the groove, the ulnar nerve enters the cubital tunnel between the underlying ulna and the overlying aponeurosis of the flexor carpi ulnaris. An articular branch to the elbow arises just above the medial epicondyle.

The most common sites of ulnar nerve injury and entrapment are in the vicinity of the elbow. The nerve may be involved acutely in association with fractures or dislocations at the elbow, particularly medial epicondylar fractures. More chronic entrapment neuropathies may occur at four sites near the elbow: (1) just above the elbow at the arcade of Struthers, (2) within the ulnar groove, (3) somewhat more distally within the cubital tunnel, and (4) between the heads of the flexor carpi ulnaris.

The ulnar nerve descends from elbow to wrist between the flexor digitorum profundus and the overlying flexor carpi ulnaris. It is joined after about one-third of its course by the ulnar artery, which lies radial to the nerve. The first major branches of the ulnar nerve arise near the elbow. There are from two to four branches to the flexor carpi ulnaris and usually one more distally to the flexor digitorum profundus. Initial branches to the flexor carpi ulnaris have occasionally been described well above the medial epicondyle. These branches must be a major concern whenever the ulnar nerve is surgically explored or transposed at the elbow. Two sensory branches arise in the forearm: the palmar cutaneous branch about midway and the dorsal cutaneous branch a variable few centimeters proximal to the ulnar styloid. The field of innervation of the former extends to the proximal hypothenar eminence, and that of the latter encompasses the dorsal ulnar aspect of the hand (Fig. 3-4).

The ulnar nerve and adjacent artery emerge medial to the flexor carpi ulnaris tendon as they approach the wrist. They lie between that tendon and that of the flexor digitorum profundus. The nerve then traverses the "ulnar tunnel," commonly known as Guyon's canal. This space is bounded medially by the pisiform bone, laterally by the hook of the hamate, below by the flexor retinaculum and the pisohamate ligament, and above by the volar carpal ligament and the palmaris brevis. Entrapment within Guyon's canal is not uncommon. It is at this point that the ulnar nerve divides into its superficial and deep terminal branches. The superficial branch is predominantly sensory, innervating the distal hypothenar eminence and contributing to the digital nerves of the fourth and fifth fingers. The deep branch innervates the hypothenar muscles, and then curves around the hook of the hamate to follow the deep palmar arch of the ulnar artery. It further innervates the interossei and ulnar lumbricals and, terminally, the adductor pollicis brevis and the deep head of the flexor pollicis brevis in the thenar group. The

course of the ulnar nerve and its innervated muscles are shown schematically in Figure 3-4.

The ulnar nerve is subject to several important anatomic variations. Anastomotic connections through which axons cross from the median (or anterior interosseus) to the ulnar nerve occur in approximately 15 to 20 percent of individuals. These connections are usually in the upper forearm, so-called Martin-Gruber anastomoses. Median and ulnar nerve injuries proximal to such connections may be associated with what appear to be complex clinical deficits. There are also many variations in hand, skin, and muscle innervation, ranging from innervation solely by one nerve or the other (so-called ulnar hand or median hand). These anatomic variations are characterized in detail in Sunderland's *Nerves and Nerve Injuries.*[1]

Median Nerve

The median nerve arises at the brachial plexus outlet, at the juncture of the lateral terminal division of the medial cord and the medial terminal division of the lateral cord. It carries axons from all roots contributing to the brachial plexus except C5; its cutaneous representation is primarily C6, while its motor representation is C6 through T1.

The median nerve descends through the arm in company with the brachial artery, medial to the coracobrachialis, then anteromedial to the brachialis and medial intermuscular septum. It reaches the antecubital fossa alongside the medial aspect of the biceps tendon, passing beneath the bicipital aponeurosis. Its first branch is to the pronator teres, sometimes arising above the elbow and sometimes within the antecubital fossa. It descends adjacent to the biceps tendon, until the nerve passes between the superficial and deep heads of the pronator teres. This is one of several potential sites of median nerve entrapment near the elbow. Further branches arising within the vicinity of the elbow joint include twigs to the pronator teres and to the flexor carpi radialis, the flexor digitorum sublimis, and the palmaris longus.

After emerging from the pronator teres, the nerve further traverses the forearm beneath the flexor digitorum sublimis after first diving under its tendinous arch (a further site of entrapment). The median nerve emerges radial to the flexor digitorum sublimis, lying between its tendon and that of the flexor carpi radialis. It is while in proximity to the flexor digitorum sublimis that the anterior interosseus branch usually arises, from 2.3 to 8 cm below the humeral articulation.[2] This branch descends and supplies, in turn, the median in-

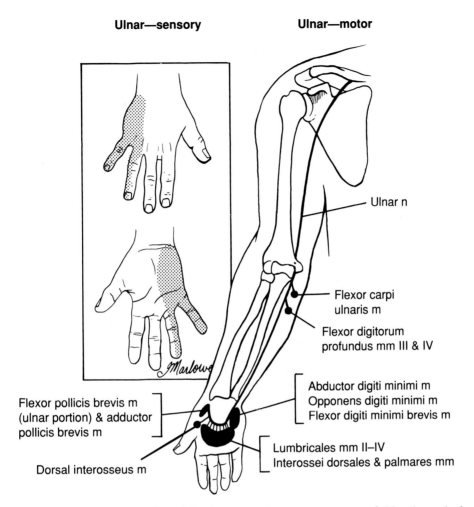

Ulnar—sensory

Ulnar—motor

Ulnar n

Flexor carpi
ulnaris m

Flexor digitorum
profundus mm III & IV

Abductor digiti minimi m
Opponens digiti minimi m
Flexor digiti minimi brevis m

Flexor pollicis brevis m
(ulnar portion) & adductor
pollicis brevis m

Lumbricales mm II–IV
Interossei dorsales & palmares mm

Dorsal interosseus m

Figure 3-4 Schematic representation of the right ulnar nerve, its cutaneous sensory field and muscles innervated
by the ulnar nerve.

nervated portion of the flexor digitorum profundus, the flexor pollicis longus, and the pronator quadratus. Anastomotic branches to the ulnar nerve arise along this same segment of the median nerve, approximately half from the anterior interosseus itself.[3]

The main trunk of the median nerve accompanies the flexor tendons, passing under the flexor retinaculum of the distal forearm and entering the carpal tunnel. Median nerve entrapment within or near the carpal tunnel is the single most common site of peripheral nerve entrapment in humans. Median nerve compression secondary to flexor muscle injury is consistent with findings of impending Volkmann's ischemic contracture. The palmar cutaneous sensory branch usually arises just above the flexor retinaculum. The median nerve emerges from the tunnel beneath the palmar aponeurosis and the thenar muscle insertions into the flexor retinaculum, where it divides into terminal branches. There are a number of reported anatomic

variations at this level of the nerve, but three terminal branches are the norm: (1) a lateral branch, which innervates the thenar muscles and gives rise to further branches to the digital nerves of the thumb and radial index finger and to the first lumbrical; (2) an intermediate branch, which contributes to the digital nerves of the ulnar index finger and the radial middle finger and sometimes supplies the second lumbrical; (3) and a medial branch, which contributes to the digital nerves of the ulnar middle finger and the radial fourth finger (see Ch. 20). Median nerve anatomy is summarized in Fig. 3-5.

Radial Nerve

The radial nerve arises in the posterior axilla from the terminal bifurcation of the posterior cord of the brachial plexus, coincident with the origin of the axil-

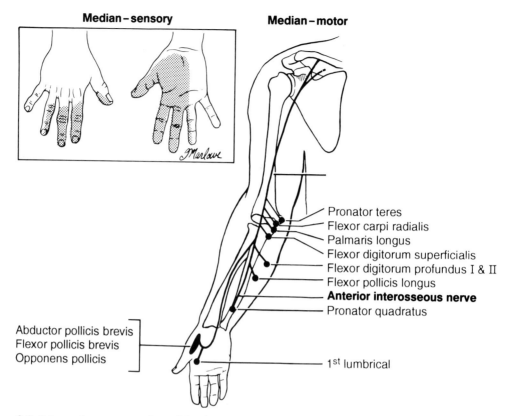

Median – sensory   **Median – motor**

Pronator teres
Flexor carpi radialis
Palmaris longus
Flexor digitorum superficialis
Flexor digitorum profundus I & II
Flexor pollicis longus
Anterior interosseous nerve
Pronator quadratus

Abductor pollicis brevis
Flexor pollicis brevis
Opponens pollicis

1ˢᵗ lumbrical

Figure 3-5 Schematic representation of the right median nerve, its cutaneous sensory field and muscles innervated by the median nerve.

lary nerve. It receives radicular contributions from C5, C6, C7, and C8 via the posterior divisions of the superior, middle, and inferior trunks. It descends within the axilla along the subscapularis muscle and the teres major tendon to the brachioaxillary angle, and then between the long and medial heads of the triceps to the spiral groove of the humerus. It winds posterolaterally around the humerus within the spiral groove, a common site of injury (fracture or impact contusion). The initial branches to the triceps arise well above the spiral groove, although the most distal branch to the triceps (and to the anconeus) often arises within the groove. Cutaneous branches to the lateral arm and posterior forearm also arise proximal to the spiral groove. Upon exit from the spiral groove, the radial nerve passes beneath the lateral head of the triceps and penetrates the lateral intermuscular septum. It passes anteriorly and descends on the lateral aspect of the brachialis muscle. Branches innervating the brachioradialis and extensor carpi radialis longus arise proximal to the lateral epicondyle, while the twigs supplying the extensor carpi radialis brevis typically arise at or distal to the epicondyle. As the nerve traverses the capsule of the elbow joint, it divides to form the predominantly motor posterior interosseous nerve and the purely sensory superficial radial nerve.

The posterior interosseus nerve immediately passes between the ulnar and humeral heads of the supinator and winds laterally around the proximal shaft of the radius. It remains in close apposition to the radius as it descends through the dorsal forearm, underlying the forearm extensors it innervates. In most instances, the posterior interosseus nerve sequentially innervates the supinator (which may also receive branches from above the origin of the posterior interosseus), the extensor digitorum communis and extensor carpi ulnaris, the abductor pollicis longus, the extensor digitorum, the extensor pollicis longus and brevis, and the extensor indicis proprius. These branches often arise in a fanlike formation fairly high in the forearm, as the nerve leaves the supinator. Lesions below the supinator, particularly penetrating lesions, may therefore appear discontinuous, affecting one or several muscles but sparing others. A terminal branch contributes to the articular innervation of the wrist.

The superficial radial branch passes distal to the forearm beneath the branchioradialis, paralleling the radial artery. Approximately two-thirds of the way along the forearm, this branch moves posteriorly to the surface, descending across the extensor retinaculum to innervate the radial dorsum of the hand and first 3 or 4 digits. There are no common anatomic variants of the

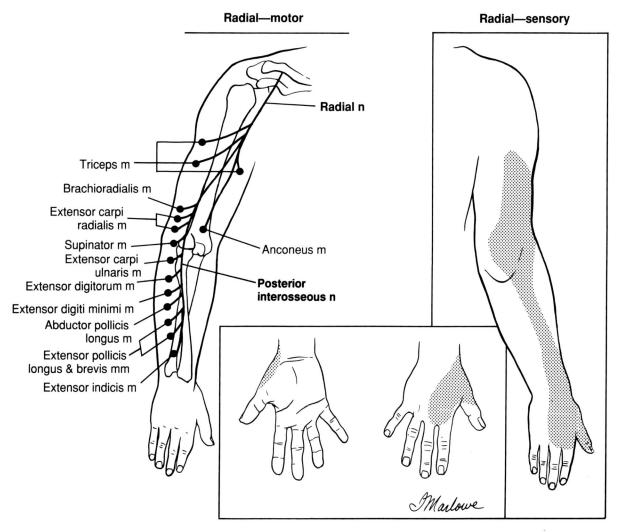

Figure 3-6 Schematic representation of the right radial nerve, its cutaneous sensory field and muscles innervated by the radial nerve.

radial nerve, although minor variations have been described at many levels. Radial nerve anatomy is summarized in Figure 3-6.

SIGNS AND SYMPTOMS OF NERVE INJURY

The clinical manifestations of peripheral nerve injuries can be functionally classified as motor, sensory, or autonomic in origin. Within each functional group, they may be further characterized as either positive or negative. Positive symptoms and signs reflect activity generated either normally or abnormally within peripheral nervous system elements, while negative symptoms and signs represent loss of normal function (Table 3-2). Accurate diagnosis of peripheral nerve in-

juries depends on recognition of such symptoms and signs and, further, on anatomic localization.

Sensory Symptoms and Signs

Numbness is the term most often used by patients and clinicians to refer to hypesthesia, a loss of normal cutaneous sensation, yet it is a term that can often be ambiguous. Many individuals will use the term *numb* to refer to mild weakness or the normally perceived sense of heaviness that may accompany limb weakness, or alternatively use the term to describe the tightness that accompanies swelling or local tissue inflammation. A useful approach is to ask patients to relate their numbness to any similar sensation they may have experienced, such as local anesthesia for a minor surgical

Table 3-2　Symptoms and Signs of Peripheral Nerve Injury

	Negative		Positive	
	Symptoms	Signs	Symptoms	Signs
Sensory	Numbness	Hypesthesia Hypalgesia	Paresthesia, Tinel's sign, pain, dysesthesia	Hyperalgesia
Motor	Heaviness, weakness, fatigue	Paresis, atrophy	Twitching, cramping	Fasciculation
Autonomic	Dryness, swelling, purple skin	Anhidrosis, edema, cyanosis	Sweating, blanching	Hyperhidrosis, pallor

or dental procedure. If their current complaint of numbness is similar, then a significant sensory deficit is likely; if it is not similar, further clarification is required.

Pain often accompanies both acute and chronic peripheral nerve lesions, but it may be a relatively nonspecific and poorly localizing symptom. Acute injuries that involve the peripheral nervous system almost invariably incur associated musculoskeletal trauma, and pain from these tissues typically predominates. Acute nerve transection or root avulsion is in and of itself rarely painful after the immediate fact.

As a general rule, pain will tend to be of greater localizing value when peripheral nerves with a significant cutaneous distribution are involved. Even then, the pain may be vague and aching in quality, rather than a sharper, neuralgic pain radiating within the cutaneous distribution of the nerve. Pain may complicate the motor examination. Apparent paresis may reflect inhibition of muscle activation secondary to pain associated with activation. Isometric muscle testing can minimize pain, but it still may be difficult to distinguish mild neurogenic weakness from apparent weakness due solely to pain. Pain accompanying injury to nerves that are predominantly motor may in fact be misleading. Many predominantly motor nerves provide innervation to associated joints; the pain arising from nerve injury may be referred to the joint, masking its nerve origin. This is characteristic of many of the nerves innervating the shoulder girdle, requiring consideration of neurologic as well as articular pathology in patients presenting with shoulder pain.

Positive sensory symptoms are also difficult for many patients to describe. "Tingling" is a term that usually indicates paresthesias, the manifestation of spontaneous activity within nonnociceptive (i.e., non-pain, sensitive) cutaneous sensory fibers. Dysesthesias reflect spontaneous activity within smaller, primarily pain-sensitive afferents, and there is a definite unpleasant or even painful quality. Patients frequently report "creeping" or "crawling" sensations, and a "hot" or "burning" quality commonly accompanies dysesthesias. The "pins and needles" sensation that follows one's "foot going to sleep" reflects spontaneous or positive activity in both pain-sensitive and nonnociceptive sensory nerve elements. Hyperalgesia refers to an apparent decrease in pain threshold, such that stimuli that are not usually painful become so. A Tinel's sign is a clinically important form of hyperalgesia, in which tapping over a nerve trunk elicits an unpleasant, electric, or spark-like sensation, which may be perceived as traveling or "shooting" along the course of the nerve. This is very similar to the "crazy bone" sensation that accompanies minor trauma to the ulnar nerve at the elbow. A Tinel's sign is a common sign of nerve entrapment, the nerve usually most sensitive at or just adjacent to the site of entrapment. It can also often be elicited from a regenerating nerve head or a neuroma, reflecting the hyperexcitability of regenerating axon terminals.

Motor Signs and Symptoms

Weakness is the most common negative symptom and sign of motor dysfunction secondary to peripheral nerve injury. The clinician must be prepared to assess each muscle's function independently of concurrent weakness in other muscles and then to apply the precise anatomy of each muscle's innervation.[4] The differentiation of a C8 root lesion versus a medial brachial plexus lesion exemplifies the precision required in performing and interpreting the motor examination. In both lesions, the pattern of weakness involving the intrinsic hand muscles and some forearm flexors will be quite similar. The only apparent difference may be the presence or absence of weakness in the portion of the C8 musculature innervated by the radial nerve. Assessment of the thumb and index extensors thus becomes crucial.

Positive motor symptoms and signs such as cramps and fasciculations are less common than weakness. Fasciculations are the result of spontaneous excitation of individual motor axons, while cramps are spontaneous mass contractions of a muscle. Both may be a manifestation of chronic denervation yet are relatively nonspecific phenomena and may accompany metabolic derangements such as calcium and thyroid imbalance, or even simple stress and fatigue. Muscle atrophy may follow peripheral nerve lesions, but may be difficult to recognize unless severe or localized. Significant neurogenic atrophy implies considerable weakness.

Deep tendon reflexes are sensitive indicators of lesions affecting either the afferent or efferent limbs of the reflex arc, the result of activation of spinal motor neurons by muscle afferents. The pattern of reflex loss may have localizing value. For example, a C5 or C6 root lesion can depress both the biceps and brachioradialis deep tendon reflexes, while a radial neuropathy in the arm will spare the biceps and may include the triceps reflex.

Autonomic Signs and Symptoms

The more obvious autonomic functions referable to the upper limb are regional circulatory control and temperature regulation. Characteristic symptoms and signs of autonomic dysfunction are therefore manifestations of altered skin temperature and color. The somesthetic and motor manifestations of peripheral nerve injuries usually predominate. Reflex sympathetic dystrophy is the major exception to this rule, a syndrome of poorly localized pain, typically burning in quality, in association with regional alterations in skin color, temperature, and sweating, and trophic tissue changes. This syndrome may follow a broad spectrum of limb injuries ranging from minor soft tissue to major orthopedic trauma. Similar sympathetic reflex changes may also follow peripheral nerve injuries, in which case the pain is often more localized within the distribution of the involved nerve. Causalgia is a more specific term for this situation.[5]

Anatomic Localization Based on Symptoms and Signs

Clinical diagnosis of peripheral nerve lesions is an attempt to localize the site of the lesion by correlating the precise anatomy of the peripheral nervous system with clinical observations. Precise localization will depend on associated sensory deficits, other musculoskeletal findings, and diagnostic studies. Generally, clinical observations should be interpreted in an attempt to localize a single lesion, which might account for the patient's findings, although two lesions or even more can occur, as can a generalized process such as a peripheral polyneuropathy. A patient presenting with sensory loss over the lateral arm and radial forearm and hand, along with weakness of shoulder abduction (deltoid), elbow extension (triceps), and wrist extension (extensor carpi muscles) can have lesions of both the axillary and radial nerves, although a posterior cord plexopathy is a single lesion with a similar presentation.

The possibility of central pathology should be considered in assessing the upper extremity in athletes, particularly following obvious traumatic episodes. It should also be kept in mind that traumatic peripheral and central nervous system injuries may coexist.

PATHOGENESIS OF NERVE INJURY

Peripheral nerve injuries involve various combinations of stretch, kinking or angulation, crush, compression or percussion, and laceration. These mechanisms rarely occur in isolation, and all are commonly accompanied by local tissue ischemia, inflammation, and edema. Radial neuropathy complicating humeral shaft fracture is an illustrative example (see Case Study I). The nerve may be stretched or kinked with diastasis of humeral fragments; it may be trapped between fragments and partially lacerated by sharp fragment edges; it may be compressed against bone secondary to local edema and hematoma; and its blood supply may be compromised by any of these insults. Relatively mild and transient compression of a nerve trunk may have no physiologic or pathologic significance, yet the same insult may become significant if prolonged or sustained repeatedly, as in the case of peripheral nerve entrapments and repetitive use injuries.

Ischemia serves to illustrate the spectrum of pathophysiologic changes. Everyone has experienced a hand or foot "falling asleep" on a positional basis. The offending posture leads to temporary loss of perfusion to the distal limb. The relative ischemia leads to numbness and weakness as axons become unexcitable. Normal circulation is restored when there is a change in position. The axons first become hyperexcitable, hence "pins and needles" paresthesias, and then normal function returns. There is no structural change or pathologic consequence following a brief episode of ischemia such as this. At the more severe end of the ischemic spectrum, however, frank infarction of a segment of nerve may occur if local perfusion is completely interrupted. The entire nerve distal to the ischemic segment will then undergo Wallerian degeneration.

Seddon[6] has classified nerve injuries into three categories combining both clinical and pathologic features within a single terminology: (1) neurapraxia, (2) axonotmesis, and (3) neurotmesis.

Neurapraxia refers to injury associated with loss of function but relative preservation of structure. Neurapractic lesions imply loss of conduction along the course of the nerve due either to loss of axon excitability or segmental demyelination. Neurapraxia can recover very quickly (e.g., in the case of positional ischemia) or within days to weeks as remyelination occurs.

Axonotmesis implies axonal degeneration, yet with preservation of connective tissue structure within the nerve and alignment between the surviving proximal axon segments and the degenerating ones. Recovery then depends upon axon regeneration, but the conditions favor earlier and more complete regeneration. A localized compression injury usually involves elements of both neurapraxia and axonotmesis.

Seddon's final category, neurotmesis, refers to nerve injuries which disrupt both axons and connective tissue elements. Extensive wallerian degeneration occurs distal to the site of injury. Nerve laceration is an example of neurotmesis. Some recovery may follow, provided the proximal and distal nerve segments are in close apposition, but it is characteristically slower and less complete. Sunderland has expanded Seddon's classification to include subcategories defined relative to the degree of connective tissue injury[1]; both classifications are summarized in Table 3-3.

Few peripheral nerve injuries fall completely within one category, with most including combinations of neurapraxia and disruption of axons and other structural elements; however, one element usually predominates. From the clinical perspective, the pathophysiologic nature of the injury is a major determinant of the rate and extent of recovery. The electrodiagnostic manifestations of various forms of myelin and axon pathology are of diagnostic and prognostic importance and are presented in the next section.

ELECTRODIAGNOSIS

Electrodiagnosis, primarily in the form of nerve conduction studies (NCS) and needle electromyography (EMG), can be invaluable in the diagnosis of peripheral nerve injury. The major limitations of electrodiagnosis reflect the experience and expertise of the technologists and physicians involved in performing and interpreting the studies. When appropriately performed, NCS and EMG may not only localize peripheral nerve pathology, but may provide clinically useful data regarding timecourse, nature, severity, and prognosis. Serial study over time can then serve to monitor recovery and thus contribute to ongoing management (see Case Study I).

Nerve Conduction Studies

Nerve conduction studies involve activation of peripheral nerve trunks at one or more sites, usually with an electrical stimulus, and measurement of the amplitude and temporal characteristics of volume-con-

Table 3-3   Classification of Peripheral Nerve Injuries

Seddon Classification	Sunderland Classification	Prognosis
Neurapraxia	1 Loss of axon excitability	Good; rapid recovery
	OR	
	2 Segmental demyelination with conduction block	Good; early recovery
Axonotmesis	3 Pure axonal degeneration	Good; recovery awaits regeneration
	OR	
	4 Axonal degeneration + endoneurial injury	May require repair
Neurotmesis	5 Axonal degeneration + endoneurial + perineurial injury	Fair; often requires repair
	OR	
	6 Axonal degeneration + endoneurial + perineurial + epineurial injury (transection)	Poor without repair

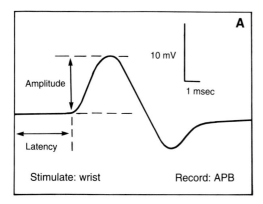

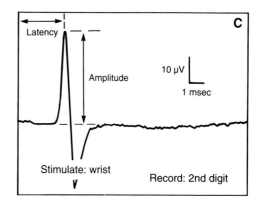

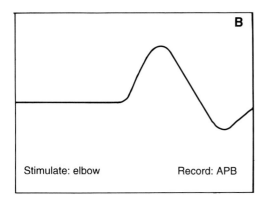

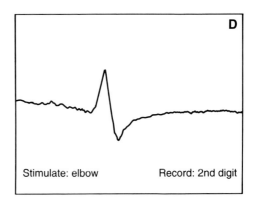

Figure 3-7 Typical **(A & B)** motor and **(C & D)** sensory responses to electrical stimulation of the median nerve at the wrist and at the antecubital fossa. The motor responses reflect orthodromic conduction from stimulus site to muscle, and are volume-conducted potentials generated by muscle fibers. The sensory responses reflect antidromic conduction from stimulus site to a recording site on the first phalynx of the index finger (2nd digit). They are volume-conducted whole nerve action potentials. Note the amplitude difference, motor responses measured in milivolts, while sensory responses are measured in microvolts.

ducted nerve or muscle responses to the activating stimulus. Figure 3-7 depicts typical sensory and motor responses to electrical stimulation of the median nerve at the wrist and antecubital fossa. In all instances, the relevant measurements are the latency between stimulus and response, the duration of the response, and the amplitude of the response. Knowledge of pathlengths between stimulus and recording sites enables further calculation of the conduction velocity along each path. "Nerve conduction velocities" are often requested by referring clinicians, although the conduction velocity is usually the least sensitive and least specific parameter. Sensory nerve action potential (SNAP) amplitudes and compound muscle action potential (CMAP) amplitudes are the parameters most sensitive to traumatic peripheral nerve injury. If even a few axons are conducting normally, velocity measurements will be normal or near normal, despite severe losses of SNAP or CMAP amplitude.

It is important to keep in mind that sensory re-

sponses are quite small (measured in microvolts), reflecting the compound action potential of the sensory nerve trunk. It is customary to measure sensory latencies from stimulus to the peak of the SNAP, these latencies therefore reflecting an average of conduction rates among axons within the sensory nerve. Motor responses are comparably large (measured in millivolts), but latencies are somewhat distorted by changes in conduction along distal axon arborizations and electrochemical transmission at the neuromuscular junction. Motor latencies are measured from stimulus to the onset of the CMAP and thus reflect the conduction rate of the fastest, largest motor axons.

Needle Electromyography

Needle electromyography (EMG) characterizes both spontaneous and voluntary electrical activity in muscle. Normal muscle is electrically silent at rest, although any movement of the electrode tip within the muscle will elicit transient electrical activity, insertional activity. The one exception is end-plate activity, but this is recorded only in small portions of the muscle and is recognizable due to its distinguishing electrical features. Voluntary activity consists of motor unit potentials, each reflecting concurrent activity in the muscle fibers innervated by a single motor axon. The EMG abnormalities most relevant to the electrodiagnosis of peripheral nerve injuries are altered insertional activity, the presence of spontaneous activity, and alterations in the number and configuration of voluntary motor unit potentials.

Insertional activity consists of an irregular burst of muscle fiber potentials in response to movement of the electrode tip within the muscle, presumably on an irritative basis. Normal insertional activity rarely persists for more than 300 ms. Insertional activity is typically increased or prolonged with denervation and decreased in the face of severe denervation atrophy.

The presence of spontaneous activity in the form of fibrillation potentials and positive sharp waves usually indicates denervation. Fasciculations (i.e., spontaneous motor unit potentials reflecting spontaneous motor axon activity) may also indicate chronic denervation and reinnervation, but constitute a less specific phenomenon (Fig. 3-8).

Normal motor unit potentials vary in amplitude and configuration both within and between different muscles. This variation reflects differences in innervation ratios (number of muscle fibers per motor axon) and the size and spatial distribution of muscle fibers within the muscle. If a portion of the muscle cannot be activated, there will be fewer than the normal number of active units for a given level of effort. Motor units recruited at any point may also be larger than normal, and most units will attain higher than normal firing rates before succeeding units are recruited. Both denervation secondary to axon degeneration and conduction block will impair recruitment. Following denervating

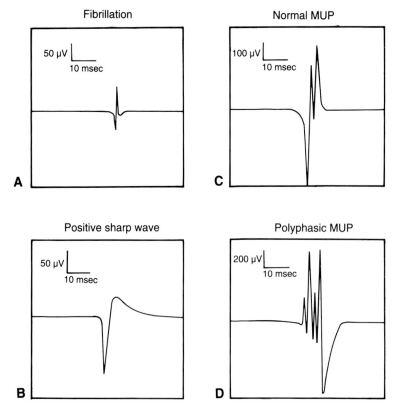

Figure 3-8 Electromyographic potentials recorded during needle examination of muscle. Note the difference in amplitude scale between Figs. A and B on the left and Figs. C and D on the right. **(A)** Fibrillation potential. Fibrillation occurs spontaneously, most commonly in denervating conditions. **(B)** Positive sharp wave. Positive sharp waves are characteristically seen on needle insertion or movement. They have the same significance as fibrillation potentials. **(C)** Normal motor unit potential (MUP), occurring with voluntary activation of muscle. **(D)** Polyphasic motor unit potential. Larger polyphasic MUPs such as that illustrated are characteristic of reinnervation; a single motor axon innervates more than the usual number of muscle fibers, distributed over a greater portion of the muscle. Small, short-duration polyphasics are characteristic of primary muscle pathology.

injuries, reinnervation by collateral sprouts from surviving axons or by regenerated axons often results in an increase in the number of muscle fibers supplied by a single motor axon, and these muscle fibers may be more variably distributed within the muscle. Motor unit potentials following reinnervation are therefore often larger and more complex (polyphasic) than normal (Fig. 3-8).

Pathophysiologic Correlation

Traumatic peripheral nerve injuries, whether acute or chronic, typically manifest some combination of conduction block along still intact axon segments, conduction delay at sites of compression, demyelination, remyelination or regeneration, and degeneration of axons distal to a site of injury. Conduction block underlies neurapraxia, while axonotmesis or neurotmesis implies a major component of axonal degeneration.

Conduction delay causes prolongation of latencies and slowing of conduction velocity. The decrease in conduction velocity along any segment will reflect not only the severity of conduction delay but also the length of the segment along which conduction is delayed. Motor (CMAP) and sensory (SNAP) amplitudes are little affected by uniform conduction delay. Pure conduction delay has little effect on voluntary activity or spontaneous activity on needle examination.

Focal conduction block along a peripheral nerve trunk typically decreases or obliterates the response to a whole nerve action potential conducted along that segment. The affected axons are in continuity, but conduction cannot pass the site of injury. Conduction block at any point between stimulation and recording sites will decrease SNAP and CMAP amplitudes. Pure conduction block will have relatively little effect on conduction velocity; there will be no denervation despite altered voluntary activity (decreased recruitment of voluntary motor units) and clinical paresis.

Decreased amplitudes with relatively normal latencies and velocities also characterize conduction abnormalities in the face of axonal degeneration. Yet, needle examination will reveal increased insertional activity, denervation potentials (except during the first 1 to 3 weeks after injury), and decreased recruitment. Reinnervation changes in motor unit activity may become apparent in time.

Table 3-4 summarizes the nerve conduction and needle examination abnormalities that are characteristic of conduction block, conduction delay, and axonal degeneration. Neither nerve conduction studies nor needle examination can be interpreted in the absence of the other. The differentiation of focal conduction block versus a focal axonal lesion exemplifies this interdependency.

Normative Data

Appropriate interpretation of electrodiagnostic studies is based in part upon comparison with normal values. Normative data must be age-matched, and comparison with normative data can only be valid when the test data and normative data are collected under identical conditions, (i.e., the same equipment, identical filter settings and stimulus parameters, comparable skin and ambient temperature conditions, and common technique in terms of factors ranging from electrode size and shape to the measurement of interelectrode distances). For example, with ulnar motor conduction studies, it is customary to initially assess

Table 3-4 Nerve Conduction and Needle Examination Abnormalities Characteristic of Conduction Block, and Delay and Axonal Degeneration

| Pathophysiology | Conduction Studies | | Needle Examination | |
	Latency (Velocity)	Amplitude	Spontaneous Activity	Voluntary Activity
Neurapraxia Conduction block	Relatively normal	Decreased	Normal	Decreased recruitment; normal motor units
Conduction delay	Prolonged	Relatively normal	Normal	Normal
Axonotmesis and neurotmesis; axonal degeneration	Relatively normal	Decreased	Denervation potentials (within 1–3 weeks)	Decreased recruitment; reinnervated motor units

ulnar motor conduction from above the elbow and from the wrist — motor latencies and amplitudes are measured following supramaximal stimulation at both sites. The motor conduction velocity is then the quotient of the distance between stimulus sites divided by the latency difference. However, the measured distance between the two stimulus sites will vary depending on whether the measurement is made with the arm straight or the elbow flexed.[7]

Case Study I

A 26-year-old major league baseball player was involved in an automobile accident that resulted in a comminuted fracture of the mid-left humeral shaft; he underwent open reduction and internal fixation with a plate and iliac crest bone graft (Fig. 3-9). The operating surgeon was uncertain whether radial nerve continuity was maintained. The patient was seen 4 weeks after the injury and surgery for evaluation of residual left arm weakness.

Examination confirmed normal strength except for muscles innervated by the left radial nerve. The triceps was weak but could easily extend the elbow against gravity. There was no obvious voluntary function in the brachioradialis or wrist and finger extensors. There was also dense hypesthesia over the dorsum of the left radial hand and fingers.

Electrodiagnostic studies were performed. The left superficial radial sensory response (SNAP) was absent. No muscle responses (CMAPs) could be recorded from the extensor digitorum communis or extensor indicis proprius in response to radial nerve stimulation in the upper arm or at the elbow. Needle examination confirmed acute denervation (increased insertional activity and spontaneous fibrillation and positive sharp waves) in all radial muscles. These findings were moderate in the triceps and severe in the other radial muscles. There was a moderate decrease in recruitment in the triceps. A single, rapidly firing voluntary motor unit was observed in the extensor carpi radialis; there were no voluntary motor units in the brachioradialis, extensor digitorum communis, or extensor indicis proprius.

Although the elecrodiagnostic studies clearly indicated a severe left radial neuropathy with extensive axonal degeneration, the preservation of even minimal voluntary activity in a distal muscle indicated some axonal continuity and suggested a neurapractic component. A decision was made not to explore the nerve, and a conservative treatment program was undertaken. By 4 months after the injury, the triceps had regained normal strength and wrist extension against gravity had returned. Repeat electrodiagnos-

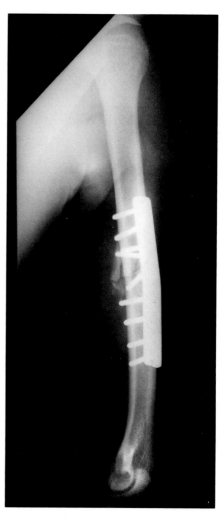

Figure 3-9 Postoperative radiograph, demonstrating fixation of the left humerus of the athlete discussed in Case Study I.

tic studies 6 months after injury confirmed extensive reinnervation of the brachioradialis and extensor carpi radialis. Early reinnervation of the extensor digitorum communis was evident, although finger extension against gravity was still lacking. Extensor pollicis longus function was the last to return (more than 7 months after injury). At 8 months postinjury, the patient began to lightly work out with a bat and glove. He was able to return to full baseball activities by 1 year postinjury and has continued to perform at the Major League level without any evidence of residual weakness or functional impairment.

Electrodiagnostic studies made it possible to monitor the return of the injured radial nerve before a physical examination demonstrated this recovery.

Somatosensory Evoked Potentials

Somatosensory evoked potentials (SEPs) are small, volume-conducted electrical potentials recorded at sites overlying peripheral and central nervous system elements that are normally activated by somatosensory stimuli. SEPs are most often utilized to assess function within central somatosensory pathways, the dorsal column-medial lemniscal systems and their projections via the thalamus to cerebral cortex. The same techniques lend themselves, however, to the evaluation of peripheral pathways, particularly proximal segments not readily accessible with more routine electrodiagnostic studies. Clinicians must keep in mind, however, that SEPs are neither highly sensitive nor highly specific; false negative tests and even positive results are possible. While a reproducible abnormality can confirm or localize a peripheral nervous system lesion, a normal study can never exclude a lesion.

There are two clinical settings in which SEPs offer distinct advantages in the evaluation of upper limb nerve injuries. SEPs may assist in localizing lesions within the brachial plexus, or at other proximal sites, especially during the immediate postinjury interval when the full spectrum of nerve conduction and electromyographic abnormalities has not evolved. SEPs can also be used to confirm some component of axonal continuity in the face of lesions sufficiently severe to obliterate routine mixed nerve and sensory nerve action potentials, although a completely absent response does not necessarily imply transection.

Case Study II

A young adult man had suffered a left shoulder fracture-dislocation in a motorcycle racing accident (Fig. 3-10), and underwent immediate surgical repair. He was noted postoperatively to have severe paresis of elbow flexion and dense hypesthesia along the radial forearm. Immobilization of the shoulder and the surgery itself prevented clinical assessment of most shoulder girdle muscles. Preoperative assessment was not possible due to the patient's pain level. Routine sensory conduction studies were not performed acutely—normal conduction is preserved for up to several days along segments peripheral to even complete transection. Conversely, preservation of a reproducible thalamocortical response to distal stimulation of a peripheral sensory nerve indicates some axonal continuity along more proximal nerve segments and excludes any possibility of complete transection or avulsion. The patient's SEPs recorded from the contralateral parietal scalp in response to

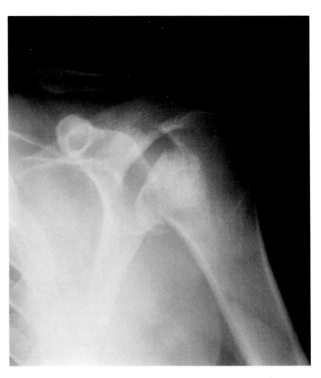

Figure 3-10 Anteroposterior view radiograph of multiple fragment fracture and posterior dislocation of shoulder that caused an injury to the musculotaneous nerve.

stimulation of the superficial radial nerve and the digital nerves of the thumb, middle finger, and fifth digit were normal and symmetric bilaterally. The SEP, in response to stimulation of the musculocutaneous sensory branch in the forearm, the lateral antebrachial cutaneous nerve of the forearm, was reduced and delayed relative to its right-sided counterpart, but still present (Fig. 3-11). This combination of observations allowed localization of the lesion to the musculocutaneous nerve, yet confirmed continuity in at least some axons. Had the musculocutaneous SEP been absent, continuity of the nerve could have been neither excluded nor confirmed.

Conservative management was elected, consisting of monitoring sensibility and maintaining elbow and forearm range of motion. Significant improvement over a several-week time frame indicated a predominantly neurapractic lesion.

These two case studies indicate the all-too-frequent association of peripheral nerve and major orthopedic injuries. They further illustrate the value of electrodiagnostic studies. Beyond localization of nerve injury, electrodiagnostic studies may provide meaningful information about the nature and severity of injury and its prognosis.

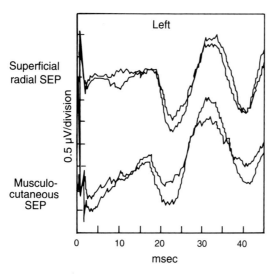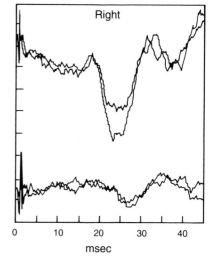

Figure 3-11 Somatosensory evoked potentials (SEPs) recorded for the patient discussed in Case Study II. These SEPs were recorded from the contralateral parietal scalp following electrical stimulation of the left and right superficial radial and musculocutaneous nerves. The superficial radial SEPs are symmetric and have comparable latencies; the right musculocutaneous SEP, while reproducibly recorded, is significantly delayed and of lower amplitude relative to its left counterpart.

Although not a typical finding in the athlete who presents with an upper extremity injury, peripheral nerve dysfunction can impact on athletic performance. Practitioners assessing the injured athlete should be aware of the related nerve anatomy and potential nerve injury. With this awareness, more significant pathology may be prevented. The individual nerves of the upper limb are considered in the following chapter, with emphasis on clinical presentation and specific athletic activities in which nerves may be at risk.

REFERENCES

1. Sunderland S: Nerves and Nerve Injuries. 2nd Ed. Churchill Livingstone, Edinburgh, 1978
2. Sunderland S, Ray LJ: Metrical and non-metrical features of the muscular branches of the median nerve. J Comp Neurol 85:191, 1946
3. Thomson A: Third annual report of the Committee of Collective Investigation of the Anatomical Society of Great Britain and Ireland for the year 1891–1892. J Anat 27:183, 1893
4. Medical Research Council: Aids to the Examination of the Peripheral Nervous System. Her Majesty's Stationery Office, London, 1976
5. Schwartzman Robert J: Reflex Sympathetic Dystrophy and Causalgia. Neurol Trauma Neurol Clin 10:4, 1992
6. Seddon HJ: Three types of nerve injury. Brain 66:237, 1943
7. Checkles NS, Russavof AD, Piero DL: Ulnar nerve conduction velocity: effect of elbow position on measurement. Arch Phys Med Rehabil 52:362, 1971.

SUGGESTED READINGS

Asbury AK, Johnson PC: Pathology of Peripheral Nerve. WB Saunders, Philadelphia, 1978
Chiappa KH: Evoked Potentials in Clinical Medicine. 2nd Ed. Little, Brown, Boston, 1990
Dawson DM, Hallet M, Millender LH: Entrapment Neuropathies. 2nd Ed. Little, Brown, Boston, 1990
Hershman EB: Neurovascular injuries. Clin Sports Med 9, 1990
Kimura J: Electrodiagnosis in Diseases of Nerve and Muscle: Principle and Practices. 2nd Ed. FA Davis, Philadelphia, 1989

4

Nerve Injuries

Randall R. Long

This chapter focuses on athletic injuries to cervical nerve roots, the brachial plexus, and the individual nerves which innervate the shoulder girdle and the upper limb. Corresponding attention is given to the details of neurologic presentation, diagnosis, and management specific to each site.

CERVICAL RADICULOPATHY

Although cervical nerve root injuries are distant from the upper limb itself, many of the symptoms and signs of cervical radiculopathy are referred to the limb. Root lesions, therefore, require inclusion in the differential diagnosis of many upper limb peripheral nerve injuries and entrapments. Trauma sufficient to cause appreciable injury to the arm or shoulder may also affect the cervical spine, and thus root and more peripheral nerve injuries may coexist. Further consideration of spinal cord injury at the cervical level, cervical myelopathy, is beyond the scope of this chapter, aside from the recommendation that it should always be considered initially in the injured athlete with either upper or lower limb symptoms. Torg[1] has provided a clear, concise discussion of athletic injuries to the cervical spine.

The most common etiology of cervical radiculopathy in athletes is acute rupture of the annulus fibrosis of an intervertebral disc and posterolateral herniation of the nucleus pulposus. The root is compressed secondarily as it exits via the neural foramen (Fig. 4-1). The

precipitating trauma typically involves asymmetric compression of the disc. Fortunately, central disc herniation with cord compression is less common than posterolateral herniation. In older athletes with acute cervical radiculopathies, there is an increased likelihood of cervical spondylosis with associated osteophytes (bone spurs) and other hypertrophic, degenerative changes that may narrow the neural foramen. In this setting, simple stretch or rotatory movement may precipitate acute root injury, although more significant trauma may lead to combinations of degenerative disease and disc herniation.

In acute cervical root lesions, pain is characteristically the presenting symptom, located proximally in the posterior cervical region and accentuated with cervical movement. Secondary spasm and tenderness within the cervical paraspinous muscles are the norm. The patient often holds the head tilted toward the painful side, and extension usually accentuates the pain (Sperling's sign). Radicular pain is also common, radiating from the cervical region into the shoulder and into the corresponding dermatome. C5 radicular pain typically radiates into the scapular and upper arm regions. C6 pain may descend as far as the radial forearm and even the thumb. C7 radicular pain may be appreciated in the triceps region and then distally into the midforearm. C8 radicular pain is experienced along the medial arm, ulnar forearm, and even into the ulnar digits. Use of the limb is usually associated with increased pain; coughing or sneezing may also be associated with radicular pain. The presumed mechanism

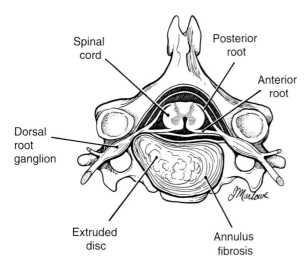

Figure 4-1 Schematic representation of an herniated cervical disc. Posterolateral extrusion of disc material is seen impinging upon the exiting nerve root on the right side.

is traction on the inflamed root secondary to expansion of the spinal subarachnoid space. Pain following voluntary Valsalva maneuver or bilateral jugular vein compression are corresponding signs that may be elicited during physical examination.

When motor or sensory deficits are present, they follow dermatomal and myotomal distributions. Careful examination relative to the distribution of motor and sensory nerve fibers exiting via a common root should reveal a root-specific pattern distinct from that of other peripheral nervous structures.

One key in differentiating cervical radiculopathies from more peripheral nerve injuries and entrapment neuropathies is cervical pain. Even distal entrapments, such as carpal tunnel syndrome and ulnar neuropathy at Guyon's canal (see later discussions), may invoke aching pain in the proximal limb, but neck pain and accentuation of pain with neck movement indicate more proximal pathology. Electrodiagnostic studies may also be very specific in differentiating root lesions. Radiologic imaging studies, particularly computed tomography (CT) scans and magnetic resonance imaging (MRI), are invaluable diagnostic tools. The high resolution of MRI technology incurs the risk of false-positive studies. Many individuals with more peripheral nerve lesions may have unrelated spondylitic findings on radiologic studies.

Cervical radiculopathies are fortunately not common in athletes. The settings in which they do occur are those in which craniocervical trauma is most likely. Football, hockey, soccer, and rugby account for most reports. Gymnasts, equestrian athletes, and skiers are also at risk for cervical spine and thus cervical root

injuries. Cumulative cervical spine injury is well recognized in American football players, and there is a study indicating accelerated cervical spondylitic disease in former soccer players.[2] Similar consequences are likely in other sports.

Initial management of cervical spine injury should focus on exclusion of skeletal injury (e.g., fracture, subluxation), conditions which could threaten spinal cord function, and further exclusion of associated head injury. If cervical root injury is suspected, rest and avoidance of strenuous physical activity are initial precautions. Nonsteroidal and even steroidal anti-inflammatory therapy has a role. Muscle relaxants are often of some benefit, although sedative side effects may be limiting, except at night. Once acute paracervical spasm begins to subside, physical therapy treatment should be offered. Any modalities that elicit radicular pain or accentuate cervical pain should be terminated.

Many individuals with acute cervical disc herniation and frank motor or sensory deficits will recover completely if conservatively managed. Recovery may require many months of restricted activity, however, and many athletes are unwilling to pursue this course. Surgical discectomy at the cervical level performed by an experienced surgeon is usually successful. Almost immediate pain relief and earlier recovery of functional deficits are the norm. Decisions regarding surgical versus conservative therapy should therefore focus on the severity of pain and clinical deficits, on individual lifestyle considerations, and risks associated with return to sports.

Case Study I

A 27-year-old major league pitcher was referred for evaluation of cervical and right scapular pain associated with pitching. He had noted pain upon awakening 4 weeks before when he had pitched five innings the previous night. These symptoms resolved with rest, heat, and use of ibuprofen, but recurred while pitching 4 days later. Symptoms again resolved quickly, but reappeared with any subsequent attempts to pitch, even warmup throwing. He also reported a vague sense of numbness over the right lateral arm.

Examination of the cervical spine revealed full range of motion, but with subjective left posterior cervical pain on lateral neck flexion to the left and rotation to the right. There was vague tenderness in the paraspinous muscles and pain on percussion over the C5 spinous process. The right shoulder examination was normal. The neuromuscular examination revealed mild infraspinatus atrophy (commonly seen in pitchers), although minimal weakness was apparent. There was hypesthesia over the upper lateral arm, the distribution approximating the C5 dermatome. The right biceps reflex was present but decreased relative to its left counterpart.

Routine radiographs of the cervical spine and right shoulder were normal. Nerve conduction studies revealed decreased right ulnar, median, radial, musculocutaneous, and medial forearm cutaneous sensory nerve action potential amplitudes (see the section on *pitcher's arm*), but otherwise were normal. Needle electromyography revealed occasional positive waves and fibrillation potentials in the right supraspinatus and infraspinatus muscles, the deltoid, and the midcervical paraspinous muscles. Magnetic resonance images (MRI) of the cervical spine, somewhat distorted by movement, suggested only a small posterior osteophyte at the C4-C5 level, but intrathecal contrast-enhanced computed tomography (CT) scans clearly defined a small posterolateral disc herniation on the right at the C4-C5 level (Fig. 4-2).

The patient received a high-dose, fast-taper course of oral corticosteroid therapy along with physical therapy consisting of heat, ultrasound, massage, and range of motion exercise. At that point he was symptom-free and advised to forego pitching for 2 months. He resumed pitching without a recurrence of symptoms. If symptoms were to recur, surgery would become a consideration.

BRACHIAL PLEXUS INJURIES

The anatomic relationships of the brachial plexus to the surrounding bone and soft tissues determine its susceptibility to injury. Sudden stretch, downward compression of the shoulder complex, or hyperabduction overhead traction are the most common form of plexus injury (see the following section). Chronic recurrent stretch and compression may occur, particularly with anatomic anomalies. Injuries related to specific athletic activities are less common to the plexus itself than to a number of proximal nerves arising from the plexus. The one probable exception is the recently recognized phenomenon of "pitcher's arm" (see p 65).

Burner/Stinger

The terms burner or stinger refer to the sudden onset of circumferential paresthesias and dysesthetic pain throughout the upper limb and hand, sometimes in association with flaccid paresis. Burners typically occur in association with downward force on the shoulder,

sometimes accompanied by lateral flexion of the head and neck to the opposite side (e.g., football tackle). The phenomenon occurs most frequently in football and rugby players following tackling. The pain rarely lasts more than a minute or two, although residual numbness and paresis may last for many minutes. Electrodiagnostic studies of individuals with residual paresis or, less commonly, sensory loss, have typically revealed mild, acute denervation or reinnervation changes limited for the most part to C5 and C6 muscles, at times indicating root injury or superior trunk injury.[3] Frank superior trunk plexopathy, so-called Erb's palsy, or even more extensive plexus injury may also result from athletic injuries, especially if motor sports are included.

An athlete who recovers quickly (within a few minutes) will usually need no further attention. Most burners are self-limited injuries, although more persistent paresis may occur, particularly in C5 and C6 muscles. Initial assessment should also focus on the cervical spine and shoulder joint; any pain or reduced mobility of either suggest the possibility of more significant orthopedic or neurologic injury. If clinical neuromuscular examination is not possible at the site of injury, return to activity should be delayed until clearance can be obtained. A persistent deficit should be fully evaluated, with special attention to the possibility of unrecognized cervical spine injury. Electrodiagnosis will not yield full diagnostic information for at least 3, and possibly 4 to 5 weeks following injury.

Case Study II

A 21-year-old college football player made an open-field tackle on a punt return. He was on the ground for a few seconds unable to move any extremity—neurogenic reflex paralysis. After this interval of immobility, he left the field with minimal assistance, but recognized his right upper extremity was weak and poorly coordinated. During the ensuing days, pain, weakness, poor coordination of upper extremity motion control, and notable deltoid atrophy were recorded. Subsequent clinical and electrodiagnostic tests demonstrated total deltoid involvement and inferior subluxation of the humeral head and weakness and electrodiagnostic changes of radial nerve-specific muscles, a combination of radial nerve and axillary nerve injury—a posterior cord injury. The treatment program included physical therapy to maintain maximum available function and close observation and repeat electrodiagnostic tests to record evidence of recovery. During this period, all function requiring strength, endurance, and fine motion control were compromised. The earliest evidence of electrodiagnostic improvement was

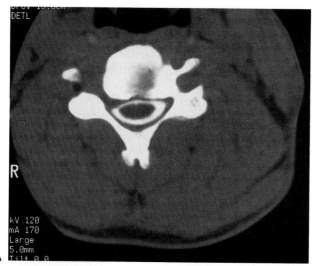

Figure 4-2 Cervical spine CT images for the right-handed pitcher discussed in Case Study I. **(A)** CT scan following intrathecal administration of radiopaque contrast medium. This image is at the level of the C4-C5 disc space, demonstrating effacement of the contrast column and a root sleeve filling defect. **(B)** CT scan coronal reconstruction of the cervical spine within a plane passing through the neural foramina. A filling defect due to extruded disc material is again seen at the C4-C5 level, impinging on the contrast column and distorting the exiting nerve root (*arrowhead*).

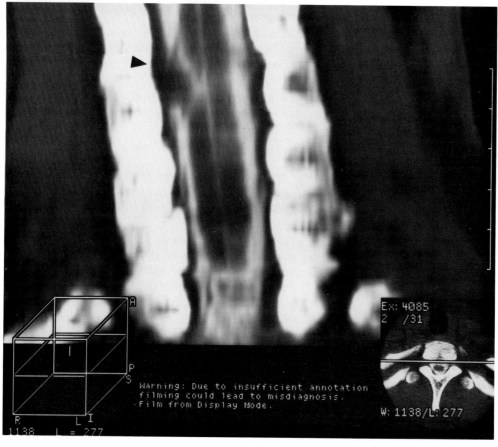

noted in the deltoid approximately 5 months postinjury. Progressive recovery continued over the next 12 months, and approximately 18 months postinjury, functional recovery was complete. During the early stages, various surgical alternatives were considered and deferred when evidence of electrodiagnostic and functional change were observed.

Recurrent burners are not uncommon, although they raise concern regarding cumulative injury and suggest a need for preventive intervention (e.g., cervical and shoulder-strengthening programs). Such an approach is reassuring to athletes, parents of younger athletes, and coaches, and may be beneficial. Various combinations of shoulder pads and neck rolls, in addition to equipment modifications, have been recommended specifically for football players[4] (see Ch. 6).

Thoracic Outlet Syndrome

Thoracic outlet syndrome refers to compression of the brachial plexus or adjacent vessels by various anatomic structures, including the scalene and subclavian muscles, the first rib, anomalous cervical ribs, the clavicle, and fibrous bands traversing these structures. Many patients with combinations of pain, paresthesias, and numbness in the ipsilateral upper limb and hand experience relief with various surgical procedures, primarily resection of the first rib.[5,6] There are far fewer patients reported who have obvious ischemic vascular changes in the distal limb (not limited to transient, postural pulse deficits).[7] An even smaller group of patients have been diagnosed with true neurogenic *thoracic outlet syndrome,* most of whom have clearly recognizable anatomic anomalies as well as objective clinical findings (neuromuscular deficits and electrodiagnostic abnormalities which localize to the inferior cord of the brachial plexus).[8,9] Occasionally, there are athletes who present acutely following falls or collisions with persistent neurologic symptoms and signs referable to the brachial plexus, particularly the medial cord.

There is a much larger group of patients who report postural paresthesias, pain, or fatigue in the arms or hands, particularly when driving or when pursuing other activities in which the arms are extended in front of the body. These individuals often slump their shoulders down and forward and often display positive Adson maneuvers on physical examination, but seldom have persistent vascular or neurologic deficits. They rarely, if ever, have abnormalities on electrodiagnostic testing. These symptoms usually respond to the classical "outlet exercises," which seek to improve shoulder and cervical muscle strength and posture.[10] Occasionally, there are athletes who present with this form of postural *thoracic outlet syndrome,* and tend to fall into two groups: The first group consists of heavily muscled individuals such as weight lifters and rowers, who develop symptoms with strenuous, repetitive use of the upper limb and shoulder girdle musculature. The second group typically presents after discontinuing training, usually in association with weight gain (see Ch. 5).

Pitcher's Arm

We have evaluated a number of baseball pitchers for upper limb neuromuscular symptoms, and have repeatedly observed abnormal sensory nerve action potential amplitudes in pitchers' throwing arms, independent of the presenting symptoms and in the absence of sensory or other findings on examination. This has been true for throwing arms even when the pitcher's symptoms have been in the nonthrowing arm.

Case Study III

Table 4-1 presents sensory conduction data for one such individual, a 37-year-old right-handed pitcher with a 12-year major league career. He has subsequently continued to pitch during frequent batting practices as a minor and major league pitching coach. He was studied following presentation with acute cervical and left radicular arm pain, reporting no symptoms or concerns about function referable to his right arm, the throwing arm. The right radial and median palmar sensory responses were unobtainable; the right ulnar and median digital sensory amplitudes were reduced in comparison with age-matched controls, and they were less than 50 percent of their normal left-sided counterparts. All obtainable sensory distal latencies and velocities were normal in both arms; all motor conduction studies, including F waves, were normal and symmetric. Needle electromyography revealed no acute denervation in either upper limb.

Although this is the most striking example of "pitcher's arm" from our clinical neurodiagnostic laboratory, it is characteristic of the generalized sensory abnormalities that we now expect to see in baseball pitchers, even in the absence of clinical symptoms or signs and in individuals at peak performance levels. Our studies have included two active, Cy Young Award

Table 4-1   Upper Extremity Sensory Nerve Action Potential Amplitudes
for a Right-Handed Pitcher

Nerve	SNAP, Right (μV)	SNAP, Left (μV)	Lower Limit of Normal (μV)
Median			
Index	4	14	14
3rd	4	18	14
Palmar	No response	70	NA
Ulnar			
5th	6	10	10
Palmar	12	30	NA
Radial (superficial)	No response	18	16

NA, not applicable

[a] Discussed in Case Study III.

[b] Sensory amplitudes were consistently decreased on the right, even though the right arm was asymptomatic at the time of study. Sensory latencies and velocities, and all motor studies were normal. (Note: SNAP amplitudes near the lower limit of normal range are expected in this 6 ft. 7 in. tall individual.

winners with qualitatively similar abnormalities despite unimpaired performance.

Conduction studies of pitchers' arms have consistently demonstrated diminished sensory amplitudes, with preservation of normal sensory latencies and conduction velocities. Motor studies (motor amplitudes, latencies, conduction velocities and F-wave latencies) have also been normal. This pattern of abnormalities would be conventionally interpreted as indicating either degeneration of sensory axons or conduction block in a portion of sensory axons in the distal limb. It would be atypical for either process to exist in a generalized distribution throughout the limb without symptoms and some degree of functional impairment. The processes that underlie the phenomenon of pitcher's arm remain unclear, although the observation of more prominent changes in more experienced pitchers suggests that it is use-related. Chronic, recurrent stretch, perhaps at a brachial plexus level, is an attractive hypothetical explanation, although the absence of more obvious motor findings is somewhat unexpected. Other chronic, traumatic mechanisms need to be considered.

Pitcher's arm imparts a further risk of overinterpretation and misdiagnosis. At least biennial baseline studies of all nerves in both arms are wise, enabling better interpretation of studies if neuromuscular symptoms should develop. Pitchers often present with elbow or ulnar nerve symptoms.[11] A too-limited study of only the symptomatic ulnar nerve without a prior study for comparison could be misinterpreted as indicating an ulnar neuropathy (see the section on *ulnar nerve injury*).

ACUTE BRACHIAL NEURITIS

The diagnosis of acute brachial neuritis in athletes poses several challenges.[12] Acute brachial neuritis is an idiopathic syndrome of shoulder pain followed by upper limb weakness, muscle wasting, and sensory loss, both sensory and motor deficits varying in degree and distribution. This syndrome has many names, including acute brachial neuropathy, brachial plexus neuropathy, paralytic brachial neuritis, neuralgic amyotrophy, and the Parsonage-Turner syndrome. Although acute brachial neuritis does not appear to result from either acute trauma or repetitive use, and while athletes do not appear to be at any greater risk than the general population, the syndrome deserves consideration in the context of sports injuries because it invariably presents with shoulder pain, weakness, and altered performance.

The presenting pain often worsens over several days and usually subsides within several weeks. Recognition of weakness may be delayed by several days or as much as 2 weeks. The distribution of weakness is characteristically "patchy," with even severe involvement of one muscle but not another, sharing a common cervical root, plexus, and nerve innervation. The muscles most commonly affected are those innervated via the superior trunk of the brachial plexus—the deltoid, spinati, serratus anterior, and biceps in order of decreasing frequency.[13] Bilateral involvement occurs in up to one-third of patients if both arms are subjected to electrodiagnostic scrutiny,[14] yet marked asymmetry is the norm. Sensory deficits are less frequent, but also tend to be patchy. Numbness in the axillary nerve distribution over the lateral arm is common. Electrodiagnostic studies indicate predominantly axonal pathology, with diminished compound muscle action potential (CMAP) and sensory nerve action potential amplitudes and acute denervation changes on needle examination of affected muscles. Conduction block or delay across the plexus is not readily demonstrable, although deficits often improve too rapidly to reflect axon regeneration.

Patients and their physicians readily associate acute pain with injury, and most patients relate the acute pain to some preceding physical activity, even though significant injury was not recognized at the time. The etiology of acute brachial neuritis remains unknown. The observation that it may follow an otherwise insignificant viral illness and may be seen with increased frequency following large-scale vaccination programs[15] has fueled speculation regarding inflammatory or immune-mediated mechanisms.

Prognosis following acute brachial neuritis is generally favorable, although it parallels the severity of clinical weakness and, in particular, the degree of muscle denervation seen on electromyographic examination. Therapy during the acute phase should consist of rest and analgesia.

Indications of acute brachial neuritis include the absence of a clearly causative injury, pain that persists or even worsens despite rest, a patchy distribution of weakness or anatomic inconsistency between motor and sensory deficits, and bilateral involvement. Acute brachial neuritis can also be quite limited in distribution, affecting only a single portion of the plexus or even a single nerve,[16] simulating a mononeuropathy. Parsonage and Turner's original series[35] included two patients who had clinical weakness limited to the anterior interosseus nerve distribution.

Case Study IV

A 23-year-old professional minor league baseball pitcher observed a significant alteration of his pitching skills following a viral-type upper respiratory infection. His coaches noted that his delivery mechanism had changed and that he was "short-arming" the ball—a lack of completing the cocking stage and a limited arc of acceleration. Within 8 weeks it was recorded that his infraspinatus and triceps were grossly atrophic and weak bilaterally with sparing of his supraspinatus. Thus the early consideration of a specific nerve entrapment was ruled out. The progressive changes were consistent with Parsonage-Turner syndrome with marked paralytic arm atrophy. Unfortunately, his recovery was not sufficient to permit his return to professional baseball.

There are several other sports in which brachial plexus injuries have been reported independent of major orthopedic injuries. These include rifle and shotgun shooting,[17] bowling,[18] and backpacking.[19,20] Again, brachial neuritis may underlie what appear to be activity-related plexus injuries in these settings.

LONG THORACIC NERVE INJURY

The classical sign of long thoracic nerve injury is medial winging of the scapula, accentuated when the patient challenges serratus anterior function (e.g., wall push-up). The presenting symptoms of long thoracic neuropathy may also be vague and nonspecific, more often soft tissue and articular in origin, secondary to glenohumeral dysfunction. Isolated long thoracic neuropathies are uncommon, but there are case reports from a number of athletic settings. Several reports involve vigorous, repetitive use of the upper limb and some forced depression of the shoulder. Electrodiagnostic studies may confirm the diagnosis of long thoracic neuropathy, although diagnosis is usually based on the clinical findings.

Management of long thoracic neuropathies is almost always conservative. Direct surgical exploration of the nerve has little value. There are various procedures for scapular stabilization with severe deficits, but the resultant loss of shoulder stability and mobility may be more limiting than the initial deficit.

SUPRASCAPULAR NERVE INJURY

The suprascapular nerve may be injured in association with shoulder trauma, particularly sudden downward depression of the shoulder, the same type of injury that can also stretch the superior cord of the plexus. In these cases, the injury to the suprascapular nerve is near its origin from the plexus. The other two common sites of injury are at the scapular and spinoglenoid notches where the nerve makes a directional change in its course, adjacent to bone. The variable presence of ligaments at both sites, the transverse scapular ligament and the spinoglenoid ligament, respectively, may further predispose to entrapment or more acute injury, as will depression and protraction of the scapula. We have also seen several patients with ganglion cysts within the supraspinatus fossa and secondary suprascapular neuropathies.[21]

Injury to the suprascapular nerve either near its origin or at the scapular notch may be associated with pain, weakness, atrophy, and shoulder dysfunction, although there may be little to distinguish it from shoulder pain of other etiologies. This presumably reflects the overlay of symptoms referable to the shoulder articulations as well as posterior scapular muscles. More distal injury at the spinoglenoid notch is typically even more vague in its presentation, any associated pain being poorly localized and weakness and atrophy limited to the infraspinatus (see Ch. 11 and Ch. 13).

Athletes in virtually any sport may injure the suprascapular nerve in association with shoulder trauma, although throwers and tennis servers appear to be at greatest risk. Ferretti and associates[22] have reported a series of asymptomatic suprascapular neuropathies in volleyball players. Bryan and Wild,[23] and Ringel and colleagues[24] have reported suprascapular nerve injuries in baseball players, particularly in pitchers.

Electrodiagnostic studies can aid in the diagnosis and localization of suprascapular nerve injuries. Confirmation of denervation in one or both of the spinati (in the absence of changes elsewhere in the C5 and C6 myotomes) supports the interpretation of a mononeuropathy; denervation only within the infraspinatus favors a more distal site of injury, usually at the spinoglenoid notch. Supramaximal electric stimulation at Erb's point activates multiple nerves, and it is also poorly tolerated by many subjects. Suprascapular conduction studies are therefore of limited value.

Acute management is similar for most proximal nerve injuries in the arm. Rest and, if needed, analgesia and anti-inflammatory agents should be used while the patient is observed closely over time. Electrodiagnostic study should be delayed for at least 3 weeks (preferably 4 weeks) as the presence or absence of denervation within the spinati and other proximal muscles will be critical to diagnosis and localization. Magnetic resonance imaging has been helpful in detecting local structural lesions within the supraspinatus fossa.[21] An apparent neurapractic lesion should be managed conservatively with gradual return to activity in conjunction with physical therapy. Even denervating lesions can be approached conservatively, unless severe, persistent, or recurrent. In such instances, surgical exploration becomes a consideration. Again, the scapular notch and the spinoglenoid notch are the more common sites of entrapment, as well as sites of possible predisposing ligamentous or other anomalies (see Ch. 11, Case Study II).

AXILLARY NERVE INJURY

The axillary nerve can be injured in conjunction with shoulder trauma, particularly shoulder dislocations. Axillary neuropathy has also been reported following blunt trauma and as a complication of axillary hematoma.[25] In contrast to acute or recurrent injury with shoulder dislocations, the most common site of entrapment in athletes is within the quadrilateral space. The "quadrilateral space syndrome" was first reported by Cahill and Palmer.[26] Again, throwing activities appear to predispose to this type of injury, and baseball pitchers may be at greatest risk. This injury is also seen in javelin throwers and rowers.

The presenting syndrome of axillary neuropathy is one of anterior shoulder pain on abduction and external rotation and inferior humeral subluxation, with a positive sulcus sign and radiograph (see Case Study II). Sensory disturbance overlying the anterior deltoid region and deltoid weakness or atrophy may be accompanying findings. Differential diagnosis should include consideration of joint and soft tissue injuries, posterior cord or superior trunk plexopathies, and C5 radiculopathy. Careful clinical examination is the key to the diagnosis, although needle electromyography is a useful adjunct. Again, the timing of the EMG is important: Early study may localize the lesion, but will not allow differentiation of a neurapractic lesion versus a more severe lesion until sufficient time has elapsed for the evolution of denervation potentials (3 to 4 weeks). Arteriographic demonstration of posterior humeral circumflex artery compression upon abduction and external rotation at the shoulder has also been considered valuable in establishing the diagnosis of the quadrilateral space syndrome (see Ch. 5).

MUSCULOCUTANEOUS NERVE INJURY

Isolated musculocutaneous neuropathies are not common. When they do occur independent of obvious shoulder or arm trauma, they follow strenuous, sustained, or repetitive use of the arm. Such deficits may reflect muscular compression as much as stretch. Most clinical reports of sports-related musculocutaneous neuropathy describe spontaneous recovery,[27,28] often within a time frame as brief as hours to days. More severe musculocutaneous lesions are typically seen in conjunction with injury to other proximal nerves or the brachial plexus itself.

The sensory manifestations of musculocutaneous nerve neuropathy are usually well-defined and localized to the radial/lateral forearm. Weakness of elbow flexion is the norm, and the biceps tendon reflex is characteristically diminished or absent. These latter signs are too often assumed to reflect C6 root lesions; musculocutaneous neuropathies should spare the brachioradialis reflex and the more distal C6 dermatome as well as other C6 muscles (see Ch. 3, Case Study I). The management of isolated musculocutaneous neuropathies is usually conservative.

ULNAR NERVE INJURY

The symptoms of ulnar nerve lesions are similar to those of other peripheral nerve lesions, with the localization and distribution of the symptoms being relatively specific. Pain, paresthesias, sensory loss, and paresis are seen, in varying degrees, dependent upon the severity of the process and upon whether it is an acute or chronic situation. Pain at the elbow may well be associated with entrapment at that level, although chronic entrapments may be painless for non-upper extremity-dominant sports. A Tinel's sign may be elicited with percussion over the ulnar groove or at the wrist, but does not always have precise localizing value. There may be a component of pain that radiates along the course of the nerve. Pain along the forearm and into the ulnar portion of the hand favors a proximal lesion, usually at the elbow; pain limited to the hand favors a more distal lesion, but exceptions are not uncommon. Sensory symptoms, either positive in terms of paresthesias or negative in terms of hypesthesia, are referred to cutaneous regions innervated by the nerve. Some anatomic variations can confuse this picture; the most common is the inclusion of the entire fourth and a portion of the third digit within the ulnar distribution. Ulnar sensory symptoms other than pain are rarely observed proximal to the wrist. The ulnar forearm is innervated by the medial cutaneous nerve of the forearm, which arises directly from the medial cord of the plexus just prior to the ulnar origin. Sensory findings that include the ulnar distribution but also the medial forearm suggest medial cord or C8 root pathology.

Ulnar motor deficits can be helpful in localizing ulnar nerve lesions, although careful examination may be required to confirm or exclude paresis in the ulnar forearm flexors in the face of significant weakness of the ulnar intrinsics. With early diagnosis, most athletes do not reach this point (see Ch. 19). Froment's and Wartenberg's signs and the so-called benediction sign all indicate severe advanced paresis of ulnar-innervated intrinsic hand muscles. Froment's sign consists of hyperextension of the first metacarpophalangeal joint and associated flexion of the adjacent interphalangeal joint of the thumb, both accentuated by thumb-index pinch. It reflects weakness of the adductor pollicis and the flexor pollicis brevis. Wartenberg's sign is flaccid abduction of the fifth digit due to weakness of the interosseus. The benediction sign, so called because it mimics the hand posture often employed voluntarily

by clerics, consists of passive "clawing" of the fourth and fifth digits due to weakness of their lumbricals in contrast to the normally posed second and third digits. The dorsal interossei are finger abductors, while the ventral or palmar interossei are primarily finger adductors. The hypothenar muscles abduct or oppose the fifth digit. The former function requires coactivation of the flexor carpi ulnaris for stabilization of the pisiform bone, while the latter also involves the ventral interossei. Preservation of fifth digit abduction in the face of weakness of other ulnar intrinsics indicates a lesion of the deep branch of the ulnar nerve. Paresis of ulnar intrinsics including the hypothenar muscles but sparing the forearm flexors tends to localize at or just proximal to Guyon's canal; such a lesion will spare sensation over the dorsal ulnar aspect of the hand, the dorsal sensory branch arising proximal to the canal.

Electrodiagnostic studies may be valuable in confirming the diagnosis of ulnar neuropathy, localizing the lesion(s), and characterizing pathogenesis and severity. Yet it is not at all uncommon, particularly with mild lesions, for conduction studies and needle examination to fall short of precise localization. Clinical examination and judgment must take precedence over diagnostic technology in such instances. Ulnar nerve conduction studies also consist of technical hazards related to limb temperature and position. Needle examination of many ulnar-innervated muscles requires a high degree of experience, skill, and patience. Even when specific abnormalities are detected, comparison with other nerves and with the contralateral ulnar nerve is necessary to exclude a more generalized phenomenon — it is not possible to confirm a mononeuropathy without excluding a polyneuropathy. The reader is referred to other sources for specific techniques.[29,30]

The most common site of ulnar neuropathy in athletes as well as others is at the elbow. Although acute nerve lesions due to direct trauma or in association with acute orthopedic injury such as epicondylar fracture are not uncommon, the majority of ulnar neuropathies at the elbow reflect chronic injury due to combinations of stretch and compression (i.e., entrapment) (see Ch. 19).

Although uncommon in comparison with the frequency of lesions at the elbow, distal ulnar lesions are encountered with a frequency sufficient to warrant inclusion within the differential diagnosis of apparent ulnar neuropathy. Again, prior trauma, ganglions, anatomic anomalies, and local inflammatory processes may be predisposing factors. The nerve can be entrapped in the vicinity of Guyon's canal or more distally as the deep branch passes the hook of the hamate and traverses the palm. Neuropathy at Guyon's canal is in some respects similar to ulnar entrapment at the elbow and even median nerve entrapment at the carpal tunnel (see the next section). In all these instances, the nerve passes through a fibro-osseous tunnel within which recurrent biomechanical trauma can occur. The relative loss of expansibility and mobility at these sites further predisposes the nerve in the event of displacing injury to any of the surrounding structures. For example, fractures of the hook of the hamate are commonly associated with ulnar nerve injury within Guyon's canal. Concussive trauma to the palm, particularly if recurrent, can also be associated with injury to the deep branch of the nerve. In this case and in the case of digital nerve injury, vascular compromise often coexists.[31]

The athletic setting in which distal ulnar neuropathies are most frequently encountered is cycling.[32,33] The combination of palmar compression against handlebars with ulnar dorsiflexion of the wrists has been suggested as the biomechanical mechanism. Fixed motor deficits are rare, and coincident median nerve symptoms may be present. Adjustments in hand position and padding often lead to improvement. More frank neurovascular trauma can be seen in baseball catchers, hockey goalies, and handball players.

The management of ulnar neuropathies in most respects parallels that of other peripheral nerve lesions. Symptoms that appear in the absence of any clearly recognized injury should first be treated with rest. If symptoms fail to respond quickly or recur with return to activity, further evaluation in the form of detailed functional examination, electrodiagnostic studies, and radiographs is indicated. If evaluation confirms entrapment at the elbow or wrist, surgical decompression becomes an option. It is unlikely that symptomatic entrapment related to a repetitive sports activity will resolve spontaneously without lengthy cessation of that activity. The severity and chronic nature of the clinical deficits, the effect of those deficits on performance, and the athlete's personal situation and attributes must be carefully weighed.

Case Study V

A 25-year-old skater fell, striking her left elbow against the ice. Initial examination revealed swelling and tenderness at the medial elbow, but the joint itself appeared stable. She complained of numbness in the fourth and fifth digits, but intrinsic hand muscle function appeared to be intact, aside from mild weakness of the abductor digiti minimi. Radiographs revealed an avulsion fracture of the medial epicondyle (Fig. 4-3). Nonoperative treatment was instituted.

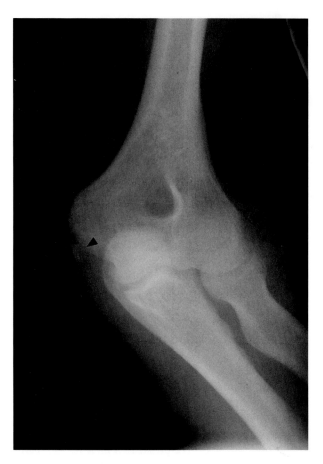

Figure 4-3 Left elbow radiograph of the skater discussed in Case Study V, demonstrating a small medial malleolar avulsion fracture (*arrowhead*).

Electrodiagnostic studies were performed 4 months after the injury. Left median and radial nerve conduction studies were normal. The ulnar sensory response from the fifth digit was markedly decreased in response to stimulation of the left ulnar nerve at the wrist, and the dorsal ulnar sensory response was absent. The ulnar motor responses from the left abductor muscle of little finger and first dorsal interosseous muscle were normal in response to stimulation at the wrist, but there was no response recorded from either muscle following stimulation of the ulnar nerve above the elbow. This could indicate a major conduction block at the elbow, although the abductor muscle of little finger and first dorsal interosseus muscle were clinically normal. These muscles also failed to respond to stimulation of the ulnar nerve several centimeters below the elbow, yet they exhibited normal responses to stimulation of the median nerve at the elbow. These observations indicated an ulnar neuropathy proximal to the wrist, but also a major Martin-Gruber anastomosis from the median to the ulnar nerve in the forearm.

The patient was managed conservatively for a further 8 months, but noted no change in sensory symptoms. At that point, she underwent anterior transposition of the ulnar nerve at the elbow. Significant scarring with traction of the nerve was noted at the level of the distal epicondyle. The sensory symptoms resolved within 2 months of the surgery.

This case demonstrates a fairly common mechanism of ulnar nerve injury at the elbow, but further underscores the importance of anatomic variants. The preservation of function in the ulnar intrinsic hand muscles falsely suggested a relatively mild ulnar nerve injury at the elbow. It is also instructive to consider the clinical presentation had this patient suffered median nerve injury at the elbow or in the arm; the apparent involvement of both median and ulnar muscles would tend to indicate a more proximal plexus lesion.

MEDIAN NERVE

Median neuropathy at the wrist in the form of the carpal tunnel syndrome is the most common human mononeuropathy. Median neuropathy is observed in athletes and may have a serious impact on athletic performance, but probably occurs with no greater incidence than in the general population. Aside from obvious local trauma, median nerve lesions may be associated with a predisposing anatomic variance, expressed clinically in association with repetitive use. Participation in sports may therefore bring an individual with predisposing anatomy to clinical presentation (e.g., physically challenged athletes) at a point earlier than more typical activities of daily living (see Ch. 7).

Median nerve injury in the shoulder and upper arm region is not common. The median nerve can sometimes be injured along with other nerves at this level and should be considered in association with more obvious axillary or musculocutaneous neuropathies. Anterior shoulder dislocation most often involves the axillary nerve, but occasionally the median nerve. Proximal median neuropathies have been reported in association with axillary and brachial artery aneurysms. Iatrogenic median neuropathies are also known to occur following shoulder procedures and with improper limb positioning during anesthesia.

Electrodiagnostic studies can be helpful in localizing proximal median nerve lesions. Key conduction abnormalities include reduced thenar CMAP amplitude and reduced median sensory amplitudes without motor or sensory conduction delays. These changes may be subtle. When median sensory amplitudes are reduced in the absence of distal conduction delay, a normal musculocutaneous sensory study helps localize the lesion distal to the brachial plexus. Needle examination of the forearm flexors is also very important. The referring clinician should keep in mind, however, that appropriate performance and interpretation of the forearm electromyogram is dependent on the skill and experience of the electromyographer. Confirmation of pronator teres denervation in conjunction with similar changes in median forearm flexors indicates pathology above the elbow.

The term *pronator syndrome* is commonly referred to as any median nerve entrapment in the vicinity of the elbow. The median nerve may actually be compressed at three potential sites as it passes through the "pronator tunnel." Compression by the pronator teres itself is just one site of entrapment. All possible sites must be considered, particularly if decompressive surgery is planned, as it may not be possible to differentiate among the potential sites except by exploration. The first site is where the nerve passes under the bicipital aponeurosis, also known as the lacertus fibrosis. Muscular hypertrophy and thickening of the aponeurosis are reported to be predisposing factors. The pronator teres itself constitutes a further site of compression, specifically at the point where the median nerve passes between the superficial (humeral) head and the deep (ulnar) head. A final site of median nerve compression distal to the elbow is the point at which the nerve passes beneath the proximal margin of the flexor digitorum superficialis. Fibrous thickening and tightening have also been reported at this site.

The clinical presentation of the pronator syndrome is quite similar to that of the more frequent and familiar *carpal tunnel syndrome.* It is thus appropriate to at least consider pronator syndrome in patients who appear to have carpal tunnel syndrome, and the two may coexist as an example of a so-called double-crush syndrome. The most specific features of pronator syndrome are tenderness or Tinel's sign in the region of the pronator teres where the median nerve passes, and the absence of the nocturnal symptoms that are so prevalent in carpal tunnel syndrome. The precipitation or accentuation of median sensory symptoms with forced pronation of the forearm against resistance is also a helpful sign. Occasionally, baseball pitchers develop a significantly swollen pronator teres secondary to eccentric injury and medial laxity that results in transient median symptomatology.

Electrodiagnostic studies should be helpful in confirming a clinical impression of pronator syndrome. Reduced median motor and sensory amplitudes in the absence of distal conduction delay, median motor conduction block or delay across the elbow, or denervation changes in median forearm flexors and thenar muscles all suggest proximal median neuropathy. Only focal conduction block or conduction delay across the elbow are clearly of localizing value, however. Most pronator syndromes, in a situation similar to the more common ulnar entrapment at the elbow (see above), cannot be clearly localized by electrodiagnostic criteria, the abnormalities only indicating pathology at some point proximal to the wrist. In fact, most of the large clinical series of patients with pronator syndrome reveal a lack of nerve conduction and EMG abnormalities.[34] Therefore, caution is advised in making what is often a clinical diagnosis. Management, in turn, should be conservative in the absence of objective, localizing symptoms. Surgical exploration of the antecubital fossa in suspected pronator syndrome should be considered only when typical symptoms have failed to respond to rest, heat, nonsteroidal anti-inflammatories, and physical therapeutic modalities, and then only when the passage of time has failed to suggest alternate diagnoses. There are patients with symptomatic pronator syndrome who do not have objective clinical deficits or electrodiagnostic abnormalities, but they are probably not at great risk of irreversible deficits if conservatively managed.

Isolated injury to the anterior interosseus nerve is also uncommon. It may follow penetrating injury to the forearm, and it may complicate fractures of the radial shaft. Both the anterior interosseous and the main branch of the median nerve may suffer ischemic or eccentric muscle injury as a part of Volkmann syndrome. Anterior interosseus entrapment near its point of origin has been reported in association with various structural anomalies, for example, thrombosed vessels, tendinous origins of the pronator teres or flexor digitorum sublimis, and accessory forearm muscles such as Gantzer's muscle and a palmaris profundus. Apparent anterior interosseus neuropathies have also been reported in association with acute brachial neuritis.[35,36] It occurs with a greater than coincidental frequency, suggesting some predilection for involvement of motor axons to the anterior interosseus muscles. It is therefore conceivable that what appears to be a spontaneous but painful anterior interosseus neuropathy may be a form of acute brachial neuritis with more proximal pathology.

The diagnosis of anterior interosseus neuropathy is based upon the expected clinical deficits and the exclusion of deficits referable to other portions of the median nerve. Any sensory symptoms in the hand direct attention to the main trunk of the median nerve. Electrodiagnostic studies should be helpful. The observation of median sensory conduction abnormalities has the same implications as sensory symptoms or signs in the hand; these are unexpected in cases of anterior inter-

osseous neuropathy. Needle examination remains the "gold standard" of electrodiagnosis of anterior interosseus neuropathy, although needle examination of the flexor digitorum profundus to the index finger and the pronator quadratus should only be performed by an experienced electromyographer. Denervation limited to the three anterior interosseus innervated muscles confirms the diagnosis.

The initial management of acute anterior interosseus neuropathies should be conservative; cases of penetrating and orthopedic trauma are exceptions. Surgical exploration becomes a consideration if deficits are progressing or if stable deficits fail to improve. A reasonable interval for reversal of neurapractic deficits would be 6 to 8 weeks, while a much longer interval is required in the face of appreciable axonal degeneration (i.e., axonotmesis). This interval should reflect the distance between the presumed site of axonal injury and the target muscles. The association between apparent anterior interosseus neuropathies and acute brachial neuritis argues for a longer course of conservative management if the presentation is clearly acute, painful, and spontaneous. In contrast, chronic deficits, particularly if appearing within the setting of repetitive, strenuous use of the forearm, may warrant early exploration.

Athletic activities that predispose the anterior interosseus nerve to injury include throwing, particularly baseball. Occasionally, there will be athletes with predisposing anatomic variants as well. Many sports involve repetitive use of the upper limbs, and thus otherwise typical anterior interosseus neuropathies may appear in athletes. There is one report of bilateral anterior interosseous neuropathies in an athlete.[37] Symptoms occurred in the dominant arm after playing tennis. Some months later, similar symptoms began in the nondominant arm after swimming. The relationship to the athletic activity is unclear; no anatomic abnormalities were found at surgery.

Despite the few athletic activities that predispose the athlete to carpal tunnel syndrome, it deserves mention (for a complete discussion, see Chs. 7 and 24). Carpal tunnel syndrome is almost always in the dominant limb when unilateral and worse on the dominant side when bilateral, indicating that use of the hands is a contributing factor. Paresthesias and pain are the typical presenting symptoms in carpal tunnel syndrome. Digital paresthesias, although presumably limited to the median nerve distribution, are often experienced and described as encompassing the whole hand. A report of paresthesias limited to the palm or ascending above the wrist should suggest other etiologies. The pain is typically aching rather than sharp, and it is less consistently use-related than sensory symptoms. Hand fatigue or clumsiness are common complaints, while actual thenar paresis is a late symptom. A sharp, electric-like pain radiating into the median fingers, Tinel's sign, may be elicited by tapping over the carpal tunnel or at its edges. Digital paresthesias may be elicited by sustained 90-degree wrist flexion, Phalan's maneuver.

The electrodiagnostic findings in carpal tunnel syndrome are more specific than presenting symptoms and signs, although various combinations of distal motor or sensory conduction delay and motor or sensory conduction block may indicate median neuropathy at the wrist. Conduction delay across the wrist segment of the nerve is the hallmark of carpal tunnel syndrome but may take many forms. The interested reader is referred to other texts for a complete discussion.[38,39]

Although demonstration of median nerve conduction delay across the carpal tunnel is the key to the electrodiagnostic confirmation of carpal tunnel syndrome, the recognition and characterization of motor or sensory conduction block further aids in diagnosis. The presence or absence of thenar denervation, indicating a component of axonal degeneration, is also a relevant finding. While it is unusual to confirm conduction delay in the absence of some degree of conduction block, major reductions in motor or sensory amplitudes or the observation of thenar denervation indicate a more severe lesion. Electrodiagnostic studies also aid in the diagnosis of carpal tunnel syndrome through recognition or exclusion of other findings, such as generalized polyneuropathies, more proximal median nerve or plexus lesions, and radiculopathies.

RADIAL NERVE INJURY

Acute traumatic injury to the radial nerve may occur at almost any level, although the most common sites are near the spiral groove of the humerus and in the proximal forearm. Injury at these sites often accompanies displaced fractures of the humerus and radius, respectively. Sunderland[40] has estimated that roughly 50 percent of all radial neuropathies are associated with fractures. Close anatomic relationship of the nerve to bone and the relative immobility of the nerve, particularly the segment between the spiral groove and the lateral intermuscular septum, are predisposing factors in these situations. The nerve may be injured by various combinations of stretch, contusion, and even laceration; entrapment between bone fragments may complicate reduction of the fracture (see Ch. 3, Case Study I).

High radial nerve lesions are associated with predominantly extensor weakness, with wrist drop usually the most obvious deficit. Lesions at the spiral groove only partially affect the triceps, although sometimes not at all. When the triceps is spared, the major issue is whether the lesion is proximal or distal to the origin of the posterior interosseus branch. A true posterior interosseous neuropathy spares the radial wrist extensors and sensation over the dorsum of the hand. The typical hand posture assumed in the presence of posterior interosseus neuropathies is that of finger flexion with radial deviation at the wrist.

True radial nerve entrapment and recurrent radial nerve trauma related to repetitive use of the limb are uncommon in comparison to ulnar neuropathies at the elbow and median neuropathies at the wrist. Isolated posterior interosseus neuropathies do, however, occur. The nerve is relatively immobile near its origin, as it penetrates the supinator muscle. There is often a fibrous arch between the two heads of the supinator, the arcade of Frohse. Any increase in soft tissue volume in the form of edema, synovitis, ganglion, lipoma, and so on can lead to nerve compression at this site. Repetitive-use injuries to the radial nerve as it penetrates the lateral intermuscular septum above the elbow or within the "radial tunnel" at the elbow are uncommon, but may be seen in association with activities involving repetitive pronation and supination.

The sensory deficit associated either with lesions of the superficial radial nerve or more proximal radial nerve lesions may be confused with a C6 dermatomal deficit. The latter should include a portion of the median nerve distribution to the volar hand and much of the musculocutaneous distribution to the radial forearm. Pain may accompany radial nerve lesions, although its localization is often vague. Local tenderness on palpation of the nerve may be of some value. This is thought by some to be a key feature in recognition of the "radial tunnel" syndrome, although local tenderness in the absence of any other nerve-specific symptoms rarely reflects a neurogenic process.

Electrodiagnostic studies often enable precise localization of radial nerve lesions, becoming particularly important if motor deficits are mild (see Ch. 3, Case Study I). In the presence of any motor deficit, an abnormal superficial radial sensory response (absent or decreased amplitude) suggests a lesion proximal to the origin of the superficial radial and posterior interosseus branches. Motor conduction studies are at times limited by volume conduction among the forearm extensors; the placement of recording electrodes more distally (over the extensor indicis) may be helpful in this respect. The optimal stimulation sites are those allowing near-nerve stimulation with surface electrodes: in the posterior axilla, at the spiral groove and at the elbow, just lateral to the biceps tendon. Some advocate the use of needle electrodes for stimulation and recording, although motor amplitude measurements are not reliable when recorded with needle electrodes. The demonstration of definite conduction delay or conduction block along any radial nerve segment has localizing value.

Assuming a component of axonal degeneration (axonotmesis), needle examination is also important for localization, extending the sensitivity of the clinical examination in cases of mild weakness. The presence of some denervation in the triceps, despite normal or near-normal triceps strength, suggests a lesion at or near the spiral groove; in such cases the anconeus may also reveal denervation. If the triceps is spared, the presence or absence of abnormality in the brachioradialis and the extensor carpi radialis group become significant, abnormality indicating a lesion proximal to the posterior interosseus origin. It may sometimes be difficult to distinguish a high radial nerve lesion from a posterior cord plexopathy. Needle examination of the deltoid should be considered. Superior trunk lesions occasionally mimic radial neuropathies; denervation in the shoulder girdle muscles as well as musculocutaneous and median sensory abnormalities can aid in this differentiation.

Most sports-related radial neuropathies are the sequela of acute traumatic injuries. Again, humeral and proximal radial fractures are often associated with radial nerve deficits; the possibility of radial nerve compromise should always be considered when assessing such fractures. Management is appropriately focused on the orthopedic injury, although if there is a significant axonal component to the nerve injury, neural regeneration may well lag behind orthopedic recovery. Once the limb is stabilized, radial motor and sensory function can be assessed in detail. Proximal radial fractures may spare the superficial radial branch, presenting as pure motor posterior interosseus neuropathies.

Compressive or contusive trauma is a further mechanism of radial nerve injury that can affect athletes. There are reports of transient deficits following strenuous muscular effort alone.[41-44] Compression just distal to the axilla or at the spiral groove can be seen with activities that require forceful adduction of the shoulder against resisting structures, such as gymnastics (parallel bars in particular) and wrestling. Contusion of the superficial radial nerve is not uncommon in "stick" sports such as field hockey and lacrosse; these are usually self-limited injuries. Compressive superficial radial neuropathy may occur at the wrist with use of constricting tape, various wrist bands, archery guards, gymnastic grips, and so on. Fortunately these are also self-limited in most instances. Bowler's thumb is the result of recurrent injury to the digital nerve on the

ulnar side of the thumb.[45] This nerve receives contributions from both the superficial radial and median nerves (see Ch. 25).

Repetitive use radial neuropathies occur occasionally in athletes. *Resistant tennis elbow* and *radial tunnel syndrome* refer to radial nerve entrapment either just above the elbow or near the origin of the posterior interosseous nerve.[46,47] The superficial radial nerve may also be entrapped as it ascends through fascial planes of the forearm to assume a superficial position. In these instances, repetitive supination or pronation activities typically precipitate symptoms (e.g., throwing, batting or swinging, rowing). There are numerous reports of relief of refractory lateral elbow pain following surgical decompression of the radial or posterior interosseous nerves at that level. However, many of these patients have not had objective radial nerve deficits or electrodiagnostic confirmation.[48]

The practitioner who treats athletic injuries should be aware of the neurologic implications of these injuries. Individual nerves in addition to the cervical nerve roots and brachial plexus can be affected. An understanding of these structures and the types of athletes who are at risk for injury will lead to an earlier diagnosis and may prevent more severe problems.

REFERENCES

1. Torg JS: Athletic injuries to the cervical spine. In Jordan BD et al (eds): Sports Neurology. Aspen Publishers, Rockville, MD 1989
2. Sortland O, Tysvaer A, Sorti O: Changes in the cervical spine in association football players. Br J Sports Med 16:80, 1982
3. Wilbourn AJ, Hershman EB, Bergfeld J: Brachial plexopathies in athletes: the EMG findings. Muscle Nerve 9(suppl):254, 1986
4. Speer KP, Bassett FH III. The prolonged burner syndrome. Am J Sports Med 18:591, 1990
5. Lord JW, Rosati LM: Thoracic outlet syndromes. CIBA Clin Symp 23:2, 1971
6. Roos DB: The place for scalenectomy and first rib resection in thoracic outlet syndrome. Surgery 92:1077, 1982
7. McCarthy WJ, Yao JST, Shafer MF et al: Upper extremity arterial injury in athletes. J Vasc Surg 9:317, 1989
8. Wilbourn AJ, Porter JM: Thoracic outlet syndrome. Spine 2:597, 1988
9. Guilliat RW: Thoracic outlet syndrome. In Dyck et al (eds): Peripheral Neuropathy. 2nd Ed. WB Saunders, Philadelphia, 1984
10. Peet RM, Henricksen MD, Anderson TP et al: Thoracic outlet syndrome: evaluation of a therapeutic exercise program. Proc Mayo Clin 31:281, 1956
11. Del Pizzo W, Jobe FW, Norwood L: Ulnar nerve entrap-

ment syndrome in baseball players. Am J Sports Med 5:182, 1977

12. Hershman EB, Wilbourn AJ, Bergfeld JA: Acute brachial neuropathy in athletes. Am J Sports Med 17:655, 1989

13. Dillon L, Hoaglund FT, Scheck M: Brachial neuritis. J Bone Joint Surg [Am] 67:878, 1985

14. Tsairis P, Dyck AJ, Mulder DW: Arch Neurol 27:109, 1972

15. Miller HG, Stanton JB: Neurologic sequelae of prophylactic inoculation. Q J Med 23:1, 1954

16. England JD, Sumner AJ: Neuralgic amyotrophy: an increasingly diverse entity. Muscle Nerve, 10:60, 1987

17. Wanamaker WM: Firearm recoil palsy. Arch Neurol 31:208, 1974

18. Shukla AY, Green JB: Letter to the editor. N Engl J Med 324:928, 1991

19. Daube JR: Rucksack paralysis. JAMA 208:2447, 1969

20. Hirasawa Y, Sakakida K: Sports and peripheral nerve injury. Am J Sports Med 11:420, 1983

21. Goss TP, Aronow MS, Coumas JM: The use of MRI to diagnose suprascapular nerve entrapment caused by a ganglion: two case reports. Orthopedics 17:4194, 1994

22. Ferretti A, Cerullo G, Russo G: Suprascapular neuropathy in volleyball players. J Bone Joint Surg [Am] 69:260, 1987

23. Bryon WJ, Wild JJ: Isolated infraspinatus atrophy: a common cause of posterior shoulder pain and weakness in throwing athletes. Am J Sports Med 17:130, 1989

24. Ringel SP, Treihaft M, Carry M et al: Suprascapular neuropathy in pitchers. Am J Sports Med 18:80, 1990

25. Mandoza FX, Main K: Peripheral nerve injuries in the shoulder of athletes. Clin Sports Med 9:331, 1990

26. Cahill BR, Palmer RE: Quadrilateral space syndrome. J Hand Surg 8:65, 1983

27. Braddon RL, Wolfe C: Musculocutaneous nerve injury after heavy exercise. Arch Phys Med Rehabil 59:290, 1978

28. Mastiglia FL: Musculocutaneous neuropathy after strenuous physical activity. Med J Aust 145:153, 1986

29. Jabre J, Wilbourn AJ: The EMG findings in 100 consecutive ulnar neuropathies. Acta Neurol Scand [Suppl] 60:91, 1979

30. Hammer K: Nerve conduction studies. Charles C Thomas, Springfield, IL, 1982

31. Rettig AC: Neurovascular injuries in the wrists and hands of athletes. Clin Sports Med 9:389, 1990

32. Eckman PB, Perlstein G, Altroochi PH: Ulnar neuropathy in bicycle riders. Arch Neurol 32:130, 1975

33. Frontera WR: Cyclist palsy: clinical and electrodiagnostic findings. Br J Sports Med 17:91, 1983

34. Hartz CR, Linscheild RL, Gramse RR et al: The pronator teres syndrome: compressive neuropathy of the median nerve. J Bone Joint Surg [Am] 63:885, 1981

35. Parsonage MJ, Turner JWA: Neuralgic amyotrophy: shoulder girdle syndrome. Lancet 1:973, 1948

36. Rennels GD, Ochoa J: Neuralgic amyotrophy manifesting as anterior interosseous nerve palsy. Muscle Nerve 3:160, 1980

37. Nakano KK, Lundergan C, Okihiro MM: Anterior interosseous nerve syndromes. Arch Neurol 34:477, 1977

38. Kimura J: Electrodiagnosis in Diseases of Nerve and Muscle: Principles and Practices. 2nd Ed. FA Davis, Philadelphia, 1989

39. Dawson DM, Hallett M, Millender LH: Entrapment Neuropathies. 2nd Ed. Little, Brown, Boston, 1990

40. Sunderland S: Nerves and Nerve Injuries. 2nd Ed. Churchill Livingstone, Edinburgh, 1978

41. Lotem M, Fried A, Levy M et al: Radial palsy following muscular effort: a nerve compression syndrome possibly related to a fibrous arch of the lateral band of the triceps. J Bone Joint Surg [Br] 53:500, 1971

42. Manske PR: Compression of the radial nerve by the triceps muscle: case report. J Bone Joint Surg [Am] 59:835, 1977

43. Mitsunga MM, Nakano KK: High radial palsy following strenuous muscle activity: a case report. Clin Orthop 234:39, 1988

44. Streib E: Upper arm radial nerve palsy after muscular effort: report of three cases. Neurology 42:1632, 1992

45. Dobyns JH, O'Brien ET, Linscheid RL et al: Bowler's thumb-diagnosis and treatment: a review of seventeen cases. J Bone Joint Surg [Am] 54:751, 1972

46. Roles NC, Maudsley RH: Radial tunnel syndrome: resistant tennis elbow as a nerve entrapment. J Bone Joint Surg [Br] 54:499, 1972

47. Ritts GD, Wood MB, Linscheid RL: Radial tunnel syndrome: a ten-year surgical experience. Clin Orthop 219:201, 1987

48. Van Rossum J, Buruma OJS, Kamphuisen HAC et al: Tennis elbow: a radial tunnel syndrome? J Bone Joint Surg [Br] 60:197, 1978

5

Vascular Problems

Michael J. Rohrer

Upper extremity vascular injury in association with acute orthopedic trauma, such as clavicular fracture, supracondylar humeral fracture, and elbow and shoulder dislocation, is well described.[1,2] In these cases, the mechanism of vascular injury involves an acute arterial stretch injury or contusion which can lead to intimal disruption and acute arterial thrombosis. Bony fragments may puncture, transect, or compress adjacent arteries and veins. The vascular pathology found in athletes, however, is fundamentally different from the vascular trauma associated with long bone fracture or dislocation. The vascular injury is a cumulative one, related to repetitive mechanical trauma. The unique repetitive actions of the competitive athlete can place unusual stress on the arterial and venous structures of the upper extremity causing intermittent vascular compression and contusion of the intima, which predisposes the vessels to thrombosis or to arterial wall degeneration and aneurysm formation.[3] The result is a series of vascular problems seen almost exclusively in the competitive athlete who performs anatomically stressful activities in a repetitive fashion.

The diagnosis of vascular problems in athletes is challenging, since the onset of symptoms is usually gradual, the complaints subtle, and the etiology of the problem often obscure. It is not unusual for arterial or venous pathology to be overlooked because the primary focus of attention is upon the musculoskeletal aspects of the presenting problem. Proper recognition of vascular compromise in the upper extremity is essential to avoid the catastrophic complication of acute arterial thrombosis and embolization, or to prevent the long-term disabling sequelae of neglected venous occlusion.

ARTERIAL PATHOLOGY

Two types of arterial injury have been defined that are related to athletic activities.[4,5] Proximal arterial injury results from intermittent compression of the subclavian or axillary artery where it is compressed by adjacent muscular and bony structures during shoulder movement. The second type of arterial lesion results from repeated blunt trauma to the distal forearm, palm, or digits, leading to arterial thrombosis and hand and finger ischemia.

Proximal Upper Extremity Arterial Disease

Pathophysiology

The repetitive mechanical trauma of overhead extremity motion, such as in baseball pitching, can cause intermittent compression of the subclavian or axillary artery at a number of anatomic locations in the proximal upper extremity. Such proximal arterial lesions can result in either arterial thrombosis or be a source of distal embolization to the hand.[6]

77

Thoracic Outlet Compression

The cords of the brachial plexus and the subclavian artery course through the thoracic outlet, which is bounded by the first rib inferiorly, by the anterior scalene muscle anteriorly and superiorly, and the middle scalene muscle posteriorly and superiorly (Fig. 5-1). Symptoms related to compression of the structures traversing the thoracic outlet are usually limited to neurologic sequelae. Pain is the usual presenting complaint, which is provoked by repetitive activity and is typically in the distribution of the ulnar nerve.

The subclavian artery can be compressed at the level of the thoracic outlet, which is the most common location for the development of arterial injury related to repetitive arterial trauma.[3] Development of the arterial complications secondary to thoracic outlet compression of the subclavian artery is almost always due to congenitally anomalous structures impinging upon the thoracic outlet, typically congenital bony abnormalities of cervical ribs.[6] Although these congenitally anomalous cervical ribs occur in only 0.5 to 1.0 percent of the population, cervical ribs are present in most patients with arterial complications of thoracic outlet syndrome.[6] Anomalous fibrous bands crossing the thoracic outlet are usually only associated with the development of neurologic symptoms, but they have also been described in patients with arterial complications of thoracic outlet syndrome.[7-10] Acquired narrowing of the thoracic outlet can be caused by malunion of a fractured clavicle or prior fracture of a first rib.[6] Compression of the structures exiting the thoracic outlet may also be caused by hypertrophy of the scalene muscles, which can occur in highly conditioned athletes such as weight lifters and swimmers.

Although the presence of bony anomalies of the thoracic outlet is an important risk factor for the development of the thoracic outlet syndrome, fewer than 10 percent of individuals with cervical ribs develop symptoms.[11] The development of the arterial injury is therefore also dependent upon repetitive activity that produces chronic intermittent compression and injury to the artery. The artery becomes thickened and fibrotic in response to the repetitive mechanical trauma to the arterial wall as it is pulled across anomalous structures of the thoracic outlet during shoulder motion. Inflammatory changes around the artery fix the vessel to surrounding structures and increase its vulnerability to further injury. This predisposes the athlete who throws or engages in other vigorous overhead activity, most typically baseball pitchers and swimmers,[12] to stenosis or thrombosis of the subclavian artery.[3,4,7] Of the 13 athletes reported by Nuber and colleagues,[7] who presented with symptoms related to thoracic outlet compression of the subclavian artery, all engaged in activity that involved vigorous overhead use of the arms, and 9 were baseball pitchers.

Arterial complications from repetitive trauma to the subclavian artery at the level of the thoracic outlet include the development of a permanent localized area of stenosis at the site of repeated injury, which may progress to arterial thrombosis. Thrombosis of the subcla-

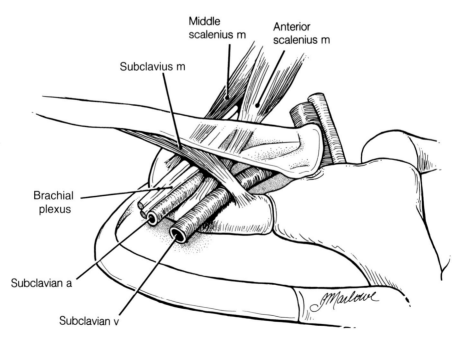

Figure 5-1 Schematic diagram of the anatomic structures defining the thoracic outlet.

vian artery at the level of the thoracic outlet has been documented in a major league baseball pitcher who suffered symptoms of arm fatigue not orginally recognized to be of vascular origin. He continued pitching and the thrombus propagated proximally back to the innominate artery. Fragments of thrombus embolized up the right carotid artery to the right cerebral hemisphere and caused a stroke.[13]

Chronic arterial injury may also lead to the development of an aneurysm of the subclavian artery secondary to poststenotic dilation.[6,14] Although these acquired subclavian artery aneurysms rarely rupture, they are still dangerous lesions because they may be a source of platelet aggregation and thrombus formation that may embolize distally to the hand and fingers, resulting in digit-threatening ischemia.[6,15]

Axillary Artery Compression

Arterial compression of the proximal upper extremity arteries may occur distal to the thoracic outlet as well. After exiting the thoracic outlet, the subclavian artery continues at the axillary artery beyond the lower border of the first rib (Fig. 5-2). The first portion of the axillary artery lies proximal to the pectoralis minor muscle, and the second portion of the axillary artery lies directly behind the muscle. Hypertrophy of this muscle, which consistently occurs in professional baseball pitchers,[16] has been implicated in the pathogenesis of effort-related axillary artery compression[17,18] and thrombosis.[4,18,19] Axillary artery thrombosis in a major league pitcher has been reported to be a result of the *hyperabduction syndrome*,[4,19] first described by Wright[17] in 1945, in which the axillary artery becomes occluded by extrinsic pressure from the overlying pectoralis minor muscle. The third portion of the axillary artery lies anterior to the head of the humerus and extends to the point where the artery crosses the lower border of the teres major muscle. Inducible compression of the third portion of the axillary artery by the head of the humerus has been demonstrated in baseball pitchers,[3,7] and has been documented to have led to repetitive episodes of thrombosis of the axillary artery in a major league baseball pitcher.[3] Shoulder instability with anterior subluxation of the head of the humerus

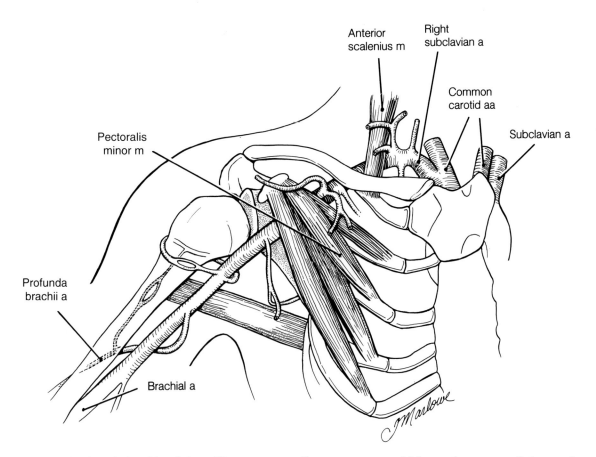

Figure 5-2 The relationship of the axillary artery to adjacent structures which may be sources of abnormal arterial compression.

has been recognized as an important factor contributing to the development of this complication.[3,7]

Clinical Presentation

Athletes with significant stenosis or occlusion of the subclavian or axillary artery will often complain of tiredness or heaviness of the arm provoked by activity analogous to claudication in the lower extremities. These symptoms occur because the blood flow through the stenotic vessel or through collateral vessels around the occluded artery is insufficient to meet the increased metabolic demands of the exercising upper extremity muscle mass.

Stenosis of the subclavian artery or formation of a subclavian artery aneurysm may only become clinically apparent after thromboembolic complications occur. The most frequent early symptoms are due to embolic occlusion of the digital arteries or palmar arch, predisposing the athlete to cold sensitivity and coolness and pain of the digits or hand.[6] Unilateral cold sensitivity, especially when noted in the athlete's dominant extremity, increases the suspicion that the symptoms are related to microembolization rather than primary Raynaud's disease.

Physical Examination

Physical evidence of significant stenosis of the subclavian and axillary arteries includes a brachial artery blood pressure differential when comparing the two extremities. A difference of greater than 20 mmHg is strong evidence of the presence of a hemodynamically significant stenosis in the subclavian or axillary artery. The presence of a pulsatile mass in the supraclavicular fossa may be evidence of a subclavian artery aneurysm. Bruits may be heard in the supraclavicular or infraclavicular areas and are indicative of turbulent blood flow in a stenotic artery. Loss of a brachial or radial pulse with the arm in an abducted and externally rotated (throwing) position is commonly seen in a very high percentage of the normal population and is therefore not a reliable sign of intrinsic arterial disease.[3] The presence of shoulder instability with anterior shoulder subluxation may be a risk factor for the development of arterial compression by the head of the humerus.[3]

Diagnostic Studies

Chest and cervical spine radiographs are essential when evaluating the athlete with symptoms of arm or hand ischemia and may demonstrate the presence of anomalous cervical ribs or evidence of old trauma to the first rib or clavicle. Unfortunately, these studies will not demonstrate the presence of congenital fibrous bands that may be the cause of the arterial compression. Although duplex ultrasound scanning can noninvasively image the presence of arterial stenoses and areas of aneurysmal dilation of the artery, the most definitive diagnostic procedure is the arteriogram, which should include the arteries of the extremity from the level of the aortic arch to the digits. This will demonstrate the location and extent of arterial occlusive lesions as well as the presence of aneurysmal dilation. Distal arterial occlusive disease or emboli can be seen on the radiographs of the forearm and hand.

Management

In general, management of the proximal arterial complications of compression involves surgically eliminating the source of abnormal arterial compression, treating the arterial lesion, and removing the distal embolization if possible. Cervical ribs, when causing compression of the subclavian artery at the level of the thoracic outlet, should be completely excised. Some authors also advocate resection of the first rib in conjunction with cervical rib excision for more complete thoracic outlet decompression. Clavicular resection should be performed in cases of malunion or hypertrophic callus formation complicating a fractured clavicle.[6] Arteriographically demonstrated compression of the axillary artery by a hypertrophied pectoralis muscle can be effectively managed by division of the pectoralis minor tendon.[4,7]

Arterial reconstruction should be performed if significant permanent intrinsic occlusive or aneurysmal disease is encountered, whether the source of compression has been the thoracic outlet, the subpectoral axillary artery, or the axillary artery anterior to the humeral head. Autogenous saphenous vein or an arterial autograft is the preferred grafting material.[6] Distal emboli may be extractable by catheter embolectomy if of recent onset. Long-standing emboli may not be removable, and arterial bypass grafting may be necessary.

Case Study I

A 22-year-old right-handed minor league baseball pitcher presented with a 24-hour history of right arm coolness and fatigue, which he noted after throwing more than 100 pitches in each of four consecutive starts over the previous 12 days. On physical examination, the systolic blood pressure was 134 mmHg in the left arm, but only 80 mmHg systolic at the brachial position on the right, and was detected only with the aid of a Doppler ultrasonic stethoscope. Axillary and more distal pulses were absent on the right, but normal on the left. The hand was cool, but motor

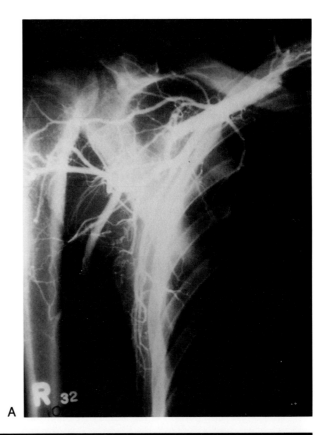

Figure 5-3 (A) Arteriogram demonstrating thrombosis of the third portion of the axillary artery immediately anterior to the humeral head. The artery is normal both proximal and distal to the area of thrombosis. **(B)** Arteriogram of the subclavian and axillary arteries following treatment with urokinase. The artery is without any evidence of intrinsic abnormality. *(Figure continues.)*

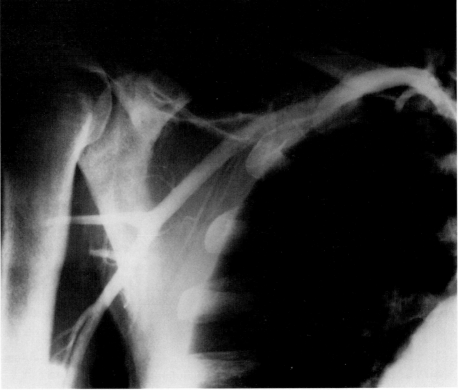

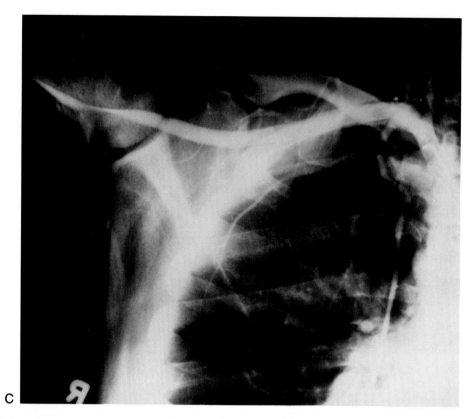

Figure 5-3 *(Continued)* **(C)** Arteriogram with the arm in the throwing position demonstrating extrinsic compression of the third portion of the axillary by the humeral head.

and sensory function was normal. There were no findings of distal embolization. Orthopedic examination of the shoulder was remarkable for the humeral head anterior subluxation.

Arteriography demonstrated thrombosis of the third portion of the axillary artery immediately anterior to the humeral head (Fig. 5-3A). He underwent a 12-hour course of urokinase infusion through the angiogram catheter, after which normal pulses were noted to have returned. Repeat arteriography revealed a normal appearing axillary artery (Fig. 5-3B). An arteriogram with the arm in the throwing position demonstrated compression of the axillary artery by the underlying humeral head (Fig. 5-3C).

An evaluation for the presence of a hypercoagulable state was normal. He was treated with 3 months of warfarin (Coumadin) anticoagulation. Although Coumadin anticoagulation was presumed to provide good prophylaxis against recurrent axillary artery thrombosis, it was thought that it was too dangerous to resume playing while still anticoagulated with Coumadin given the possibility of injury from a batted ball or collision between players. After stopping the Coumadin he resumed pitching effectively without further thrombotic complication on an antico-

agulant regimen of 5,000 units of heparin injected subcutaneously after each pitching inning and every 12 hours afterward for a total of 4 doses.

Distal Upper Extremity Arterial Disease

Vascular lesions of the hand or fingers may follow embolization from proximal arterial sources. However, vascular injury of the distal forearm, palm, and digital arteries can also be seen in athletes exposed to repetitive blunt trauma of the hands and forearms.[20]

Pathophysiology

The radial artery is found on the lateral aspect of the arm and continues into the hand as the deep palmar arch. The ulnar artery courses on the inner aspect of the forearm to the level of the wrist where it leads to the superficial palmar arch (Fig. 5-4). The anatomic location of the ulnar artery in the area of the hypothenar eminence is in a vulnerable position. The superficial palmar arch arises in a groove called Guyon's tunnel, bounded medially by the pisiform and the hook of the hamate bone and dorsally by the transverse carpal liga-

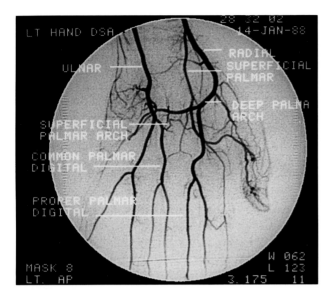

Figure 5-4 Normal arteriogram of the distal forearm and wrist showing the radial and ulnar arteries, the superficial and deep palmar arches, and the digital arteries.

ment. Over a distance of 2 cm, the ulnar artery lies quite superficially in the palm where it is covered by only skin, subcutaneous tissue, and the palmaris brevis tendon.[5] When this area is repeatedly traumatized, ulnar or digital arterial spasm, aneurysm formation with distal embolization, and arterial thrombosis may all contribute to palmar or digital ischemia.[5] Although ulnar arterial injury may be asymptomatic because of collateral perfusion through a patent palmar arch, approximately 20 percent of people do not have a complete palmar arch.[21] In these individuals, interruption of any of the arteries supplying the hand may compromise the vascular supply to one or more digits.

Injury to the ulnar artery is well recognized in workers who use the palm of the hand to strike tools, and is known as the *hypothenar hammer syndrome*.[5,22,23] Professional baseball players, particularly catchers, are exposed to this type of repetitive palmar trauma.[5] In a review of 13 athletes with hand ischemia by Nuber's group,[20] 11 patients were baseball players, including 9 catchers. Bartel and coworkers[24] examined 10 baseball catchers and noted that 40 percent had interrupted palmar arches. A survey of baseball players by Sugawara and coworkers[25] identified an increasing incidence of digital ischemia with increasing years of baseball-playing. The digit most commonly involved was the index finger of the gloved hand.[25] Other athletes who were reported as having had arterial trauma of the hand, followed by digital ischemia, include Frisbee[4] and handball players.[26]

Blunt trauma to both the radial and ulnar arteries has been demonstrated in three volleyball players who have repeated injury to the distal forearms and palms from repeated ball and floor impacts.[27] This pattern of injury has been called the *antebrachial-palmar hammer syndrome.*

Clinical Presentation

The chief complaints of those who present with forearm, hand, and digital arterial occlusive disease are ischemic digits, finger coolness and numbness, and cold hypersensitivity.[5,20,25]

Physical Examination

Clinical clues should be sought to identify possible proximal arterial lesions that could be a source of distal embolization. Symmetrical brachial artery blood pressures eliminate the possibility of significant proximal arterial occlusive disease. The presence of normal radial and ulnar pulses help to localize the vascular lesion to the distal forearm or palm. The Allen test, which demonstrates the patency of the superficial and deep palmar arch, will be demonstrably abnormal if ulnar artery cross-filling is absent when the radial artery is compressed.

Diagnostic Studies

Normal segmental arm blood pressures obtained using Doppler pressure measurements at the level of the antecubital fossa and wrist can localize the site of vascular injury to a site distal to the wrist. Digital arterial pressure measurements document the presence of palmar or digital occlusive disease. Arteriography typically demonstrates distal ulnar artery occlusion, interruption of the palmar arch, and distal artery occlusive disease.[5] The proximal subclavian and axillary arteries should be imaged during the angiographic study to identify any potential sources of arterial emboli.

Management

In general, the management of hand and digital ischemia due to local hand trauma is nonoperative and includes cessation of the traumatizing activity, smoking and the use of tobacco products, and avoidance of cold exposure.[5,20] Vasodilating drugs may provide some symptomatic relief.[27] A stellate ganglion sympathetic block may also prove to be of some benefit.

The athlete who returns to participation in the sport that provoked the vascular injury must be made aware of the pathophysiology of the digital ischemia so that precautions can be taken to avoid further trauma, such as increasing the padding in the catcher's mit or handball glove. A return of symptoms after resuming participation in the offending sport is a sign of further arterial injury which threatens the viability of the ischemic digit. The inciting activity must then be stopped.

Case Study II

A 24-year-old right-handed avid recreational handball player presented with intermittent right hand coolness and cold sensitivity, which had progressed in severity over 4 months. There were no arm or forearm symptoms. His left hand was asymptomatic. On physical examination, the blood pressures were equal in both arms, and axillary, brachial, and radial pulses were all normal, but the ulnar pulse was absent. The right hand was cooler than the left. The Allen test demonstrated interruption of the collateral flow to the hand from the ulnar artery.

An arteriogram demonstrated interruption of the superficial and deep palmar arches and retrograde thrombosis of the ulnar artery proximally above the level of the wrist, findings characteristic of the hypothenar-hammer syndrome (Fig. 5-5).

It was recommended that the patient stop playing handball to avoid further injury to the hand. His symptoms generally improved over the course of several months after abstaining from handball.

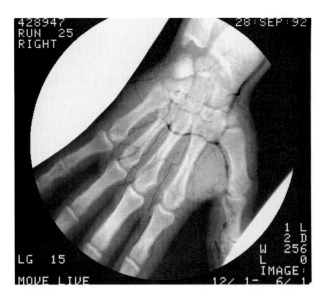

Figure 5-5 Arteriogram demonstrating interruption of the superficial and deep palmar arches and ulnar artery thrombosis. (Courtesy of Elias J. Arous, M.D., the Medical Center of Central Massachusetts.)

UPPER EXTREMITY VENOUS THROMBOSIS

Upper extremity deep venous thrombosis associated with strenuous physical activity was first reported in the medical literature in 1875 by Sir James Paget and in 1884 by von Schroetter, and is commonly referred to as Paget-Schroetter syndrome.[28] The condition has also been referred to as primary thrombosis,[29] spontaneous thrombosis,[30] traumatic thrombosis,[31] and effort thrombosis[32,33] of the subclavian vein.

Upper extremity deep venous thrombosis can be classified as either primary or secondary. Primary thrombosis is attributed to venous trauma brought about by repetitive shoulder movement in the setting of abnormal thoracic outlet anatomy. Secondary thrombosis is associated with the presence of indwelling venous catheters such as central lines or pacemaker leads, although thrombosis secondary to local compression, radiation, and hypercoagulability also occur.[34]

Upper extremity deep venous thrombosis is an important clinical entity, not only due to the 12 percent risk of pulmonary embolization,[35] but also because of the long-term postphlebitic sequelae that can often lead to disabling arm symptoms.

Pathophysiology

Effort thrombosis is an unusual presentation of thoracic outlet compression. The overwhelming majority of patients with anomalies of the thoracic outlet present with neurologic symptoms, while only 3 to 5 percent of patients have symptoms related to venous obstruction.[36,37]

Effort thrombosis of the subclavian vein is caused by the anatomic relationship of the thoracic outlet to the axillary and subclavian veins which are bounded by the anterior scalene muscle posteriorly, clavicle and costoclavicular ligament and subclavius muscle posteriorly and superiorly, and the first rib inferiorly (Fig. 5-1). The vein may be compressed by any of these structures as well as the presence of anomalous structures of the thoracic outlet, such as cervical ribs,[38,39] anomalous musculofascial bands,[35] or a prevenous phrenic nerve.[35]

Effort thrombosis of the subclavian vein is usually secondary to unusual or excessive use of the arm in addition to the presence of one or more compressive elements.[33,40] The athlete whose activity involves upper extremity hyperabduction and repetitive or excessive motion of the shoulder may stretch or subsequently injure the wall of the subclavian vein at the level of the thoracic outlet initiating venous thrombosis.[38]

Clinical Presentation

Effort thrombosis typically occurs in young healthy individuals with an athletic build and is usually noted in the dominant extremity.[39-41] It is often seen in hikers who carry backpacks. Patients usually complain of abrupt-onset swelling involving the entire arm and cyanotic discoloration. A recent history of upper extremity exertion such as weight lifting, tugging, or other stressful activity is noted in at least 50 percent of cases.[12,40] Exertion of the extremity typically results in a dramatic exacerbation of the symptoms of swelling and pain in the arm as the extremity becomes further engorged with venous blood.

Inquiry should be made regarding symptoms of pulmonary embolization such as episodic shortness of breath, pleuritic chest pain, hemoptysis, or a new nonproductive cough. Upper extremity deep venous thrombosis is associated with pulmonary embolization in up to 12 percent of cases.[35]

Physical Examination

The physical examination is most remarkable for the finding of swelling of the involved extremity from the level of the hand to the upper arm. Prominent superficial venous collaterals are usually seen across the shoulder and anterior chest wall.[40]

Diagnostic Studies

Although the diagnosis of upper extremity deep venous thrombosis is often clinically obvious, objective documentation of the presence and extent of thrombosis is important. Duplex ultrasound scanning is a noninvasive modality that is frequently able to accurately define the presence of upper extremity deep venous thrombosis.[42] False-negative examinations can occur, however, and are related to the mistaken identification of a large collateral vein as the axillary or subclavian vein.

The diagnosis of upper extremity deep venous thrombosis is best made by venography. Venography defines the presence and extent of the upper extremity thrombus and demonstrates the presence of collateral venous drainage. Furthermore, venography is essential to accurately define the anatomic detail necessary to identify the etiology of thrombus by demonstrating the site of compression.

Once a diagnosis of upper extremity deep venous thrombosis is made, chest and cervical spine radiographs should be obtained to identify the presence of abnormalities of the first rib, clavicle, or anomalous cervical ribs.

Management

The management of deep venous thrombosis in the lower extremities has been standardized, but there is no consensus regarding treatment of effort thrombosis of the upper extremities. Initial management of effort thrombosis involves heparin anticoagulation to prevent propagation of thrombus, maintain patency of venous collaterals, and to help prevent pulmonary embolization.[35,38] Supportive care involves elevation of the extremity to reduce swelling and relieve some of the associated discomfort. Coumadin anticoagulation is generally instituted and maintained for at least 3 months after the initial thrombotic event. Unfortunately, anticoagulation with Coumadin prohibits participation in sports where violent contact is possible because of the inherent risk of bleeding.

The natural history of primary upper extremity deep venous thrombosis is controversial. Ameli and colleagues[43] treated 15 patients with primary upper extremity deep venous thrombosis with anticoagulation alone. In a 40-month follow-up, they noted that 73 percent of patients were asymptomatic, and the remaining patients had only minimal symptoms. Based on this data, they have concluded that conservative management of axillary vein thrombosis is safe and effective with good long-term results. Other authors report a much more morbid natural history of upper extremity deep venous thrombosis treated with anticoagulants alone, with long-term symptoms and disability rates ranging as high as 90 percent with complaints of arm pain, fatigue, swelling, weakness, and discoloration.[9,33,40,44-46] Compared to secondary axillary vein thrombosis, primary thrombosis has been observed to result in more frequent disability.[35]

This high rate of chronic disability has prompted many surgeons to intervene more aggressively to attempt to prevent the long-term sequelae of effort thrombosis. Although some authors have recommended surgical thrombectomy of the axillary vein,[40] the recent availability of thrombolytic agents has permitted the dissolution of venous thrombus using pharmacologic means.[12,38,47] When instituted within 3 days of thrombus formation, clot dissolution can be achieved 95 percent of the time.[48] After 5 weeks, thrombolysis can be achieved in only 14 percent of cases.[48]

Following successful dissolution of the axillary and subclavian deep venous thrombosis, a discrete area of stenosis within the vein may be identifiable at the time of repeat venography. Some authors have advocated balloon angioplasty of these focal areas of venous stenosis.[38,41] Since the area of stenosis is generally due to extrinsic compression from anatomic structures at the

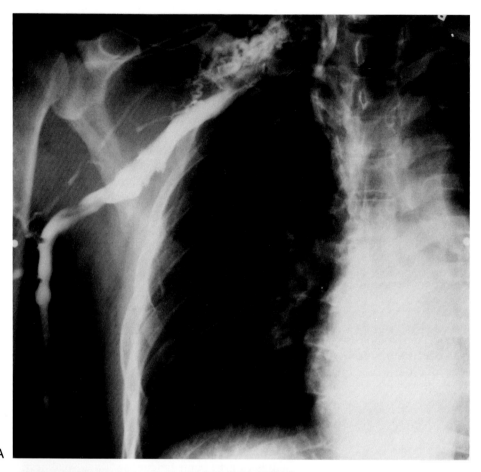

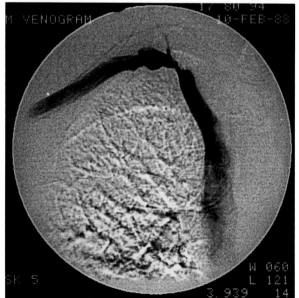

Figure 5-6 (A) Venogram showing thrombosis of the subclavian vein at the level of the thoracic outlet. Collateral veins around the occluded vein are prominent. **(B)** Venography following treatment with urokinase shows dissolution of the thrombus within the subclavian vein. An area of residual stenosis is demonstrated at the level of the thoracic outlet.

thoracic outlet, most authors have felt that angioplasty is inadequate treatment and have recommended decompression of the structures exiting the thoracic outlet by first rib resection to eliminate the extrinsic compression.[46,47]

Case Study III

A 20-year-old right-handed college baseball player presented the morning after throwing hard for the first time in spring training with a swollen, painful right arm. On physical examination, his blood pressures were equal bilaterally, and pulses were normal in both arms. His right arm was swollen from the hand to the shoulder, and the fingers were cyanotic. A prominent superficial venous pattern was obvious in the upper arm and shoulder. A venogram showed subclavian vein thrombosis (Fig. 5-6A). Urokinase was started through the venogram catheter that had been impacted in the thrombus. Venography was repeated 18 hours later, and thrombus dissolution was noted. A residual stenosis of the subclavian vein was noted where the vein crosses the first rib (Fig. 5-6B). Three days later he underwent resection of the first rib from an axillary approach without complication. He has resumed pitching with no further thrombotic episodes.

CONCLUSION

Arterial occlusive disease should be suspected in any athlete who presents with complaints of upper extremity fatigue or hand or finger ischemia who experiences repetitive arterial trauma while participating in their sport. Proper recognition of vascular compromise in the upper extremity and intervention is essential to avoid the catastrophic complications of arterial thrombosis and embolization. The athlete who presents with arm swelling and heaviness should undergo objective testing to identify the presence of upper extremity DVT. Aggressive intervention is indicated to achieve recanalization and prevent recurrence of DVT to avoid the long-term morbidity associated with chronic upper extremity venous thrombosis.

ACKNOWLEDGMENTS

I thank Bruce S. Cutler, M.D. for his review of the manuscript and helpful suggestions. Elias J. Arous, M.D. generously provided material for a case study.

REFERENCES

1. Zuckerman JD, Flugstad DL, Teitz CC, King HA: Axillary artery injury as a complication of proximal humeral fractures. Clin Orthop 189:234, 1984
2. Hayes JM, Vanwinckle GN: Axillary artery injury with minimally displaced fracture of the neck of the humerus. J Trauma 23:431, 1983
3. Rohrer MJ, Cardullo PA, Pappas AM et al: Axillary artery compression and thrombosis in throwing athletes. J Vasc Surg 11:761, 1990
4. McCarthy WJ, Yao JST, Schafer MF et al: Upper extremity arterial injuries in athletes. J Vasc Surg 9:317, 1989
5. Yao JST: Occupational vascular problems. p. 898. In Rutherford RB (ed): Vascular Surgery. 3rd Ed. WB Saunders, Philadelphia, 1989
6. Kieffer E, Ruotolo C: Arterial complications of thoracic outlet compression. p. 875. In Rutherford RB (ed): Vascular Surgery. 3rd Ed. WB Saunders, Philadelphia, 1989
7. Nuber GW, McCarthy WJ, Yao JST et al: Arterial abnormalities of the shoulder in athletes. Am J Sports Med 18:514, 1990
8. Roos DB: Congenital anomalies associated with thoracic outlet syndrome. Am J Surg 132:771,1976
9. Dorazio RA, Ezzet F: Arterial complications of the thoracic outlet syndrome. Am J Surg 138:246, 1979
10. Simon H, Gryska PF, Carlson DH: The thoracic outlet syndrome as a cause of aneurysm formation, thrombosis, and embolization. South Med J 70:282, 1977
11. Pollak EW: Surgical anatomy of the thoracic outlet syndrome. Surg Gynecol Obstet 150:97, 1980
12. Machleder HI: Thoracic outlet disorders: thoracic outlet compression syndrome and axillary vein thrombosis. p. 687. In Wilson SE, Veith FJ, Hobson RW II, Williams RA (eds): Vascular Surgery: Principles and Practice. McGraw-Hill, New York, 1987
13. Fields WS, Lemak NA, Ben-Menachem Y: Thoracic outlet syndrome: review and reference to stroke in a major league pitcher. Am J Neuroradiol 7:73, 1986
14. Short DW: The subclavian artery in 16 patients with complete cervical ribs. J Cardiovasc Surg 16:135, 1975
15. Judy KL, Heymann RL: Vascular complications of thoracic outlet syndrome. Am J Surg 123:521, 1972
16. Tullos HS, King JW: Lesions of the pitching arm in adolescents. JAMA 220:264, 1972
17. Wright IS: The neurovascular syndrome produced by hyperabduction of the arm. Am Heart J 29:1, 1945
18. Dijkstra PF, Westra D: Angiographic features of compression of the axillary artery by musculus pectoralis minor and the head of the humerus in thoracic outlet compression syndrome: case report. Radiol Clin 47:423, 1978
19. Tullos HS, Erwin WD, Woods GW et al: Unusual lesions of the pitching arm. Clin Orthop 88:169, 1972
20. Nuber GW, McCarthy WJ, Yao JST et al: Arterial abnormalities of the hand in athletes. Am J Sports Med 18:520, 1990

21. Coleman SS, Anson BJ: Arterial patterns in the hand, based upon a study on 650 specimens. Surg Gynecol Obstet 113:409, 1961
22. Pineda CJ, Weisman MH, Brookstein JJ et al: Hypothenar hammer syndrome: form of reversible Raynaud's phenomenon. Am J Med 79:561, 1985
23. Conn J, Bergan JJ, Bell JL: Hypothenar hammer syndrome: posttraumatic digital ischemia. Surgery 68:1122, 1970
24. Bartel P, Blackburn D, Peterson L et al: The value of noninvasive tests in occupational trauma of the hands and fingers. Bruit 8:15, 1984
25. Sugawara M, Toshihiko O, Minami A, Ishii S: Digital ischemia in baseball players. Am J Sports Med 14:329, 1986
26. Buckout BC, Warner MA: Digital perfusion of handball players: effect of repeated ball impact on structures of the hand. Am J Sports Med 8:206, 1980
27. Kostianen S, Orava S: Blunt injury of the radial and ulnar arteries in volleyball players: a report of three cases of the antebrachial-palmar hammer syndrome. Br J Sports Med 17:172, 1983
28. Hughes ESR: Venous obstruction of the upper extremity (Paget-Schroetter's syndrome): a review of 320 cases. Int Abstr Surg 88:89, 1949
29. Matas R: So-called primary thrombosis of axillary vein caused by strain: report of a case, diagnosis, pathology, and treatment. Am J Surg 24:642, 1934
30. French GE: Spontaneous thrombosis of axillary vein. Br Med J 2:271, 1944
31. Roelsen E: So-called traumatic thrombosis of the axillary and subclavian veins. Acta Med Scand 98:589, 1939
32. Kleinsasser LJ: "Effort" thrombosis of the axillary and subclavian veins. Arch Surg 59:258, 1974
33. Adams JT, DeWeese JA: "Effort" thrombosis of the axillary and subclavian veins. J Trauma 11:923, 1971
34. McCarthy WJ, Vogelzang EL, Bergan JJ: Changing concepts and present-day etiology of upper extremity venous thrombosis. p. 407. In Bergan JJ, Yao JST (eds): Venous disorders. WB Saunders, Philadelphia, 1991
35. Horattas MC, Wright DJ, Fenton AH et al: Changing concepts of deep venous thrombosis of the upper extremity: report of a series and review of the literature. Surgery 104:561, 1988
36. Selke FW, Kelly TR: Thoracic outlet syndrome. Am J Surg 156:54, 1988
37. Stanton PE Jr, Vo NM, Haley T et al: Thoracic outlet syndrome: a comprehensive evaluation. Am Surg 54:129, 1988
38. Nemmers DW, Thorpe PE, Knibbe MA, Beard DW: Upper extremity venous thrombosis: case report and literature review. Orthop Rev 19:164, 1990

39. Daskalakis E, Bouthoutsos J: Subclavian and axillary vein compression of musculoskeletal origin. Br J Surg 67:573, 1980
40. Rutherford RB, Piotrowski JJ: Axillary-subclavian vein thrombosis. p. 883. In Rutherford RB (ed): Vascular Surgery. 3rd Ed. WB Saunders, Philadelphia, 1989
41. Druy EM, Trout HH III, Giordano JM, Hix WR: Lytic therapy in the treatment of axillary and subclavian vein thrombosis. J Vasc Surg 2:821, 1985
42. Falk RL, Smith DF: Thrombosis of upper extremity thoracic inlet veins: diagnosis with duplex doppler sonography. AJR 149:677, 1987
43. Ameli FM, Minas T, Weiss M, Provan JL: Consequences of "conservative" conventional management of axillary vein thrombosis. Can J Surg 30:167, 1992
44. Swinton NW Jr, Edgett JW Jr, Hall RJ: Primary subclavian-axillary vein thrombosis. Circulation 38:737, 1968
45. Tilney NL, Griffiths HJG, Edwards EA: Natural history of major venous thrombosis of the upper extremity. Arch Surg 101:792, 1970
46. Urschel HC, Razzuk MA: Improved management of the Paget-Schroetter syndrome secondary to thoracic outlet compression. Ann Thorac Surg 52:1217, 1991
47. Shuttleworth RD, Vandermere DM, Mitchell WL: Subclavian vein stenosis and axillary vein "effort thrombosis." South Afr Med J 71:564, 1987
48. Theiss W, Wirtzfeld A, Fink U, Maubach P: The success rate of fibrinolytic therapy in fresh and old thrombosis of the iliac and femoral veins. Angiology 34:61, 1983

SUGGESTED READINGS

Kieffer E, Ruotolo C: Arterial complications of thoracic outlet compression. p. 875. Rutherford RB (ed): Vascular Surgery. 3rd Ed. WB Saunders, Philadelphia, 1989
Machleder HI: Thoracic outlet dosorders: thoracic outlet compression syndrome and axillary vein thrombosis. p. 687. In Wilson SE, Veith FJ, Hobson RW II, Williams RA (eds): Vascular Surgery: Principles and practice. McGraw-Hill, New York, 1987
McCarthy WJ, Yao JST, Schafer MF et al: Upper extremity arterial injuries in athletes. J Vasc Surg 9:317, 1989
Nuber GW, McCarthy WJ, Yao JST et al: Arterial abnormalities of the hand in athletes. Am J Sports Med 18:514, 1990
Nuber GW, McCarthy WJ, Yao JST et al: Arterial abnormalities of the hand in athletes. Am J Sports Med 18:520, 1990
Rutherford RB, Piotrowski JJ: Axillary-subclavian vein thrombosis. p. 883. Rutherford RB (ed): Vascular Surgery. 3rd Ed. WB Saunders, Philadelphia, 1989

6

Protective Equipment

Lisa A. Schulz
Brian D. Busconi
Arthur M. Pappas

Protective equipment guards athletes from injury, allows for an early return to competition postinjury, and prevents reinjury. For example, protective braces may prevent reinjury by providing extra mechanical support and through proprioceptive feedback from the braces points of attachment.[1] With new materials and technology, protective equipment has become better fitting, more durable, lighter in weight, and easier to maintain. Adaptations to existing equipment may provide stability for healing tissues and protection of surgical repairs (e.g., a skier or biker who has sustained an ulnar collateral ligament rupture may be able to return to skiing sooner with a thumb splint that fits securely in the glove). Health care providers who treat athletes should be familiar with the protective equipment available and the rationale for its usage. Equipment misuse or disuse may lead to litigation if injury or reinjury occurs.[2]

The design of protective equipment ensures that forces are channeled away from an anatomic structure. Through these designs, the equipment protects the body part while allowing the athlete to function with minimal restriction. If the protective equipment does not fit properly, it will not allow the athlete to meet his or her functional goals. Athletes generally prefer to wear smaller and less restrictive equipment so that it is less of an impediment to functional performance; however, this may lead to an increased risk of injury. Equipment is either commercially premade (with minor adjustments if necessary) or can be custom-made for the athlete. Protective equipment is designed according to the nature of the athletic activity. Sports can be classified as contact/collision, limited contact/impact or noncontact, (i.e., strenuous, moderately strenuous, and nonstrenuous).[3] The following areas should be assessed to determine the protective equipment needed:

1. Classification of the injury and the anatomy requiring protection
2. Similar previous injuries
3. Age of athlete and level of competition
4. Length of time since injury/what phase of rehabilitation (Table 6-1) (see also Ch. 2)
5. Clinical evaluation of healing and functional recovery
6. Participatory demands associated with the athlete's position
7. Psychological effect/perception

Equipment needs will change as the athlete progresses through the five phases of rehabilitation. As discussed in Chapter 2, the five phases of rehabilitation are (1) acute injury, (2) initial rehabilitation, (3) pro-

Table 6-1 Protective Supports: Examples of Progression of Protection Through Phases of Rehabilitation

Injury	Phases of Rehabilitation				
	Acute Injury	Initial Rehabilitation	Progressive Rehabilitation	Integrated Functions	Return to Sport
Phalanx fracture	Rigid cast or splint	Rigid cast or splint	Hand based resting splint	Finger-based splints	Splint or buddy taping
Ulnar collateral ligament rupture (thumb)	Splint	Thumb spica cast	Spica cast	Thermoplastic splint	Soft splint Soft splint/short opponens
Metacarpal fracture	Splint	Gutter cast splint 3 pt pressure	Forearm based gutter splint 3 pt pressure	Hand-based gutter splint	Protective glove
Scaphoid fracture	Splint	Spica cast	Spica cast	Thermoplastic splint	Splint/bivalve cast Protective glove
Radial or ulnar fracture, or both	Splint/cast	Cast	Bivalve cast or volar wrist splint	Volar wrist splint	Padded bivalve or forearm splint (prefab or custom)
Epicondylitis	Splint	Splint	Splint/counter force brace	Counterforce brace	Counterforce brace
Elbow hyperextension	Rigid splint-common or custom	ROM adjustability Long arm common splint	ROM adjustability Long arm common splint	Check rein tape	Check rein tape
Olecranon contusion	Long arm rigid support (cast, brace, splint)	Long arm rigid support (cast, brace, splint)	Hinged brace	Variable secondary to sport	Taping/padding Commercial
Anterior shoulder instability	Sling/swathe	Sling/swathe	Sling	Shoulder subluxation inhibitor brace	Shoulder subluxation inhibitor brace
AC disruption	Sling/swathe	Sling/swathe	Sling	Sponge support Tape	Shoulder pad Adaptations Sponge Support Tape
Cervical burners/neurologic	Semirigid collar soft collar	Soft collar	Soft collar	Soft collar	Neck roll
Soft tissue sprains/ strains	Compressive dressing and splint	Compressive dressing	Compressive dressing	Protective pad	Protective pad

gressive rehabilitation, (4) integrated functions, and (5) return to sport. Protection progresses from maximum protection whereby the structures remain immobile to less restrictive protection so the athlete can participate through the five phases of rehabilitation (Table 6-1). Unnecessary involvement of adjacent structures can increase the risk of additional injury as well as impede the athlete's performance. As structural stability improves, there is less need for restrictive protection.

During the acute injury and initial rehabilitation phases, the athlete will often benefit from rigid immobilization and protection of injured structures, since this will reduce pain, swelling, and tissue damage (Fig. 6-1). It is too early for the athlete to return to athletic activity, and therefore selection of the ultimate adaptation of equipment is not yet warranted, but the immediate needs of protection should be addressed.

It is during the latter phases of rehabilitation, that is, the return to sport skills and ultimate competition, that the need for adapted equipment, which permits participation, is determined. Selection is based on functional needs, with specific equipment chosen that allows for motion, function, and performance. Practice along with simulated and actual competition will provide the athlete the opportunity to adapt to the equipment and/ or suggested activity modifications. Once an athlete has been prescribed with the appropriate support and/or protection, performance should be assessed while the equipment is being used. This assessment should include the positive or negative psychological impact the equipment may have on the athlete. Some athletes with protective equipment feel more secure during athletic activity, while others feel impaired. Still others believe that the appearance of the equipment not only puts them at a disadvantage with their opponents but that their public image may be damaged as well.

The athlete's performance requirements will determine what equipment is necessary as well as practical. The football linebacker who has sustained an anterior shoulder subluxation may be allowed to return to competition using a shoulder subluxation inhibitor brace (Fig. 6-2) once he has regained his general strength and desired range of motion. This brace limits shoulder abduction, extension, and external rotation, the motions associated with potential recurrence of anterior shoulder subluxation and dislocation. A baseball catcher or pitcher with the same injury could not participate with a shoulder subluxation inhibitor brace because it would limit the necessary motions required for athletic performance.

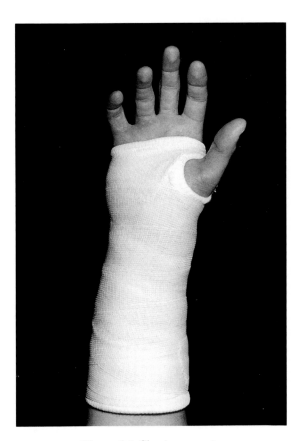

Figure 6-1 Short arm cast.

SELECTION OF PROTECTIVE EQUIPMENT

There is a considerable range of type and quality of equipment available to the athlete. Selection of equipment should be a collaborative effort involving the coaching staff, trainer, equipment manager, health care practitioner, rehabilitation staff, athlete, and, with younger athletes, parents.

External support materials consist of (1) splints, (2) commercially available braces, (3) tape, and (4) pads. Some of the materials are only used to protect athletes from injuries, while others are used postinjury or to protect vulnerable areas. The following should be considered before selecting specific equipment:

1. Inherent safety factors and goals of protection
2. Design and fabrication of the protective equipment
3. Maintenance of the equipment
4. Quality in workmanship and cost
5. Availability of supplies and service

Splints

Splints provide external support and limit motion, and can be used alone or incorporated into other supports or the athlete's standard equipment. Splints can

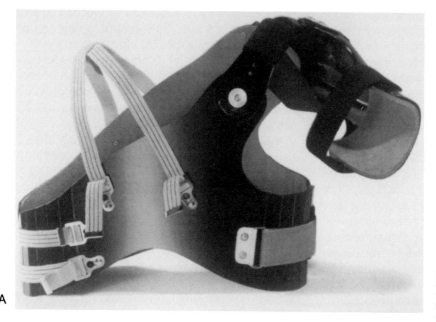

A

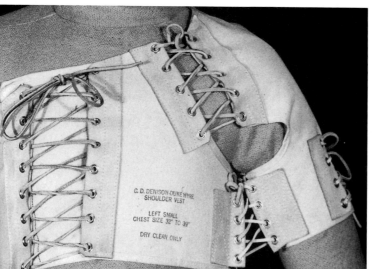

B

Figure 6-2 Shoulder subluxation inhibitor brace. **(A)** SSI. **(B)** C.D. Denison-Duke Wyre Shoulder Vest. The SSI is more rigid than the shoulder vest.

be categorized as rigid, semirigid, and soft, with rigid materials obviously providing the most support to injured structures.

Rigid splints are primarily used in the acute injury and initial rehabilitation phases, offering more immobilization and protection. The most commonly used materials are the ⅛-in. low temperature thermoplastics including Orthoplast, Multiform, Aquaplast, Polyform, Polyflex, and Ezeform (Table 6-2). Each type of material has unique handling qualities but all provide rigid protection. Extra care must be taken in the fabrication of these splints to guarantee minimal pressure on neurovascular structures, full clearance of unin-

volved joints, and secure splint fit (Fig. 6-3). Rigid splints can also be padded to decrease the risk of injury to other athletes. Wrist and thumb immobilization can be provided with thumb spica splints (Fig. 6-4). There are numerous prefabricated splints also available for upper extremity protection during the early phases of rehabilitation.

A semirigid splint provides light support to a given structure but maintains some pliability. It protects the anatomic site, while decreasing the potential for injury to other structures or other competitors. This type of splint is used in the later phases of rehabilitation and sometimes during athletic activity. Semirigid splints

Table 6-2 Trademark Information: Low
Temperature Thermoplastic Materials

Orthoplast and Orthoplast II
    Johnson & Johnson Orthopedics, Inc., New Bruns-
        wick, NJ
Multiform
    Alimed, Inc., Dedham, MA
Aquaplast
    WFR/Aquaplast Corp., Wykoff, NJ
Polyform
    Smith & Nephew Rolyan, Inc., Menomonee Falls,
        WI
Polyflex II
    Smith & Nephew Rolyan, Inc., Menomonee Falls,
        WI
Ezeform
    Smith & Nephew Rolyan, Inc., Menomonee Falls,
        WI
Aliplast
    Alimed, Inc., Dedham, MA

are less bulky than elastomer (soft) splints, and the fit is usually less conforming without the shock-absorbing quality of the soft splints. Aliplast is an example of a cross-linked, polyethylene foam material with variable firmness that can be used to fabricate a semirigid splint (Fig. 6-5). Information on the optimal temperature, best method for heating, and tips for working with the material are generally included or available from the manufacturer or vendor.

Soft splints are gaining wider recognition in the field of sports medicine, particularly with hand and wrist injuries. These splints are typically fabricated with a combination of a silicone-based elastomer product (e.g., Roylan silicone elastomer) and gauze. The joint/area to be protected is first wrapped with gauze, then an elastomer layer is applied. Using more gauze, the elastomer layers are added until the desired thickness is achieved.[4] The use of silicone splints following thumb sprains, wrist sprains, and for postcast immobilization with scaphoid fractures has been reported.[4]

Custom protective splints may be necessary (during the later phases) to provide the appropriate support or adaptation to ensure an athlete's safe return to competition. For example, an athlete's hand may be too big to obtain adequate support with a prefabricated wrist splint. Splint inserts can be fabricated for use within standard gloves. An opponens splint can be easily used in a catcher's mitt or skier's glove to protect the thumb from lateral stresses. It is helpful to fabricate the splint around any objects the athlete may need to manipulate (e.g., ski poles or bicycle handlebars) (Fig. 6-6). Following the initial use of any insert, the fit and the athlete's ability to function should be evaluated, and modifications made if the splint is causing skin irritation on pressure areas or inadequate protection/performance. Mallet splints and alumifoam splints can be used for digit protection following tip crush injuries or a mallet finger (see Ch. 25).

Braces

Braces help prevent reinjury by restricting joint motion and limiting muscle excursion. A hinged elbow brace may be used to protect the joint from excessive motion during the recovery stages of rehabilitation (initial and progressive rehabilitation) following an

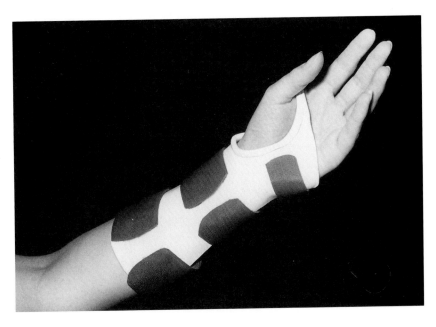

Figure 6-3 Volar wrist splint fabricated using a low-temperature thermoplastic material.

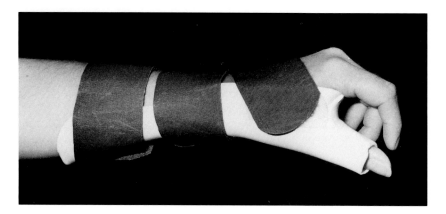

Figure 6-4 Thumb spica splint.

elbow subluxation or dislocation as well as a significant hyperextension injury (perhaps a subluxation). A shoulder subluxation inhibition brace would be used in the latter stages of rehabilitation (integrated functions) to restrict glenohumeral motion, limit muscle action, and prevent excessive abduction, extension, and external rotation (the usual positions associated with anterior inferior instability). The counterforce braces limit muscle excursion, constrain muscular expansion, and limit axial stress on musculotendinous origins, thereby decreasing symptoms. For example, there are various types of braces for tennis elbow (lateral epicondylitis) such as the Epitrain, Nirschl, and Aircast counterforce forearm braces[5] (Fig. 6-7). These braces are also used to limit axial muscle excursion in other anatomical sites (e.g., biceps).

Tape

Adhesive tape consists of two components, the backing and the adhesive substance. The backing is usually composed of fabric. There are instances, however, when an elasticized fabric backing is used for protection and is most beneficial when combined with pad-

ding to protect soft tissue injuries (e.g., a muscle contusion). The elasticized backing accommodates for the expansion and contraction of the muscle mass yet continues to hold the appropriate padding in place. More rigid tape is used in association with felt padding or plastic sponge to protect the acromioclavicular joint under shoulder pads (Fig. 6-8). In this case, the padding is designed to protect the acromioclavicular joint, and during motion, the adhesive with a more rigid backing will hold it in place to provide the necessary protection to the injured joint.

Taping is also used to physically limit available range of motion (which prevents overstretch of tissues), or to stabilize an injured soft tissue part or intra-articular injury (e.g., to avoid reinjury of a hyperextended elbow by limiting maximum extension) (Fig. 6-9). In these cases, the tape is utilized to provide an anterior stop or check-rein, thereby protecting the anterior structures from sudden extension. Taping is most beneficial in cases where less support but some function is needed, and its success is often dependent on the trainer's experience and technique.

Buddy taping is used to protect a recently reduced dislocation of an interphalangeal joint. The digits should be wrapped side by side with two pieces of tape

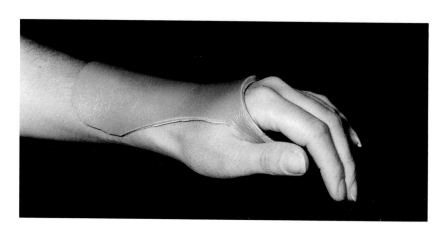

Figure 6-5 Dorsal wrist extension block splint fabricated from Aliplast.

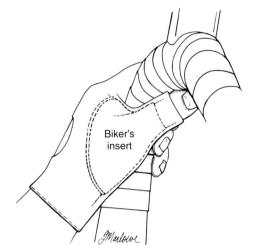

Figure 6-6 Splint around bicycle handlebar.

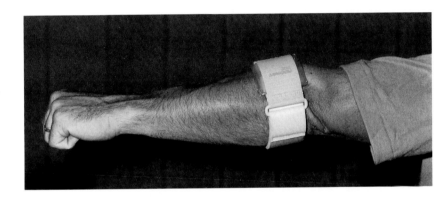

Figure 6-7 Aircast, used for the treatment of lateral epicondylitis.

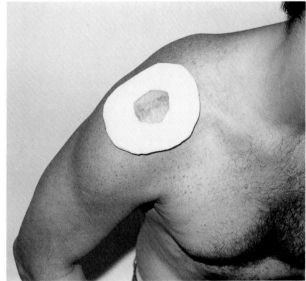

Figure 6-8 Self-adhesive foam padding "donut" to protect the acromioclavicular joint.

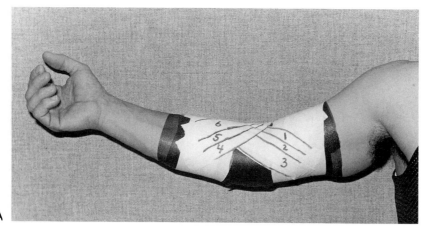

A

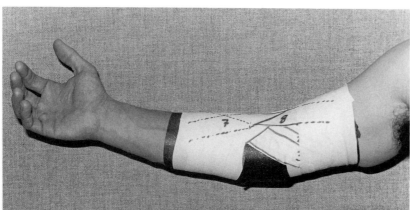

B

Figure 6-9 (A & B) Taping technique for prevention of hyperextension injury at the elbow. Numbers indicate different anchors. (Photograph courtesy of Karolyn Busconi.)

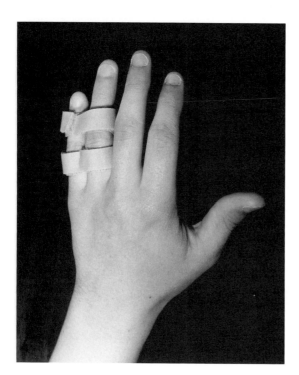

Figure 6-10 Velcro digit buddy tapes.

applied—one piece at the proximal phalanx and one piece at the middle phalanx, keeping the PIP (proximal interphalangeal) joint free (Fig. 6-10). Other examples of when tape is appropriate include taping the wrist to provide additional support during a gymnastic competition (Fig. 6-11).

Pads

Pads help in the protection of the shoulder, elbow, forearm, and hand from direct and indirect trauma. The shoulder is exposed to constant trauma in contact sports such as ice hockey, lacrosse, or football. The trauma can result from the bumping action of contact sports or following a landing on hard surfaces. Indirect trauma may be transmitted from direct forces, from the hand or elbow, or sports requiring a throwing or swinging motion. Injuries resulting from many of these mechanisms can either be acute or chronic. Protective devices in the shoulder area are designed to reduce these forceful contacts and to prevent injuries (Fig. 6-12).

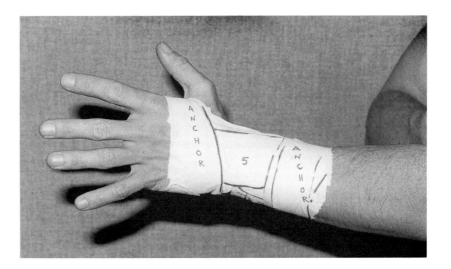

Figure 6-11 Taping technique for prevention of hyperextension injury at the wrist. Numbers indicate different anchors. (Photograph courtesy of Karolyn Busconi.)

Designers and manufacturers of shoulder pads have made great strides toward protecting the player against direct forces of the shoulder girdle. This has been accomplished by fitting the front and back panels and adding cantilevers over the top of each shoulder to protect the acromioclavicular joint.

Hockey and lacrosse shoulder pads are primarily designed to protect direct contact to the clavicle, acromion, and the acromioclavicular joint. Football shoulder pads are generally larger and expected to protect more components of the shoulder girdle, depending on the position of the player (e.g., linemen are larger than quarterbacks and will require more protection).

For correct fitting, the shoulder should be measured to determine what size pad is needed. When a football shoulder pad is fit correctly, the pads should not slip or move on contact; the base of the cantilever system should extend approximately 1- to 1½-in. over the acromium; there should be flaps to cover the deltoid; the scapula should be covered, and the neck opening should enable the athlete to have a full range of shoulder flexion and abduction. Drapes and lacing should be as snug as possible without constricting breathing, and there should be the potential to add cervical motion restriction collars or drop-down pads as adjuncts to neck, shoulder, and arm protection. The design of the

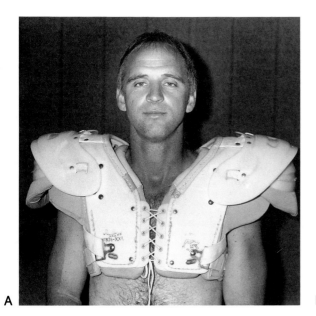

A

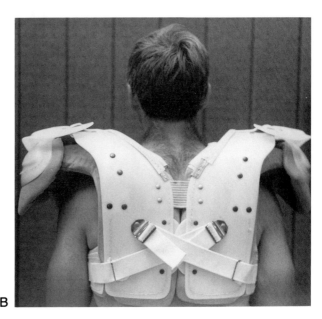

B

Figure 6-12 (A & B) Football shoulder pads.

cervical restraint padding should be considered in light of the symptomatology, that is, whether there is a need to limit extension, flexion, or lateral motion. This supplementary equipment will often be incorporated or attached to other standard protective equipment (i.e., shoulder pads and helmet) (Fig. 6-13).

Additional padding can be added beneath commercial pads (Fig. 6-14). The acromioclavicular joint is the most common site for the use of supplemental padding and is accomplished by a donut-type cutout and some form of shock-absorbing material (i.e., thick felt or moderately dense sponge material) either attached to the conventional shoulder pad to protect the acromioclavicular area or individually taped over the acromioclavicular joint. If the area needs to be protected on a long-term basis, it is preferable to attach it within the shoulder pad, thus avoiding the daily fitting of the protective equipment and the potential for secondary skin problems from repetitive adhesive applications. Soft padding (felt or sponge) with overlying rigid or elasticized tape is used to protect contusions of soft tissue as well as areas of bony prominence (e.g., padding and tape either as focal or general protection for a forearm bruise in a football lineman; an olecranon prominence in hockey players and football players).

Protection for the elbow and forearm is necessary because of the direct blows imposed on this area. Often

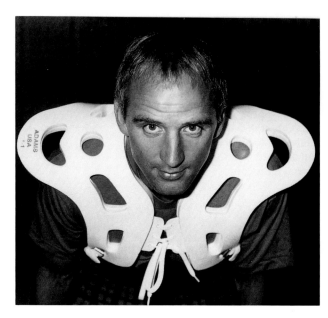

Figure 6-14 Shoulder pad to protect acromioclavicular joint.

well-fitting prefabricated arm pads can be used to protect against repeated contusions. Protective foam elbow pads have excellent contour design, enabling the athlete adequate protection and good range of motion at the elbow (Fig. 6-15). Elbow protection is necessary to prevent contusions and fractures in athletes who have repeated falls on athletic surfaces (e.g., football players on artificial surfaces), contact with opponents, ice hockey players, or diving volleyball players. High-impact materials are often needed for forearm protec-

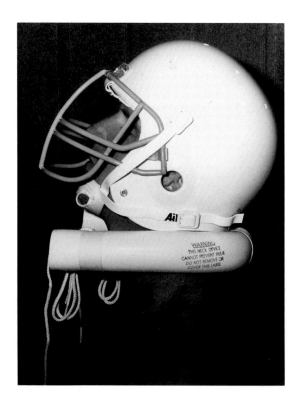

Figure 6-13 Helmet with supplementary cervical collar to limit cervical spine extension.

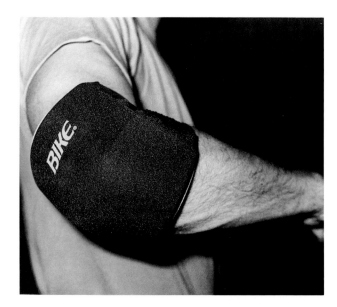

Figure 6-15 Foam elbow pad to protect olecranon and ulnar nerve from impact forces.

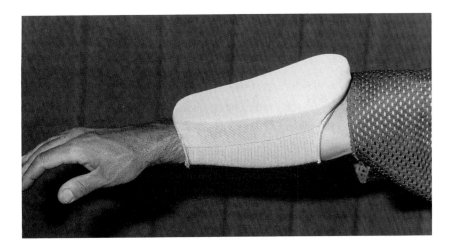

Figure 6-16 Forearm pad to provide shock absorption and padding to the radius, ulna, and soft tissues.

tion in sports such as lacrosse, football, or ice hockey (Fig. 6-16).

The athlete's hands are constantly exposed to various types of force movements and direct trauma. For example, wrist and hand pads, as well as gloves, are used to protect the dorsum of the hand (Fig. 6-17). Gloves provide wrist support and protection and thus have become the standard equipment for many sports such as hockey, football, golf, bowling, archery, and biking (Fig. 6-18). With lightweight and synthetic materials now available, athletes can maintain the dexterity needed in their specific sports while protecting their hands from further damage.

REGULATORY CONCERNS

Regulations for noncontact sports often allow increased latitude with respect to the types of equipment and equipment modifications used during competition. Equipment specifications for contact sports are regulated by the governing bodies for each specific sport. The regulations will vary depending on the age group of the participants and the type and level of competition. The agencies governing each sports should be contacted for specific information (Table 6-3).

One of the primary concerns of the governing bodies is an athlete's use of equipment as a "weapon" during

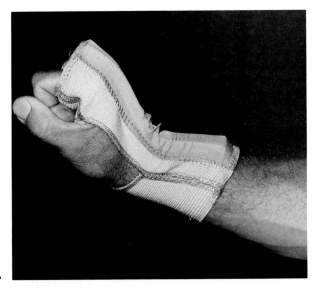

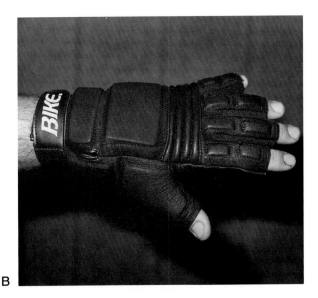

A   B

Figure 6-17 (A) Pad allows wrist extension and full digit range of motion. **(B)** Dorsally padded glove providing wrist, hand, and digit protection.

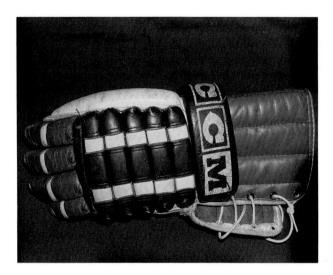

Figure 6-18 Hockey glove.

competition, resulting in injuries to other athletes. Another regulatory issue is the possibility of the equipment providing an unfair advantage to the athlete. The physical demands of specific athletic activities will also influence the type of equipment to be used, modified, or fabricated. For example, the upper extremity demands of a soccer player returning to competition will

Table 6-3   Rules and Regulation Information

Tennis
    NELTA
    P.O. Box 587
    Needham Heights, MA 02194
    (617) 964-2030
Football and Lacrosse
    NCAA
    P.O. Box 7347
    Overland Park, Kansas 66207
    (913) 339-1906
Volleyball
    AAHPERD
    P.O. Box 704
    Waldorf, Maryland 20601
Baseball
    Sporting News
    P.O. Box 44
    St. Louis, Missouri 63166
    1-800-825-8508
Basketball, fieldhockey, ice hockey, soccer, swimming,
    track, wrestling
    National Federation
    P.O. Box 20626
    Kansas City, Missouri 64195
    (816) 464-5400 (Publications Department)

vary greatly from those of a football quarterback or of a gymnast performing on the parallel bars. More specifically, a football player's upper extremity demands will vary with the position played (e.g., a quarterback or receiver needs fine motor control and manipulation ability versus upper extremity motion used by an interior lineman).

Problem-solving between the athlete and the rehabilitation staff (particularly the athletic trainer who has extensive experience in this area) may be necessary to design splints or modify equipment for athletic performance. A balance can usually occur between the protection used and the effect it has on performance. An illustrative example is the baseball catcher who has an unstable ulnar collateral ligament in his catching thumb. His glove does not provide adequate stability to prevent reinjury of the thumb. A lightweight, thermoplastic splint can be designed to fit into his glove, providing rigid metacarpophalangeal joint stability yet allowing for normal hand function. Additionally, metacarpophalangeal joint support may be necessary when batting—accomplished by taping under the hitting glove or padding the glove or bat, since a splint cannot be used. Similarly, the football offensive guard who sustains a distal radius fracture may be allowed an early return to competition with a covered, padded, rigid splint.

Any structural changes made to the standard equipment should be carefully evaluated to ensure that adequate support and protection are maintained. Standard protective equipment as well as any supplemental items that may be indicated are effective only if they are consistently used by the athlete. Careful assessment of the athlete, the injury, and the position demands are critical to providing appropriate adaptive or protective equipment. Use of protective equipment is essential for preventing injury and guarding against reinjury.

REFERENCES

1. Rovere GD, Curl WW, Browning DG: Bracing and taping in an office sports medicine practice, Clin Sports Med 8:3, 1989
2. Ellis TH: Sports protective equipment. Primary Care 18:4, 1991
3. Paul G. Dyment: Sports Medicine: Health Care for Young Athletes. 2nd Ed., American Academy of Pediatrics, 1991, Elk Grove Village, IL
4. Athletic Training and Sports Medicine. 1st Ed. American Academy of Orthopaedic Surgeons, Chicago, IL, 1984
5. Rettig A, Alexy C, Malone K: Protective devices for hand and wrist injuries in athletes, J Musculoskeletal Med December, 9:62, 1992

7

Physically Challenged Athletes

Brian D. Busconi
Kathleen A. Curtis

Of the current population in the United States, approximately 43 million (17 percent) are mildly or severely physically challenged (Fig. 7-1). Each year, 6,000 to 10,000 Americans sustain an injury to their spinal cord, with 40 to 50 percent of these rendered quadriplegic or paraplegic. Before World War II, 80 percent of quadriplegics and paraplegics died within 3 years of injury due to complications. Today, however, 80 percent of paraplegics have a longer life expectancy.

Historically, physically challenged athletes have had limited access to physical education and competitive athletics. It was not until the pioneering efforts of Dr. Ludwig Guttman from the National Spinal Cord Injury Centre at the Stoke Mandeville Hospital in Aylesbury, England, that sports and recreational activities for the physically challenged became popular. Dr. Guttman recognized the importance of the rehabilitative values of sports and in 1948 organized an informal competition of spinal cord-injured World War II veterans. In the following years, more sports were included in these competitive events. Today the Stoke Mandeville Games represent one of the largest international athletic competitions for physically challenged athletes.

In the United States, at approximately the same time as the British movement, competitive sports were being organized for the physically challenged by the Veterans Administration Hospitals under the auspices of the Paralyzed Veterans of America (PVA). In 1949, the National Wheelchair Basketball Association (NWBA) was formed, thereby rendering a definitive form and character to the growing sports movement for the physically challenged in the United States.

The National Wheelchair Athletic Association (NWAA) was formed in 1957. Through this legislative body, new sports were introduced to the physically challenged athlete beyond basketball, such as track and field, table tennis, archery, weight lifting, and swimming. In 1960, the NWAA established a formal affiliation with the International Stoke Mandeville Games Committee. In the same year, following the Olympic Games in Rome, the first Paralympic Games were held.

Due to the eagerness of the physically challenged population to engage in competitive sports, the development of sport-related technology, and marked performance improvement, the emphasis has changed from a "rehabilitative endeavor" to a "competitive event," which has generated an increase in sport-related injuries.[1] All sports health professionals should become informed of the needs of physically challenged athletes, with the understanding that these participants are serious and elite-level competitive athletes. They should consider sports for their physically challenged patients as they would for their nonchallenged patients and should not discourage certain sports.[2]

Both recreational and competitive sports have been shown to provide significant psychological and physio-

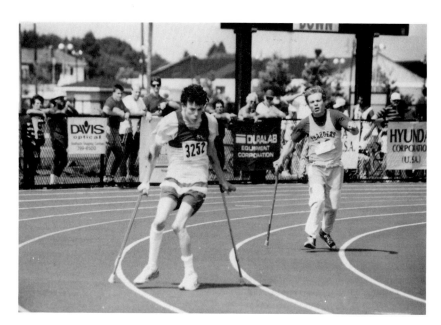

Figure 7-1 Physically challenged athlete at a cerebral palsy competition.

logic benefits for the physically challenged athlete.[3] Participation in recreational or competitive sports has been shown to decrease the negative psychosocial reactions to being physically challenged, such as self-pity, rejection, depression, and poor self-image, which lead eventually to social isolation.[3,4] Physical activity has been shown to have significant positive effects on all

aspects of general health. In Table 7-1 the effect on function of various systems throughout the body in response to exercise is documented.[3-7]

The improved strength, endurance, range of motion, and cardiovascular and respiratory capacity facilitates routine activities such as dressing, bathing, transfers, wheelchair mobility, and mobility with other orthotic aids. With these obvious physiologic benefits also come the previously mentioned psychological benefits of a better self-image and the self-perception of being in control. Physically challenged athletes have demonstrated their ability by continued achievements in national and international competition as well as limitless participation in recreational activities with the use of adaptive equipment (Figs. 7-2 and 7-3).

Classification systems categorize the extent of an athlete's physical challenge and ensures equitable competition, so that athletic ability and skills and not the degree of physical challenge are the factors that differentiate competitors. Thus, athletes with a similar level of function are grouped to compete against each other rather than against athletes with lesser or greater degrees of physical challenge (Table 7-2).

Classification systems are changing and should develop further as sports for athletes with physical challenges evolve and as we gather experience in sport-specific functional classification. Table 7-2 summarizes the classification systems used in various competitive sports.[8-11]

Published reports have documented that the injury rate of physically challenged athletes appears to be within the same range as for their able-bodied counterparts.[12] Although the number of injuries sustained by physically challenged athletes is not greater, the types of

Table 7-1   Benefits of Exercise

Organ System	Benefits
Cardiac	Increased cardiac output
	Increased stroke volume
	Decreased heart rate
Vascular	Increased blood volume
	Increased venous return
	Decreased deep venous thrombosis
	Decreased peripheral edema
Respiratory	Increased oxygen uptake
	Increased lung volume
Renal	Decreased urinary tract infection
	Decreased pyelonephritis
	Decreased renal stones
Skin	Decreased pressure sores
Musculoskeletal	Increased muscle mass
	Increased coordination
	Decreased spasticity
	Decreased ankylosis
	Decreased osteoporosis
	Decreased blood lactate levels
Gastrointestinal	Increased metabolism
	Decreased constipation

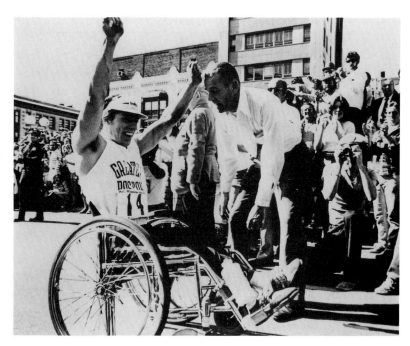

Figure 7-2 Bob Hall, winner of the first official Wheelchair Marathon race in Boston, Massachusetts. Time: 2 hours, 40 minutes, 6 seconds. (Photograph courtesy of Bob Hall.)

injuries that occur are different. In studies conducted by Ferrara and colleagues[13] and Curtis and Dillon[14] on paraplegic wheelchair athletes, the nature, type, extent, and frequency of athletic injuries were documented by a positive survey. In both studies the largest number of

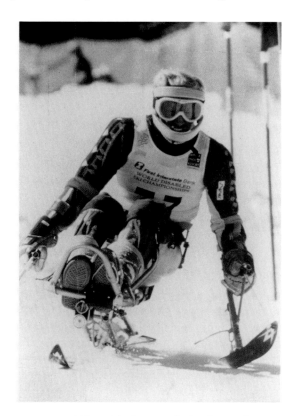

Figure 7-3 Skier with the use of adaptive equipment.

injuries was associated with track events, followed by basketball and road racing.

Curtis and Dillon noted that 72 percent of athletes in their series reported an injury that involved the upper extremity.[12] Both reports show that soft tissue injuries were most frequently noted with blisters, lacerations, abrasions, and cuts, followed by joint disorders and fractures. In the examination of 83 pediatric competitors at the 1990 Wheelchair National Games, Wilson and Washington[15] noted that 97 percent of the track athletes and 91 percent of the swimmers reported injury. Unlike the adult population, bruising blisters/abrasions were more common than soft tissue injuries. All of these studies concluded that prevention and education can help optimize performance and safe participation.

THE WHEELCHAIR ATHLETE

In the evaluation of the wheelchair athlete, one must look at the level of injury and the ability of the athlete to use his or her trunk muscles. There is a significant difference in the trunk involvement of the paraplegic and quadriplegic athlete. If the athlete lacks trunk musculature, the trunk must be stabilized in the chair for the athlete to have a maximum push. This is accomplished by strapping and/or customizing seat positioning. By stabilizing the trunk, the athlete will increase the lever arm by use of the upper extremity muscles, which help increase momentum for the push.

Table 7-2 Various Classification Systems

Physically Challenged Group	Sport	Classification System
2, 3, 4, 5, 6, 7	Alpine skiing	10 classifications, LW 1-10, based on type of ski equipment used
3, 4, 7	Basketball (wheelchair)	3-class system, USA based on neurologic function; 4-class international system based on functional trunk movement in wheelchair; combined classification points of players on court limited by rules
3	Cycling	3-class system, based on limb involvement
2, 3, 4, 5, 7	Powerlifting	Competition by weight classes
2, 3, 4, 7	Swimming	10-class integrated system, with different classifications for breast stroke, back stroke, and freestyle
3, 7	Table tennis (standing)	5-class system for standing athletes
3, 4, 7	Table tennis (wheelchair)	5 seated classes, based on upper extremity and trunk function
3	Track and field (amputees standing) (*Note:* Bilateral above knee amputees can compete in wheelchair or standing)	9-class system based on upper vs lower extremity involvement and level of amputation
3, 4, 7	Track and field (wheelchair)	4 classes for track events; 7 seated classes for field events; one standing class for field events
3, 7	Volleyball (sitting)	All players must sit
3	Volleyball (standing)	8-class system played by combined classification points of players on court
1	All sports for AAAD	Must have hearing loss greater than 55 dB in best ear
2	All sports for DAAA	Eligibility based on height less than 5 ft. 0 in.
5	All sports for USABA (in cycling, athletes ride tandem)	3-class system, based on visual field and acuity
6	All sports for USCPAA Swimming competition internationally is done in integrated system	8-class system, based on level of function of extremities and ambulatory status
7	All sports for USLASA Most athletes compete under sport-specific functional classifications for wheelchair or ambulatory athletes	6-class system, based on extremity and trunk function in sitting and standing for competition

1, American Athletic Association for the Deaf (AAAD); *2*, Dwarf Athletic Association of America (DAAA); *3*, National Handicapped Sports (NHS) (amputees); *4*, National Wheelchair Athletic Association (NWAA/NWBA) (wheelchair); *5*, United States Association for Blind Athletes (USABA) (blind); *6*, United States Cerebral Palsy Athletic Association (USCPAA) (cerebral palsy); *7*, United States Les Autres Sports Association (USLASA) (other physical challenges).

Although there is still no consensus as to the ideal sport or racing wheelchair, body and leg length, neuromuscular control and posture, and strength of the athlete should be considered in the selection of a wheelchair. Today's designs have reduced the weight of conventional wheelchairs by two-thirds of the earlier models by utilizing different metals such as aluminum, titanium, and aircraft steel. Instead of a more standard fit, the current models can be customized according to the size of the user and level of physical challenge (Fig. 7-4).

The goal of the wheelchair-racing athlete is to cover a specific distance in the least amount of time possible. The speed at which this distance is covered is a product of three factors: (1) the athlete's ability to generate power in exerting force on the push rim, (2) the amount of time the athlete is applying this force to the push rim, and (3) the frequency at which a push stroke occurs. By evaluating these three factors, an athlete's performance can be maximized.[16] The push stroke has been divided into six phases: (1) preparation, (2) a drive forward and downward, (3) push rim contact/squeeze, (4) movement of the hand along the rim, (5) push-off in normal or pronation flick, and (6) elbow lift and recovery (M. Morse and T. Milihan, personal communication, 1994).

In the *first phase,* the body prepares itself for optimizing the pushing stroke (Fig. 7-5). The position in the preparation phase is thoracic extension, shoulder extension, and minimal abduction, elbow flexion, and wrist neutral. In this position, there is maximal stretching, reversal of normal kyphosis, and eccentric contraction of the pectoralis major muscle and the deltoid muscle, which maximizes potential energy for the creation of force toward the push ring.

In the *second phase,* described as a drive forward and

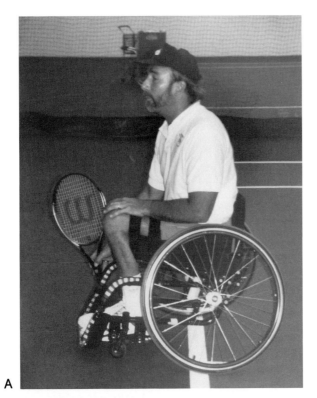

A

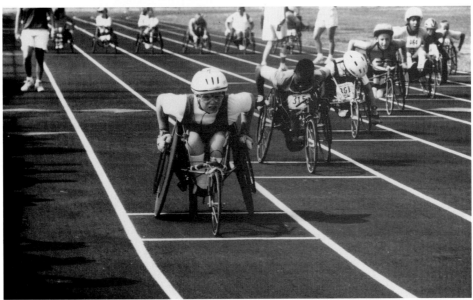

B

Figure 7-4 (A) Sports wheelchair. **(B)** Racing wheelchairs.

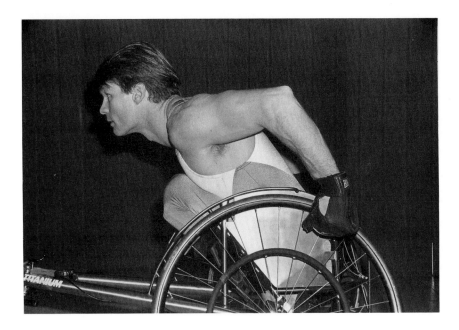

Figure 7-5 Preparatory phase of the wheelchair push stroke. (Photograph courtesy of Bob Nichols.)

downward, there is a strong concentric contraction of the pectoralis major muscle and the anterior deltoid muscle, which accelerates the forearm and hand toward the push ring (Fig. 7-6). Investigations have determined that a lower seating position (approximately 4.4 to 7.6 cm behind the main axles) facilitates smoother kinematic motion of the upper limb joints in this phase of the push.[17] Proper positioning of the seat should enable the hand to approach the push ring at approximately 10 degrees to the horizontal, enabling the hand to strike the ring at approximately the 12 o'clock position.

In the *third phase* of the push, as the hand hits the push ring, the elbow is extended, and a transfer of kinetic momentum is generated from the body to the wheel (Fig. 7-7). There is firm wrist and hand flexion in the glove as it contacts the push ring. The main contact area should be along the surface between the distal interphalangeal joints and the cuticles of the index and middle finger (Fig. 7-8). The momentum is maximized by three variables: (1) the angle at which the hand hits the push ring; (2) friction between the glove and the push ring (a slippery push ring surface will allow the hand to slip, and subsequently there will be a loss of

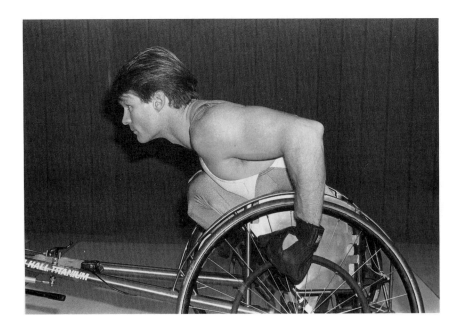

Figure 7-6 Acceleration toward the push ring. The force is directed forward and downward. (Photograph courtesy of Bob Nichols.)

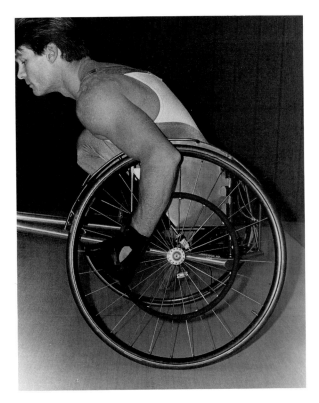

Figure 7-7 Elbow extension and transfer of momentum. (Photograph courtesy of Bob Nichols.)

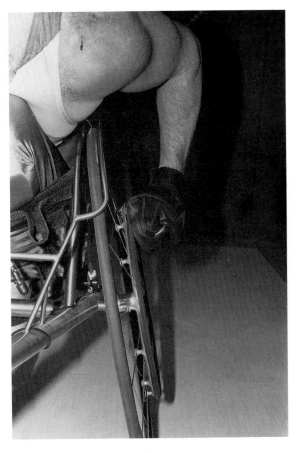

Figure 7-8 Push rim contact–hand squeeze. (Photograph courtesy of Bob Nichols.)

momentum; and (3) the speed at which the hand is hitting the push ring.

During this phase, it should be noted that the hand and wrist are in neutral slight ulnar deviation (Fig. 7-8). By being in a neutral position, described as the position of power, the hand will also stabilize the wrist and subsequently decrease wrist injuries. The quadriplegic's mode of push ring contact is very similar but depends upon the level of injury. High quadriplegics (C6–C7) may stroke the push ring with the wrist in more volar flexion. It is important that these athletes receive proper glove fittings and that their wrist mechanics are regularly checked to prevent wrist damage.

In the *fourth phase,* the elbow is fully extended as it follows the ring out to its lowest point. The athlete efficiently transfers the resulting momentum to the push ring (Fig. 7-9). Contact along the ring should be with the outermost portion of the ring to efficiently utilize mechanical advantage.

The *fifth phase,* an applied push at the bottom of the wheelchair rim, occurs if the wheelchair is viewed at approximately the 6 o'clock position (Fig. 7-9). In this sequence, as the hand is following around the push ring, there is a hyperpronation of the forearm and ulnar deviation of the wrist and hand (Fig. 7-10). This serves as a final push and is also used as the recovery phase

when the arms are driven back up to their original starting position. Repetitive hyperpronation is reflected in complaints of lateral epicondylitis of the elbow and wrist tendonitis. In an attempt to decrease these problems, practitioners at the University of Illinois recommend finishing the push with the forearm and wrist in neutral or slight supination (Fig. 7-11). Repetitive injuries in the wrist and elbow have been reduced by a change in this part of the stroke pattern (M. Morse and T. Milihan, personal communication, 1994).

The *sixth phase* is a return to the preparatory phase (Fig. 7-5). The athlete will strive to get the elbow as high as possible to maximize momentum for the next push. With minimal shoulder abduction, the extremity is brought up in the plane of the push ring (Fig. 7-12).

HISTORY AND PHYSICAL EXAMINATION

The history and physical examination of the physically challenged athlete is important not only for the

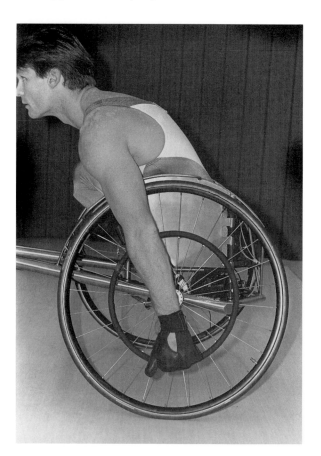

Figure 7-9 Movement of the hand along the ring to its lowest point. (Photograph courtesy of Bob Nichols.)

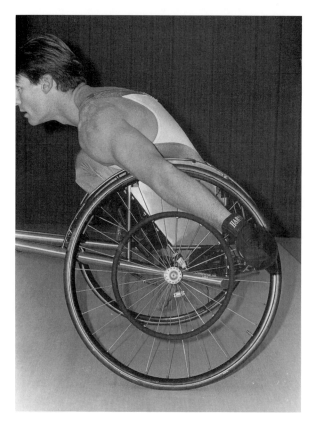

Figure 7-10 Push-off with forearm and wrist in pronation. (Photograph courtesy of Bob Nichols.)

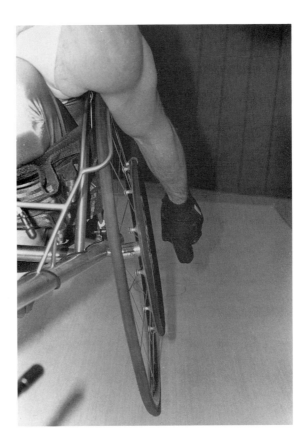

Figure 7-11 Push-off with forearm and wrist in neutral. (Photograph courtesy of Bob Nichols.)

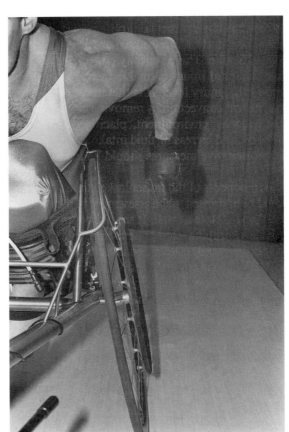

Figure 7-12 Elbow lift and recovery. (Photograph courtesy of Bob Nichols.)

documentation of the injury but also to ensure that the participant is able to safely compete. Many of these athletes have additional medical conditions, such as hypertension, cardiopulmonary disorders, renal disease, or endocrine abnormalities. The health professional should be aware of the types of medications prescribed to the participant, and dosages may require adjustment for the athletes to compete at an optimal level.

Athletes need to be thoroughly questioned and educated on personal hygiene. Issues of nutrition, bladder and bowel management, hydration, and temperature regulation must be specifically addressed. The sports medicine professional must be especially aware of the specific autonomic dysfunctions to the physically challenged athlete, including dysfunctions of neurogenic bowel/bladder, autonomic dysreflexion, and problems with temperature regulation. Impaired vascular function, decreased muscle mass, absence of active muscles, and restricted innervation of sweat glands will tend to render the physically challenged athlete susceptible to extremes in environmental temperature and dehydration.

In colder climates (i.e., for the physically challenged skier or ice hockey player), excessive heat loss and hypothermia must be prevented. It is important to provide athletes with dry insulated clothing and to warm parts below the level of spinal injury and vascular-deficient areas. In warmer environments, problems with hyperthermia and dehydration can lead to subsequent heat exhaustion or stroke. The physically challenged athlete with a spinal cord injury is unable to rely on evaporation below the injury level. It is therefore imperative to assist in heat convection by removing clothing, moving to a cooler environment, placing cool towels over the body, and increasing fluid intake. If it is hot, the above resuscitative measures should be initiated.

The specific components of the musculoskeletal examination should be addressed in the assessment of the physically challenged athlete as well. It should be understood that the level of spinal cord or neuromuscular involvement of the physically challenged athlete often determines expected functional goals. Individuals with spinal injuries at T1 or above and many athletes with cerebral palsy, postpolio paralysis, and neuromuscular disease have some type of upper extremity neuromuscular involvement. Athletes with injuries from T1 to T11 have poor postural and scapular stability, which has adverse effects on their upper extremity function (Fig. 7-13). Muscular imbalance, muscle tone, spasticity, flexibility, fixed contractures, and spinal deformities must be documented.

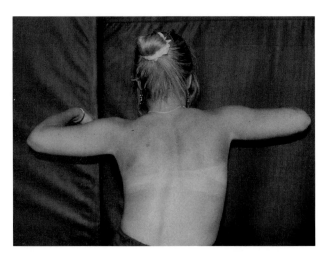

Figure 7-13 Poor postural and scapular stability secondary to high thoracic neuromuscular involvement.

INJURIES TO THE PHYSICALLY CHALLENGED POPULATION

There are three main mechanisms of injury incurred by the physically challenged athlete: the first is direct impact, which usually results in soft tissue skin trauma (e.g., abrasions, lacerations, contusions, or fractures); the second involves various injuries secondary to repetitive stress, such as overuse syndromes and blisters; the third concerns muscular imbalances and repetitive stresses. It has been shown that most injuries are secondary to repetitive impact and not acute direct impact.[17-19] The need for adjunct or supportive equipment (i.e., wheelchair, ambulatory aids, and orthotics and prosthetics) may also be directly or indirectly associated with athletic injuries in the physically challenged population. In the following sections, specific injuries to the physically challenged athlete as well as prevention and specific treatment are highlighted. Many of the injuries listed are common to the nonphysically challenged as well as the physically challenged and the reader should refer to other chapters for history, physical examination, and treatment.

THE SHOULDER

The most common soft tissue injury in the upper extremity of the physically challenged athlete is injury to the shoulder complex.[13] The physically challenged athlete has several predisposing factors that make the shoulder vulnerable to injury: (1) congenital or acquired musculotendinous conditions leading to improper, poor, or nonexistent neuromuscular control; (2) the abnormal stresses experienced from weight-bearing transfers or crutch use or from wheelchair-pushing leading to repetitive abnormal musculotendon and intra-articular stress[20,21]; and (3) the frequent overhead positions of the arm for sports. These factors can lead to problems of shoulder imbalance, inflexibility, and impingement overuse syndromes, which can ultimately result in chronic shoulder dysfunction. Burnham and coworkers[22] have reported the significance of the risk of muscular imbalance as a factor in the development of rotator cuff impingement in wheelchair athletes. We have observed that physically challenged athletes will often have poor flexibility and muscular imbalance around the shoulder. We have many physically challenged athletes presenting with either injuries to the rotator cuff and/or shoulder instability. Wheelchair athletes often have well-developed flexors, internal rotators, and adductors. They will have an imbalance secondary to poor development of their external rotators and thoracoscapular muscles. Because of the repetitive nature of the wheelchair push in positions 1, 2, and 3 (as stated earlier), the increase in adduction and internal rotation predisposes the rotator cuff to impingement between the greater tuberosity and coracoacromial arch (see Ch. 16).

The athletes who present with anterior shoulder instability at our clinic all have some degree of rotator cuff tendonitis. It is our belief that repetitive axial loading and significant adduction of the scapula, both of which occur in the first three phases of the pushing cycle, cause the anterior capsule and ligaments to stretch. As the rotator cuff muscles weaken, the imbalance of joint stabilizers occurs and subluxation symptoms increase.

Stretching and strengthening programs must be initiated in these athletes to help promote a well-balanced shoulder to prevent further harm. It is our experience that physically challenged athletes need to be better educated in preventive measures to help curtail the incidence of shoulder pathology (see Ch. 16).

ELBOW

Irritation of the lateral epicondyle of the wheelchair-racing athlete or tennis player is very common, most often resulting from progressive repetitive grasping of objects with the elbow extended and a hyperpronated wrist and hand, which are positions needed for wheelchair propulsion. Discomfort is increased with any stress or repetitive eccentric contractions of the extensor musculature.

Tennis players develop lateral epicondylitis secondary to overuse or a lack of adjustment to the racquet: weakness in the extensor mechanisms, a racquet that is too heavy, excessive tension in racquet stringing, or a grip that is inadequate or difficult for grasp. Of special note are the quadriplegic athletes who often have difficulty with wrist control. The tennis racquet should be placed onto the arm with the use of a special glove and taping (Fig. 7-14). Often adjustments of this support must be made to modify the lateral epicondylitis stress and pain.

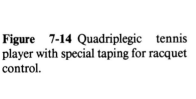

Figure 7-14 Quadriplegic tennis player with special taping for racquet control.

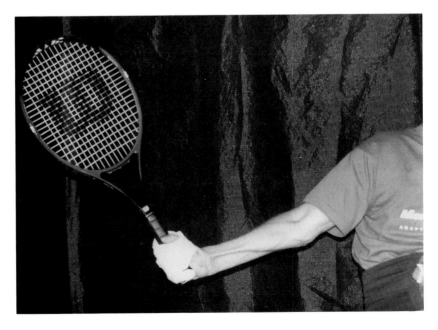

Long-distance wheelchair racers will often develop lateral epicondylitis. These athletes often complain of symptoms when they extend their elbows and hyperpronate their arms at the end of the stroke, causing eccentric stress for the extensor muscles.

In the cerebral palsy crutch-ambulating population, ulnar nerve entrapment neuropathies at the cubital tunnel and distally have been observed in our clinic for cerebral palsy athletes. It is generally secondary to repetitive use of crutches with elbows in flexion. The ulnar nerve can be entrapped proximal to the elbow, in the cubital tunnel, or as it passes under the two heads of the flexor carpi ulnaris muscle. In physically challenged athletes, the latter is the most common etiology. The spastic pattern of the flexor carpi ulnaris muscle contributes to the compression at the two heads of the muscle. These athletes will present with weakness in the hand, numbness, and dysesthesias in the ulnar nerve distribution. Treatment usually consists of crutch alterations and periods of rest, allowing the athlete to fully extend the elbow (see Ch. 19).

WRIST

Carpal Tunnel Syndrome

Carpal tunnel syndrome is a common entrapment neuropathy of the median nerve at the wrist (for a complete discussion of this subject, see Chs. 23 and 25). In athletes who compete with crutches (e.g., individuals with cerebral palsy), the wrists are often in an extended or hyperextended position while ambulating. This constant hyperextension results in decreased volume, and compressive stress to the carpal tunnel often causes bilateral carpal tunnel symptoms. This syndrome is also seen with wheelchair racers or athletes in whom there is compression at the carpal tunnel structures secondary to the constant repetitive trauma when the wrist is hyperextended and pressure is directed to the heel of the hand with each hand stroke on the push rim. These athletes will often present with significant night pain paresthesias, decrease in their grip strengths, and lack of dexterity (see Ch. 23).

Treatment for carpal tunnel syndrome requires a recognition of unique demands for functional performance in the physically challenged athlete. When examining the physically challenged wheelchair athlete, it is important that the competitive and repetitive stresses put on each wrist are closely reviewed. In our experience with crutch walking and wheelchair propulsion, extrapalmar padded gloves and/or orthoplast splints, along with rest, often decrease symptoms (Fig. 7-15). An evaluation of the biomechanical perform-

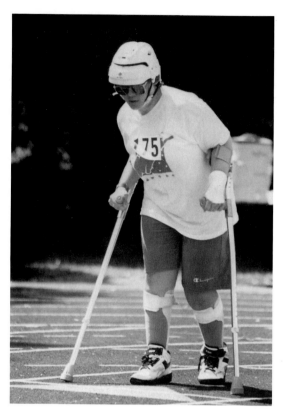

Figure 7-15 Preventive orthoplast splint for carpal tunnel syndrome.

ance of wheelchair-pushing athletes should be undertaken in relation to the exact mechanism of wrist contact to the rim. Often adjustments in trunk and seating position will help the athlete to diminish the symptoms. If carpal tunnel syndrome continues after conservative care, operative care may be considered (see Ch. 23).

Soft tissue and tendonitis disorders of the wrist commonly occur in physically challenged athletes due to the combined strains put on the wrist with normal activity and the stress of sports. Tendonitis is generally localized to a specific area, is aggravated by use, and will generally improve with rest. Impairment is based on the tendon involved and the pain threshold of the athlete. Common tendonitis problems about the wrist include de Quervain's tenosynovitis; extensor digitorum longus, extensor carpi ulnaris, flexor carpi ulnaris, and abductor pollicis longus tendonitis; and intersection syndrome. These are frequently associated with the same repetitive use and overuse disorders seen in the able-bodied athlete, and the treatments for both the physically challenged and able-bodied are parallel (see Ch. 23).

HAND

The hand is also a common area for repetitive or overactive use in the physically challenged athlete. Prior to the development of the well-padded glove, athletes taped their hands to protect them from injury. The glove has become an integral part of the regular athletic gear for many physically challenged wheelchair athletes. Gloves are now manufactured for sport-specific events. For example, there are specific gloves manufactured for the pushing of wheelchairs, both for the paraplegic and quadriplegic athlete. In wheelchair-racing events gloves have made significant differences in decreasing the frequency of hand injuries while maximizing an athlete's performance (Fig. 7-16). Gloves decrease the incidence of blisters, abrasions, contusions, and fractures.

In sports involving racquets, gloves along with proper taping, have enabled athletes who have a weak grip to compete (Fig. 7-14). If an athlete suffers an acute or chronic injury, modifications to the glove may be needed. When padding gloves, foam should be positioned over the area of contact (i.e., for the wheelchair racer: thenar eminence, distal cuticles, and phalanges). If a manufactured glove is not purchased, the athlete must make modifications to a glove if there is a chronic problem. The most common types of tape used are white athletic tape, elastic adhesive bandage, or friction tape. The maintenance of the athletic glove should be

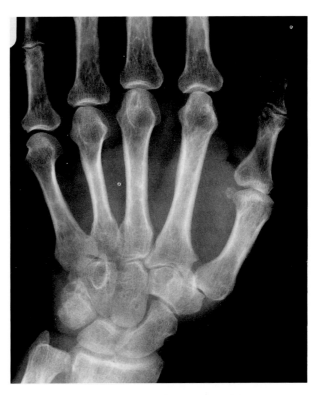

Figure 7-17 Chronic degenerative changes of the thumb carpometacarpal joint secondary to repetitive stress.

part of every athlete's program before the event. Often advice from more experienced athletes is helpful.

The thumb remains a common area of complaint and concern for the wheelchair sports population and crutch ambulator. Thumb problems typically occur at the carpometacarpal and the metacarpophalangeal joints. Often degenerative changes at this joint, accompanied by laxity, will be present (Fig. 7-17). It should be remembered that whatever treatment and splint are recommended, splinting should be devised to accommodate functions for daily activities (Fig. 7-18). At the metacarpophalangeal joint, injuries to the ulnar collateral ligaments are common. These injuries can occur in sports such as amputee skiing,[23] when the thumb is placed in a forced abducted position (see Ch. 25).

BLISTERS

Blisters account for the second most common injury in the upper extremity of the adult physically challenged population.[14,24] In the pediatric wheelchair population, this is the most common source of injury.[15] Blisters most commonly occur on the hands and fingers, followed by the inner aspects of the forearm and arm, and in areas of strapping or contact with the

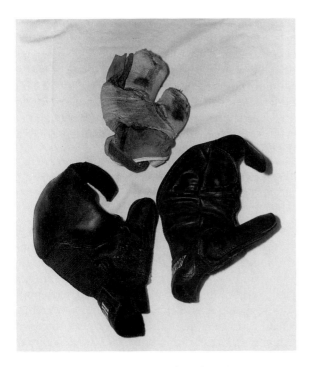

Figure 7-16 Wheelchair racing gloves.

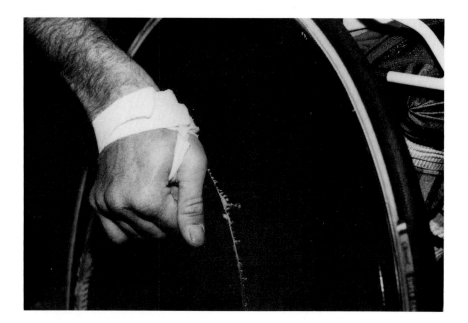

Figure 7-18 Protective thumb splinting for daily activities.

wheelchair seats. Athletes who participate in road racing, basketball, track, and tennis are at the highest risk for blisters, while athletes who participate in field events are not as susceptible.[14] The mechanism of the injury appears to be the repetitive trauma to the affected areas. Prevention of blisters includes the training and development of callus formation of the hands, taping the fingers, and wearing gloves. Occasionally, excessively calloused areas may require filing to prevent cracking.

If blisters are on the athlete's back, rearrangement of the padding and seat positioning as well as wearing a shirt have been found to prevent the problem. Blistering may lead to or accompany pressure sores, which, if not recognized and treated, may progress to chronic ulcerations and secondary infections. These conditions often necessitate an interruption of all athletic activity. This is often the case when the wheelchair participant is in a new chair, in a chair designed to raise the knees higher than the buttocks, or in a chair or wearing clothes that increase sweat production. Adequate cushioning and padding are needed in areas of pressure. It is important for the athlete to make frequent skin checks and intermittently shift weight, in addition to not remaining in the wheelchair for an excessive period of time other than during competition.

ABRASIONS, CONTUSIONS, AND LACERATIONS

Abrasions, contusions, and lacerations represent approximately 17 percent of the injuries seen in adult competitive wheelchair athletes and almost 40 percent

of pediatric wheelchair racers.[13,15] These injuries occur most often from falls or contact with equipment (either the athlete's own or a teammate's). Abrasions, contusions, and lacerations of fingers, thumbs, and arms may be caused by contact with brakes or sharp edges of the athlete's own wheelchair or by contact with larger tires of track chairs, by fingers being trapped between wheels, or by repetitive overuse. One common injury to the wheelchair athlete is upper arm and forearm friction burns on the inner surfaces of the arm, secondary to contact with the wheelchair tire during the push stroke. Preventive methods consist of padding of the upper extremity, correct seat positioning, proper stroke mechanics, cantering of the wheelchair's wheels, or a protective guard covering the tire.

Strapping of the trunk and legs of the individual into the wheelchair can also result in contusions or friction burns. The sports practitioner should inspect and advise the athlete regarding the dangers of insensate areas.

PREVENTIVE STRETCHING AND STRENGTHENING OF MUSCLES

As with able-bodied athletes, stretching exercises are done to improve flexibility, to achieve a complete range of motion, and to reduce the risk of injury to muscles, tendons, and ligaments surrounding the joint. It is especially important for the physically challenged population to adhere to strict protocols for stretching. Stretching can be done alone but is best performed with assistance. If stretching is done in a wheelchair, the wheelchair should be stabilized to prevent the athlete from tipping (Fig. 7-19) (see Ch. 16).

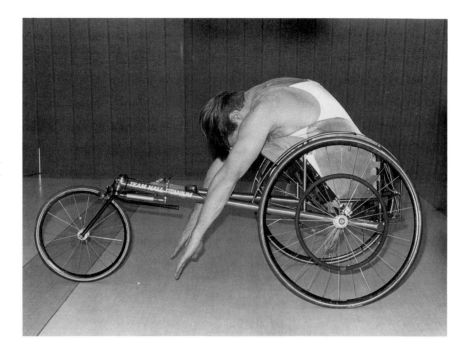

Figure 7-19 Trunk stretching of an athlete in racing wheelchair. (Photograph courtesy of Bob Nichols.)

The full length of the muscle must be stretched. When muscles cross two joints there should be a combination of movements to attain the best flexibility. Stretching should be done both before exercise and after a competition or workout and cool-down.

As with the able-bodied athlete, the purpose of the warm-up phase is to begin muscular contraction and increase blood flow to the muscles at a low intensity of work. The warm-up may facilitate a peak performance; omission may lead to muscle cramping, postexercise soreness, and severe injuries to muscles and tendons.

Following strenuous exercise, there should be a short period of less intense exercise to prevent muscle cramping and aid in circulatory return from the exercising muscles. Cool-down should be carried out at a medium pace with low resistance, and should last from 5 to 10 minutes. The same stretching routine should be carried out as a final phase of the workout, and should take from 5 to 8 minutes.

REFERENCES

1. Madorsky JGB, Curtis KA: Wheelchair sports medicine. Am J Sports Med 12:128, 1984
2. Hamel R: Getting into the game: new opportunities for athletes with disabilities. Phys Sports Med 20:121, 1992
3. Shephard RJ: Review articles: sports medicine and the wheelchair athlete. Sports Med 4:226, 1988
4. Stotts KM: Health maintenance: paraplegic athletes and nonathletes. Arch Phys Med Rehabil 67:109, 1986
5. Davis GM, Shephard RJ: Cardiorespiratory fitness in highly active versus inactive paraplegics. Med Sci Sports Exerc 20:463, 1988
6. Holland LJ, Streadward RD: Effects of resistance and flexibility training on strength, spasticity/muscle tone, and range of motion of elite athletes with cerebral palsy. Palaestra Summer:27, 1990
7. Figoni SF: Perspectives on cardiovascular fitness and SCI. J Am Paraplegia Soc 13:63, 1990
8. Curtis KA: Sport-specific functional classification for wheelchair athletes. Sports Spokes 17:45, 1991
9. Weiss M, Curtis KA: Controversies in medical classification of wheelchair athletes. In Sherrill C (ed): Sport and Disabled Athletes. Human Kinetics, Champaign, IL, 1986
10. International Stoke Mandeville Wheelchair Sports Federation: General and Functional Classification Guide: IX Paralympic Games, Barcelona, 1992
11. Strohkendl H: A new classification system for wheelchair basketball. In Sherrill C (ed): Sport and Disabled Athletes. Human Kinetics, Champaign, IL 1986
12. Bloomquist LE: Injuries to athletes with physical disabilities: prevention implications. Phys Sports Med 14:97, 1988
13. Ferrara MS, Davis RW: Injuries to elite wheelchair athletes. Paraplegia 28:335, 1990
14. Curtis KA, Dillon DA: Survey of wheelchair athletic injuries: common patterns and prevention. Paraplegia 23:170, 1985
15. Wilson PE, Washington RL: Pediatric wheelchair athletics: sports injuries and prevention. Paraplegia 31:330, 1993
16. Robertston RN, Cooper RA, Baldini F: Biomechanics of racing wheelchair propulsion. NWAA Newslett Fall, 1992

17. Masse LC, Lamontagne M, O'Riain MD: Biomechanical analysis of wheelchair propulsion for various seating positions. J Rehabil Res 29:12, 1992

18. McCormack DAR, Reid DC, Steadward RD, Syrotuik DG: Injury profiles in wheelchair athletes: results of a retrospective survey. Clin J Sport Med 1:35, 1991

19. Burnham R, Newell E, Steadward R: Sports medicine for the physically challenged: the Canadian team experience at the 1988 Seoul Paralympic Games. Clin J Sport Med 1:193, 1991

20. Bayley JC, Cochran TP, Sledge CB: The weight-bearing shoulder. J Bone Joint Surg [Am] 69:676, 1987

21. Wing PC, Tredwell SJ: The weightbearing shoulder. Paraplegia 21:107, 1983

22. Burnham RS, May L, Nelson E, Steadward R: Shoulder pain in wheelchair athletes: the role of muscle imbalance. Am J Sports Med 21:238, 1993

23. Ferrara MS, Buckley WE, Messner DG, Benedict J: The injury experience and training history of the competitive skier with a disability. Am J Sports Med 29:55, 1992a

24. Ferrara MS, Buckley WE, McCann BC et al: The injury experience of the competitive athlete with a disability: prevention implications. Med Sci Sports Exerc 24:184, 1992

8

Sport Injuries in the Skeletally Immature

Arthur M. Pappas
Nancy M. Cummings

Unique injuries occur in the skeletally immature athlete, although they are the result of similar biomechanic and performance forces that the mature athlete encounters. The primary differences are associated with growth and maturation and the development of bone, tendon, and muscle attachments. For example, the shoulder complaints presented by the skeletally immature athlete may mimic the complaints of a skeletally mature athlete; however in the skeletally immature, the complaints may be related to a congenital abnormality or variance in skeletal development, whereas in the skeletally mature, the complaints may be related to glenohumeral instability or rotator cuff inflammation. The senior athlete may present with similar complaints caused by attritional changes of aging. The clinical and radiographic findings among these groups, however, are quite distinct. Within this chapter, the development of the skeletal system in relationship to specific anatomic areas of the upper extremity (e.g., shoulder, elbow, wrist, and hand) is presented, followed by a series of typical sport-related problems.

GENDER-SPECIFIC DIFFERENCES IN SKELETAL MATURATION

It is important to recognize the differences in skeletal maturation between boys and girls. Until age 10, children grow and develop size and strength on a near equal basis. After age 10, there is a rapid and significant variation in growth. This rapid growth and maturation is associated with menarche and other physiologic changes for girls at age 12 to 13 approximately, while boys on average are 1.5 to 2 years later in experiencing their peak maturational growth period. During the accelerated growth period, the average boy will experience more growth than the average girl, and therefore it should be kept in mind that many of the skeletal changes occur at different developmental ages for girls versus boys. Although similar problems occur in both sexes, the specific injuries or complaints will depend on the stage of growth and development in addition to the athletic endeavors undertaken. Involvement of skeletally immature individuals in unorganized free play compared to highly organized year-round single athletic events correlates with many of the problems seen in this developmental period. Growing athletes who participate on a year-round basis to achieve maximum skill performance without recovery periods experience year-round stress to areas of growth and development, whereas growing athletes who vary their athletic events or have scheduled periods of rest or time away allow for physiologic recovery.

DEVELOPMENTAL CONSIDERATIONS

The epiphysis is most vulnerable during times of rapid maturational growth (i.e., physiologic change).[1] If the peripheral epiphysis is the origin or insertion of a muscle or tendon, it may be identified as an apophysis or traction epiphysis. Repetitive physical stress during this developmental stage results in traction and distraction at the epiphyseal metaphyseal junction, contributing to discomfort and a higher incidence of physeal stress symptoms. Compressive palpation over the physis or apophysis causes acute discomfort. The radiograph reveals an image of a widened physeal area that is similar to the findings of an undisplaced Salter-Harris type I injury. Examples of this syndrome at various anatomic sites are presented later in this chapter. The radiographic appearance of the secondary ossification center is usually homogeneous and any variations in size or density (similar to the fragmentation appearance of osteochondroses) most likely indicates changes that will be associated with discomfort[2] (Fig. 8-1).

Recognized bone growth factors present four variables to be considered: (1) the longitudinal growth of a long bone from its physes; (2) the progressive change of the secondary ossification center from a cartilage model, associated with the induction of angiogenesis and the progressive ossification; (3) the area of the peripheral epiphysis where the articular surface is developing or the apophysis where muscles and tendons attach; and (4) in the dorsal/volar plane where remodeling tends to correct malalignment (more so near a physis and less than diaphyseal) but has no effect on rotational malalignment. An injury to any of these four components will present different clinical problems to consider. A fracture through the physis may result in growth alteration, either longitudinal or angular. An interruption secondary to trauma or abnormal function in the development of the secondary ossification center may cause an abnormal configuration of the articular structures and surfaces, while an injury to the periphery may cause articular damage or a muscle or tendon micro- or macroavulsion injury. Repetitive

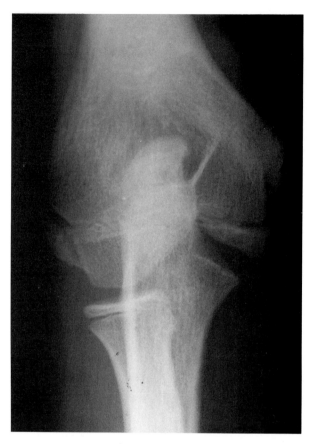

Figure 8-1 The apophyses and epiphyses. The distal humerus and proximal radius and ulna are seen in their normal radiographic appearance. The osseous development of these areas is frequently affected by athletic activity. An area of irregularity can be seen on the inferior border of the medial epicondyle that is consistent with a recent avulsion injury and will later be evident as an osteophyte or spur.

stress or specific injury can result in an altered configuration of the entire epiphysis.

Each physis contributes a known percentage to the longitudinal growth of each long bone. For example, the proximal humeral physis contributes approximately 80 percent of growth and the distal humeral physis approximately 20 percent of the growth. It is possible to interrupt longitudinal growth without significantly changing the development of the articular surface (unless there is an asymmetrical change of growth patterns, that is, one side arrests while the other side continues). The distal humeral physis contributes less longitudinal growth potential but is more involved in elbow articular configuration. There are six sites of secondary ossification where epiphyseal growth contributes to the complex articular surfaces of the distal elbow (Fig. 8-2). An injury to an area of the distal humeral physis is more likely to result in a disabling de-

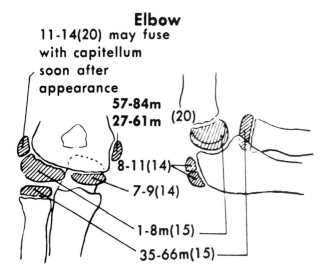

Elbow
11-14(20) may fuse
with capitellum
soon after
appearance
57-84m
27-61m (20)
8-11(14)
7-9(14)
1-8m(15)
35-66m(15)

Figure 8-2 Anterior and lateral view of secondary ossification centers about the elbow. The ages reflect the range of time that these ossification centers appear. The numbers in parentheses represent the age at time of fusion. M, age in months.

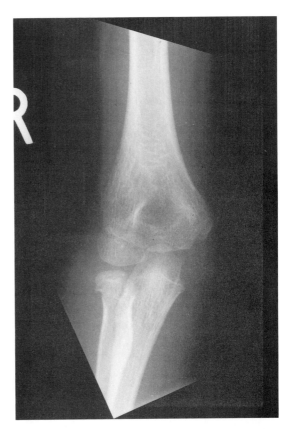

Figure 8-4 A displaced fracture of the radial neck. This fracture presents the potential for both altered longitudinal growth and maldevelopment of the radial head capitellum articulation.

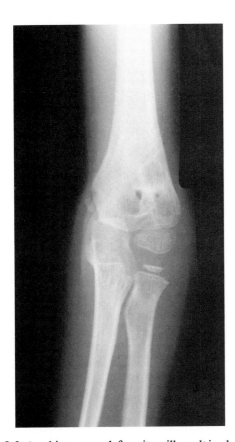

Figure 8-3 A cubitus varus deformity will result in abnormal elbow function: a typical residual deformity of an incompletely reduced and malunited supracondylar fracture.

formity secondary to an abnormal articular configuration of the elbow joint[3] (Fig. 8-3). The multiple sites of distal humeral development also account for a number of potential elbow problems in the skeletally immature athlete, which are discussed later in this chapter.

The proximal physes at the radius and ulna contribute 20 percent of the overall length, while the distal physes contribute 80 percent. As with the humerus, any injury or disturbance to the proximal physes of the forearm bones is more likely to result in a significant interarticular deformity at the elbow than disturbance of longitudinal growth (Fig. 8-4), although the latter is not to be disregarded.[4] If there is disproportionate growth of both bones (Fig. 8-5), articular wrist alignment and function will be affected, leading to angular forearm/wrist deformity and abnormal wrist biomechanics. Both of these situations will result in major malalignment, instability, and significant functional impairment.

The immature carpal bones are an epiphyseal complex equivalent (there is no accompanying diaphysis). Injury to these individual carpal bones will affect inter-

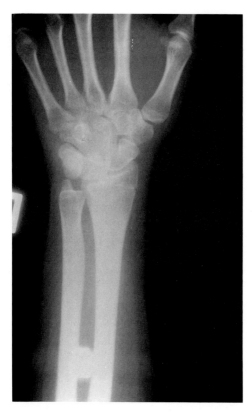

Figure 8-5 A shortened ulna resulting from premature closure of the distal ulna physis secondary to an injury incurred during a gymnastic maneuver. The resultant deformity associated with a shortened ulna caused an unstable wrist and pain with stressful wrist function.

articular alignment and wrist dynamics, thereby altering ultimate wrist function. Due to the ligamentous attachments, most physeal fractures of the metacarpals and phalanges are on the metaphyseal diaphyseal portion of the bone. An avulsion of an extensor tendon insertion may appear to be associated with a physeal fracture. A major crush injury through a physis of the hand will result in a growth deformity either longitudinally or angularly, although the majority of metacarpal injuries are more likely to result in disability caused by abnormal angular and/or rotational malalignment.

Apophyseal disorders of growth are often related to a particularly sensitive stage of skeletal development and the impact of repetitive force during this sensitive stage. Repetitive stresses may cause an epiphyseal stress syndrome or an avulsion injury: (1) the physeal area may be avulsed similar to a classic physeal metaphyseal separation fracture, or (2) a series of microfractures at the periphery may result in local discomfort. The periphery of the medial epicondyle of the humerus, which is the origin of the flexor muscles and the ulna collateral ligament, may sustain a series of microavulsion frac-

tures during later stages of development, causing discomfort and deformity (Fig. 8-6). This will be the origin of disability and impairment of athletic performance, as exemplified by the "Little League elbow." (Specific case examples are presented in the subsection *Elbow* below.)

Thus, many of the problems seen in skeletally immature individuals are in part related to repetitive stress as well as to overdemand on developing structures at this vulnerable stage in skeletal development. During earlier years, the apophyses and epiphysis can tolerate more activity than during a sensitive stage of growth and development (e.g., a growth spurt). Once these young athletes are beyond this skeletal stage of accelerated growth and development, they will be able to return to their previous level of athletic commitment unless overemphasis of a sport has resulted in residual anatomic changes. There must be a recognition of the sensitive biologic phase of development and possible need to alter athletic performance. This is a difficult concept to convey to parents and coaches who typically believe that decreased participation equals skill regres-

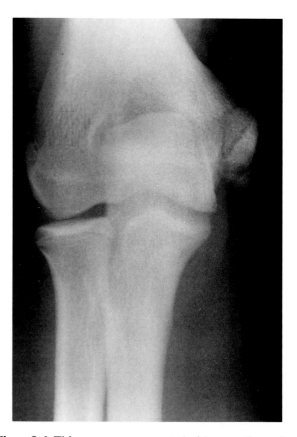

Figure 8-6 This young man presented with acute discomfort and swelling of his medial elbow at the end of a baseball season. He had experienced an avulsion of the inferior aspect of the medial epicondyle.

sion and less athletic achievement. In fact, if musculoskeletal problems can be avoided, the short-term inactivity will provide the skeletal foundation for long-term sports participation, whereas functional damage to a developing area may result in residual deformity and an altered athletic career. An understanding of normal development and the impact of repetitive stress or trauma provides guidance for advising skeletally immature athletes during periods when less participation in a particular event is wise.

CLINICAL CONSIDERATIONS

The remainder of this chapter is devoted to clinical problems recognized in the skeletally immature athlete. In most instances, these problems relate to specific developmental stages of the musculoskeletal system. There is an apparent association between excessive ligamentous laxity and increasing stress on musculotendinous bone interfaces. The repetitive forces of sports in individuals who have more lax ligaments will increase stress on physeal areas, resulting in more problems during specific developmental stages.

Shoulder

The postnatal development of the shoulder complex includes the scapula, clavicle, and proximal humerus. The scapula is formed both by intramembranous and enchondral ossification. At birth, the body of the scapula has been ossified by intramembranous ossification but later areas of epiphyseal secondary enchondral ossifications occur (i.e., for the acromion, coracoid, and the vertebral and inferior borders). Of clinical significance related to the skeletally immature athlete are the acromial and coracoid centers of ossification. There are two centers of secondary ossification in the acromion, which develop independently. These centers of ossification demonstrate a progressive enlargement and fuse to form the bony acromion during the period of adolescent growth; at times, however, there is an incomplete or lack of osseous fusion, and one section (os acromiale) will remain a source of discomfort and occasional rotator cuff irritation and inflammation.[5] The discomfort associated with incomplete fusion usually follows either a major injury or repetitive athletic stress such as a direct blow or repetitive overhead activity.[6] The diagnosis is made from the combination of clinical palpation and an axillary view radiograph (Fig. 8-7). Aside from recognition, the treatment is limited activity and maintenance of balanced muscle control about the shoulder. There is minimal value in the use of anti-inflammatory medications and injections. A third ossi-

fication center of the acromion may appear in adolescence, although it is unclear whether this is truly a third ossification center or perhaps an avulsion injury with subsequent ossification of an avulsed peripheral section of cartilage — in effect, an ununited fracture (Fig. 8-8). In most instances, a modification of activity will resolve the problem; however, in certain instances a persistent fragment may require surgical intervention.

The coracoid develops a secondary ossification center in its mid- to distal portion early in life. At a later period, (approximately age 10 in girls and age 12 in boys), a second ossification center appears at the base of the coracoid. The original ossification center is rarely the source of discomfort, except when there is an acute fracture in this area; however, the later-appearing ossific nucleus may be the origin of local pain. Typically, the physis at the base of the coracoid area is the focus of a stress syndrome, since it is a combination of an area undergoing rapid growth, along with the impact of the coracoid serving as the major anchor for the pectoralis minor. Thus, this area receives extraordinary stress from any individual using repetitive upper extremity activity. The key to the diagnosis is the radiographic recognition of a widened physeal line at the base of the coracoid and the associated clinical finding of exquisite sensitivity on compression of the coracoid (Fig. 8-9). The treatment is directed to the cause of the discomfort and appropriately modifying the pain-inciting activities as well as advising and reassuring parents that this clinical problem will be self-limited without functional or long-term implications. If an apparent third ossification center at the tip of the coracoid appears (similar to such found with the tip of the acromion), the same concerns are raised as for the tip of the acromion. Is this truly a third ossification center, or is it an avulsion injury that has ossified? This may be the source of discomfort in skeletally immature athletes who undertake repetitive stressful activity (e.g., baseball pitchers, swimmers, and tennis players) (Fig. 8-10). Again, the treatment is recognition and modification of activity. In rare instances, if the ossification at the tip of the acromion or coracoid does not fuse, it will act as an ununited avulsion fracture, and excision of the fragment and reattachment of the muscle may be indicated. Injuries that result in acromioclavicular ligamentous disruption in the skeletally mature athlete are more likely to result in fractures in the skeletally immature athlete.[6] (Fig. 8-11).

The separate ossification centers of the glenoid are usually not the source of discomfort associated with repetitive activities. When there is major trauma to the shoulder, however, it is possible for these ossification centers to be disturbed, resulting in altered subsequent growth and development of the glenoid (Fig. 8-12).

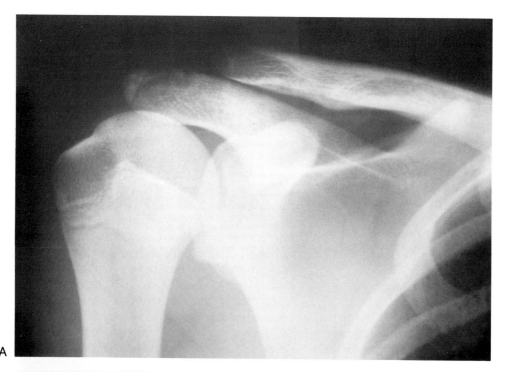

A

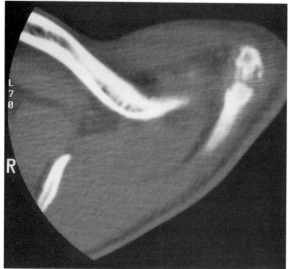

B

Figure 8-7 (**A**) Radiograph and (**B**) computed tomographic image of an abnormal and symptomatic os acromiale in a 14-year-old nationally ranked tennis player (note the irregular ossification pattern).

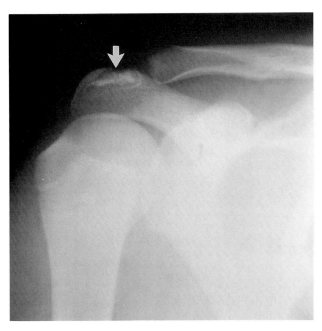

Figure 8-8 The osteosclerotic appearance *(arrow)* of the distal acromion associated with persistent discomfort in an adolescent baseball pitcher, possibly an ununited portion of the acromion.

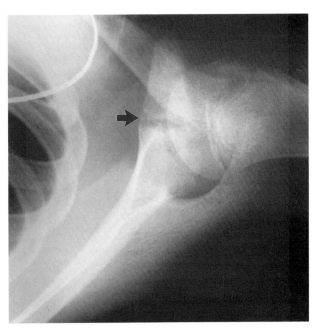

Figure 8-9 An unfused physis *(arrow)* at the basis of the coracoid secondary to overstress that was the cause of pain in a year-round competitive 11-year-old male swimmer. One year of limited competitive swimming was necessary to provide relief.

Figure 8-10 An irregular ossification pattern at the tip of the coracoid that may be the effect of continued repetitive stress of pitching on this physis or possibly a true avulsion injury of the muscles that originates from this site.

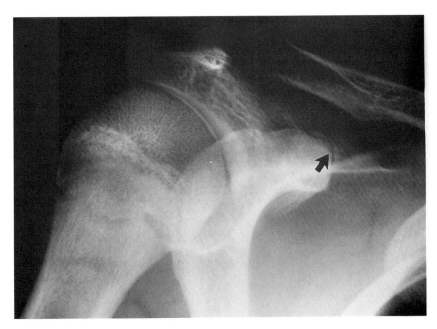

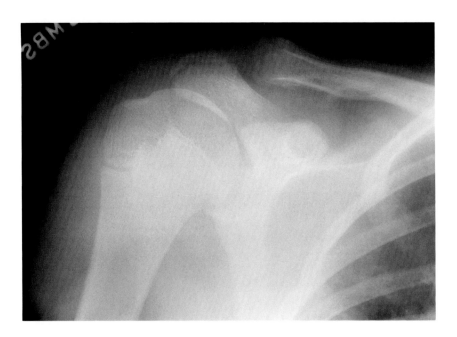

Figure 8-11 A severe board check to an adolescent hockey player caused multiple sites of injury of the clavicle acromion and coracoid. This injury demonstrated a double disruption and required extensive postinjury physical therapy treatment to achieve satisfactory shoulder motion function and stability.

Humerus

The proximal humerus forms from three separate ossification centers. Only one may be present at birth—the secondary ossification center for the humeral head. From age 3 until puberty, there is secondary ossification and growth of both the greater and lesser tuberosities (Fig. 8-13). Physeal injury of the tuberosities is unusual; however, the insertion of the supraspinatus may be associated with supraspinatus tendon traction stress on the secondary ossification center, resulting in discomfort with repetitive function. The radiographic appearance of the greater tuberosity in these instances is one of an irregular pattern of bone development and/or widening of the physis. The clinical examination demonstrates significant local sensitivity to compressive palpation. This relationship is akin to the majority of apophyseal syndromes frequently grouped as osteochondroses and individually identified by an eponym.[7] The greater tuberosity may be avulsed in the skeletally immature adolescent athlete subjected to biomechanical forces, resulting in an acute glenohumeral dislocation.

Figure 8-12 The centers of ossification that contribute to the development of the glenoid.

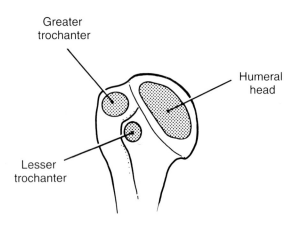

Greater trochanter

Humeral head

Lesser trochanter

Figure 8-13 The centers of ossification that contribute to development of the proximal humerus, the physis of the humeral head, and the epiphyses of the greater and lesser trochanters.

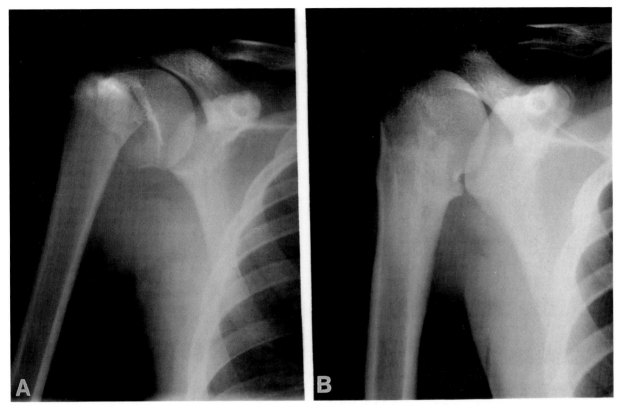

Figure 8-14 (A & B) A displaced physeal fracture of the proximal humeral physis in a 14-year-old boy who fell from a horse. Although the fracture remained displaced, the ultimate result was a well-healed site of fracture and full range of motion and normal strength of the shoulder. This individual ultimately continued with his athletic career, and 7 years postinjury became captain of his college football team.

Most injuries to the proximal humeral physis are related to three mechanisms: (1) macrotrauma causing a Salter-Harris type 2 fracture (Fig. 8-14); (2) an epiphyseal stress syndrome without osseous displacement, associated with repetitive overhead athletic activity (generally seen in adolescent individuals focusing on one sport such as tennis, baseball, swimming, or gymnastics) (Fig. 8-15); or (3) injuries to the physis secondary to a metabolic or neoplastic lesion, such as a solitary unicameral bone cyst (Fig. 8-16). Many metabolic or

Figure 8-15 Chronic stress syndrome in the proximal humeral physis—"Little League Shoulder." Note the associated denser margin on the physeal side and the widening of the humeral physis. These findings along with some observed changes on the tip of the coracoid were present in this overworked adolescent baseball pitcher.

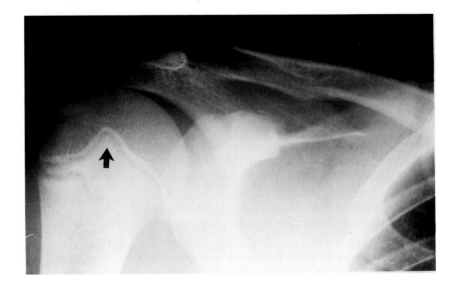

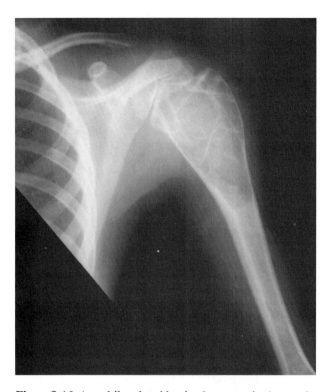

Figure 8-16 A multiloculated benign bone cyst in the proximal humerus of a young man who presented with pain secondary to a minimal cortical infraction sustained during a basketball game. A bone cyst in this location is especially worrisome because 80 percent of the growth of the humerus occurs from the proximal physis and interruption of this growth in a younger child will result in a significantly shortened upper extremity.

neoplastic lesions of the proximal humerus are initially diagnosed following some form of athletic activity associated with a major or minor traumatic event. For example, it is not uncommon for a benign unicameral bone cyst or malignant tumor to be diagnosed from a pathologic fracture secondary to throwing a ball. Thus, radiographic findings about the proximal humerus must be carefully evaluated, particularly when there is recent evidence of new bone formation.

Differentiating between a benign periosteal bone reaction to repetitive trauma and a tumor will challenge even the most experienced clinician. Fractures of the metaphysis and diaphysis of the humerus are generally associated with specific injury, repetitive use, or underlying pathologic diagnosis. The evaluation and treatment of these conditions are discussed in other texts and are not discussed here. Complaints in the arm area may be associated with local reaction to athletic injury (e.g., myositis ossificans, local benign lesions) (Fig. 8-17), or referred pain from shoulder or elbow problems (Fig. 8-18).

For some skeletally immature athletes, the glenohumeral articulation itself will be the site of clinical complaints. The three most common situations which are associated with instability of the glenohumeral articulation in the skeletally immature athlete are (1) congenital abnormal development of the glenohumeral joint associated with chronic dislocation (Fig. 8-19); (2) performance-related glenohumeral instability secondary to acquired capsular ligamentous laxity associated with repetitive motions; and (3) those who are functionally unstable on the basis of acquired capsular laxity or muscular imbalance, who then become voluntary subluxators and dislocators (Fig. 8-20). The latter group must be carefully evaluated and analyzed. The combination of physiologic ligamentous laxity and acquired muscle imbalance may raise clinical concerns that range from multidirectional instability to psychogenic patterns of instability (see Ch. 11).

Residual deformities of the distal humerus secondary to a malunion of a supracondylar fracture will result in abnormal function of the entire upper extremity. The most complex deformity will include three components: cubitus varus, hyperextension, and internal rotation. If all components of the deformity are not corrected, there will be residual abnormal function.[8]

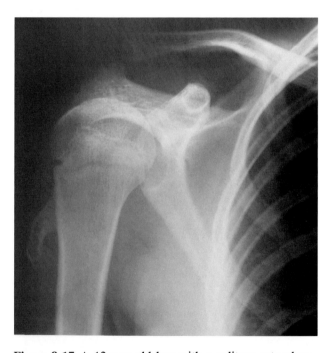

Figure 8-17 A 12-year-old boy with a solitary osteochondroma of the proximal humerus that caused discomfort associated with all overhead activities and ultimate weakness of his deltoid. The surgical removal of this osteochondroma resulted in relief of discomfort and a return to full unrestricted activity.

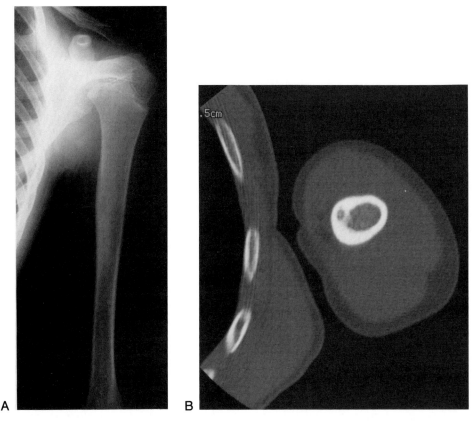

Figure 8-18 (A & B) This 10-year-old boy experienced persistent pain and secondary weakness of his upper extremity. The radiograph **(A)** reflects the lesions observed in the diaphysis of the humerus and the computed tomographic scan **(B)** localized the typical osteoid osteoma defects. The surgical excision of these lesions provided immediate relief of pain and the ability to regain muscle strength and return to unrestricted athletic activity within a few months.

Figure 8-19 The lack of anterior glenoid development in this 5-year-old boy was associated with recurrent dislocations whenever he attempted overhead activity. Prior to the recognition of the problem and secondary surgical intervention, he had developed a tendency to become ambidextrous.

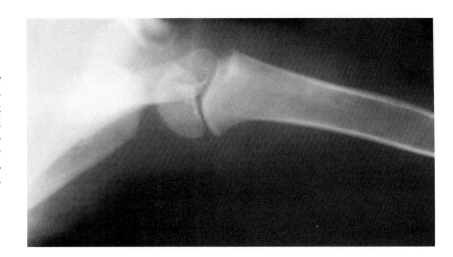

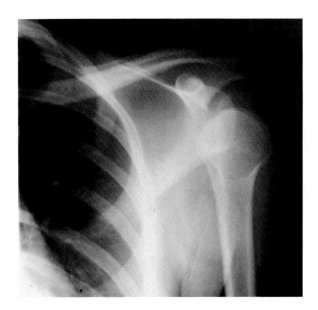

Figure 8-20 This 15-year-old female athlete sustained an injury to her shoulder while diving for a ball. Her instability developed into a multidirectional instability that she was able to voluntarily reproduce. This radiograph demonstrates her voluntary ability to "put her shoulder out"—the sulcus sign.

Elbow

The elbow region is the most frequent source of upper extremity problems in the skeletally immature athlete. Pain with performance is the most typical presenting complaint, although other complaints include local sensitivity or swelling, decreased range of motion, a progressive flexion deformity, or intermittent locking. The factors that most often contribute to these problems include the musculoskeletal development of the elbow, the biomechanical demands of the specific sport, the frequency of performance, and the genetic history of the individual.

The skeletal development of the distal humerus and proximal radius and ulna present six different secondary ossification centers. These ossification centers appear and develop at different times in addition to the known differences in female and male maturation. It is important to recognize these variables and in certain

cases obtain a plain radiograph of the opposite elbow for comparison of developmental variances.

The biomechanical forces associated with different sports potentially may determine the problematic area of development (see Ch. 17). For example, in analyzing the pitching mechanism, the forces involved in the late cocking and early acceleration phases when correlated with the developmental stages of ossification often determine the etiology of elbow discomfort. In the transition from maximum cocking stage (Fig. 8-21A) to the acceleration stage, significant force is directed toward the medial side of the elbow, presenting a distraction valgus force that produces tension across all of the components of the medial elbow, the medial epicondyle, muscles attaching to the medial epicondyle, ulnar medial collateral ligament, ulnar nerve, and the triceps insertion on the medial olecranon. This valgus traction mechanism will focus stress on the most sensitive and physically weakest site, and repetitive overload may

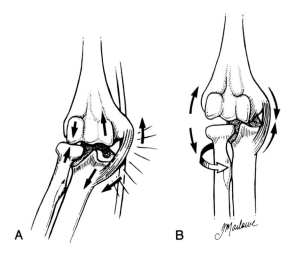

A   B

Figure 8-21 **(A)** Stresses during the period of maximum cocking to early acceleration stage where there is evidence of valgus stress on the medial side of the elbow and compression on the lateral side of the elbow. **(B)** Changes at the final stages of acceleration to deceleration. After ball release, there is actual varus distraction on the lateral side of the elbow with compression on the medial side, and rotation of the radius to pronation with compression on the medial and posterior aspects of the capitellum.

result in local changes that cause discomfort with performance. For example, stress on the developing medial epicondyle while in the stages of middle to late secondary ossification will cause minor or total avulsions (discussed in more detail in the next subsection, *Medial Elbow*). It is necessary to consider the biomechanical forces involved in each athletic event to understand presenting complaints for other skeletally immature athletes.[9]

The "Little League elbow" is a classic example of the need for limiting the amount of throwing during a particular stage of development. It was initially recognized as a problem in skeletally immature baseball players who were throwing more often than most of their peers and experiencing progressive discomfort and deformity.[8] The recognition of this entity has resulted in the development of advisory regulations by the Little League Association of America. While some view this as restricting the development of the pitcher, it actually preserves the athlete for a more significant expression of ability later in his or her career.

In certain instances, there is a genetic tendency toward mild anatomic variances, most commonly seen in the radiocapitellar area, that predispose to discomfort and limited motion in the preadolescent period of development. These individuals typically complain of discomfort and never achieve maximum performance. In other instances, there may be a genetic predisposition to an osteochondrosis that results in earlier symptoms of discomfort.

Medial Elbow

The medial elbow is the area most frequently associated with problems in the skeletally immature athlete. Within this region, the most common source of complaint is the medial epicondyle of the distal humerus.

The problems associated with the medial epicondyle can present as four different entities (Fig. 8-22).

The first entity may be a physeal fracture that may be partially or totally separated with distraction and/or rotation. This usually occurs with a forceful contraction of the muscles attaching to the medial epicondyle either through an active sport performance or through a fall on the outstretched hand (Fig. 8-23). The characteristics of the epiphyseal separation will determine treatment as discussed in many standard texts on pediatric fracture treatment.

The second entity is again within the physeal area, where frequent repetitive throwing results in the development of an epiphyseal stress syndrome or a permanent ununited physeal area and becomes the source of persistent discomfort (Fig. 8-24).

The third area of involvement is a typical irregular ossification pattern of the secondary ossification center most often associated with an osteochondrosis (Fig. 8-25). This is most likely related to excessive repetitive activity and an alteration of the angiogenesis pattern (Fig. 8-26). In addition, there will be a potential overgrowth (resulting in a larger medial epicondyle) associated with secondary hyperemia.

The fourth circumstance causing discomfort is the avulsion of small osteochondral fragments from the medial epicondyle, and the avulsion of small chondral sections of the medial epicondyle with sudden muscle contractions that later ossify. In certain instances, these will present as spurs off the inferior medial epicondyle that may not be symptomatic long term or may remain as free unattached ossicles that develop a secondary reaction similar to an ununited avulsion fracture.

It is unusual for skeletally immature athletes to develop ulnar nerve or medial collateral ligament symptoms and pathology. The medial epicondyle is the most susceptible anatomic area during this developmental period.

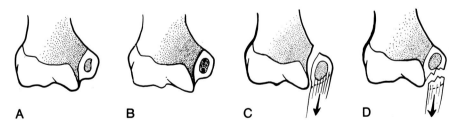

Figure 8-22 Different types of injury that may occur to the medial epicondyle, secondary to baseball pitching in the young athlete. **(A)** Normal appearance of the secondary ossification center in relation to the medial epicondyle. **(B)** Stress area of the physis of the epiphysis and the potential for a complete avulsion injury of the medial epicondyle. **(C)** Stress area of the physis of the medial epicondyle where repetitive action results in a widening and probably incremental traumatic separation of the physis without displacement. **(D)** Avulsion of the inferior portion of the periphery of the epiphysis associated with forceful activity of the common flexors.

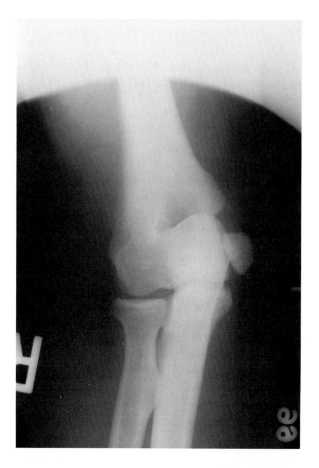

Figure 8-23 This avulsion of the medial epicondyle occurred when this young man was 14 years old. He had been an outstanding pitcher and after throwing one pitch experienced sudden pain that terminated his successful pitching career. The injury was not diagnosed at that time; however, later he complained of recurrent medial elbow pain associated with all athletic activities. He had an avulsed and un-united medial epicondyle.

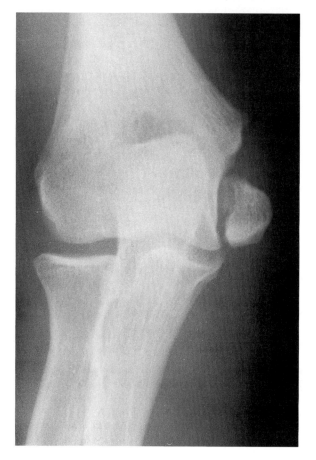

Figure 8-24 A 17-year-old baseball pitcher complained of aching on the medial side of his elbow after completing a game. His repetitive stress on the medial epicondyle resulted in a nonunion of the physis of his medial epicondyle. He elected to terminate his baseball career and did not experience significant changes in his life activities or athletic endeavors following his decision.

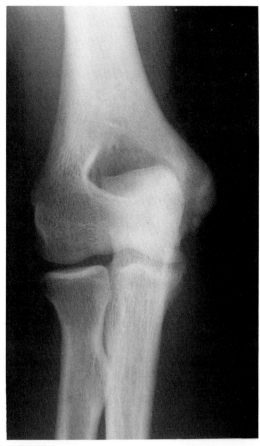

Figure 8-25 This young man experienced onset of pain in his elbow after a single pitch approximately 2 years prior to this visit. The pain persisted whenever he attempted to throw a ball and the radiographs demonstrate an avulsed portion of the inferior section of his medial epicondyle. A secondary reaction developed around this ossicle that created a symptomatic bursa. The excision of the ossicle and the reattachment of the muscle permitted him to return to pain-free athletic activity.

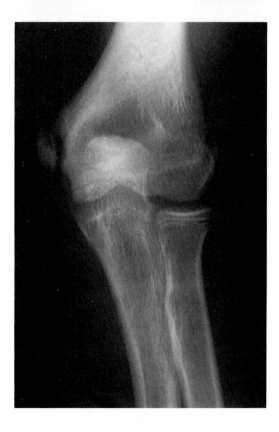

Figure 8-26 This successful young baseball pitcher experienced continual pain in the region of his medial epicondyle for 3 months after having completed a championship season when he pitched more frequently than advised. The observed widening of his medial epicondyle physis and the irregularity in the ossification pattern of the medial epicondyle are consistent with the typical findings associated with overactivity and overuse in this age group—the classic Little League elbow.

Lateral Elbow

During the time interval from late cocking and early acceleration, the forces within the elbow include the valgus medial force and a varus compressive lateral force as elbow extension and pronation occur (Fig. 8-21B). During the phases of rapid pronation, there is the combination of compression and rotation with particular stress during maximum pronation of the medial and posterior components of the radial head and capitellum. These forces are associated with changes observed in the radius/capitellum articulation and will result in changes contributing to the development of osteochondrosis (Panner's disease)[10] or osteochondritis of the capitellum or the radial head.[2]

Young athletes with these problems are likely to complain of arthralgia with associated discomfort, effusion, progressive flexion deformity, limited motion,

and occasionally a loose osteocartilaginous fragment. The radiographic finding is a typical subchondral lucency with or without sclerosis and with or without overlying subchondral bone (Fig. 8-27). If these are identified at a very early stage of puberty/adolescence, limited activity may decrease the causative forces and provide time for repair. At a later stage of adolescence or if there is sclerosis observed in the osseous crater, then arthroscopic and/or open surgical intervention should be considered, otherwise the process contributes to the formation of loose osteocartilaginous fragments and progressive degenerative joint disease may occur.[11] These problems are most frequently seen in baseball players and gymnasts, although they are also seen in a host of other athletes[12] (Fig. 8-28).

Posterior Elbow

The forces that affect the olecranon vary with each stage of throwing. During the cocking stage, the medial valgus force on the olecranon contracts to traction

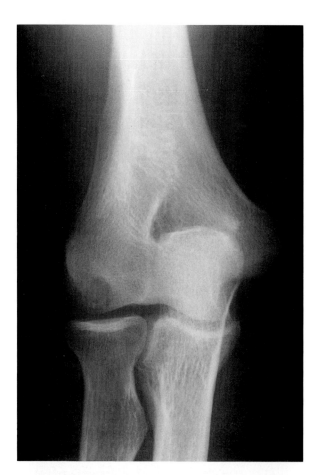

Figure 8-27 Typical radiographic changes of an osteochondrosis of the capitellum: Panners disease. A period of rest may help this problem in the skeletally immature child. However, in a skeletally mature athlete who continues participation, the risk of the articular component becoming a partially detached or totally detached osteochondral fragment may require either open or arthroscopic surgical intervention.

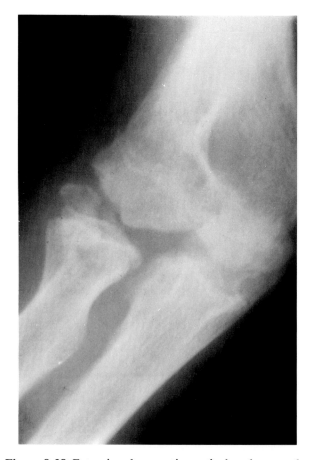

Figure 8-28 Extensive degenerative articular changes observed in this 15-year-old baseball pitcher. The changes are both on the radial head and capitellum surfaces of the elbow.

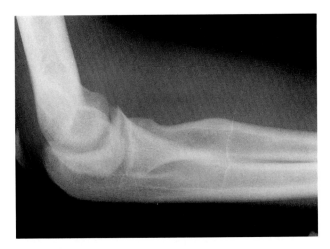

Figure 8-29 This 16-year-old football player sustained an avulsion of his triceps when he landed on a partially flexed elbow after diving for a pass. This triceps avulsion was treated with open surgical repair with a result that permitted a return to full unrestricted athletic activity.

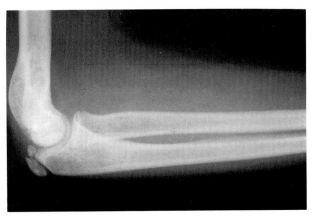

Figure 8-30 This 12-year-old baseball pitcher was seen for persistent posterior elbow discomfort. The repetitive activity of pitching was associated with an irregular pattern of ossification of the olecranon epiphysis. These findings are considered consistent with an osteochondrosis that is most likely related to the repetitive stress of his triceps on the olecranon physis.

valgus on the triceps and medial olecranon. This will create an asymmetrical force that can result in partial avulsion or osteophyte formation. During the acceleration phase, the forceful extension of the triceps may result in three different problems in the olecranon: (1) an acute avulsion of the triceps with a portion of the olecranon (Fig. 8-29); (2) an irregular pattern of development of the entire secondary ossification center demonstrating characteristic radiographic changes of

an osteochondrosis (Fig. 8-30); and (3) repetitive forces contributing to an epiphyseal stress syndrome with failure of physeal fusion (Fig. 8-31). During the deceleration phase of throwing, the combined antagonist-protagonist triceps-biceps relationship results in more posterior triceps-olecranon traction; when the olecranon extends into the posterior lateral humerus, there may be reactive compressive changes along the lateral olecranon and the adjacent synovium.

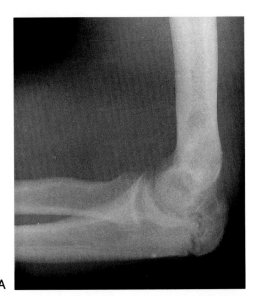
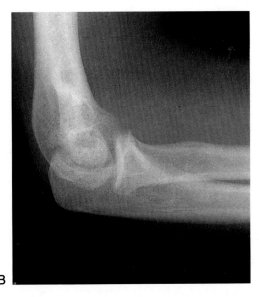

A   B

Figure 8-31 View of both elbows in an 18-year-old baseball pitcher who complained of persistent elbow discomfort. The radiograph on the left represents his throwing side and the incomplete union of his olecranon epiphysis to the ulna that was the cause of his discomfort. Surgical procedure was performed to graft this incompletely united area and the ultimate result was a pain-free return to athletic activity.

Anterior Elbow

During the final stages of cocking and in the early stages of acceleration, there is compressive force on the trochlea and traction on the capsular insertion and the coronoid process. The classical effect of these forces may be recognized as an irregular ossification pattern of the trochlea (Fig. 8-32) and a traction overgrowth of the coronoid.[13] In late adolescence, stress fractures of the coronoid have been recognized. These athletes generally present with a mild (10- to 15-degree) elbow flexion deformity and complain of discomfort with athletic performance. After the appropriate examinations for diagnosis, the treatment is usually event-performance modification and symptomatic treatment, with observation and the repeat of tests until return can be advised. Surgery, open or arthroscopic, is usually not necessary.

There are four grades of functional severity that provide guidelines for treating the skeletally immature athletes who present with growth-related problems[9] (Table 8-1). Grade I problems generally improve with restricting play for a minimum of 4 to 6 weeks. Grade II will generally improve after a short break or limited participation, and in some cases, a temporary change in position (e.g., from pitcher to first base). Grade III problems are more severe, with a minimum of 12 weeks of treatment and rest, and in certain cases, a permanent change in position or performance. Athletes with grade IV problems will not be able to play for a minimum of 6 months, and should be advised to consider surgery. Other sports are often recommended.[9]

There are specific congenital abnormalities in the elbow area that have a significant impact on athletic performance. A congenital variance in the relationship of the radial head to the capitellum may limit forearm rotation and cause elbow arthralgia that limits function and performance (Fig. 8-33). In some instances, the inability to perform certain athletic activities may be the presenting complaint that points to the diagnosis of an intrinsic deformity, such as a radioulnar synostosis (Fig. 8-34).

The majority of fractures seen about the elbow in the growing child are not discussed here as they are well described in standard texts on pediatric orthopedic fracture treatment. There are two fractures that should be noted, however, since they may contribute to potential elbow problems in the skeletally immature athlete: (1) residual deformities associated with a proximally displaced epiphysis fracture (Fig. 8-35); and (2) unrecognized recurrent radial dislocation of the Monteggia fracture, associated with disruption of the annular ligament (Fig. 8-36).

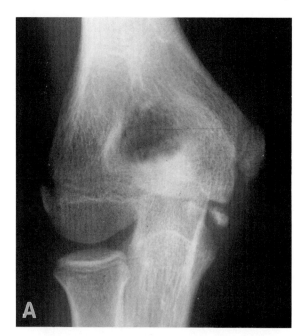 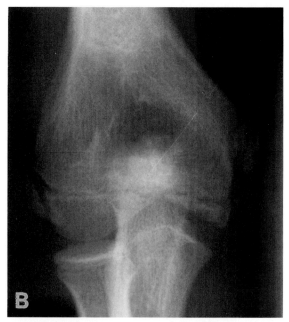

Figure 8-32 (A & B) This 12-year-old tennis player presented with elbow pain and a 20-degree elbow flexion deformity. The radiograph demonstrated irregular ossification pattern of his trochlea. Following a period of relative inactivity and limited tennis playing, the elbow flexion deformity improved, as did the ossification pattern of the trochlea that ultimately developed to a normal-appearing trochlea. This is an example of a developmental osteochondrosis of the trochlea.

Table 8-1   Grades of Functional Severity of
Elbow Injuries

Grade I
    Ache during performance
    No limitation of performance
    No residual pain after performance
    No physical examination changes
    No radiographic changes
Grade II
    Ache/minimal pain during performance
    Mild limitation of performance
    Mild ache after performance
    Minimal local tenderness
    Presents with mild deformity and limited motion
    Early radiographic changes (comparison views)
Grade III
    Pain during performance
    Obvious change of performance
    Pain after performance
    Presents with flexion deformity and limited motion
    Definite radiographic change
        Osteochondritic defect
        Asymmetry of articulation
Grade IV
    Pain during performance
    Major change of performance
    Physical examination change
        Muscle atrophy
        Decreased motion
        Crepitation
        Intermittent locking
    Advanced radiographic changes
        Articular degeneration
        Osteocartilaginous fragments

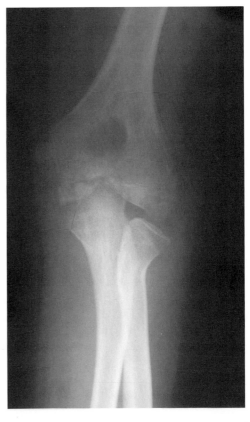

Figure 8-33 This 13-year-old young man presented with elbow discomfort, a mild flexion deformity, and inability to completely rotate his forearm. The multiple changes of the elbow include the abnormal development of the proximal radius as well as the osteochondrotic changes of the capitellum and trochlea.

Figure 8-34 A 10-year-old girl with a congenital synostosis of her proximal radius and ulna. This deformity remained unrecognized until her parents became aware that she was unable to perform certain athletic maneuvers such as throwing a ball normally and performing some early-stage gymnastic maneuvers. The recommendation was not to attempt any surgical takedown of such a synostosis but to observe the functional development for normal activities of daily living and to advise regarding selected athletic activities.

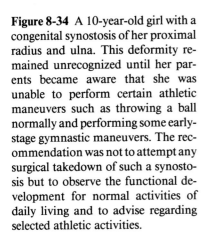

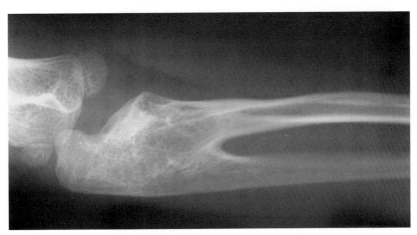

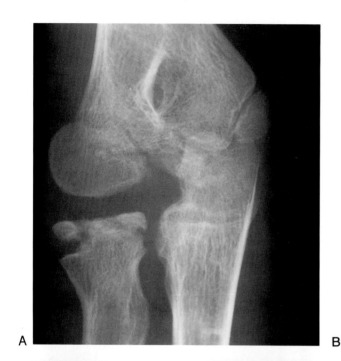

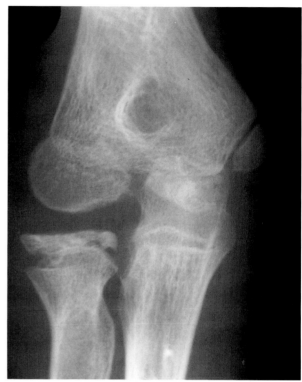

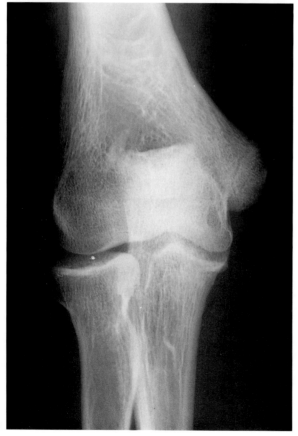

Figure 8-35 (A–C) This 11-year-old boy sustained a displaced fragmented fracture of his radial head. He was treated without surgery and monitored regarding his selection of athletic activities to limit stress as much as possible on his elbow. The ultimate result 5 years postinjury was a normal-appearing radiograph and a normal-functioning elbow.

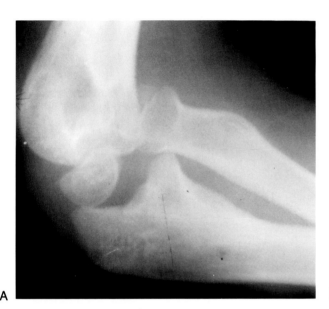 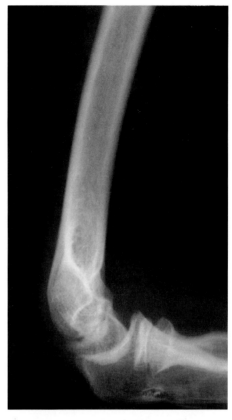

A   B

Figure 8-36 (A & B) This 7-year-old boy sustained a dislocation of his radial head in addition to a forearm fracture. The radial head remained unstable. It was observed during fluoroscopic examination that his radial head could be completely reduced with supination; however, it became unstable with forearm pronation. The annular ligament was disrupted and was reconstructed using a fascia lata graft. **(B)** At 4 years follow-up, showing a stable elbow and a normal range of motion, although the secondary changes in the neck of the radius, the location of the reconstructed annular ligament, should be noted.

Forearm

Fractures of the forearm are common in skeletally immature athletes. The mechanism is usually a direct blow or fall on the outstretched hand. The treatment for these injuries is discussed in other textbooks. Three areas of concern in the long-term complications of these injuries and the skeletally immature athlete should be noted: (1) the residual deformity that limits forearm rotation (Fig. 8-37); (2) the premature closure of either the distal ulna or radius physis resulting in discomfort and instability; and (3) the asymmetrical incomplete physeal arrest that ultimately causes progressive pain, limited function, and deformity (Fig. 8-38). The earlier these problems are recognized, the better the long-term athletic outlook. Unfortunately, many of these problems are not recognizable for a number of months or years postinjury. Thus, it is important to advise the family and other health care professionals on the need for periodic examination and the

clinical concerns that may follow all fractures and physeal injuries.

Wrist

Injuries to the wrist area in skeletally immature athletes usually are associated with a fall on the outstretched hand with varying degrees of axial and rotational forces. If the forces are mild, the usual presentation will be a grade I (mild) sprain and treatment is as outlined. If the forces are greater, the most likely injury will be a physeal fracture of the radius and/or ulna with possible long-term results noted. Identifiable injuries to the carpal bones are rare but do occur. The most likely focus for a carpal injury is the scaphoid-lunate complex. These injuries rarely present as isolated cases and related combination injuries should be evaluated (Fig. 8-39). A fractured scaphoid may be the obvious presentation of a more complex

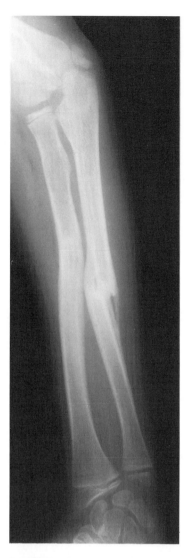

Figure 8-37 This young man sustained a fracture of both bones of his forearm when he fell during a soccer game. The incomplete reduction has resulted in a bony block that limits forearm rotation.

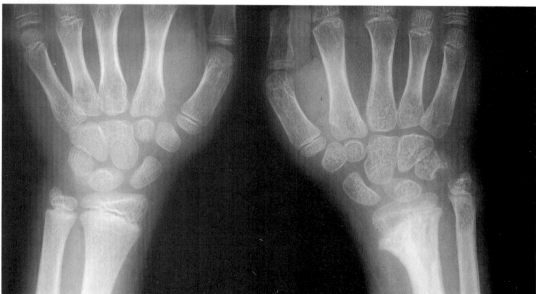

Figure 8-38 This 9-year-old boy fell on his outstretched hand during a soccer game, and sustained an open fracture on the volar aspect of his wrist with secondary infection in the area of the displaced radial physis. The cessation of growth in the radial physis and the continued growth of the ulna physis have resulted in asymmetrical wrist mechanics. The treatment recommendation included a shortening of the ulna with a concurrent resection of the distal ulna physis.

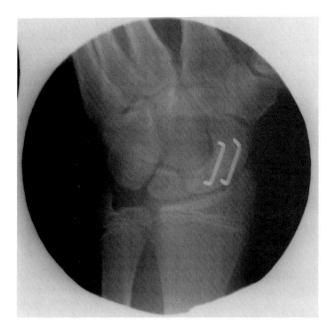

Figure 8-39 A 14-year-old football player sustained a fracture of his scaphoid with an associated ligamentous disruption of the scapholunate complex. To perform the open reduction, the scaphoid was stapled and the ligamentous disruption repaired. Carpal fractures and ligamentous disruptions can occur in skeletally immature athletes.

perilunate dislocation, including a scapholunate ligamentous injury.

In young athletes who perform forceful repetitive wrist motions (gymnasts, volleyball players) and have relative ligamentous laxity (inherent or acquired), wrist pain is a frequent complaint. This may represent instability secondary to excessive motions or a true anatomic variant. If excessive motion is evident, then the etiology of the pain may be associated with performance hypermobility, instability with subluxation, or perhaps secondary to cartilage compression trauma. If there is a variance in the length of the ulna or radius, the dynamics of the wrist will be altered, and athletic activity will likely cause wrist pain, secondary to instability or impingement. For example, if the ulna is shortened on a congenital or postinjury basis, the carpus will tend to drift in that direction with each forceful function. It has been suggested that both hypermobility and an ulna minus (shortened ulna) may contribute to the etiology of Kienbock syndrome. These factors along with forceful and/or repetitive dorsiflexion contribute to instability and the effect on vascularity or cartilage compression. It is unusual to diagnose Kienbock syndrome by radiograph in the skeletally immature athlete; however, persistent or recurrent wrist pain may be the prodrome of the syndrome (see Ch. 24).

Hand

Injuries to the hand are usually associated with direct trauma. The concerns in many instances are similar to adults regarding alignment and function, but the major differences are physeal involvement and the presence of an underlying pathogenic condition. The physeal involvement must be specifically evaluated in all metacarpal and phalangeal fractures, dislocations, and apparent tendon avulsions. The typical interphalangeal dislocation in the skeletally mature athlete most likely represent a physeal fracture in the skeletally immature athlete (Fig. 8-40).

The typical baseball (mallet) finger in the skeletally mature athlete is secondary to an avulsion of the extensor tendon, whereas an injury in the skeletally immature athlete is most likely associated with a physeal injury of the distal phalanx (Fig. 8-41). Fractures involving the base of the proximal phalanx are commonly seen in sports such as football and basketball, where forced compression, extension, and adduction or abduction occur. Tolerance for fracture malalignment is the same as those for the adult athlete. (See the discussion of these parameters in Ch. 25).

Fractures of the distal phalanx deserve special mention because of the deforming forces of the terminal extensor tendon and the flexor digitorum profundus, often resulting in a characteristic deformity. Due to these forces, these fractures are frequently unstable.

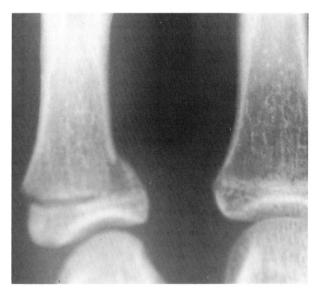

Figure 8-40 AP radiographic view of a displaced Salter III fracture of the base of the proximal phalanx of the index finger.

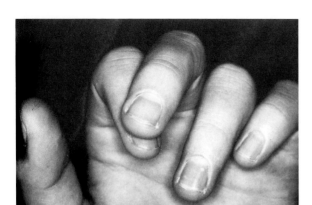

Figure 8-41 Clinical photograph of the patient in Figure 8-40 with a malrotation of the index finger manifested by the criss-crossing of the index and middle fingers.

Often, there is associated injury to the nail matrix from the angulation of the fracture, which needs to be addressed. The threshold for removing the nailplate (to inspect the matrix) should be quite low. If there is a subungual hematoma associated with this fracture, then the likelihood of an associated matrix injury is

high. If the matrix has been lacerated, it should be repaired under loupe magnifications. Careful consideration should be given to pin fixation of this fracture because of its unstable configuration. If internal fixation is utilized, a smooth, nonthreaded wire can be placed transfixing the fracture as well as the distal interphalangeal joint. Central placement of a smooth wire across the physis for a short period of time (3 weeks) will have minimal adverse effects on physis growth. The pin should be removed as early as possible, and therapy to begin range of motion should begin at this time. However, mobilization of the adolescent digit should commence earlier—at approximately 3 weeks because of the usual vigorous healing in these fractures.

Special mention should be made of the concept of remodeling in pediatric fractures. The two major long-term concerns in the skeletally immature relate to rotational deformity and physeal damage. If possible, these problems should be included in the early treatment phase. Often the treating physician will accept less of an

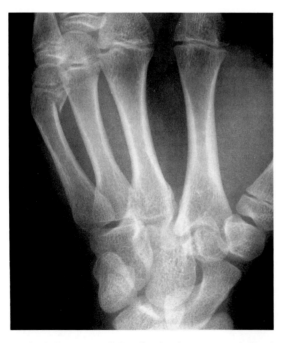

Figure 8-42 Fracture of the distal 5th metacarpal that has resulted in both angular and rotational deformities. The early evaluation of this combination of deformities permits for the manipulative reduction necessary to avoid the residual rotational deformity.

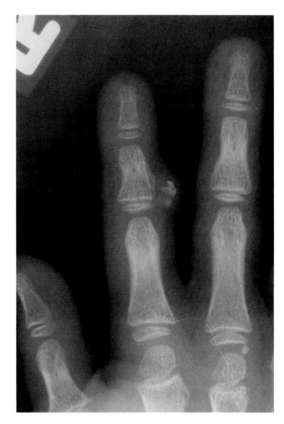

Figure 8-43 This active young woman experienced progressive deformity and discomfort with functional activity. An epiphyseal dysplasia is evident in the region of her middle phalanx. One must be careful to minimize surgical trauma to the existing physis to avoid asymmetrical closure.

anatomic alignment in the child because of the concept of bone remodeling over time. Rotational malalignment is perhaps the most worrisome and most frequently seen deformity in metacarpal and phalangeal fractures. Therefore, concerns about maintenance of rotational alignment and the thresholds for operative intervention should be the same for the child as for the adult (Fig. 8-42).

Metacarpal and phalangeal fractures are often secondary to a predisposing pathologic origin. In these instances, minimal trauma or discomfort with athletic performance may cause the young athlete to limit activity and seek medical advice (Fig. 8-43).

REFERENCES

1. Pappas AM: Epiphyseal injuries in sports. Phys Sports Med 11:140, 1983
2. Pappas AM: Osteochondroses: diseases of growth centers. Phys Sports Med 17:551, 1989
3. Peterson HA: Physeal fractures of the elbow. p. 248. In Morey BF (ed): The Elbow and Its Disorders. 2nd Ed. WB Saunders, Philadelphia, 1993
4. Wedge JH: Fractures of the neck of the radius in children. p. 266. In Morrey BF (ed): The Elbow and Its Disorders. 2nd Ed. WB Saunders, Philadelphia, 1993
5. Mudge MK, Wood VE, Frykman GK et al: Rotator cuff tears associated with os acromiale. J Bone Joint Surg [Am] 66:427, 1984
6. Eidman DK, Shift SJ, Tullos HS: Acromioclavicular lesions in children. Am J Sports Med 9:150, 1981
7. Siffert RS: The osteochondroses. Clin Orthop 158:2, 1981
8. Adams JE: Injury to the throwing arm: a study of traumatic changes in the elbow joints of boy baseball players. California Med 102:127, 1965
9. Pappas AM: Elbow problems associated with baseball during childhood and adolescence. Clin Orthop 164:30, 1982
10. Shaughnessy WJ, Bianco AJ: Osteochondritis dissecans. p. 282. In Morrey BF (ed): The Elbow and Its Disorders. 2nd Ed. WB Saunders, Philadelphia, 1993
11. McManama GB, Micheli LJ, Berry MV et al: The surgical treatment of osteochondritis of the capitellum. Am J Sports Med 13:11, 1985
12. Singer KM, Roy SP: Osteochondrosis of the humeral capitellum. Am J Sports Med 12:351, 1984
13. Osebold WR, El-Khoury G, Ponseti IV: Aseptic necrosis of the humeral trochlea. Clin Orthop 127:161, 1977

<table>
<tr><td>9</td></tr>
</table>

Shoulder Anatomy and Function

Arthur M. Pappas

Athletic functions attributed to the shoulder complex cannot be discussed without an understanding of the individual and coordinated anatomy that make these functions possible. This understanding is critical for the evaluation and treatment of clinical problems of the upper extremity in the athlete. Although the focus of this chapter is anatomy and function, the potential of other anatomic interactions contributing energy and precision to the shoulder complex should be kept in mind as well.

Athletic functions that demand upper extremity action require more than single-joint motion, and all functions described as single-joint motion (e.g., shoulder, elbow, wrist) in fact represent multiple joint interactions. Interference in the total interaction of movements resulting in shoulder motion potentially influences an apparent specific pattern of function. A single distant anatomic variance can negatively impact comprehensive shoulder motion (e.g., hamstring strain, lumbar nerve root irritation, thoracic intercostal muscle strains, cervical neuropathy) and will result in altered function and increased stress to the shoulder to compensate for the varied pattern of function. Pain and dysfunction of the shoulder complex may occur as a result of this compensation. The cervical spine is a frequent site of pathology that is either referred or reflected as a shoulder problem. Thus, apparent problems of the shoulder may reflect variances of anatomy and function at a different site in the total sequence of functions.

Likewise, abnormal shoulder function will contrib-

ute to other problems at distal locations (e.g., shoulder dysfunction in baseball pitchers or javelin throwers, resulting in altered elbow function and pain). Within the shoulder complex, limited glenohumeral motion requires increased scapulothoracic activity, resulting in muscle fatigue, pain, and dysfunction.

The anatomic basis of the biomechanics and function of the shoulder complex is discussed in the sequence of joints—sternoclavicular, acromioclavicular, glenohumeral, and scapulothoracic. Within each of the following sections, the relevant osteology and arthrology is presented as is the complementary myology associated with specific motions. The last part of this chapter is devoted to a more detailed examination of function and how the anatomic parts coordinate for a highly specialized pattern of motion.

The advent of shoulder arthroscopy, careful evaluation of athletic performance, recent laboratory investigations, image studies (e.g., computed tomography with arthrography, magnetic resonance imaging, ultrasound), new electroneurodiagnostic techniques, contrast arteriography, and noninterventional studies of angiographic patterns have all contributed to our current understanding of shoulder anatomy and dysfunction. Despite these advances, there is still minimal information on the central neurologic control and microanatomy that allow one individual to have extraordinary skill in an upper extremity-dominated sport, while others with apparently similar anatomy do not have this capability. An analysis of each component of shoulder anatomy, however, does yield information on the known intricacy that makes function possible. The anatomy presented here focuses on structures that most frequently contribute to athletic functions and performance. Other comprehensive details of anatomy are well described in many textbooks and should be referred to for details.

ANATOMY

Sternoclavicular Joint

The sternoclavicular joint, the connection between the manubrium portion of the sternum and the clavicle, is a diarthrodial joint and the only true skeletal articulation that exists between the shoulder complex and the axial skeleton. The joint is saddle-shaped, with the longer axis in the superoinferior direction, the concavity more on the sternal side, and the convexity on the clavicular side. The clavicular end is larger than the sternal component, and there is a cartilaginous disc between the clavicle and the sternum. The ligamentous stability is primarily accounted for by four ligaments: superior, inferior, anterior, and posterior (Fig. 9-1). The anterior ligament is generally considered the strongest ligament. The inferior portion of the sternoclavicular joint is further stabilized by the costoclavicular ligament that attaches from the medial clavicle to the first rib. These fibers are primary limiters of superior displacement, whereas anterior and posterior fibers are contributors to joint stability. The motion at the sternoclavicular joint is variable in the four anticipated directions and contributes a universal-type rotation critical for accommodating clavicular rotatory motion required for internal and external rotation of upper extremity sports function.[1] Although the clavicle is an important link in the skeletal continuity, the midportion is a major external protector of the underlying axillary artery and brachial plexus. The major vascular and neural structures posterior and lateral to the sternoclavicular joint offer a greater potential for catastrophic injury (see Chs. 14 and 15).

The rotation of the clavicle at the sternoclavicular joint presents a rotation of approximately 10 degrees with internal rotation and approximately 50 degrees with the extreme position of elevation, external rotation, and extension.[2,3] The greater amount of clavicular motion at the acromioclavicular articulation is a factor in the significantly higher rate of acromioclavicular joint injuries compared to sternoclavicular joint injuries. The major muscle attachments to the clavicle include the sternocleidomastoid medially, the pectoralis major and the subclavius in its midportion, and the trapezius and deltoid laterally.

Acromioclavicular Joint

The acromioclavicular joint is a diarthrodial and plane-type joint that has a slight anterior effacement. The articular surface of the acromion is slightly concave to accommodate the articular surface of the distal clavicle, which is a convex broad surface directed anteriorly and inferiorly.[4] The shape of the distal clavicle and the acromion may vary as to the angle of the acromioclavicular joint configuration. The acromioclavicular ligaments are strongest in the anterior and posterior aspects of the joint, and there is an intricate association of these ligaments to the intra-articular disc and the synovial cavity that may be associated with the proprioceptive control of the acromioclavicular joint. These acromioclavicular ligaments are more involved

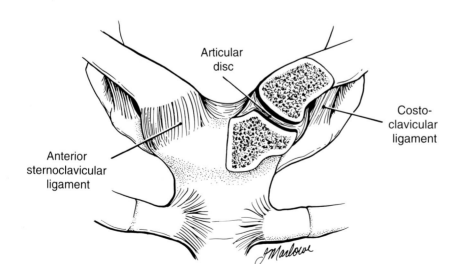

Articular disc

Costo-clavicular ligament

Anterior sternoclavicular ligament

Figure 9-1 The sternoclavicular joint, emphasizing the relationship of the clavicle and manubrium with the ligamentous relationships that provide the major stability and the intra-articular relationships that contribute to mobility.

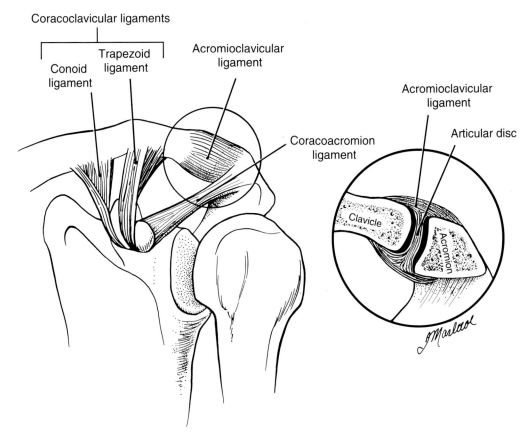

Figure 9-2 The acromioclavicular joint with identification of the ligaments that provide the stability to the joint: coracoclavicular ligaments, acromioclavicular ligaments, and coracoacromial ligament.

in the anteroposterior movement and rotatory control of the joint. At 2 cm medial to the distal end of the clavicle is the attachment site for the coracoclavicular ligament, which includes the trapezoid and the conoid ligaments (Fig. 9-2). These ligaments control the superoinferior motion of the acromioclavicular joint and will be indirectly programmed with the acromioclavicular and coracoclavicular ligaments-discs relationship. The trapezoid component is larger, and, together with the conoid, limits anterior, posterior, and superior displacement of the clavicle. This ligamentous linkage is the strongest direct connection between the scapula and the clavicle. The peripheral capsule and ligaments of the acromioclavicular joint are not as tight as those at the sternoclavicular joint. They are associated with the required greater range of motion at the acromioclavicular joint than the sternoclavicular joint and emphasize the significance of the coracoclavicular ligaments for clavicular and scapular stability. The coracoacromial ligament is a part of the shoulder complex and a border of the impingement space. The motion at the acromioclavicular joint is primarily one of rotation and secondarily one of gliding.[3] The rotation is necessary as

a contributor to accommodate scapular motion, thereby providing the direction and effacement of the glenoid for coordinated glenohumeral motion.[1]

The variety of motions and the relative laxity of capsular ligamentous structures associated with the acromioclavicular joint contribute to the rate of injury. Concurrent fracture of either the distal clavicle or acromion, and disruption of the articular disc and variable degrees of ligamentous injury of the conoid and trapezoid ligaments, help determine both the severity of the injury and the goals of anticipated treatment[1,2,5] (see Ch. 14).

Glenohumeral Joint

The osteology of the glenoid and proximal humerus, the minimal containment of the humerus by or within the glenoid, and the extreme global mobility attributed to this joint, emphasize the uniqueness and anatomic importance of the capsule, ligamentous structures, and rotator cuff.

The proximal humerus is retroverted approximately

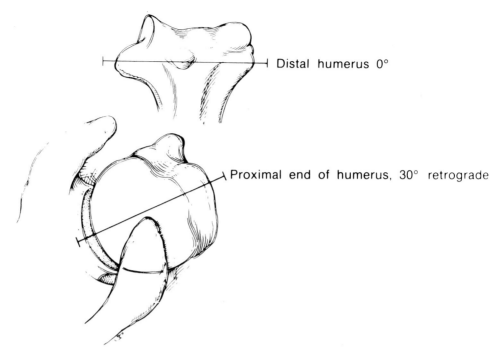

Distal humerus 0°

Proximal end of humerus, 30° retrograde

Figure 9-3 Anatomic alignment of the humerus with the position of the humeral head retroverted approximately 30 degrees in relation to the epicondylar alignment of the distal humerus.

30 degrees in relation to the epicondylar alignment of the distal humerus (Fig. 9-3). The angle of inclination between the shaft and head of the humerus is approximately 45 degrees (Fig. 9-4). The articular surface of the proximal humerus encompasses approximately two-thirds of the head. Saha[6] has reported that the articular surface of the humeral head and the receptive articular surface of the glenoid reveals a relationship of

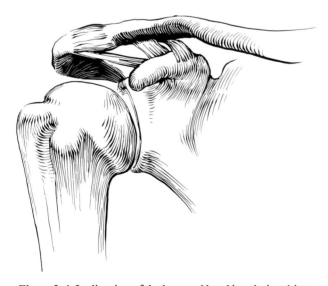

Figure 9-4 Inclination of the humeral head in relationship to the shaft of the humerus, an angle and inclination of approximately 45 degrees.

0.8 in the coronal plane and 0.6 in the horizontal-transverse plane. This observation is consistent with others who note that less than one-half the articular surface of the humeral head is in contact with the glenoid at any specific point in motion. The position of the scapula on the thorax presents a 30 degree forward direction of the glenoid cavity (Fig. 9-5). The glenoid is directed from the body of the scapula with a slight tilt posteriorly of approximately 5 degrees and in approximately a 5 degree inferior effacement, providing more posterior and inferior bony stability.

The glenohumeral joint is not a true ball-and-socket joint. The configuration of this joint places the retroverted humeral head in position with the posterior and inferior osseous alignment of the glenoid, resulting in minimal bony constraint in the anterior and superior planes. The glenoid is part of the scapula and therefore imparts significant motion to coordinate with the humeral head; it is not analogous to the relatively immobile acetabulum. The primary containment in the anterior and superior planes is provided by the soft tissue structures: glenoid labrum, superior glenohumeral ligament, biceps tendon, middle glenohumeral ligament, inferior glenohumeral ligament, coracohumeral ligament, and rotator cuff.

One significant difference between shoulders and other joints is the visible capsular thickenings (i.e., the glenohumeral ligaments) involvement in shoulder function. These structures are critical for maintaining

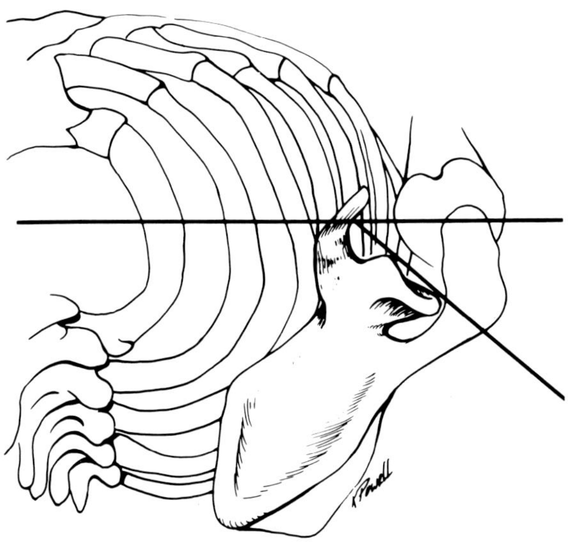

Anterior

Posterior

Figure 9-5 Position of the scapula on the thorax. The three-dimensional view emphasizes the multidirectional potential of the scapular motion and highlights the effacing anatomy of the glenoid and the minimal anterior bony containment.

the balanced centralization of the humeral head in or on the glenoid. To achieve this remarkable articular relationship and stability, these structures must be interactive and dynamic in their individual and collective actions. The changes in appearance and function of the glenohumeral ligaments will depend upon the position and anatomic relationship of the humeral head to the glenoid. Through currently unknown neuroproprioceptive mechanisms, these structures coordinate the neuromusculotendinous interactions that direct for the synchronized rhythm between the scapula and the humerus.

The glenoid should not be considered a static receptacle within which the humeral head moves. The glenoid and scapula must move in relationship to the humeral head. It is functionally deepened by the glenoid labrum to accept and provide containment for the humeral head. The glenoid labrum is a fibrous and fibrocartilaginous structure, histologically similar to the meniscus of the knee[7,8] (Fig. 9-6). The labrum mechanically increases the potential containment of the humeral head within the glenoid. Its anterior and inferior peripheral attachment is histologically and intricately related to the glenoid, and its superior portion is histologically combined with the origin of the long head of the biceps.[7]

The superior glenoid labrum-biceps tendon relationship represents an important anatomic site for clinical problems often observed in throwing athletes.

The looseness of the labrum and its conjoined anatomy with the biceps tendon provides less constraint to superior and rotational motion of the humeral head in the maximum portions of external rotation/abduction and extension.[9] If the humeral head is not centralized within the glenoid, the superiorly directed force will contribute to superior instability and will have a shearing impact on the undersurface of the rotator cuff (see Ch. 13).

The histologic and physiologic features of the anterior and inferior labral glenoid relationship indicate that this junction is significant as a mechanical stabilizer. The glenoid labrum anatomic relationship changes with age and contributes to various shoulder problems.[4] A disruption of this labral glenoid interface will contribute to instability. The degree of disruptions and the related integrity of the middle and inferior glenohumeral ligaments as well as the subscapularis tendon containment will determine the clinical degree of anteroinferior instability (see Ch. 11). Yet just as important is the presumed proprioceptive relationship of the labrum anteriorly and inferiorly to the dynamic activity of the glenohumeral ligaments. This relationship is significant, since it provides a coordinated constraint force, making this inherently unstable joint, which provides multidimensional motion, more stable. The ligamentous structures of the shoulder are closely associated with the capsule and labrum in providing support, constraint, containment, control, and a proprioceptive response for glenohumeral joint function.

Anteriorly, there are the superior glenohumeral, middle glenohumeral, and inferior glenohumeral ligaments with these arrangements simplified into one **Z** pattern[10] (Fig. 9-7). O'Brien and colleagues[11] have noted that the inferior ligament has an anterior and a posterior component. When these structures are observed from the anterior vantage, the **Z** pattern includes the coracohumeral ligament combined with the superior glenohumeral ligament — the cross of the **Z** is the middle glenohumeral ligament, and the inferior bar is the inferior glenohumeral ligament.[10] The inferior glenohumeral ligament has an anterior and posterior attachment, and each of these attachments provides different functional aspects.[11]

The superior glenohumeral ligament has been identified as a constant structure over 90 percent of the time. When the shoulder is arthroscopically approached from the posterior, the opening of the subscapularis bursa is easily seen. The superior portion of this opening is the superior glenohumeral ligament, which appears to resist external rotation in the first 60 degrees of glenohumeral abduction, contributes to humeral suspension, and resists inferior translation.[9,12]

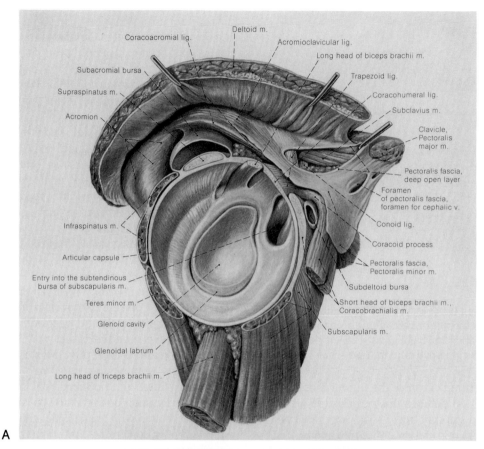

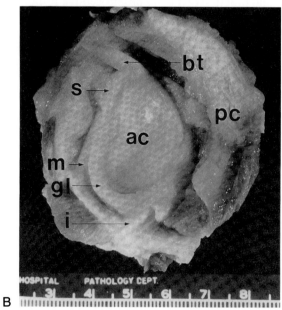

Figure 9-6 **(A)** Glenoid effacement and relative location of intra- and extra-articular structures. **(B)** Glenoid anatomy in a skeletally immature boy. The size and configuration of the labrum are demonstrated as more significant structures than in Fig. A.

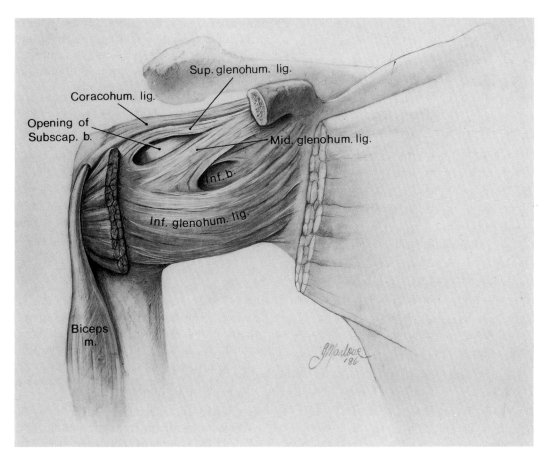

Figure 9-7 Relationship of the major ligaments of the glenohumeral joint form the anterior advantage demonstrating the position of the ligament with the shoulder at rest.

The relationship between the superior glenohumeral ligament, the origin of the biceps tendon, including its shared relationship to the glenoid labrum, and the rotator cuff constitute an anatomic meeting point where problems in the overhead-throwing athlete are often identified.

The middle glenohumeral ligament has greater variability of presentation and is identified as significantly attenuated or absent in approximately 8 to 30 percent of anatomic observations.[4,10] The middle glenohumeral ligament originates from the labrum immediately below the superior glenohumeral ligament and passes across the subscapularis tendon. It inserts just medial to the lesser tuberosity, contributes to support of the extremity, and restrains external rotation from 0 to 90 degrees in conjunction with the superior glenohumeral ligament. It is a primary restraint at 45 degrees but can go up to 90 degrees.

The inferior glenohumeral ligament has been reportedly identified in the 80 to 90 percent range; however, if the area of the ligament is palpated, a thickening will be appreciated 100 percent of the time. The consistent presence of the ligament has been confirmed microscopically by O'Brien and colleagues.[11] The inferior glenohumeral ligament is a contributor to the containment in abduction, with the majority of the dynamic component related to the anterior portion in conjunction with the middle glenohumeral ligament for containment in extension and external rotation. The posteroinferior glenohumeral ligament contributes inferior and anteroinferior stabilization of the glenohumeral joint, particularly in the extreme position of cocking (Fig. 9-8). The close interaction of the middle glenohumeral ligament and both the anterior and posterior portions of the inferior glenohumeral ligament contribute to the limitation of humeral head mobility in abduction, extension, and external rotation. Acquired ligamentous laxity or an avulsion of the middle and/or the inferior glenohumeral ligaments are often associated with anterior instability and recurrent dislocation (Bankart lesion).[12,13]

The shoulder has multidimensional range of motion with the humeral head staying centered within the glenoid in its (near) 360 degree rotations. If there is a

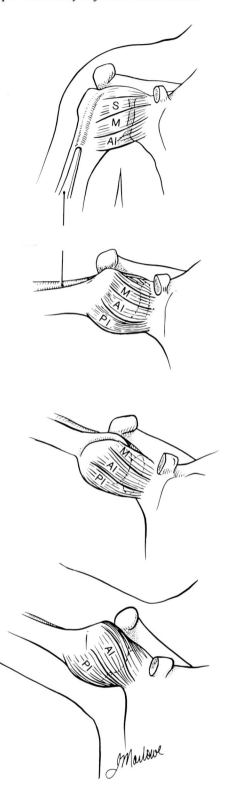

Figure 9-8 Changing relationship of the major glenohumeral ligaments during the cocking phases of pitching. The position of the ligaments must be integrated with a changing position of the humeral head in relationship to the glenoid and scapular motion.

variance of more than a few degrees in the centering of the humeral glenoid relationship, symptoms of instability will be manifested. The symptoms and dysfunction depend on the degree of decentralization and functional demands.[14,15] (see Ch. 11).

Scapulothoracic Joint (Articulation)

As compared to the sternoclavicular, acromioclavicular, and glenohumeral joints, the scapulothoracic joint is not a diarthrodial joint. The scapulothoracic joint represents scapular motion as it moves about the rib cage (Fig. 9-9). There is a bursa mechanism that facilitates this jointlike function. The undersurface of the scapula is concave and moves in a gliding fashion about the convex rib cage. The motion of the scapula on the thorax is multidimensional and intricately associated with combined humeral motion. The overall pattern of motion includes an integration of scapulothoracic and glenohumeral motions. When multidimensional shoulder motion is discussed, it is implied that both components are critical and balanced.

The skeletal connection of the scapula to the axial skeleton is through the clavicle to the sternum and the supportive coracoclavicular ligaments. The osseous processes include the coracoid, glenoid, and acromion (Fig. 9-10). The coracoid process is the attachment for three muscles: the short head of the biceps, the coracobrachialis, and the pectoralis minor. The area above the scapula spine, the supraspinatus recess, contains the body of the supraspinatus muscle and the suprascapular notch through which pass the supraspinous nerve and artery. The notch is covered by the superior transverse ligament, an important anatomic area for throwing athletes.[16] The spinoglenoid notch, inferior to the glenoid scapula junction, is the continuation of the

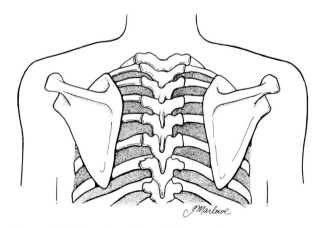

Figure 9-9 Normal position of the scapulae.

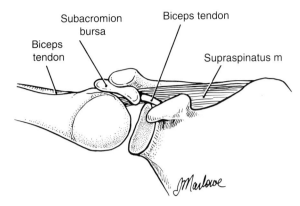

Subacromion bursa

Biceps tendon

Biceps tendon

Supraspinatus m

Marlowe

Figure 9-10 Relationship of the humeral head in 90 degrees of abduction and external rotation to the glenoid with the associated change in position of the biceps tendon and supraspinatus muscle. These changes are related to commonly observed clinical problems reported by overhead performance athletes.

suprascapular nerve and artery. These structures then continue to the infraspinatus muscle and the posterior glenohumeral joint capsule. The acromion is the superior portion of the shoulder that accounts for proximal coverage of the glenohumeral articulation and stability of the shoulder complex through the acromioclavicular joint and the clavicle to the axial skeleton. The mobility that occurs through the acromioclavicular joint directs and coordinates the glenoid motion, especially in the phases requiring abduction and external rotation.

There is considerably more information on glenohumeral motion than scapulothoracic motion.[15,17] However, unless they are considered as a unified and combined motion, the information is incomplete when applied to clinical situations. When the scapula is fixed, the forces associated with humeral motion on the glenoid cannot be considered equivalent to the forces of combined glenohumeral motion.[17] The reported humeral scapular motion ratio varies from 2 : 1 to 3 : 2.[18,19] However, these motions reflect scapular pendulum motion and do not represent other more complex three-dimensional scapular motions. The scapula may elevate, depress, adduct (retract), abduct (protract), and pivot with the fulcrum in the neck of the glenoid[6,20] (Figs. 9-11 and 9-12).

The multiple complex movements of the scapula must be coordinated and integrated with the multiple complex movements of the humerus and clavicle to achieve the ultimate function. The studies performed usually have focused on only one aspect of total shoulder functional anatomy. Thus, we are not able to provide as broad a scholarly scientific basis for shoulder function compared to experiential clinical observa-

tions. There are various groups of muscles that interactively result in this motion, including the thoracoscapular, vertebroscapular, scapulohumeral, thoracohumeral, and clavicular; these are listed in Table 9-1. The activities of these individual muscles have been comprehensively discussed by several authors.[18,21-25] Although individual motions are basic to the primary functions, comprehensive patterns of anatomic interactions are essential for the understanding and evaluation of normal and abnormal function and athletic performance.

In clinical situations, direct or indirect dysfunction[26] of any of the muscles involved in glenohumeral motion may produce two results: (1) a change in the relative relationship or interaction of the glenoid with the hu-

Table 9-1 The multiple muscles involved in all comprehensive shoulder motions

Vertebrao scapular
  Trapezius
    Middle
    Lower
  Rhomboid
    Major
    Minor
  Levator scapulae
Thoracoscapular
  Serratus anterior
  Pectoralis minor
Thoracohumeral
  Latissimus dorsi
  Pectoralis major
Scapulohumeral
  Subscapularis
  Supraspinatus
  Infraspinatus
  Teres minor
  Teres major
  Deltoid
    Anterior
    Middle
    Posterior
  Biceps
    Long head
    Short head
  Coracobrachials
  Triceps
    Long head
    Lateral head
    Medial head
Clavicular
  Sternocleidomastoid
  Omohyoid
  Scalenae
  Deltoid
  Trapezius
  Pectoralis major

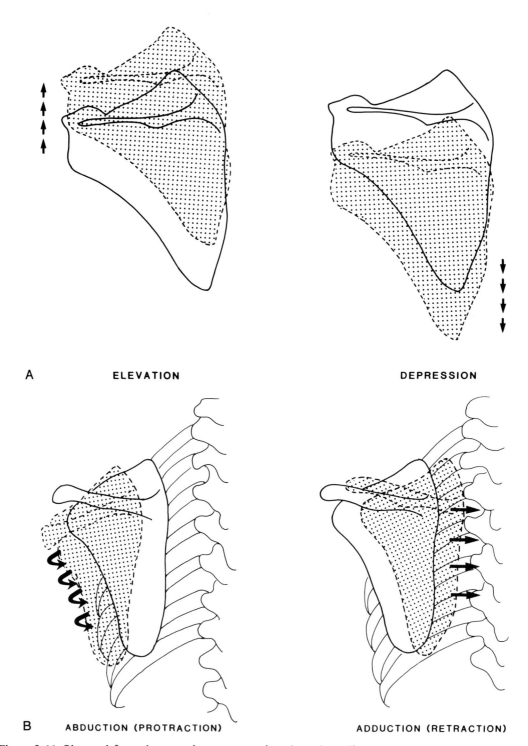

A   ELEVATION   DEPRESSION

B   ABDUCTION (PROTRACTION)   ADDUCTION (RETRACTION)

Figure 9-11 Observed from the posterior vantage point, these three diagrams document the resting position of the scapula and the dynamic motion of the scapula during the assessment of comprehensive shoulder motion. **(A)** The superior elevation and the depression of the scapula. **(B)** The abduction (protraction) or adduction (retraction) of the scapula in relationship to the spinous processes, as well as the third dimension of motion about the thorax. *(Figure continues.)*

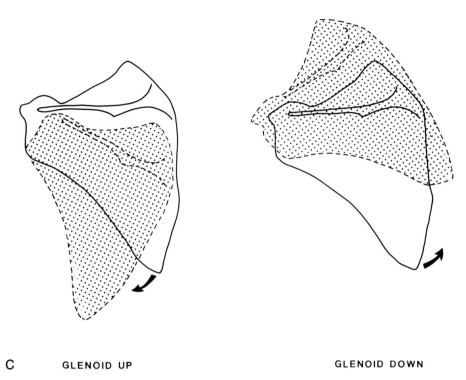

C   GLENOID UP   GLENOID DOWN

Figure 9-11 *(Continued)* **(C)** The rotation of the total scapula and repositioning of the glenoid, with the peak fulcrum of this rotational angle just medial to the spinoglenoid region.

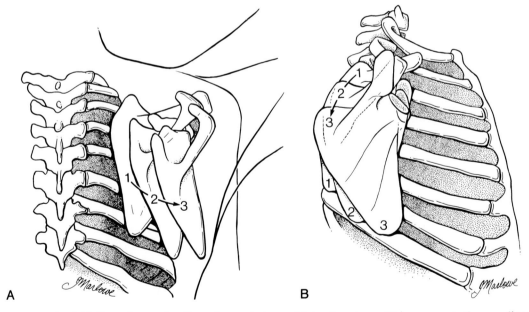

Figure 9-12 (A & B) Scapular motion from the posterior and lateral vantages. This represents the coordinated motion of the scapula in relationship to the thorax, requiring integration of the motion of the humeral head in relationship to the glenoid.

meral head, and (2) disruption of the coordinated synchronous scapulohumeral motion. If either of these events occurs, there undoubtedly will be pain, altered motion, and dysfunction.

The integrative action of these various muscles results in multidimensional activity of comprehensive shoulder motion. The coordinated function of this entire pattern can be compared to a well-rehearsed symphony. If each musculotendinous interaction is not properly orchestrated, an altered performance will result. The change may be very gradual (e.g., a slight alteration of ligamentous capsular laxity, traction injuries of certain ligamentous tendon structures, neurovascular variations, and/or shearing changes of the labrum) (*Dynamic Instability* in Ch. 11). This interaction of multiple units must act in a desired synchrony of concentric and eccentric contractions of the musculotendon units, coordinated with appropriate flexibility and balanced strength. These should result in the appropriate multidimensional control of both scapulothoracic and glenohumeral rhythm.[18,23]

There is not yet a comprehensive understanding of how this multidimensional activity occurs with minimal skeletal stabilization. The shoulder has anatomically and functionally evolved over many centuries to its functional human status today. Evolution has contributed to specific adaptations necessary for athletic performance, but related research studies in other species as well as opportunities for laboratory input are extremely limited. Most laboratory investigations have been confined to individual and limited aspects of shoulder motion and stability. In most instances, the humeral head and scapula-glenoid relationship is not integral to the evaluation—either the scapula is stabilized or static observations are recorded.[17] These techniques often direct the attention away from the potential significance of the interaction of the anatomic contributions.

Additional information on various anatomic contributions to comprehensive shoulder motion has been provided by clinical observations of abnormal shoulder function with certain congenital abnormalities and acquired problems. These observations provide an opportunity to evaluate the effect of specific anatomic alterations on "shoulder motion."

The child with an abnormal scapula or occasionally a total fixation to the cervical and thoracic vertebra by an omovertebral bone, and limited or absent scapulothoracic motion associated with Sprengel's deformity or Klippel-Feil syndrome, will demonstrate abnormal or no scapulothoracic motion (Fig. 9-13). This limitation of scapulothoracic motion results in excessive force on

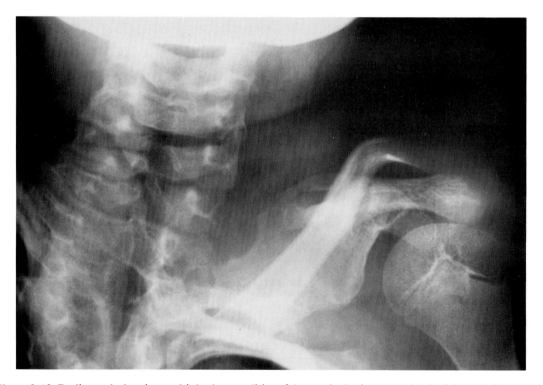

Figure 9-13 Radiograph showing multiple abnormalities of the cervical spine, scapula, clavicle, and rib cage of a young man. He develops his entire range of motion without any scapula contribution, resulting in a weak and limited range of motion entirely of the humeral head in relation to the other abnormal anatomy.

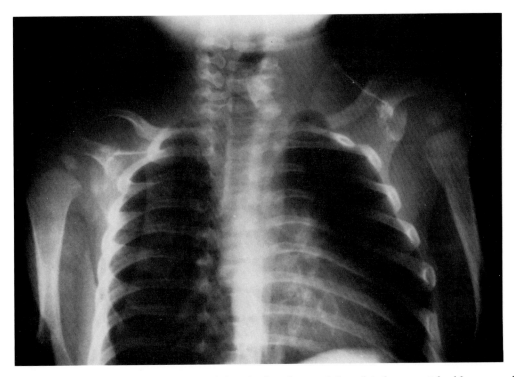

Figure 9-14 Radiograph showing Sprengel's deformity in a boy and the related omovertebral bone providing complete fixation of the scapula to the cervical thoracic spine. The lack of scapular motion is associated with unusual stress with any attempts at humeral motion, which resulted in a dislocation of the humerus in relationship to the glenoid.

the glenohumeral articulation. Humeral head motion within the glenoid and without scapular contribution will result in total shoulder motion that develops into a subluxation and/or a frank dislocation of the humeral head in relation to the glenoid. The totally immobile scapula requires the dislocation as a necessary adaptation to achieve any shoulder motion, and demonstrates the required integration of scapulothoracic and humeral motion for comprehensive shoulder function (Fig. 9-14).

The child with typical Erb's obstetric palsy will progressively develop an internal rotation and adduction deformity of the humerus. If this deformity is untreated, the progressive unbalanced forces on the humerus will result in posterior subluxation or dislocation of the humeral head in relation to the glenoid, with associated secondary overgrowth of the acromion and coracoid. This demonstrates the impact of an acquired muscle imbalance on the development of a progressive humeral and scapular deformity.

The child with a congenital nonunion of the clavicle or a cleidocranial dysostosis demonstrates the importance of the clavicle as the only true skeletal connection of the upper extremity to the axial skeleton. Such a clavicular deficiency influences scapula and acromio-

clavicular joint function, and results in limited shoulder motion as well as abnormal patterns of function. These children are unable to throw a normal pitch mechanism and tend to push it instead (Fig. 9-15).

An individual with neuromuscular function interruption will present various patterns of abnormal function, which may result from trauma or viral infections. For example, an individual with a long thoracic nerve palsy will demonstrate scapular "winging" and will not be able to adequately control the scapula due to serratus anterior paralysis. The effect of the lack of scapular control clearly creates the abnormal location of the glenoid in relation to the humeral head, as well as the inability of other muscles to function properly.

PATTERN OF FUNCTION

Knowledge of the individual anatomic components directly involved in comprehensive shoulder motion is a necessary requisite for a complete shoulder evaluation, and the successful treatment of various abnormal patterns of shoulder motion.[27] Although the anatomy is usually similar in all athletes, the patterns of function may be vastly different (e.g., baseball pitcher, gymnast,

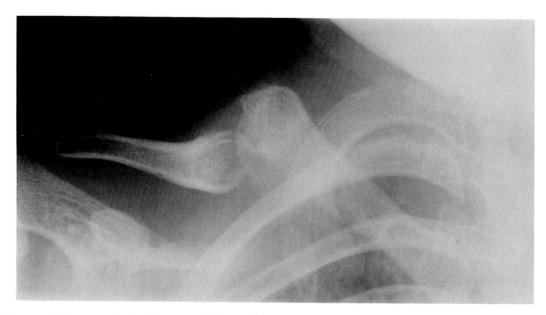

Figure 9-15 Radiograph showing congenital nonunion of the clavicle in a young boy. This abnormality resulted in a limited ability to perform normal upper-extremity activities.

power weight lifter, swimmer).[26] Thus, an understanding of the biomechanical demands resulting from the integrated functions of individual anatomic structures is required.

The experienced coach is often capable of advising an athlete of an undesirable or less effective pattern of motion without knowledge of the underlying anatomy. The challenge to health professionals is to combine anatomic knowledge with the experiential observations of the coach to better condition, train, and rehabilitate the athlete with specific problems. The nuances of each pattern of upper extremity function is not discussed in this section; however, the baseball pitch is discussed as an example.

Analysis of Pitching Sequence

Analysis of a baseball pitch provides the most studied pattern of integrated comprehensive shoulder motion.[26] The baseball pitch is divided into four phases: wind-up, cocking, acceleration, and deceleration.[28-31] These phases are important in relation to the anatomy of the articulations, their related ligaments, and the contributions of various interactive muscle groups that have an impact on ultimate function, possibly leading to dysfunction (Fig. 9-16).

The pitch begins with the push-off power of plantar flexion and rotation on the great toe and ankle and proceeds through the kinetic energy chain to the shoulder complex. It has been estimated that in the best

biomechanical pitch, approximately one-half of the velocity of the overhand throwing is contributed by the lower extremity and trunk.[29,32] Any impairment in the earlier components of the kinetic energy chain sequence will have a significant impact on the integrated pattern of the shoulder complex motion. The remainder of the discussion describing the pitch is limited to the details of shoulder motion.

Wind-Up

The wind-up is the pitching phase between the initiation of motion and the moment at which the ball is removed from the glove.[29-32] It is by far the most individualized and variable of the four pitching phases, dependent on and reflective of a pitcher's personal style. This phase lasts from 500 to 1,500 ms and generally presents more complex total body motion than high-demand shoulder complex motion. There is generally not a consistent identifiable pattern for the wind-up, since each pitcher is unique. The purpose of the wind-up is threefold: (1) to place the body at a biomechanical advantage so that all segments appropriately contribute to the propulsion of the ball; (2) to establish a rhythm in order to achieve appropriate positioning and timing of subsequent movements; and (3) to conceal the ball and distract the hitter. The personal style variables may include trunk rotation, a high leg kick, or variable arm motions, yet these variables are not universal characteristics of the baseball pitch.

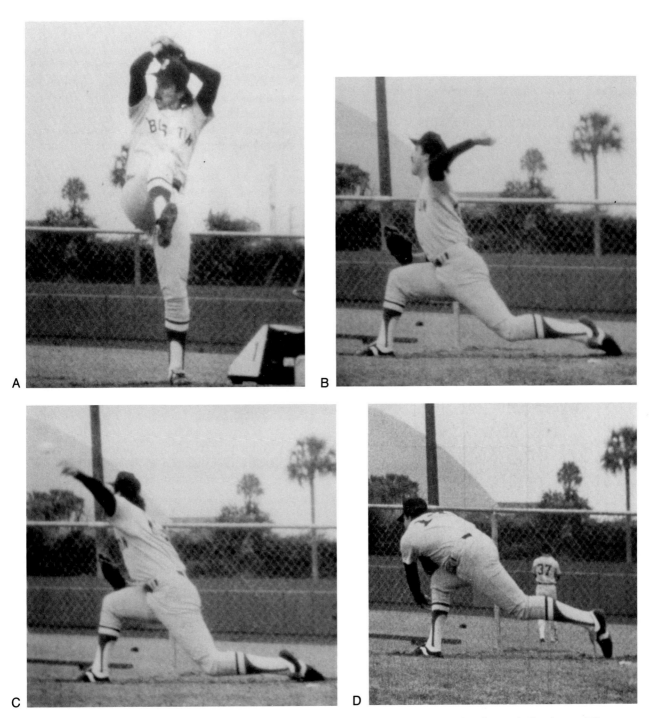

Figure 9-16 The four phases of pitching. **(A)** Wind-up. **(B)** Cocking. **(C)** Acceleration to ball release. **(D)** Deceleration. It is important to consider these four phases not only for the relationship of arm-shoulder position but for their sequential relationship to the total body movement.

Cocking

The cocking phase begins as the ball leaves the glove, and the shoulder complex moves into 90 degrees of abduction and maximum horizontal extension. The maximum horizontal extension of at least 30 degrees is then reduced to neutral horizontal extension (Fig. 9-17) and maximum external rotation to 180 degrees occurs. This sequence terminates the cocking phase and prepares for the beginning of the acceleration phase. The cocking phase lasts for 500 to 1,000 ms and the combination of the wind-up and cocking phases accounts for 80 percent of the pitching sequence.

During the cocking phase, there is concurrent movement of all shoulder articulations. The sternoclavicular and acromioclavicular joints externally rotate to accommodate for clavicular rotation. The humeral head changes from its initial position of 35 degrees of retroversion (or internal rotation) to approximately 135 degrees of external rotation, bringing the greater tuberosity well under and posterior to the acromion, positioned toward the posterior glenoid. The humeral head proceeds into a position of 90 degrees of abduction and 30 degrees of extension, and external rotation to 180 degrees, with the center of the humeral head

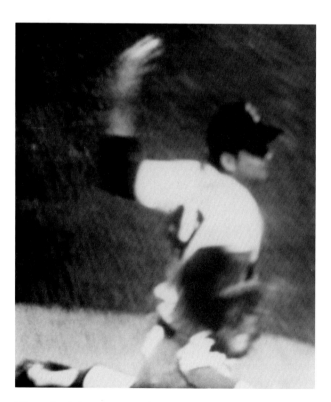

Figure 9-17 In the phase of cocking, prior to achieving maximum external rotation, there is a definite component of maximum extension of the shoulder.

directed anteriorly with minimal skeletal containment (Fig. 9-18). The direction and function of the glenohumeral ligaments must change significantly. The superior glenohumeral ligament follows the humeral head and reaches from its anterosuperior position adjacent to the biceps tendon on the scapula glenoid, while the humeral insertion of the superior glenohumeral ligament is directed posteriorly, since the position of the humeral head is now directed posteriorly. The middle glenohumeral ligament extends from its point of origin on the glenoid and labrum and is directed at an angle to an area of the superoposterior position on the humerus under and slightly posterior to the anterior edge of the acromion. The anterior component of the inferior glenohumeral ligament extends from the anteroinferior glenoid origin across the anterior portion of the glenohumeral joint to an area near the acromion. The posteroinferior glenohumeral ligament is directed from its glenoid position toward the anteroinferior area of the humerus, providing a fan-shaped containment of the anterior and inferior aspects of the glenohumeral joint and, with the subscapularis, provides the primary anterior buttress of the glenohumeral joint[11] (Fig. 9-19).

It is difficult to perceive these ligamentous structures as static, although specific dynamic functions have not been attributed to them. Yet the maintenance of stability, with the extremes of motion demanded by specific athletic functions, indicates the probable dynamic interactive function of these soft tissues. The ligamentous, labral, and glenoid relationships will be a source of continuing investigation to determine their contribution to the dynamic patterns.

The overhead-throwing pattern, which includes external rotation, extension, and most likely a slight superior migration of the humeral head, results both in compression of these structures as well as traction on the glenohumeral ligament-labral relationship. This motion is also associated with traction and compression on the bicipital origin superior labral area. This combination of forces often contributes to a wearing of the anterosuperior labrum, fraying and/or reactive tissue about the biceps, and partial or incomplete tears and fraying on the undersurface of the rotator cuff. If there is damage to these structures and probable rotator cuff weakness, there will be excessive humeral head mobility, resulting in a variety of clinical symptoms—anterosuperior and posterosuperior discomfort with overhead activity, bicipital tendonitis, supraspinatus tendonitis, and clinical evidence of an impingement syndrome (see Ch. 13).

This rotation of ligament directions becomes an important consideration when analyzing injuries. The ligamentous avulsion associated with the acute disloca-

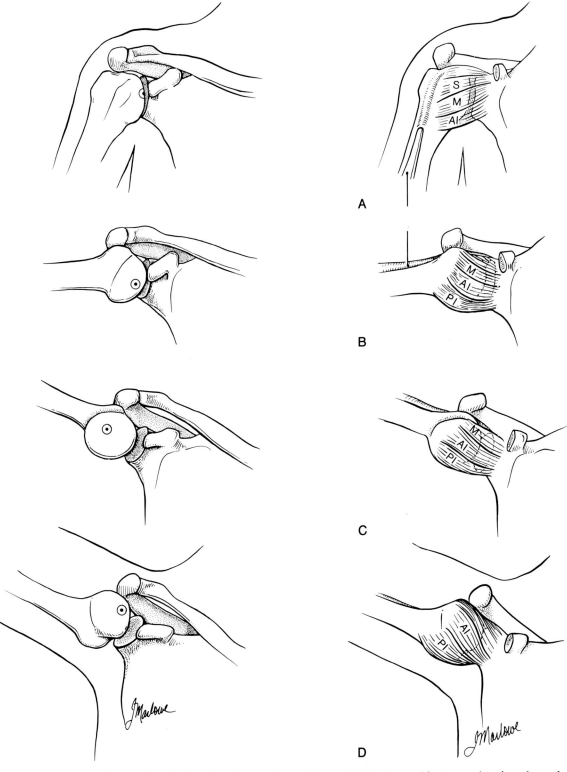

Figure 9-18 Osseous and articular relationship changes in the phases of pitching. The changes include the relative position of the humeral head, scapular glenoid, and the acromioclavicular relationship. The integration of each of these changes must be coordinated for an evaluation of comprehensive shoulder motion.

Figure 9-19 In the cocking to acceleration phase, the altered position of the major ligaments must be considered when analyzing pathologic function. **(A)** Neutral. **(B)** 90° abduction with limited external rotation. **(C)** With midexternal rotation of cocking. **(D)** With maximum external rotation and extension.

tion in the football arm tackle identifies the avulsion of the middle glenohumeral ligament or the anterior portion of the inferior glenohumeral ligament from the glenoid. The more common problem seen in the overhand pitcher is in the area of the superior portion of the joint—from the middle glenohumeral origin to the anterior superior labrum to the superior glenohumeral ligament to the biceps tendon and the adjacent rotator cuff (see Ch. 12). This damage is more likely a combination of traction secondary to the maximum extension, external rotation, and mild superior migration of the humeral head compressing and shearing the above-mentioned structures, as well as the anterior glenoid labrum shearing force of the rotating and anterior motion of the humeral head.

The scapulothoracic motion during the cocking phases directs the scapula through adducting (retracting) to the midline by concentric contraction of the serratus anterior, the three units of the trapezius, and the two rhomboid muscles.[33] During the cocking phase, the deltoid, supraspinatus, infraspinatus, and teres minor muscles are active concentric contractors, directing and maintaining the humeral head to its central position within the glenoid.[28,33] The subscapularis, pectoralis major, teres major, and latissimus dorsi muscles must eccentrically contract to serve as a protective mechanism to the external rotation motion.[31,33,34] The biceps tendon is positioned toward the posterior directing a traction force to the biceps/glenoid origins. This will account for the distraction and separation of the superior labrum frequently seen in baseball pitchers. The eccentric contraction of these muscles protects the anterior joint structures, which are placed under tension by the extreme degree of humeral head external rotation. At this point, the scapula has adducted and rotated the glenoid to efface as superior as possible, and the lower tip of the scapula is positioned at or beyond the midaxillary line, anterior to the position of the glenoid contributing to and accounting for "external rotation" of the arm. The thoracic spine also extends, decreasing kyphosis, and rotates as part of comprehensive shoulder external rotation (Fig. 9-20). Balanced action of the rotator cuff musculature is of prime importance in maintaining the humeral head centralized in and on the glenoid.

Acceleration

The acceleration phase begins with forward motion from the maximum position of external rotation and neutral horizontal extension and terminates with the moment of ball release. This phase averages 50 ms and is the most consistent phase of throwing in major

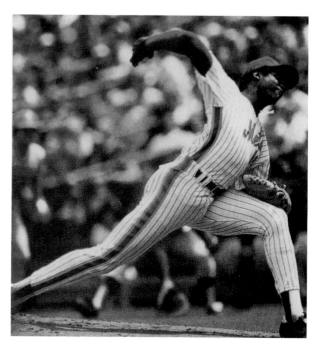

Figure 9-20 The motion of the thoracic spine reversal of normal kyphosis.

league pitchers.[29] It accounts for only 2 percent of the pitching sequence, and the forceful internal rotation of the shoulder generally changes from more than 160 degrees of external rotation to neutral at point of ball release (Fig. 9-21A). This will generate a peak shoulder velocity of 6,000 to 8,000 degrees per second (Fig. 9-21B).

During this phase, there is a powerful derotation of the humerus in the horizontal plane at 90 degrees of abduction. There is an associated scapular position change to gradual abduction or protraction (away from the midline) as well as a slight elevation, gradually redirecting the glenoid in relation to the humeral head as the reduction in external rotation is occurring. The body of the scapula returns to its more customary position on the thoracic cage, the lower tip of the scapula returns to a plane behind the glenoid, and the medial scapula border is parallel to the vertebral spine. This is most likely accounted for by contraction of the serratus, limiting the motion of the scapula; also a concentric contraction of the latissimus dorsi, pectoralis major, teres major, and the subscapularis muscles produces the internal rotational force. The majority of the effort appears to be directed toward derotation of the humerus within the glenoid.

The middle trapezius and rhomboid muscles eccentrically contract, while the lower and upper trapezius and serratus anterior muscles concentrically contract to stabilize the scapula and permit the distal tip to rotate on the rib cage. While the scapulohumeral motion occurs, there is concurrent change in both the spine-thorax and scapula-clavicle-sternum relationships. The sternoclavicular joint derotates, and the scapular acromion (in effect, the acromioclavicular joint) changes from external rotation to neutral. If the scapula-acromion unit is laterally displaced on the thorax secondary to muscle weakness and postural change, the medial compression and rotatory motion of the acromioclavicular articulation can result in increased acromioclavicular compression and articular change causing osteophyte formation that can result in secondary bursal inflammation and bursal side rotator cuff changes. Also, the lack of electromyogram activity observed in most muscles during the explosive acceleration phase must indicate some other controlling neurologic mechanism.[33] The spine motion change includes a combined motion of extension to normal kyphosis and derotation of the costovertebral complex. The recognition of these motion requirements contributes to the definition of the trunk aspect of conditioning/rehabilitation programs.

If there is a disruption in the rhythm of the pitch or stability of the shoulder during this phase, a pitcher usually becomes less effective and loses velocity, location, and ball motion (Fig. 9-22).

If a pitcher is unable to experience a complete and coordinated acceleration phase (approximately 90 degrees of combined scapulohumeral motion), there will be a loss of force directed to ball delivery. The cause of this functional impairment can be either anterior contracture and loss of flexibility or thoracoscapular scapulohumeral muscle imbalance. These are two basic concerns in the conditioning and rehabilitation of the throwing athlete.

Deceleration (Follow-Through)

The deceleration after ball release (or follow-through) phase allows for a comfortable deceleration of the entire throwing arm. The deceleration phase begins at the moment of ball release, a few degrees of external rotation and 90 degrees of shoulder flexion abduction, and continues through the completed motion.[29] This phase lasts approximately 350 ms and accounts for 18 percent of the pitching sequence. The shoulder complex moves into a position of horizontal flexion and internal rotation. There is intense activity in all muscle groups during this phase. The deceleration and derotation of the humeral head relative to the glenoid accounts for intense eccentric activity in the deltoid, supraspinatus, infraspinatus, teres major and minor, latissimus dorsi, and pectoralis major.[29] The posterior muscle groups controlling the scapula, trapezius, rhomboids, levator scapula, and serratus anterior are all eccentrically contracting to limit the rate and degree of the rotation and lateral migration of the scapula about the rib cage. The concentric contraction of the

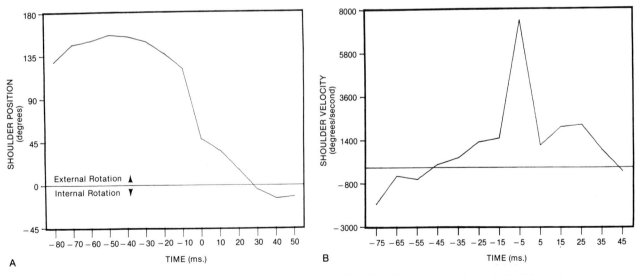

Figure 9-21 Excursion of shoulder rotation during the acceleration phase in a single pitch. Positive values are external rotation. Ball release occurred at zero on the time scale. **(A)** Derotation of approximately 150 degrees that occurs in approximately 40 ms is shown. **(B)** Extreme peak of shoulder velocity to more than 5,000 degrees per second during that same approximately 40-ms interval. These explosive changes cannot be duplicated with any of the exercise equipment currently available.

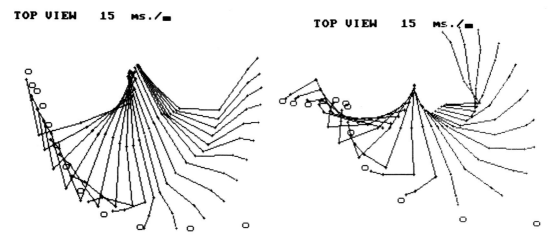

Figure 9-22 Computer-generated analysis of a good pitch on the left and an abnormal pitch, or a biomechanically poor pitch, on the right, demonstrating an interrupted sequence that is ultimately reflected in a loss of velocity and control. This reflection of a poor pitch may represent a number of potential problems, ranging from specific muscle weakness, abnormal positions and motions of the scapula, instability the glenohumeral joint, inflammation, or injury to any of a number of contributing musculotendinous units.

subscapularis muscle contributes to the early components of internal rotation and then becomes a more neutral factor. If these muscles have not been appropriately conditioned, or if they are injured, there will be progressive fatigue and an inability to control the scapula.

While the scapulohumeral change occurs, there is a change in the spine-thorax and scapula (acromion)-clavicle-sternum relationship—the spine increases its relative kyphosis, and the costovertebral complex increases its rotation to follow the upper extremity. The total deceleration process derotates the clavicle and increases the compressive forces on the acromioclavicular and sternoclavicular joints. If the muscular component is not properly balanced to control deceleration, the increase in compression on the acromioclavicular joint may contribute to discomfort and degeneration (see Ch. 14).

The purpose of this phase is to decelerate the throwing limb. It is during the transitional phase of acceleration to deceleration that the triceps and biceps become active. It is unclear if these are more active in their relationship to comprehensive shoulder motion or elbow acceleration and deceleration. They are probably involved in both areas but more likely contribute to the elbow biomechanics.[29]

The total range of motion throughout the pitching sequence represents more than 200 degrees of shoulder motion, ranging from a combined 170 degrees of external rotation at the maximum cocking phase and internally rotating to more than 45 degrees. This motion is not achieved only within the glenohumeral joint. The

contribution of the thoracic spine, scapula, and clavicle must be considered as significant parts of the total motion. The contribution of the scapulothoracic and glenohumeral motion is generally discussed in ratios that are more often determined on a two-plane model, as 2 : 1 or 3 : 2. However, these ratios do not reflect the multidimensional nature of scapular motion, the peripheral rotation of the scapula around the rib cage, or the directing and coordinating of the glenoid to the humerus and the acromioclavicular contributions to these motions. The importance of the scapula is much greater than generally considered in its contribution to comprehensive shoulder motion.

REFERENCES

1. Goss TP: Double disruptions of the superior suspensory shoulder complex. J Orthop Trauma 7:99, 1993
2. Fukuda K, Craig EV, An K, Cofield RH: Biomechanical study of the ligamentous system of the acromioclavicular joint. J Bone Joint Surg [Am] 68:434, 1986
3. Conway AM: Movements at the sternoclavicular and acromioclavicular joints. Phys Ther Rev 41:421, 1961
4. DePalma AF: Surgery of the Shoulder. JB Lippincott, Philadelphia, 1973
5. Rockwood CA, Matsen FA: The Shoulder. 1st Ed. WB Saunders, Philadelphia, 1990
6. Saha AK: Dynamic stability of the glenohumeral joint. Acta Orthop Scand 42:491, 1971
7. Cooper DE, Arnoczky SP, O'Brien SJ et al: Anatomy, histology, and vascularity of the glenoid labrum. J Bone Joint Surg [Am] 74:46, 1992

8. Prodromos CC, Ferry JA, Schiller AL, Zarins B: Histologic studies of the glenoid labrum from fetal life to old age. J Bone Joint Surg [Am] 72:1344, 1990

9. Bowen MK, Warren RF: Ligamentous control of shoulder stability based on selective cutting and static translation experiments. Clin Sports Med 10:757, 1991

10. Ferrari DA: Capsular ligaments of the shoulder. Am J Sports Med 18:20, 1990

11. O'Brien SJ, Neves MC, Arnoczky SP et al: The anatomy and histology of the inferior glenohumeral ligament complex of the shoulder. Am J Sports Med 18:449, 1990

12. Turkel SJ, Panio MW, Marshall J: Stabilizing mechanisms preventing anterior dislocation of the glenohumeral joint. J Bone Joint Surg [Am] 63:1208, 1981

13. Terry GC, Hammon D, France P, Norwood LA: The stabilizing function of passive shoulder restraints. Am J Sports Med 19:26, 1991

14. Howell SM, Galinat BJ, Renzi AJ, Marone PJ: Normal and abnormal mechanics of the glenohumeral joint in the horizontal plane. J Bone J Surg [Am] 70:227, 1988

15. Poppen NK, Walker PS: Normal and abnormal motion of the shoulder. J Bone Joint Surg [Am] 58:195, 1976

16. Ringel SP, Treihaft M, Carry M et al: Suprascapular neuropathy in pitchers. Am J Sports Med 18:80, 1990

17. Harryman DT, Sidles JA, Clark JM et al: Translation of the humeral head on the glenoid with passive glenohumeral motion. J Bone Joint Surg [Am] 72:1334, 1990

18. Inman UT, Saunders JC, Abbott LC: Observations on the function of the shoulder joint. J Bone Joint Surg 26:1, 1944

19. Kibler WB: Role of the scapula in the overhead throwing motion. Contemp Orthop 22:525, 1991

20. Saha AK: Mechanics of elevation of glenohumeral joint. Acta Orthop Scand 44:668, 1973

21. Basmajian JV, Bazant FJ: Factors preventing downward dislocation of the shoulder joint. J Bone Joint Surg [Am] 41:1182, 1959

22. Basmajian JV: Muscles Alive: Their Function Revealed by Electromyography. 3rd Ed. Williams & Wilkins, Baltimore, 1974

23. Freedman L, Munro RR: Abduction of the arm in the scapular and glenohumeral movements. J Bone Joint Surg [Am] 48:1503, 1966

24. Kent BA: Functional anatomy of the shoulder complex. Phys Ther 51:867, 1971

25. Perry J: Anatomy and biomechanics of the shoulder in throwing, swimming, gymnastics, and tennis. Clin Sports Med 2:247, 1983

26. Atwater G: Biomechanics of overarm throwing movements and throwing injuries. Exerc Sport Sci Rev 7:43, 1979

27. Dempster WT: Mechanisms of shoulder movement. Arch Phys Med Rehabil 46:49, 1965

28. Jobe FW, Moynes DR, Tibone JE, Perry J: An EMG analysis of the shoulder in pitching. Am J Sport Med 12:218, 1984

29. Pappas AM, Zawacki RM, Sullivan TJ: Biomechanics of baseball pitching. Am J Sport Med 13:216, 1985

30. Tullos HS, King JW: Throwing mechanism in sports. Orthop Clin North Am 4:709, 1973

31. Pappas AM, Zawacki RM, McCarthy CF: Rehabilitation of the pitching shoulder. Am J Sports Med 13:223, 1985

32. Pappas AM: Injury of the shoulder complex and overhand throwing problems. In Grana WA, Kalenak A (eds): Athletic Injuries. WB Saunders, Philadelphia, 1991

33. Jobe FW, Tibone JE, Perry J: An EMG analysis of the shoulder in throwing and pitching. Am J Sports Med 11:3, 1983

34. Townsend H, Jobe WB, Pink M, Perry J: Electromyographic analysis of the glenohumeral muscles during a baseball rehabilitation program. Am J Sports Med 19:264

10

Assessment of the Athlete's Shoulder

Arthur M. Pappas
Claire F. McCarthy
Richard Diana

Shoulder coordination and strength are necessary for all athletic function. In certain sports (e.g., baseball pitching) the shoulder may be the primary location for functional demand, while in other instances, it may serve to enhance the balancing mechanism (e.g., running, cycling, skating). The shoulder complex has a unique structural design, resulting in more mobility than any other area of the body while sacrificing some intrinsic stability. The mobility of the glenohumeral joint is facilitated by the sternoclavicular, acromioclavicular, and scapulothoracic components, which add significantly to the degrees of freedom of the upper extremity and thus to the variety of movement patterns in the athlete. Functional stability at the glenohumeral joint is achieved by the addition of the glenoid labrum, the 30 degrees retroverted position of the humeral head, and the scapulothoracic component, which optimally positions the glenoid fossa for the humeral head. To withstand the stresses placed on the shoulder complex by a variety of athletic function, joint integrity, muscle balance, and the integration of movement patterns must be maintained.

The clinical evaluation, as presented in this chapter, will result in a summary of information gained from three components: observation of the patient, historical review, and physical examination. Appropriate ancillary tests are determined after the clinical evaluation. Each component of the assessment is presented separately, although in clinical practice, integration of these components frequently occurs.

OBSERVATION OF THE PATIENT

The examiner's clinical observations begin with the athlete en route to the treatment room. The examiner's impression of the athlete's posture, such as a sloping shoulder and protective position of the arm, carriage of the shoulder and upper extremity while walking, and facial expression while exchanging greetings and initial interactions (e.g., a grimace or other dramatic demonstration) often determines the tone and direction of the interview.

Critical observation of the athlete continues throughout the assessment. How comfortably are positions changed? Is the involved arm used for support?

Are there spontaneous voluntary movement patterns? What are the patterns used in undressing and dressing? How do the observations made by the examiner compare with information supplied by the athlete and ultimately become integrated with findings of the clinical examination?

HISTORY

Some of the history can be obtained from the patient prior to the actual visit (Fig. 10-1); however, the conversation that occurs between introductions and the beginning of the physical examination is integral to diagnosis. A positive relationship and rapport can be established during discussions of the presenting problems associated with the athlete's activity. The age of the patient will also influence the evaluation. The same symptoms of discomfort in the physically mature athlete will involve different diagnostic considerations from the skeletally immature athlete. Detailed information on the presenting problem, other relevant history (e.g., medical status, other injuries, hand preference), and any treatment used (both in the past and the present) should be considered.

Pain is an important element in any musculoskeletal assessment. The presence or absence of pain, whether it is acute or chronic in nature, and levels of pain intensity should be addressed during all aspects of the clinical examination. Observations of body language while the pain is described may alert the examiner to the voluntary dislocator. The examiner's observation of the athlete's affect in describing the pain provides certain clinical impressions on the intensity and disability associated with the pain. For example, the athlete may point to a specific area and grimace when attempting to abduct his or her arm. Identifying the onset of pain with a specific incident (arm tackle, basketball rebound, volleyball spike, seizure), a repetitive action (e.g., overhead lifts in pairs skating, serves in tennis), or one component of a specific pattern (e.g., the point of contact with a ball during a forehand tennis stroke) should also be noted and reviewed in detail.

Assessment of the pain affect or how the athlete "feels" about the injury, its impact on participation, self-esteem, and peer relationships is as important to an evaluation and the rehabilitative process as is the assessment of the sensation of pain. Although considered subjective, an attempt to evaluate pain is relevant when based on the examiner's visual observations and impressions along with the patient comparing the degree of current pain with other painful or pain-inducing experiences. Numerical and comparative pain scales

are helpful. The Visual Analog Scale (VAS)[1] is both a valid and reliable method of assessing the sensation and affect of pain. A verbal numerical scale similar to the VAS is also frequently used[2] (Fig. 10-2). In athletes with special needs, the Faces Method[3,4] can be used as an alternate method of pain measurement. The self-report ratings provided by the athlete are helpful evaluative factors and important as outcome measures. In addition, the examiner's experience with other patients, pain comparison with other injuries, and contrasting individual responses and performance modifications provide a guide for pain interpretation.

It should also be remembered that pain may be used as a gracious way to withdraw from an event that is undesirable to the athlete. For example, an adolescent who no longer wants to compete often presents with undiagnosable pain in a location that is prominently involved in the athletic event. Likewise, an athlete whose performance is recognizably depreciating may introduce pain as the apparent problem in order to gracefully exit. In these situations, it is sometimes impossible to diagnose the source of pain, since there are no objective or physical findings. As a result, conflicts may occur between the patient, the parents (if the patient is a child), and health care professionals, resulting in numerous tests and consultations, and, in some instances, surgery.

Does the athlete describe a certain part of a recognized performance pattern as abnormal? For example, does the basketball player limit rebound performance because of anterior instability apprehension or symptoms? Does the swimmer limit or alter stroke mechanisms because of acute pain? Additional questions should focus on painful experiences at times other than during athletic performance (i.e., positions and motions in daily activities that are painful or uncomfortable, the presence of night pain, and necessary alteration of sleeping positions). Does the athlete have a known seizure disorder or a history of posterior dislocation or subluxation? If so, is it difficult or painful to reach across the body to grasp an object? Are there changes in dressing habits (e.g., elimination of overhead sweaters, a change to a front-closing bra) or in personal hygiene (e.g., showering, shaving, or hair care)?

For a baseball pitcher, the chronic pain described may be associated with several symptoms, including instability of the glenohumeral joint, a weak or inflamed rotator cuff, or dysfunction of scapular control musculature. These symptoms may be reflected by one or more performance measures: in fewer innings pitched per game; decreased velocity; an increase or decrease in the use of certain pitches; an inability to throw and locate the ball accurately; or an alteration in

PATIENT SCREEN (PREVISIT):

Name:_____
Date: _____ MR#: _____

Completed by patient:

Sport(s): _____   _____
Competitive   Recreational

Hand used in eating/writing: _____R _____L

Describe (injury, condition, problem); be specific: How: Major problems:
                                                        When: Major limitations:

Pain (with activity): _____Yes _____ No. If yes, complete below.
    Location (pain and activity):   Level
                                                     None   Worst
    _____   0 _____ 10
    _____   0 _____ 10
    _____   0 _____ 10

Pain (without activity): _____Yes _____ No. If yes, complete below.
    Location: Level
    _____   0 _____ 10
    _____   0 _____ 10
    _____   0 _____ 10

Pain on touch/pressure: _____Yes _____ No. If yes, complete below.
    Location: Level
    _____   0 1 2 3 4 5 6 7 8 9 10
    _____   0 1 2 3 4 5 6 7 8 9 10
    _____   0 1 2 3 4 5 6 7 8 9 10

Changes in sensation (numbness, dullness, etc.):
    _____Yes _____No
    If yes, describe (location, type, level):

Impact on/interference with athletic participation:
    _____Yes _____No
    If yes, describe (amount of time, intensity level,
    ability to perform, etc.):

On the scale below, rate how you "feel" about your injury.
    0 _____ 10
    (Best)   (Worst)

Medications taken: _____Yes _____No
    If yes, _____ Prescription   _____ Nonprescription
            _____ Name   _____ Name
            _____ Dosage   _____ Dosage
            _____ Frequency   _____ Frequency

    Side effects: _____Yes _____No
        If yes, describe:

    Impact on performance: _____Yes _____No
        If yes, describe:

Daily activities affected in order of rank (worst/most painful = 1):
    _____ Putting on shirt, jacket, blouse
    _____ Taking off shirt, jacket, blouse
    _____ Tucking in shirt/blouse
    _____ Putting on overhead sweater/shirt
    _____ Taking off overhead sweater/shirt
    _____ Eating/drinking
    _____ Combing hair
    _____ Brushing teeth
    _____ Pulling off bed sheets/spreads
    _____ Rectal cleaning
    _____ Opening doors
    _____ Pushing doors/objects
    _____ Reaching for objects overhead
    _____ Other, describe

Assistive equipment used: _____Yes _____No
    If yes, describe (type, frequency/duration of use,
    affect):
Other concerns:

    _____
    _____
    _____

Figure 10-1 Evaluation form to be completed by the patient before the visit.

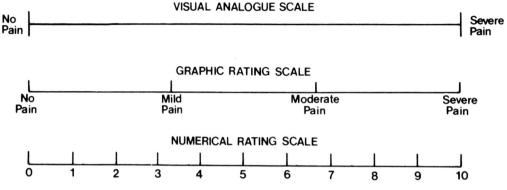

Figure 10-2 Various scales for rating patient's pain levels.

the motion of the pitched ball. Reviewing the pitcher's earned run average (ERA) statistic, innings pitched, ball motion, and velocity changes provides information and measures functional outcome.

The following is a suggested sequence of questions to answer when obtaining the history:

1. The length of time the symptoms have been noted and whether there was a specific precipitating event (a description and demonstration of the event is important).
2. The presence (past or present) of changes to touch, and pressure or sensations (e.g., burning, "pins and needles").
3. Whether there is a perception that the shoulder is coming out of place, slipping (if so, in what direction(s)), or locked? What maneuvers cause these symptoms?
4. Does fear (apprehension) of the problem limit any activities, e.g., swimming, throwing, skiing?
5. Does a particular position of the arm cause symptoms and, if so, what position? An anteriorly unstable shoulder will generally be symptomatic when the arm is above the horizontal, extended, and externally rotated. A posteriorly unstable shoulder will generally be symptomatic when the arm is below the horizontal, adducted, and internally rotated. An inferiorly unstable shoulder will generally be symptomatic when the arm is dependent, especially with attempts to lift heavy objects. Symptoms associated with a multidirectionally unstable shoulder are variable and depend upon the predominant direction(s) of instability.
6. Does the clinical problem or pain occur during sleep?
7. Is there pertinent general medical history, e.g., convulsions, arthritis, other hospitalizations, injuries.
8. What diagnostic tests have been performed and are available to review?
9. What treatment (including medication, surgery, physical therapy) has been used in the past? Both prescribed and self-determined care should be considered.
10. How does the athlete feel about the injury? How has it

affected him/her personally? Have relationships with the coach and with team members changed?

Information on medication should also be obtained:

1. The type, frequency, and effect of medication use for pain relief (e.g., analgesic, anti-inflammatory, steroidal, and nonsteroidal); injections, frequency, dosage, subsequent rehabilitation, and ultimate response should be documented along with intercurrent injuries or episodes of disability.
2. An accurate record of usage for both prescription and nonprescription medication.
3. The perception of the value of medication on motion and performance.
4. Any side effects of medication (e.g., gastrointestinal, headache, hepatic, renal, and secondary treatment for side effects).

The historical information may be expedited if the patient prerecords the answers to many of these questions (Fig. 10-1). Although in certain cases, evaluating the athlete's verbal responses to these questions can be used to elicit more questions, direct or focus the examination, and determine the need for supplemental tests.

When the historical component of the examination is completed, the transition to the physical examination should be performed with the clinical evaluator present. Significant information is missed if the evaluator leaves the area, although in certain instances it may be socially inappropriate to remain. It is beneficial to specifically observe how a patient physically rises from a chair as well as the method of moving an outer garment such as a coat or shirt. The impression of discomfort as well as motions included or avoided provide clinical indicators. When maximum information has been gathered and assimilated by the examiner, a carefully planned physical examination should be performed.

PHYSICAL EXAMINATION

The physical examination of the shoulder should be performed with maximum exposure of both shoulders. The male athlete should disrobe to the waist and the female athlete should be prepared with a halter top or an appropriate gown that allows for complete visibility and freedom of motion of the glenohumeral joint and scapulae of both extremities. The examiner should follow a planned sequence (comfortable for the patient, efficient for the examiner) and utilize the standing, sitting, and recumbent positions as needed for completion of the comprehensive physical examination. Our preferred sequence for the examination is as follows:

1. Inspection
2. Palpation
3. Active motion
4. Passive motion
5. Individual muscle examinations
6. Sensation tests
7. Neurovascular tests
8. Standard tests or specific clinical tests

Following this sequence, the need for supplemental examinations or tests such as radiography, arthrography, computer tomography, magnetic resonance imaging, electroneurodiagnosis, Doppler ultrasonography, and/or arteriography is determined.

Inspection

Inspection of specific areas begins with the athlete assuming either a standing or sitting position. Sitting is a good starting position, particularly if this is a first

injury and the examination is a new experience for the athlete. Conversation is generally more relaxed and resting postures can be easily observed. For the adolescent or younger patient, the sitting position provides a feeling of security and a degree of control of the situation (Fig. 10-3).

Inspection should be made by comparing the contralateral side, which is assumed to be normal. However, in bilateral sports, such as swimming and gymnastics, comparison may be difficult and reliance on anatomic relationships becomes a necessity. Information on observed surface irregularities such as asymmetry of specific anatomic area surfaces, obvious atrophy, contusions, local swelling, scars, and variations of color (representing vascular variations or potential sources of infection) is obtained through inspection and can be enhanced through a continuing dialogue with the athlete. A decrease in muscle volume of either the supraspinatus or infraspinatus will alert the examiner to likely rotator cuff dysfunction. Atrophy of these muscles may be secondary to neurapraxia of the suprascapular nerve or intramuscular injury or inflammation and secondary disuse/pain atrophy.

A relaxed resting posture should be observed and alignment compared with ideal posture (Fig. 10-4). If there is acute pain, the shoulder is likely to be held slightly elevated and forward—a combination of scapular protraction, elevation, and humeral internal rotation. This is easily observed from either the anterior or posterior vantage. If there is a chronic problem, such as with a baseball pitcher, the shoulder and scapula may be depressed, partially protracted, and anteriorly positioned (Fig. 10-5).

From the side, a forward head and rounded forward-

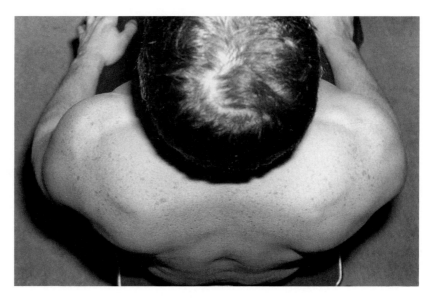

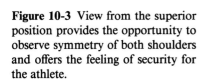

Figure 10-3 View from the superior position provides the opportunity to observe symmetry of both shoulders and offers the feeling of security for the athlete.

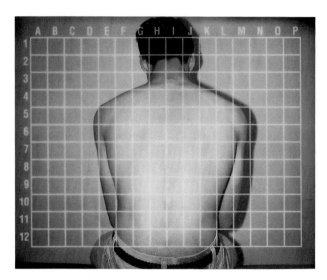

Figure 10-4 Relaxed resting posture observed and alignment compared with ideal posture. Grid film allows for a more objective evaluation of shoulder symmetry. (Photograph courtesy of Polaroid.)

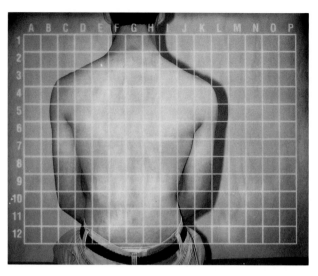

Figure 10-5 Upright posture using grid film to evaluate the relative elevations of the shoulders. Note the right shoulder is depressed and protracted and anteriorly positioned. (Photograph courtesy of Polaroid.)

positioned shoulders can be easily seen and any asymmetry carefully noted. Roundness (more kyphosis) of the thoracic spine or widely separated scapulae indicate a possible overstretch of scapula retractors and a potential source of dysfunction.[5]

Standing in front, the examiner can observe a decrease or a comparative difference in muscle volume of the deltoid, pectoralis major, and biceps. An abnormal appearance of the deltoid contour may reflect either a neurologic injury to the axillary nerve from a dislo-

cated shoulder, direct blow, or a brachial plexus injury. A depressed humeral head can also be observed and may be secondary to a glenohumeral capsule incompetency, associated with a sulcus sign (defect or abnormality) (abnormal contour of muscle outlines consistent with disruption of biceps and pectoralis) (Fig. 10-6). Additional observations should be made as to the position and alignment or configuration of the clavicles, and the prominence of the sternoclavicular and acromioclavicular areas.

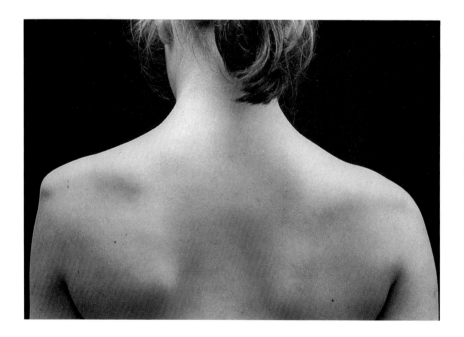

Figure 10-6 Sulcus sign. Subacromial depression consistent with anterior and inferior displacement of the humerus frequently observed with multidirectional instability.

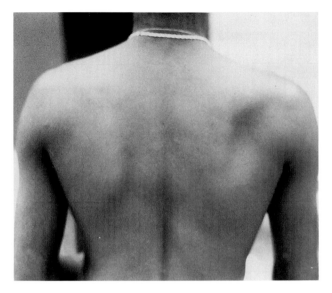

Figure 10-7 Remarkable atrophy of the infraspinatus musculature of a professional baseball player.

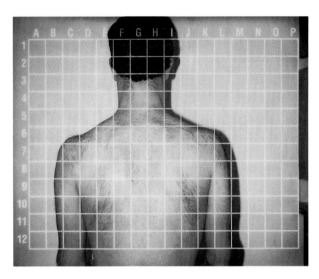

Figure 10-9 Grid film provides opportunity to evaluate cervical spine-shoulder relationship. Spine of scapula on right at normal level; left is below the third thoracic spine. (Photograph courtesy of Polaroid.)

Posteriorly, a decrease in muscle volume of either the supraspinatus or infraspinatus will alert the examiner to likely rotator cuff dysfunction (Fig. 10-7). From the posterior vantage, the position of the scapulae in relation to the spinous processes of the thoracic vertebra is observed. In normal posture, the spine of the scapula is directed to the spinous process of the third thoracic vertebra (Fig. 10-8). The medial borders of the scapulae are flat against the thorax and equidistant from the vertebral spinous processes.[6] Since some muscular imbalance is likely, the individual muscle examinations should be specific and diagnostic. If one scapula is malpositioned, either the spine is located lower or higher than the third thoracic spine or the medial border is more distant from the spinous processes (Fig. 10-9).

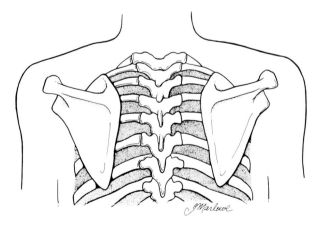

Figure 10-8 Normal posture. Spine of scapula directed to spinous process of third thoracic vertebra.

From this vantage, asymmetries in the cervical spine can be assessed, and, if observed, a cervical spine examination should be performed.

Palpation

The palpation component of the physical examination should be done with a gentle but firm hand and follow a planned sequence: (1) the individual joints, (2) local regions of change in muscle volume, (3) the course and insertion of various tendons (particularly those of the rotator cuff and biceps muscles to note focal sensitivity), and (4) identified areas of discomfort.

Palpation of each joint (acromioclavicular, sternoclavicular, and glenohumeral) should include a review and a recording of congruity, symmetry, discomfort, stability, ballotability, and crepitation (palpable and audible). The acromioclavicular joint is readily accessible for examination and the history of a previous injury will be critical to correlate with residual physical findings. In general, the more severe the prior injury, the more impressive are the abnormal findings. Grades III to V acromioclavicular disruptions will usually result in a permanent elevation of the clavicle in relation to the acromion (i.e., discomfort and crepitation or compression; excessive motion and ballotability; pain with certain motions). Such a significant alteration is frequently associated with other functional changes recorded in both the history and physical examination.

The clavicle should be palpated for a congenital anomaly or the residual of early trauma, an asymmet-

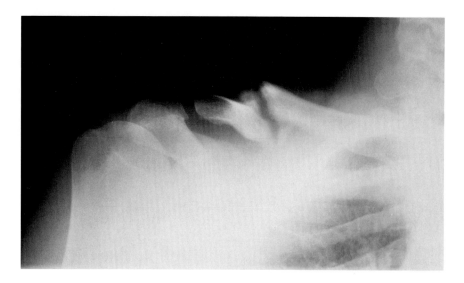

Figure 10-10 Ununited clavicle fracture presents as irregular configuration with palpation of clavicle.

rical configuration, and focal sensitivity (Fig. 10-10). The sternoclavicular articulation should be palpated for the same comparative findings of ballotability, discomfort, stability, and crepitation. In addition, there should be a specific evaluation of peripheral neurologic and vascular findings that may be secondary to posterior instability of the sternoclavicular joint (see Chs. 4 and 5). Palpation of the glenohumeral joint will focus on specific areas: the joint line (anterior, superior, posterior, inferior), biceps tendons, and the insertions of the rotator cuff tendons on the greater and lesser tuberosities.

The full length of each muscle is palpated in a comfortable resting length position and, if possible, in a lengthened position as well. Palpation of specific musculotendon units will assist in identifying areas of local spasm and inflammation. Tenderness in the region of the supraspinatus insertion on the greater tuberosity is often consistent with inflammation or tissue damage. Sensitivity at the junction of the musculotendinous portion or within the muscle of the infraspinatus and/ or teres minor is often consistent with an eccentric injury or local inflammation (common in baseball pitchers) (Fig. 10-11).

Palpation of the muscle bodies provides information on relative volume, with atrophy especially noted. Specifically, the changes in muscle volume and/or nodules within a muscle may be reflective of focal areas of injury, inflammation, or neurapraxia (the suprascapular nerve). Baseball pitchers frequently demonstrate painful nodules medial to the border of the scapula in the middle trapezius and rhomboid muscles the day after they have pitched. It is believed that these nodules represent a metabolic response to the microinjury and fatigue resulting from repetitive high-speed reciprocal concentric and eccentric activity. Recognition and continued observation of these nodules on a timely basis is critical for any active overhand functioning athlete (see Ch. 16). Persistence of these nodules could be associated with muscle weakness and earlier fatigue —a reflection of the excessive demand placed on muscles and supporting structures for a maximum performance.

During palpation, the examiner should be alert to changes in temperature and the potential need for additional tests. An increase in temperature may be indicative of an inflammatory process, while a decrease may be indicative of vascular compromise. Shoulder

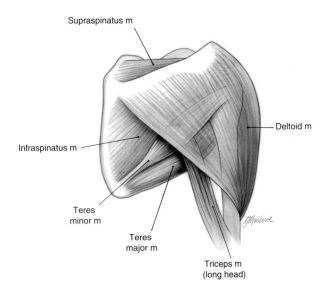

Figure 10-11 Sensitivity at junctions of musculotendinous portion or within muscle of infraspinatus and/or teres minor. Relative position of these muscles is presented with overlay of the deltoid.

dysfunction is commonly manifested by weakness or spasm of the trapezius, atrophy of either the supraspinatus or infraspinous muscles, and decreased volume of the deltoid. The decreased muscle volume of the supraspinatus/infraspinatus areas will impact on rotator cuff function and is often associated with local inflammatory damage or neurologic injury.

Active Movement

Injuries to the cervical spine are frequently reflected in the shoulder complex and upper extremity as pain, discomfort, weakness, or changes in sensation.[5] Prior to proceeding with the examination of the scapulae and shoulders, an assessment of active movement of the cervical spine in flexion, extension, lateral flexion, and rotation is important. In addition to range, the ease and smoothness of movement, symmetry of range and pattern, and the presence or absence of pain during movement should also be noted. If differences are observed or pain is experienced, then a more extensive skeletal and neural assessment of the cervical spine should be performed.

The normal relationship between the humeral head and the glenoid cavity of the scapula at rest and during motion is maintained by a coordinated balance of all muscles acting on the shoulder complex. Clinically, the accepted ratio of scapular to humeral motion is either 2:1 or 3:2, although this can vary slightly with individuals as well as with degrees of resistance.[7,8] These ratios are described as a pendulum arc and do not reflect the three-dimensional or multidimensional concept of scapulothoracic motion. Yet what is important to the examiner is the development of a three-dimensional conceptual image of the shoulder and dynamic visualizing of the glenoid and the humeral head in a continuous congruent relationship.

The initial examination of active movement and active range of motion is best performed bilaterally and in the standing position. Unless pain is obvious, the examiner should request the athlete to perform five maneuvers of an incomplete range of motion: (1) forward flexion; (2) external rotation with arms at the side; (3) abduction to 90 degrees and external rotation; (4) horizontal adduction; and (5) internal rotation at shoulder level (Fig. 10-12). Photographs taken at the end position of the described five maneuvers may be helpful to document asymmetries in contour and positions. Discolorations and other markings can be monitored for intensity of color and size. These photographs are also useful in educating the injured athlete and documenting changes over time. If specific variances are noted, the examiner should refer to the AAOS

manual for a description of motions and planes.[9] The patient's responses to these maneuvers need to be recorded on a form, in a narrative, or through a diagram (Table 10-1).

If these maneuvers are performed slowly through a 50 percent range of motion, the examiner is able to observe contraction of specific muscle groups and the basic pattern of scapulohumeral rhythm of the individual. The contribution of the individual joints to the coordination of shoulder motion, particularly the scapulothoracic articulation, can also be observed. Signs or complaints of pain or discomfort should be noted and the location, type, and intensity identified by the athlete. If pain or weakness necessitates assistance, the examiner should stand in front with a mirror placed behind the athlete for continued observation of scapular movements. In the presence of pain, stress across the glenohumeral joint can be minimized by having test maneuvers performed in the "plane of the scapula" (Fig. 10-13). This position is best estimated by following the direction of the spine of the scapula.

Following the incomplete range of motion examination, an attempt at complete active range of motion in the five previously noted positions is initiated. The inability to do a complete range of motion could be noted, and a polaroid grid (Fig. 10-14) film should be used for documentation. The athlete should again be asked if there is any local sensitivity during or after these motions. If pain-free, the same motions are repeated with moderate hand resistance by the examiner and again the presence of pain, discomfort, or abnormal motions should be noted. With moderate hand resistance, the area of pain and thus pathology will be localized (i.e., the insertional area of the supraspinatus tendon). During this sequence, the examiner also needs to be alert to postural adjustments in alignment, particularly if adjustment occurs with each attempted active movement. For example, posterior lean of the upper body during forward flexion or abduction indicates an inability of the shoulder musculature to meet the force requirements demanded by the test motions.

The motion of the scapula should be observed and recorded with the same five maneuvers. One of the most sensitive indicators of shoulder dysfunction is the initial positioning of the scapula in the early stages of abduction. If the athlete initiates abduction with the slightest elevation of the scapula, other findings consistent with supraspinatus weakness and shoulder dysfunction will undoubtedly be found. This part of the examination is best observed from the back. Associated with this finding is the inability of the humeral head to descend and glide under the acromion at the initiation of movement and then remain centralized within the glenoid fossa throughout the full motion—an indica-

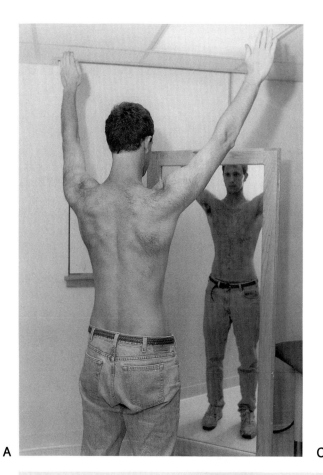

A

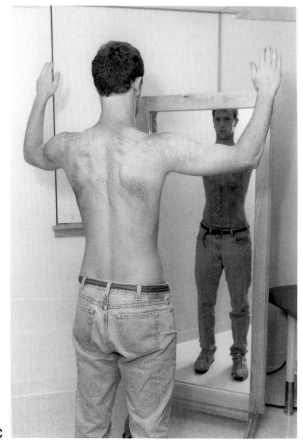

C

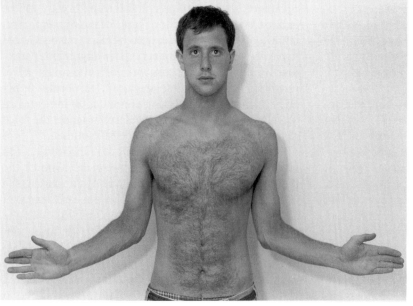

B

Figure 10-12 **(A)** Forward flexion. **(B)** External rotation with arms at the side. **(C)** Abduction to 90-degrees and external rotation. (Photographs courtesy of James Koepfler.) *(Figure continues.)*

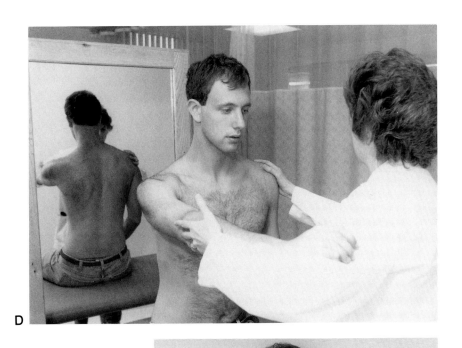

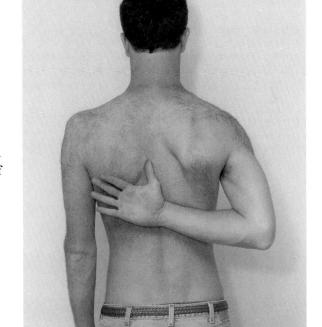

Figure 10-12 *(Continued)* **(D)** Horizontal abduction. **(E)** Internal rotation at shoulder level. (Photographs courtesy of James Koepfler.)

Table 10-1   The Society of American Shoulder and Elbow Surgeons Basic Shoulder Evaluation Form

Name _____

Shoulder: R/L
Hospital No. _____

Date of Examination: _____
(Circle choice)

I. Pain: (5 = none, 4 = slight, 3 = after unusual activity, 2 = moderate, 1 = marked, 0 = complete disability, and NA = not available) _____
II. Motion
  A. Patient sitting (enter motion or NA if not measured):
    1. Active total elevation of arm: _____ degrees
    2. Passive internal rotation:
       (Circle segment of posterior anatomy reached by thumb)
       (Enter NA if reach restricted by limited elbow flexion)

1 = Less than trochanter	8 = L2	15 = T7
2 = Trochanter	9 = L1	16 = T6
3 = Gluteal	10 = T12	17 = T5
4 = Sacrum	11 = T11	18 = T4
5 = L5	12 = T10	19 = T3
6 = L4	13 = T9	20 = T2
7 = L3	14 = T8	21 = T1

    3. Active external rotation with arm at side: _____ degrees.
    4. Passive external rotation at 90° abduction: _____ degrees.
       (enter "NA" if cannot achieve 90° of abduction)
  B. Patient supine:
    1. Passive total elevation of arm: _____ degrees.*
    2. Passive external rotation with arm at side: _____ degrees.
III. Strength (5 = normal, 4 = good, 3 = fair, 2 = poor, 1 = trace, 0 = paralysis, and NA = not available) (Enter numbers below)
  A. Anterior deltoid _____
  B. Middle deltoid _____
  C. External rotation _____
  D. Internal rotation _____
IV. Stability (5 = normal, 4 = apprehension, 3 = rare subluxation, 2 = recurrent subluxation, 1 = recurrent dislocation, 0 = fixed dislocation, and NA = not available) (Enter numbers below)
  A. Anterior _____
  B. Posterior _____
  C. Inferior _____
V. Function (4 = normal, 3 = mild compromise, 2 = difficulty, 1 = with aid, 0 = unable, and NA = not available) (Enter numbers below)
  A. Use back pocket (if male); fasten bra (if female) _____
  B. Perineal care _____
  C. Wash opposite axilla _____
  D. Eat with utensil _____
  E. Comb hair _____
  F. Use hand with arm at shoulder level _____
  G. Carry 10 to 15 lb with arm at side _____
  H. Dress _____
  I. Sleep on affected side _____
  J. Pulling _____
  K. Use hand overhead _____
  L. Throwing _____
  M. Lifting _____
  N. Do usual work _____ (Specify type of work) _____
  O. Do usual sport _____ (Specify sport) _____
VI. Patient Response:
   (Circle choice)
   (3 = much better, 2 = better, 1 = same, 0 = worse, and NA = not available/applicable)

* Total elevation of the arm is measured by viewing the patient from the side and using a goniometer to determine the angle between the arm and the thorax.

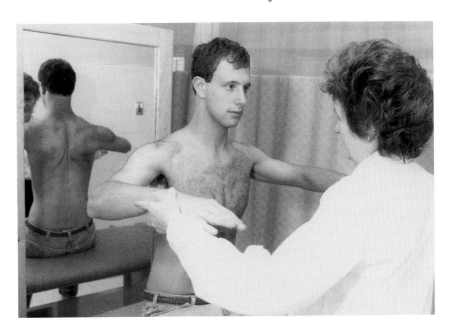

Figure 10-13 Test maneuvers performed in plane of scapula when pain is present. (Photograph courtesy of James Koepfler.)

tor of potential instability. The use of a mirror by the athlete to observe a change in early shoulder or scapular elevation and the descent of the humeral head is most beneficial (Fig. 10-15). Such observations can become a guide for later therapeutic recommendations. The maximum overhead position of both arms provides an opportunity to evaluate the "scapula profile" (Fig. 10-16). The scapular profile or prominence is best observed with the athlete either sitting or supine and both arms in the maximal overhead positions. The scapular position as observed in the subaxillary area will present symmetrically if shoulder complex motion is unim-

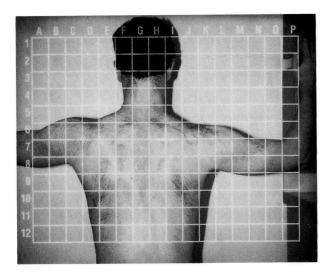

Figure 10-14 Grid film provides opportunity to show inability to perform a complete range of motion. (Photograph courtesy of Polaroid.)

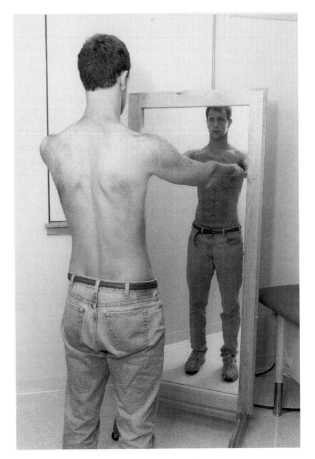

Figure 10-15 Use of mirror so athlete can observe changes in early shoulder or scapular elevation and descent of humeral head. (Photograph courtesy of James Koepfler.)

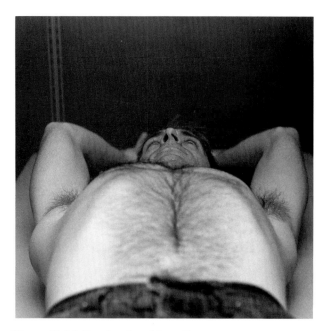

Figure 10-16 Overhead position offers opportunity to evaluate scapular profile. Note the excessive projection of the scapula on the right indicating abnormal scapulohumeral motion.

paired or asymmetrically if shoulder complex motion is abnormal. If there is any contracture of the glenohumeral capsule and ligamentous structures, there will be less potential glenohumeral motion, and substituted scapulothoracic motion is demonstrated by the prominent scapular profile.

Lowering of the arm from overhead or from the abducted position requires eccentric control by the serratus anterior and upper and lower trapezius to maintain optimal position of the glenoid. Loss of dynamic synchrony at the end of the movement pattern can also be a cause of dysfunction and thus deserves the examiner's attention. Other movements (i.e., adduction or retraction, abduction or protraction, elevation and depression) of the scapulae should also be assessed for relative position and motion on the thorax (Fig. 10-17) and compared with the opposite shoulder. In some sports, such as in rowing, the associated movements are primary. Changes in rhythm, timing, and coordination that result in asynchronous scapulothoracic movement will likely be reflected in functional incompetence, clinical dysfunction, or discomfort.[5] During observations of scapular motion, the dynamic synchrony of both scapulae should be compared (Fig. 10-18).

Throughout the active motion examination, there should be an alertness to potential audible findings that would indicate intra-articular derangement (e.g., torn labrum, acromioclavicular crepitation), or impaired tendon function, (e.g., supraspinatus crepitation).

Passive Range of Motion

If complete unmodified active range of motion is not possible, passive testing is performed to differentiate between contractile and noncontractile tissue problems and establish the cause—from muscle weakness, soft tissue contractures, or a bony or other intra-articular restriction. Passive motion is particularly important in the evaluation of the independent contribution of the glenohumeral and scapulothoracic articulations to shoulder motion. The use of a goniometer is recommended and the recording of motions according to the 0 to 180 degree method is suggested.[9,10] Many examiners also include descriptors of the "end-feel" of a passive movement, as proposed by Cyriax.[11] The evaluation of true glenohumeral motion as well as subsequent monitoring of prescribed therapy is best performed in the supine position and can only be achieved by deleting scapular motion[5] (Fig. 10-19). Documentation of the plane used, frontal or scapular, is important. This position restricts scapular motion, thus allowing true glenohumeral motion to be assessed. Maneuvers that delete scapular motion are most helpful, and require that the examiner stabilize the scapula by blocking motion with his or her hand on the lateral border of the scapula. The degree of motion possible when the arm is placed overhead and then across the chest can then be observed (Fig. 10-20). If it is not possible to position the arm in a near complete overhead position, this is indicative of some tightness or contracture in the capsule of the glenohumeral articulation, most likely anteriorly and inferiorly. If it is not possible to achieve approximately 45 degrees of horizontal adduction with the scapula stabilized, most likely there is a contracture of the posterior capsule.

An analysis of internal and external rotation with the arm at the side, in 45 and 90 degrees of abduction, and in the across-the-chest positions should follow (Fig. 10-21). Finally, there should be assurance that the arm with the elbow extended can rest at the side without a forward or lateral tipping of the scapula.

While in the supine position, passive ranges of motion of the cervical spine can be reviewed. In this position, the examiner can stabilize the shoulders and support the head throughout all the movements.

Scapula mobility is an important component of shoulder function. If a restriction is suspected, passive motion of the scapula can be assessed with the patient in a sidelying position. With a firm grip on the scapula, the examiner can move the scapula on the thorax approximately 15 cm in abduction-adduction and 10 to 12 cm in elevation/depression[6] (Fig. 10-22).

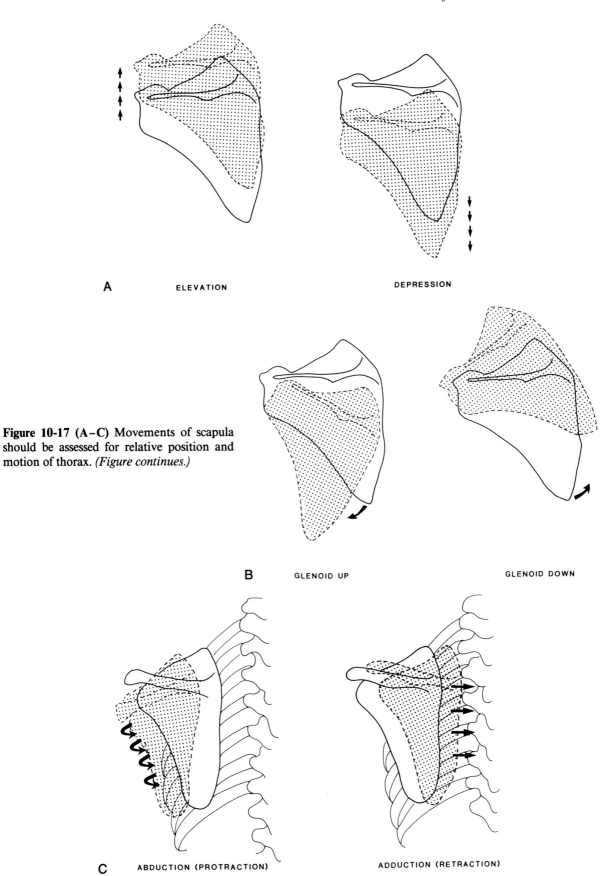

Figure 10-17 (A–C) Movements of scapula should be assessed for relative position and motion of thorax. *(Figure continues.)*

A   ELEVATION   DEPRESSION

B   GLENOID UP   GLENOID DOWN

C   ABDUCTION (PROTRACTION)   ADDUCTION (RETRACTION)

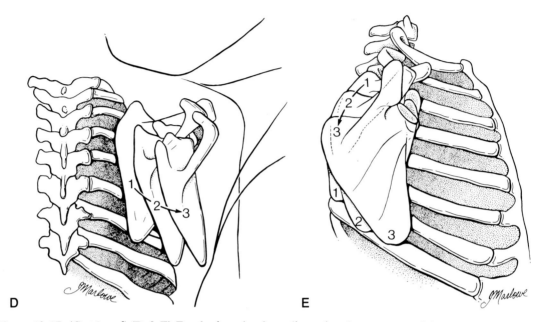

Figure 10-17 *(Continued)* **(D & E)** Emphasizes the three-dimensional movement of the scapula around the thorax.

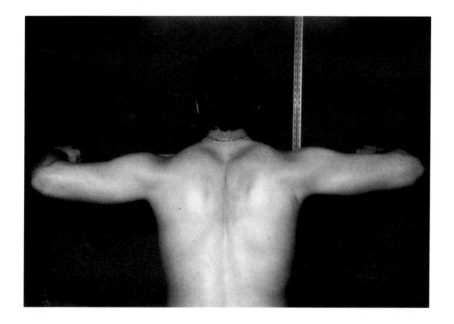

Figure 10-18 During observation of scapular motion, dynamic synchrony of both scapulae should be compared.

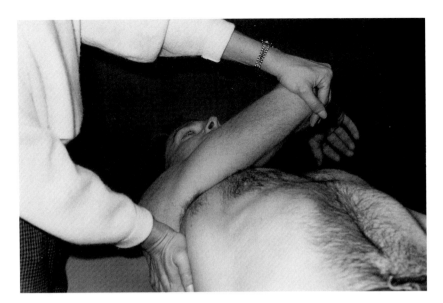

Figure 10-19 Evaluation of the glenohumeral motion. Note examiner blocking scapular motion in flexion abduction.

Muscle Examination

As an initial screen, information from the athlete's history along with the observations made during the physical examination (i.e., diminished muscle mass, limited active joint range versus passive joint range, asynchrony in glenohumeral rhythm, and winging of the scapula) can focus and direct the muscle examina-

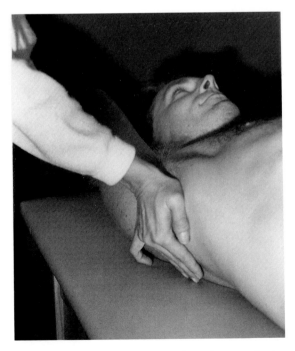

Figure 10-20 Degree of motion possible when arm is placed overhead in flexion abduction and scapular motion blocked.

tion (Fig. 10-23). To the extent possible, the examination of individual muscles should be included. The use of such a screen is beneficial, particularly in the presence of acute pain or suspected joint instability.

When the status of an injury permits, the examination of individual muscles should be completed. Five groups of muscles interact during shoulder motions (Table 10-2). In a detailed examination, each of these muscles is individually activated for performance by using the movement pattern for which the muscle is identified as a prime mover. For example, the upper trapezius muscle both elevates the scapula and contributes to upward rotation of the scapula during abduction; it is tested as an elevator of the scapula. Likewise, the serratus anterior muscle both abducts the scapula and contributes to upward rotation and is tested as the primary muscle in abduction of the scapula. When applied, resistance is directly opposite to the line of the pull of the muscle or tendon. For consistency in serial examination, and as a means for monitoring the effectiveness of therapeutic interventions, the positions and methods described in Manual Muscle Testing (MMT) are recommended.[12,13] Although there have been additions to the original description by Lovett,[14] the basic principles of MMT—the arc of motion, gravity as a standard, and the role of resistance—have remained the same. Proficiency in MMT requires a comprehensive and detailed knowledge of anatomy and muscle function in order to palpate muscle, recognize degrees of atrophy, and to identify position and movement abnormalities.

The various grading systems identified with MMT (see Appendix 10-1) use similar criteria for assignment of performance and can be compared. The use of posi-

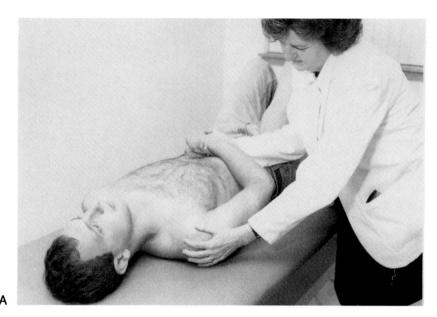

A

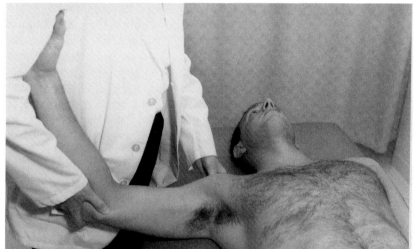

B

Figure 10-21 Analysis of internal and external rotation **(A)** with the arm at the side, **(B)** in 45 and 90-degrees of abduction. (Photographs courtesy of James Koepfler.)

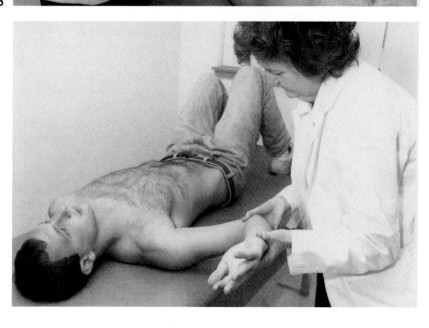

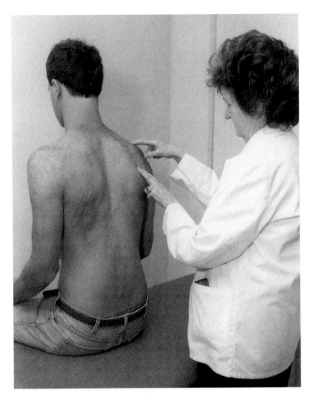

Figure 10-22 Careful evaluation of the plane of the scapula position and motion. (Photograph courtesy of James Koepfler.)

tive (+) and negative (−) with each grade, although more descriptive for each system, is less comparable. Except in severe peripheral nerve injuries, such detail is not generally required in the examination of the shoulder; however, the positive or negative sign can be used to indicate slight differences between shoulders. Regardless of which grading system is used, it should be remembered that the scale is an ordinal one, particularly the percentage scale. For example, the difference between the muscle tension needs for a grade change between "trace" and "poor" is not equal to the tension needed for a change between a "fair" and a "good" grade.

For the examiner, attention to the individual's position, stabilization of the part being examined, and the method of applying resistance is necessary. Resistance can be applied in three ways: (1) through the range; (2) during an isometric contraction at a selected point in the range; or (3) for a "break"-type test. Placement of the resistance can also be different. With the arm as the moving segment, resistance is applied above the elbow, on the forearm, or at the wrist. With the scapula as the moving segment, resistance is applied directly on the scapula and/or on the arm or forearm. Standardization of technique by individual examiners, particularly when evaluating the shoulder, will add to their own reliability and general understanding of the shoulder complex sequence. Our preference is to apply re-

Table 10-2 "Shoulder" Muscles

Vertebroscapular	Thoracoscapular	Thoracohumeral	Scapulohumeral	Clavicular
Trapezius Upper Mid Lower	Serratus	Latissimus dorsi	Subscapularis	Sternocleidomastoid
Rhomboid Major Minor	Pectoralis minor	Pectoralis major	Supraspinatus	Deltoid
Levator scapulae			Infraspinatus Teres minor Terea major Deltoid Anterior Middle Posterior Biceps Long head Short head Coracobrachialis Triceps Long head Lateral head Medial head	Trapezius Pectoralis major

Name:_____

Date:_____ MR#:_____

SHOULDER ASSESSMENT SCREEN

Presenting problems:
_____
_____

Associated problems:
_____
_____

Pre-examination observations:
    Difficulty with general activity: _____Yes _____ No
        If yes, describe:
    Arm symmetry when walking: _____Yes _____ No
        If no, describe:
    Pain or discomfort in evidence: _____Yes _____ No
        If yes, describe:

History (past and present):
    What happened: _____   Medication: _____
    How it happened: _____   Pain:_____
    When it happened: _____   Treatment: _____

Physical examination—positive findings:
    Observations:
        Posture (head, shoulders, scapulae):
        Asymmetries:
        Areas of concern:
    Palpation:
        Pain/discomfort: _____Yes _____ No   Location: _____
        Joint/muscle/tendons: _____Yes _____ No   Location: _____
    Active motion (range and asymmetries):
        Movement patterns:
            Forward flexion:
            Arm abduction:
            Arm abduction with external rotation:
            Horizontal adduction/abduction:
        Overhead scapula profile:
        Scratch tests:
    Passive motion:
        Glenohumeral joint:
        Scapula-thoracic articulation:
        Combined movements:
    Muscle performance:
        Asymmetries in strength:
        Functional tests:
            Wall push-ups:
            Seated push-ups:
            Selected movements related to sport:
    Sensation:
    Reflexes:
    Other comments:
Impression: _____
_____

Other tests considered:
    _____
    _____
    _____

_____   _____
Signature   Date

Figure 10-23 Shoulder assessment screen.

sistance throughout the range with an isometric "hold" test but not a "break" test. Resistance applied at the elbow or on the scapula is also preferred.

When planning a muscle examination, the need to change positions is an important consideration for the comfort of the patient as well as for the examiner's efficiency. A suggested order of testing is shown in Table 10-3. Prior to initiating the shoulder examination, an explanation of the test with a demonstration of a familiar muscle and motion such as the quadriceps and knee extension may be beneficial. Also helpful to the examiner is a mirror placed behind the seated patient to observe the overall movement of the scapula. For example, winging of the vertebral border of the scapula if observed would alert the examiner to a need for manual stabilization for a valid deltoid test. Throughout a MMT, attention to detail such as position, test motion, and application or resistance is required to assure accuracy not only for reliability in serial testing, but also for a true analysis of the presenting problem.

At the end of the examination and within the limits of pain, some functional tests should be attempted. The examiner can observe the serratus anterior in its role as scapular stabilizer by having the patient perform a wall pushup (Fig. 10-24). It is important to observe eccen-

tric as well as concentric control. The role of the latissimus dorsi and lower trapezius in scapular depression can be observed during a seated pushup (Fig. 10-25). In addition, observations of functional motions directly related to the athlete's sport can be informative. For example, the wind-up of a baseball pitch is different from a javelin thrower or volleyball spike, which in turn is different from a hockey slapshot.

When completed, a review of the MMT and functional data should provide the examiner with a clinical picture of the patient, and together with other clinical information will be the basis for a critical evaluation of the athlete's presenting problem.

Sensation Testing

Throughout the clinical examination, comments by the athlete on changes in sensation should be noted. Frequently in shoulder dislocation, the axillary nerve is involved and a feeling of anesthesia is felt in the anterior and middle of the deltoid muscle. A systematic assessment of the dermatome of both shoulders should be performed with a sharp and dull instrument such as a pin and a brush or soft material. Differences between

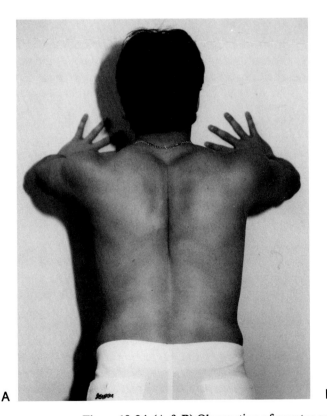 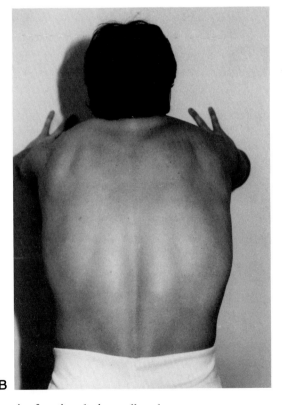

A   B

Figure 10-24 (A & B) Observation of serratus anterior function during wall push-ups.

Table 10-3   Suggested Order of Tests

Sitting
   Upper trapezius
   Anterior and middle deltoid
   Serratus anterior
   Supraspinatus[a]
Supine
   Biceps
   Triceps
   Corabrachialis
   Pectoralis major (sternal and clavicular)
   Pectoralis minor
   Sternocleidomastoids
Prone
   Posterior deltoid
   Internal rotation
   External rotation
   Middle trapezius
   Lower trapezius
   Rhomboids
   Latissimus dorsi
   Teres major[a]
   Teres minor[a]
   Infraspinatus[a]
   Subscapularis[a]
   Upper trapezius (neck extension)
   Functional tests
      Wall push-ups
      Seated push-ups
      Overhead reach and return
      Scratch test
      Pull sheet from table
      Selected sport-specific

[a] For identification and palpation muscle/tendon only.

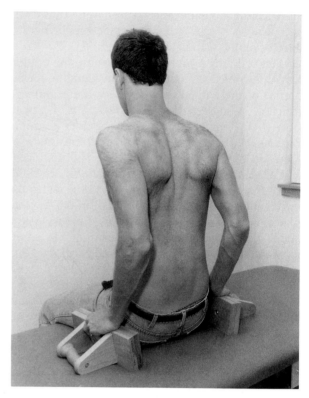

Figure 10-25 Evaluation of latissimus dorsi and lower trapezius while performing a seated push-up. (Photograph courtesy of James Koepfler.)

shoulders should be noted. A review of positive sensory findings with the manual muscle examination can be helpful in directing or confirming a diagnosis (see Ch. 3).

General Assessment of Glenohumeral Stability

If glenohumeral instability is suspected, the following tests will contribute to an evaluation but do not solely determine a diagnosis of instability. They should be performed initially in a sitting or standing position with the other shoulder then examined for a comparison. Subsequently the patient can be examined in the supine position. Stability of the glenohumeral joint must always be initiated with the humeral head in a reduced position (Fig. 10-26). Stabilization of the glenoid fossa of the scapula is accomplished by first grasping the coracoid and scapular spine with the

thumb and fingers, respectively, in order to control the glenoid/scapula. With the opposite hand, the humeral shaft is held as proximal to the humeral head as possible. A force is applied to the humeral head in order to appropriately move the joint (Fig. 10-27). Degrees of anterior and posterior translation can then be assessed as the anterior and posterior forces are applied to the humerus—known as the load and shift test. Assessment of the inferior translation can be accomplished by providing an inferior distracting force to the elbow and observing for a sulcus sign.

Apprehension and Relocation Test

The apprehension test can be performed with the patient remaining supine or sitting. With the elbow directed at a 90-degree right angle and the arm abducted 90 degrees, the shoulder should be externally rotated slowly. The patient may show signs of apprehension due to fear of the shoulder subluxing anteriorly. The potential re-creation of symptoms is a positive test.

Posterior apprehension can be tested as described in the general assessment section or by forward flexing the arm to 90 degrees and applying a posterior force. Poste-

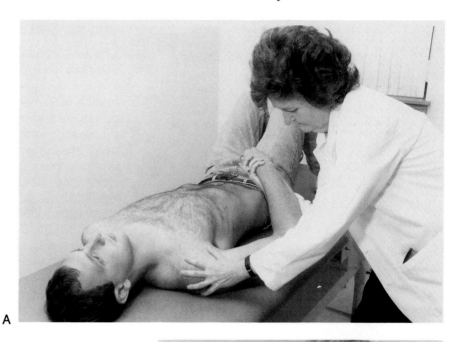

A

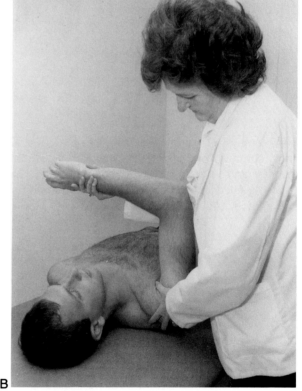

B

Figure 10-26 Stability of glenohumeral joint must be initiated with humeral head in reduced position. (Photographs courtesy of James Koepfler.)

rior translation palpated in thin, less muscular patients can be felt easily; the diagnosis is more difficult in more muscular patients and patients with more soft tissue.

The relocation test is performed to confirm the presence of anterior instability as determined by a positive apprehension test. With the patient supine, the arm abducted 90 degrees and externally rotated, the patient with anterior instability will have apprehension of impending subluxation-dislocation. To perform the relocation test, the physician applies a force in a posterior direction intended to relocate to the humeral head. With true subluxation, apprehension should be relieved as the posterior force relocates the humeral head.

Multidirectional instability refers to instability in

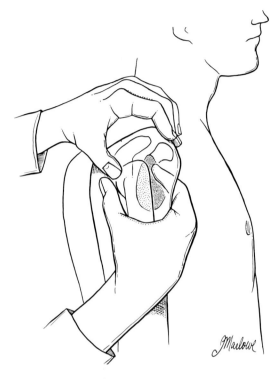

Figure 10-27 Relocation test.

combinations of anterior, inferior, and posterior. The most common multidirectional instability combines anterior and inferior instability. These patients may exhibit a sulcus sign (anterior and posterior) and positive apprehension and relocation tests.

Impingement

While Neer and Welch[15] popularized the impingement test, there have since been many modifications. Classical elevation of the arm was described as causing impingement of the supraspinatus tendon. The impingement test actually reproduces the compression of the supraspinatus tendon and subacromial bursa between the humeral head (greater tuberosity) and the acromion process and/or coracoacromial ligament. In an attempt to effectively position the greater tuberosity against the acromion, health care examiners more often abduct the arm 90 degrees and then internally rotate the arm. Pain and apprehension above 90 degrees is consistent with a diagnosis of impingement and should direct the examiner to the possibility of superior instability or dysfunction (see Ch. 11). A position of forearm flexion should be used to impinge on the coracoacromial ligament. If the diagnosis is questionable after an impingement test, an injection of local anesthesia into the subacromial bursa can be given to determine if the pain associated with impingement maneuvers is from compression of the soft tissue structures or another cause. In true impingement, pain should be alleviated by the injection. In patients under the age of 35, there is a question if impingement is ever primary. Instability and muscle imbalance have been noted to be a cause of impingement.

Biceps Tendon Pathology

A ruptured biceps is more common in middle-aged athletes and is readily diagnosed by the distal positioning of the contracted flexed biceps (Fig. 10-28). More

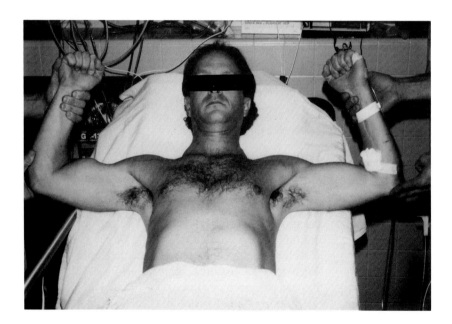

Figure 10-28 Distal positioning of biceps muscle mass after rupture of the long head of the biceps (right arm).

typically, overhand athletes develop biceps tendon pathology, with tendonitis and fraying affecting the superior labrum and biceps origin. Palpation in the biceps groove through the overlying anterior deltoid often leads to discomfort. Speed has described a test whereby the extended arm held in supination is forward-flexed to 60 degrees.[16] Resistance is then provided by the physician and anterior shoulder pain in the bicipital groove is monitored. A similar test has been made popular by Yergason[17] whereby the examiner grasps the elbow and the wrist, and provides resistance to supination. In the past 10 years, biceps tendon pathology has been considered a more complex entity, since it is often associated with instability or other intra-articular lesions. If the tests are indicative of pathology, the physician should pursue additional evaluation with these conditions in mind.

ACROMIOCLAVICULAR JOINT EVALUATION

Athletes involved in collision sports, arm overhead activities, and weightlifting often sustain injury to the acromioclavicular joint. Primary evaluation starts with palpation of the joint. If depression of the distal clavicle causes pain, primary degenerative disease is probable. Adduction of the arm across the chest may also cause discomfort to the patient with an acromioclavicular pathology. Patients with acromioclavicular pathology will have pain if asked to perform an adduction resistance test.

VASCULAR EXAMINATION

A vascular examination should be performed on each athlete. In addition to the traditional pulse evaluation, a standard component of the examination should be to rule out thoracic outlet syndrome. In a modified Adson test, the radial pulse is palpated while the shoulder is extended and abducted to approximately 60 degrees. The head is then rotated to the opposite shoulder and the athlete is asked to take a deep breath. A reduction or obliteration of the radial pulse suggests thoracic outlet syndrome. A negative test, however, does not fully exclude thoracic outlet syndrome (see Ch. 5 for a full discussion on thoracic outlet syndrome).

REFLEX TESTING

Reflex testing is not performed on the shoulder. The biceps reflex, C5, the brachioradialis reflex, C6, and the triceps reflex, C7, however, can be helpful in the presence of potential neurologic pathology.

After the musculoskeletal examination, the evaluation should be extended to a complete neurologic and vascular assessment. The details of these neurologic and vascular examinations are discussed in Chapters 3 and 5.

SPECIAL TESTS

After the entire clinical evaluation is completed, the need for appropriate ancillary tests is then determined. These may include radiography, electrophysiologic tests, arthrography, computed tomography, magnetic resonance imaging, Doppler ultrasonography, and arteriography. The need for additional tests such as an isokinetic evaluation should also be considered at this time and specifically planned. An analysis of functional performance can also be scheduled. Home or team videotapes of an athlete's actual performances described as "good" or "usual" may be helpful in understanding the presenting problem and later used during the rehabilitation process.

REFERENCES

1. Price DD, McGrath PA, Rafil A, Buckingham B: The validation of visual analogue scales as ratio scale measures for chronic and experimental pain. Pain 17:45, 1983
2. Chapman DD, Casey KL, Dubner R, et al: Pain measurement: an overview. Pain 22:1, 1985
3. Whaley L, Wong D: Nursing Care of Infants and Children. 3rd Ed. p. 1070. CV Mosby, St. Louis, 1987
4. Wong DL, Baker CM: Pain in children: comparison of assessment scales. Pediatr Nurs 14:9, 1988
5. Cailliet R: Soft tissue pain and disability. In: Neck and Upper Arm Pain. FA Davis, Philadelphia, 1989
6. Kapandji IA: The Physiology of the Joints. Vol 1. Upper Limb. Churchill Livingstone, New York, 1970
7. Inman VE, Saunders JB, Abbott LC: Observations on the function of shoulder joint. J. Bone Joint Surg 26:1, 1944
8. Saha: Theory of shoulder mechanisms. Charles C Thomas, Springfield, IL, 1961
9. American Orthopedic Association Manual of Orthopaedic Surgery, 6th Ed. Chicago, IL, 1985
10. Moore ML: Clinical assessment of joint motion. In Basmajian JV (ed): Therapeutic Exercise. 3rd Ed. Williams & Wilkins, Baltimore, 1978
11. Cyriax J: Textbook of Orthopaedic Medicine. Williams & Wilkins, Baltimore, 1975
12. Daniels L, Worthingham C (eds): Muscle Testing: Technique of Manual Examination. 4th Ed. WB Saunders, Philadelphia, 1980

13. Kendall FP, McCreary EK (eds): Muscles: Testing and Function. 4th Ed. Williams & Wilkins, Baltimore, 1993
14. Lovett RW: The Treatment of Infantile Paralysis. 2nd Ed. p. 135. Blakiston's, Philadelphia, 1917
15. Neer CS II, Welsh RP: The Shoulder in Sports. Orthop Clin 8:583, 1977
16. Crenshaw AH, Gilgore WE: Surgical treatment of bicipital tenosynovitis. J. Bone Joint Surg [Am] 48:1496, 1966
17. Yergason RM: Supination Sign. J Bone Joint Surg 13:160, 1931

SUGGESTED READINGS

Brunnstrom S: Clinical Kinesiology. 3rd Ed. [Revision by R Dickinson]. FA Davis, Philadelphia, 1983
Kent BE: Functional anatomy of the shoulder complex. Phys Ther 51:867, 1971
Lamb RL: Manual muscle testing. In Rothstein JM (ed): Measurement in Physical Therapy. Churchill Livingstone, New York, 1985

Appendix 10-1

Robert W. Lovett, MD., introduced a method of testing and grading muscle strength, using gravity as resistance. A description of the Lovett system was published in 1932 and listed the following definitions:

Gone: no contraction felt

Trace: muscle can be felt to tighten, but cannot produce movement

Poor: produces movement with gravity eliminated, but cannot function against gravity

Fair: can raise part against gravity

Good: can raise part against outside resistance as well as against gravity

Normal: can overcome a greater amount of resistance than a good muscle

While symbols may vary, the movement and weight factors set forth by Lovett form the basis of most present-day muscle testing. The Kendalls introduced the 0 to 100 percent scale of grading in order to use numbers for computing the amount of change in muscle strength when doing research with patients recovering from poliomyelitis. They had used the word and letter symbols prior to using numerals and it was possible to translate grades from one scale to the other.

The authors of the 4th edition of *Muscles, Testing and Function* believe that it is in the best interest of those who engage in manual muscle testing that an effort be made to standardize as much as possible the descriptions of the tests and the symbols used. There is increasing use of numerals, and such use is needed for research that involves muscle test grades.

The *Key to Muscle Grading* on the following page is basically the same as the Lovett system with added definitions for the minus and plus grades. The Poor plus grade provides for movement in the horizontal plane and for partial arc against gravity. Both methods for grading Poor plus are in common use.

In the 4th edition, the percentage sign has been dropped, the normal minus grade has been eliminated, and the scale changed to 0 to 10. Leaving zero as 0 and trace as T, the word and letter symbols translate directly as indicated by the *Key to Grading Symbols* below. The scale of 0 to 10 consists of whole numbers, and does not involve the use of fractions or decimals. If computations were to be made using the scale of 5, the minus and plus symbols would translate as indicated below.

As noted in the *Key to Muscle Grading*, there is no movement involved with the O and T grades, and the numerals 1 to 10 refer to Test Movement and Test Position grades.

Key to Grading Symbols

Normal	N	10	5	(5)	(5.0)	++++
Good+	G+	9	4+	(4½)	(4.5)	
Good	G	8	4	(4)	(4.0)	+++
Good−	G−	7	4−	(3⅔)	(3.66)	
Fair+	F+	6	3+	(3⅓)	(3.33)	
Fair	F	5	3	(3)	(3.0)	++
Fair−	F−	4	3−	(2⅔)	(2.66)	
Poor+	P+	3	2+	(2⅓)	(2.33)	
Poor	P	2	2	(2)	(2.0)	+
Poor−	P−	1	2−	(1½)	(1.5)	
Trace	T	T	1	(1)	(1.0)	
Zero	0	0	0	(0)	(0.0)	0

Key to Muscle Grading

Function of the Muscle	Grade Symbols		
No movement			
No contraction felt in the muscle	Zero	0	0
Tendon becomes prominent or feeble contraction felt in the muscle, but no visible movement of the part	Trace	T	T
Test movement			
Gravity eliminated in horizontal plane			
Moves through partial range of motion	Poor−	P−	1
Moves through complete range of motion	Poor	P	2
Moves to completion of range against resistance			
or			
Moves to completion of range and holds against pressure	Poor+	P+	3
Test movement against gravity	Poor+	P+	3
Moves through partial range of motion			
Gradual release from test position	Fair−	F−	4
Holds test position (no added pressure)	Fair	F	5
Holds test position against slight pressure	Fair+	F+	6
Holds test position against slight to moderate pressure	Good−	G−	7
Holds test position against moderate pressure	Good	G	8
Holds test position against moderate to strong pressure	Good+	G+	9
Holds test position against strong pressure	Normal	N	10

11

Glenohumeral Instability

Arthur M. Pappas
Thomas P. Goss

The glenohumeral joint is the most mobile as well as the most potentially unstable articulation in the body. Glenohumeral instability is excessive movement or abnormal displacement of the proximal humeral and glenoid articular surfaces relative to each other, producing symptoms and functional impairment. Glenohumeral instability can result from muscle imbalance, contracture, ligamentous and capsular laxity, and/or deficiency to the bony and periarticular soft tissue-retaining structures.

The pathology responsible for instability may be on the glenoid/scapular or humeral sides of the articulation, on both sides, or within the retaining structures. The anterior retaining structures include the anterior bony glenoid rim, the anterior labrum, the anterior capsule, and the superior-middle-inferior glenohumeral ligaments. The posterior retaining structures include the posterior bony glenoid rim, the posterior glenoid labrum, and the posterior capsule. The muscle structures that influence shoulder stability include those muscles that attach to the scapula and the humerus (see Ch. 9).

Prior to 1970, instability was equated with a dislocated shoulder proven by radiograph, and, if unresponsive to nonoperative treatment, the physician's favorite surgical repair was performed. During the past two decades, it has become clear that shoulder instability is a far more complex clinical entity requiring a compre-

hensive approach if diagnosis is to be accurate and treatment successful: restoration of stability as well as preservation of maximum glenohumeral motion, flexibility, strength, and overall functional use.

In both the general and athletic populations, shoulder instability is one of the most difficult clinical entities to diagnose due to several variables that characterize the type of instability: (1) there may be no identifiable precipitating event; (2) the patient's signs and symptoms may be subtle; (3) plain radiographs as well as various image studies may be negative or equivocal; and (4) the distinction between excessive physiologic mobility and pathologic instability may be difficult to evaluate due to the functional demands of the sport (e.g., baseball pitching) and mobility of the glenohumeral joint.

The athlete presents additional diagnostic and therapeutic challenges. The varied forces associated with certain sports make shoulder dislocations most common (arm tackling in football), while the lesser but repetitive stresses associated with other sports (gymnastics, swimming) can result in milder, less anatomically obvious, shoulder instability that can be just as disabling during athletic activity. Minor muscle imbalances, capsular contractures or laxity, and intra-articular derangements may become functionally disabling for high-demand events but not for daily activity. In addition, some athletes develop compensatory motions that cause an alteration of the normal biomechanics, contributing to development of abnormal function but later noted as instability (e.g., baseball pitching).

Accurate diagnosis requires a detailed history and physical examination supplemented by defined tests (both subjective and objective) and observations of expected performance, in addition to the physician's subjective judgment and experience. The majority of cases of glenohumeral instability should initially be treated nonoperatively. If nonoperative treatment is unsuccessful, surgery to restore stability must be considered. Arthroscopic and open surgical procedures may resolve intra-articular pathology and restore stability but compromise specific motion necessary for athletic function. The patient's postoperative management and rehabilitation is critical to an optimal end result. Accordingly, this chapter provides an outline of the various instability variables that must be considered when dealing with an athletic population, offers a diagnostic approach, and includes therapeutic options.

ETIOLOGY AND CLASSIFICATION

Instability is defined as excessive movement or abnormal displacement of the proximal humerus and glenoid articular surfaces relative to each other. A dislocation is an instability in which the apex of the humeral head circumference moves beyond the glenoid rim and the head remains displaced out of the glenoid fossa for a variable period. A subluxation is an instability in which the apex of the humeral head circumference moves out toward but not beyond the glenoid rim and then back into its "normal" anatomic position. There is a wide spectrum of glenohumeral subluxation, and the signs and symptoms are usually more stable than those of shoulder dislocation.

Traditionally, the labels *acute* and *recurrent* and *traumatic* and *atraumatic* have been used to define glenohumeral instability—from an obvious dislocation to the more subtle symptoms of subluxation. Yet this range of symptoms and findings, due to the variability of physiology and athletic function, calls for a series of subclassifications that reflect this spectrum (Table 11-1).

At one end of the spectrum are individuals who remember a specific traumatic event in which a significant direct or indirect force was applied to the shoulder, resulting in a dislocation (e.g., a football arm tackle, a ski pole jam). The label acute is used when this type of instability occurs for the first time. Usually, variable degrees of injury to the capsule, ligamentous, and labral tissues, and possibly the glenoid rim and subscapularis

Table 11-1   Classification of Shoulder Instability

Etiology and types of dislocations and subluxations
    Acute-traumatic
    Congenital-inherent-atraumatic
        Physiologic
        Overt
        Subtle-high performance
        Dynamic-attritional
    Functional
    Neurologic
Direction
    Anterior
    Posterior
    Superior
    Inferior-multidirectional
        Inherent-atraumatic
        Post-traumatic
Control
    Involuntary
    Voluntary

occur, which create multiple sites of laxity, weakness, and altered soft tissue containment. With this type of instability, males outnumber females by a 3:1 margin and sports-active individuals in the second and third decades of life are most susceptible.

In general, the younger the person at the time of the initiating event, the greater the chance of a recurrent instability: dislocation.[1,2] Traumatic recurrent dislocating shoulders are generally unidirectionally unstable and involuntary (e.g., capsular ligamentous laxity, labral ligamentous avulsion, bone deficiency).[3-5] They are usually more symptomatic than those with voluntary instability and less responsive to nonoperative treatment.

Individuals sustaining an anterior dislocation during the second decade of life have a near-90 percent chance of recurrence; those in the third decade have a 40 to 60 percent risk of recurrence; those in the fourth decade have a 10 to 30 percent chance of recurrence; and those over the age of 40 have a less than 10 percent risk of a subsequent event.[6] If the dislocation is associated with a fracture of the proximal humerus (see Ch. 15), the chance of recurrence is significantly reduced, approximately 2 percent in all age groups. *Chronic instability* is when the shoulder has remained in a fixed dislocated position for an extended period of time (rarely seen in athletes).

Case Study I

A 35-year-old man who made a diving catch with his gloved left hand positioned across his chest experienced immediate discomfort and was taken to a nearby emergency facility for evaluation. Since his pain was severe, only one radiographic view was attainable and was interpreted to demonstrate a normal humeral head glenoid relationship (Fig. 11-1A). The athlete continued to experience pain and limited motion after 12 weeks of therapy for his rotator cuff injury and presented for additional consultation. Physical findings and two plain radiographs at 90 degrees to each other were consistent with a chronic posterior dislocation of his shoulder (Fig. 11-1B). He underwent an open repair that required both anterior and posterior approaches to reestablish the humeral head-glenoid relationship. After an extended period of closely supervised physical therapy, he regained near-normal motion but elected not to return to the inciting athletic activity.

At the other end of the spectrum are individuals with a less obvious or so-called atraumatic instability.[7] They may or may not experience a single specific traumatic incident but rather note the gradual development of symptomatic excessive or abnormal glenohumeral mobility. Physiologically, these individuals' ligaments are often inherently more lax, thus making it easier for the humeral head to be displaced and leaving the individual more susceptible to symptoms of instability ranging from subluxation to multidirectional dislocations.

There are four types of glenohumeral subluxation instability seen in the athletic population: (1) congenital, inherent physiologic-anatomic or tissue structure variance, (2) overt, (3) subtle or high performance, and (4) dynamic-attritional. Although these are separate entities, they can change from one category to the other (particularly high performance and dynamic to overt), creating a diagnostic challenge.

In each category, there may be congenital variances of the humerus, glenoid, labrum, and ligaments, muscle strength, and microalteration of the collagen structure of the capsule and ligaments. The range that is within this subclassification is often considered atraumatic, implying lesser force is necessary to cause instability, and in some instances only provocative motion. The treatment for these individuals is determined by careful analysis of the defects causing the underlying problem[8-10] (Fig. 11-2).

The athlete who presents with subluxation after a single traumatic incident is usually demonstrating an overt subluxation, that is, typically an individual who has sustained trauma to the soft tissue containment mechanism, resulting in the subluxation.[11,12] In heavily muscled athletes, a strong subscapularis muscle may provide the mechanism that prevents dislocation. An overt subluxation comes close to a dislocation—the shoulder is almost "out." Diagnosis is less difficult in individuals with an overt recurring subluxation, since the clinical tests are usually positive (e.g., relocation, apprehension) as are the anatomic findings (e.g., the labrum may be torn, the ligaments may be disrupted but usually not avulsed from the glenoid, and there is normal muscle control). Occasionally, after many episodes, these patients can voluntarily demonstrate their instability.

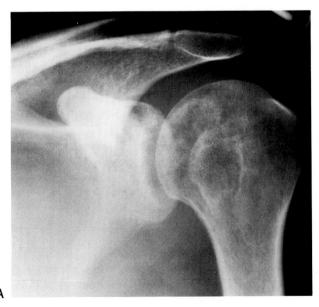
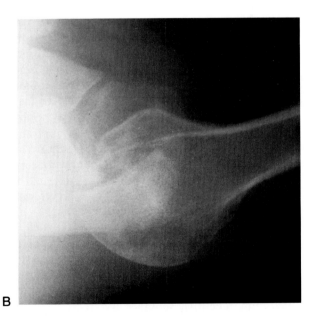

A   B

Figure 11-1 **(A)** Anterior view of posterior dislocation. A single view in this projection is frequently interpreted as a nondislocated shoulder. **(B)** Axillary view confirming posterior dislocation 3 months postinjury.

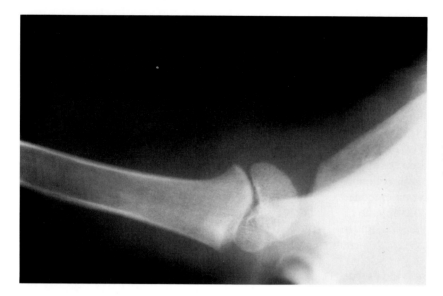

Figure 11-2 Five-year-old boy with congenital deficiency of the glenoid resulting in congenital instability and recurrent dislocations.

Case Study II

An 18-year-old lacrosse and football player first experienced shoulder problems during a lacrosse game when he was checked while passing the ball. His top hand (right) and his shoulder were forcibly extended and externally rotated while in a position of abduction. He was able to describe the immediate discomfort of his "shoulder slipping out." After a few days rest, he continued his season without difficulty. Approximately 5 months later, while playing as a defensive back in a football game, he attempted an arm tackle and experienced a similar sensation of his shoulder slipping. Although he was able to return to football when his arm was in a position of abduction, external rotation, and extension, he experienced recurrent symptomatology. He was able to demonstrate his instability by positioning his arm in the susceptible position. A physical therapy program did not cause significant improvement in his symptoms. He underwent an open capsular labral reconstruction. The findings at surgery included a moderate disruption within his anteroinferior labrum and a significantly loose patulous capsule. He returned to lacrosse after a rehabilitation program with slightly limited extension-external rotation. Although this did not interfere with his specific sport, it would probably limit a baseball pitcher.

Athletes with high-performance subluxation constitute the most difficult group to diagnose because these individuals have a microinstability that generally becomes symptomatic for a brief period only during maximum repetitive shoulder use (e.g., a baseball pitcher's symptoms reported after 15 to 20 pitches). These athletes usually do not recall one specific incident, and they are not able to demonstrate their insta-

bility. The apprehension tests are occasionally positive in the extreme position, while the relocation test is usually not positive, as the degree of excessive mobility is limited.

For these athletes, repetitive motion most likely has attenuated the capsule and the ligaments, and their labrum may be smaller and looser but not necessarily disrupted (versus the athlete with a frank dislocation or overt subluxation). This is an instability that causes discomfort and possibly altered performance but not severe pain, and does not always result in muscle weakness and significant contracture (i.e., scarring in the capsule and ligaments). This type of instability may be due to inherent tissue characteristics (i.e., the athlete's ligamentous tissues are more lax) or from abnormal mechanics (i.e., humeral head position changes due to altered anatomy or improper athletic function).

If the problem relates to inherent tissue laxity, an operative procedure will provide short-term success. However, after cellular tissue remodeling is complete and a primary tissue type has been reestablished, the laxity will most likely recur, and the athlete will not be able to achieve maximum performance. If associated with improper functional performance, a rehabilitation program should include specific advice and coaching to correct skill requirements to avoid repetitive high-performance subluxations.

Case Study III

A highly skilled professional 21-year-old major league baseball player experienced progressive shoulder discomfort. The ultimate result was an inability to participate for more than 15 pitches without pain and altered performance. Various image studies were of minimal value in identifying the underlying problem. An arthroscopic examination confirmed the laxity of the capsular ligamentous structures and some anterior and inferior fraying of the labrum. The frayed tissues were resected and an intensive therapeutic regimen was initiated. When he attempted a return to professional baseball 6 months later, he continued to experience similar symptomatology. Although an open capsular labral repair was performed at a later date, he was unable to regain the necessary skills to become a major league pitcher.

In numerous athletes' overhead performances, scapulothoracic dysfunction is the key to many shoulder difficulties and, in particular, causes glenohumeral instability. Contracture of the anterior or posterior capsule will result in an altered performance and secondary weakness of the opposite musculotendinous function. A contracted anterior capsule is frequently associated with weaker superoposterior muscles, limited motion, and altered function. Baseball pitchers who do not abduct and externally rotate normally experience an inhibition of the cocking to acceleration transition, causing them to "short-arm" the baseball or "push" instead of pitch.

A dynamic-attritional subluxation may be the earliest phase of a gradual sequence that causes more symptoms with continued performance and ultimately becomes an overt subluxation with a typical characteristic physical examination and clinical tests. This process can continue to the ultimate—involuntary and voluntary overt subluxation. We have termed this *dy-namic* instability, demonstrated by a clear progression and significant changes in mechanics of performance and muscle interactions. An athlete who has an inflamed capsule or tendonitis in the rotator cuff can progress to tightness in the capsule and weakness in the rotator cuff, creating a gradual change in mechanics of performance. This progressive alteration causes the scapula to laterally protract and inferiorly drop down (Fig. 11-3), which in turn alters the glenoid direction, scapular synchrony, and acromioclavicular joint compression, and creates scapuloglenohumeral dysfunction. Although the symptoms may present as other problems such as bicipital tendonitis or supraspinatus tendonitis, in reality it is dynamic instability causing the symptoms of tendonitis. Abnormal scapular position and atrophy of the infraspinatus and supraspinatus muscles associated with abnormal scapulothoracic synchrony are usually the initial findings. Additional findings may include neurodiagnostic changes in the suprascapular nerve and there may be discomfort of the acromioclavicular joint.

Individuals with dynamic-attritional instability who fail to receive adequate rehabilitation may develop a progressive instability from: (1) residual weakness/imbalance of the scapular, glenohumeral muscle groups (i.e., failure to properly rehabilitate the rotator cuff and, in particular, the supraspinatus muscle, leading to anterosuperior instability with secondary impingement; (2) a soft tissue contracture of the capsule, ligament, or tendon may cause an abnormal relationship of the humeral head to the glenoid (see Chs. 13 and 16);

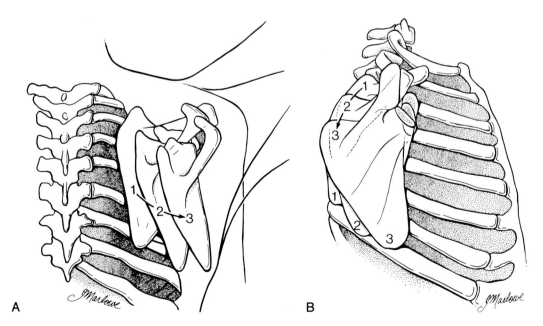

Figure 11-3 (A & B) Position 1 is the normal position of the scapula. Position 3 indicates a position of dynamic attritional malposition, protraction rotation, and depression of the scapula, resulting in abnormal position of the glenoid affecting glenohumeral function.

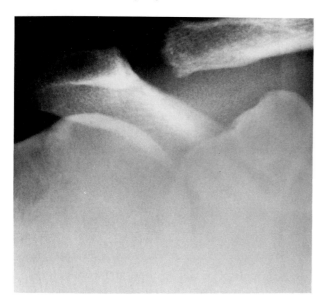

Figure 11-4 Clavicular osteolysis secondary to chronic attritional displacement of scapula and secondary compression of the acromioclavicular joint.

or (3) the continued scapular malposition, protraction and rotation on the thorax, will cause compression of the acromioclavicular articulation and result in joint pain, osteophytes, and clavicular osteolysis (Fig. 11-4). Thus, the process and symptoms of dynamic instability are initially different from other types of instability, but they may gradually change and become overt.

Case Study IV

A 26-year-old successful major league pitcher who was a Cy Young Award winner developed progressive shoulder discomfort and an inability to pitch as frequently or as well as in the past. He had significant infraspinatus atrophy and a decompression of his suprascapular nerve had been considered. The findings at the time of his clinical examination included an abnormal scapular position (i.e., depressed and protracted), notable atrophy of his infraspinatus muscle mass, and lesser but definite atrophy of his supraspinatus. There was abnormal asynchronous scapulothoracic motion and irregular scapulohumeral and thoracoscapular muscle integration. He described symptoms of impingement and instability when he attempted to pitch. The motion of his pitch had also changed — he no longer achieved the maximum cocking position that had been observed in videos at his peak performance, and he now pitched in a "short-arm" or pushing style. Neurodiagnostic studies revealed changes in his supraspinatus consistent with muscle damage and denervation; how-

ever, only one-third of his infraspinatus presented evidence of electrical activity, the other two-thirds were permanently damaged. He pursued a recommended therapy program focusing on achieving normal scapulothoracic as well as scapulohumeral function and improving the strength of all "shoulder" muscles. His pitching mechanics were evaluated and instruction on performance changes were recommended to resemble those of his peak performances. All aspects of his shoulder function improved, although he never regained any evidence of muscle activity in the two-thirds of his infraspinatus. His skills were sufficient for him to return and remain at the major league level for an additional 10 years with a continued commitment to his therapy program but without surgical intervention.

Functional instability-internal derangement of the glenohumeral joint results when a portion of tissue (e.g., a labral fragment, a cartilaginous body, etc.) is loose or partially attached within the joint and becomes intermittently interposed between the articulating surfaces. This causes the shoulder to catch, slip, or lock — symptomatology similar to that of the torn meniscus of the knee.[13] Removal of the tissue causing the symptoms will often resolve the symptoms and functional impairment. This clinical entity has been increasingly recognized with the advent of sophisticated imaging techniques and arthroscopy. In some cases, there may be an associated injury resulting in classical instability (e.g., Bankhart lesion) (see Ch. 12).

Case Study V

A 24-year-old professional football linebacker and wrestler experienced acute shoulder symptomatology after an arm tackle. He was not able to define symptoms of frank dislocation or overt subluxation; however, he did describe his arm getting stuck or locking when in the position of abduction external rotation and extension during various athletic activities. Due to this athlete's inability to continue his career, surgery was performed. The significant finding at surgery in this heavily muscled individual was a bucket-handle tear of his anteroinferior glenoid labrum. Following an excision of the torn fragment, and without any specific capsular ligamentous reconstruction, he returned to his professional athletic activities without symptoms of functional impairment.

Athletes whose instability is from a neurologic origin may have developed a traction neurapraxia following an acute traumatic glenohumeral dislocation. Axillary nerve dysfunction resulting from a traumatic anterior glenohumeral dislocation is a frequent problem, resulting in deltoid paralysis and/or secondary inferior displacement of the humeral head (see Ch. 3). If neurologic dysfunction is suspected, neurodiagnostic testing may be indicated to obtain objective documentation of either primary muscle injury or neurologic pathology. Nonoperative treatment is usually the norm, with a closely supervised physical therapy program. It usually takes 6 to 12 months for evidence of nerve recovery. Impairment of suprascapular nerve function may cause impingement of the supraspinatus and/or infraspinatus muscles, with resultant dynamic instability (see Case Study V and Ch. 4).

Case Study VI

A 17-year-old high-school athlete sustained a dislocation while playing as a defensive halfback in a football game. His shoulder was relocated, but he noted persistent dysfunction and weakness about his shoulder. A neurodiagnostic study 6 weeks postinjury demonstrated a severe axillary nerve neuropathy as well as some slight changes in his teres minor. In addition to the physical evidence of remarkable deltoid atrophy, a radiograph of his shoulder demonstrated inferior displacement of his humeral head in relationship to the glenoid. Repeat neurodiagnostic studies demonstrated a gradual return of activity approximately 5 months postinjury. Shortly thereafter, there was clinical evidence of recovery and a continued physical therapy program was developed to parallel the recovery of his neurologic improvement. One year postinjury, he demonstrated muscle strength that equaled his other shoulder. He returned to playing baseball and continued at the collegiate level without any impairment of function.

DIRECTION

The glenohumeral joint may be unstable in different directions: anterior, posterior, superior, and multidirectional-inferior. The shoulder is most inherently unstable anteriorly—95 percent of traumatic dislocations and the majority of all instabilities occur in this direction. Depending on the anatomic disruption or pathology present, the direction of instability may be specific, for example, the athlete with an anteroinferior glenohumeral ligamentous avulsion is usually anteroinferiorly unstable.

With an anterior instability, the humeral head moves excessively anterior relative to the glenoid. Anterior instability is usually the result of an external rotatory force applied to the shoulder with the arm in midabduction and extension. Anterior instability can cause traction damage to the posterior glenohumeral-retaining structures, resulting in increased posterior instability[14] (see Ch. 12).

If the joint is unstable posteriorly, the humeral head moves excessively in the posterior direction relative to the glenoid. Posterior instability is usually the result of a force applied along the long axis of the arm with the shoulder adducted, internally rotated, and in midforward flexion, and is common with seizure convulsive disorders. Posterior instabilities are less common than anterior; however, as more information is gathered on shoulder instability, it is evident that posterior instability is more common than previously acknowledged.[15]

Superior instabilities have been diagnosed in the athletic population but are difficult to demonstrate or reproduce on physical examination; they may also exist and be associated with rotator cuff injuries, particularly supraspinatus weakness in overhead athletic activities. An acute superior instability occurs when an upward force is applied to a flexed elbow, and the athlete experiences acute shoulder pain, possibly associated with AC joint pain[16,17] (see Ch. 12).

Case Study VII

A 26-year-old multiathletic woman was playing hockey and checked into the boards. She recalled that when her elbow struck the boards she experienced immediate superior shoulder discomfort. She was assisted from the ice and the radiographs obtained did not reveal any evidence of bony injury or articular malalignment. After 6 months of rest and rehabilitation she was still unable to perform any overhead functions, and she desired to return to basketball and baseball. Image studies identified abnormalities of her superior shoulder region and the findings on arthroscopy included a disruption of her superior labrum and a partial to midthickness tear of the rotator cuff. Following her arthroscopic procedure and rehabilitation she returned to unrestricted participation in baseball, basketball, and ice hockey.

In general, multidirectional unstable shoulders are less traumatic than unidirectional unstable shoulders in etiology. The causes of this type of instability are several: laxity, hypermobility, weakness, a smaller mobile labrum (usually not torn), an enlarged capsule, weakened subscapularis, and altered proprioception. Symptoms generally appear during adolescence or early in the third decade of life. These patients usually have milder symptoms yet more physical findings (as opposed to other directions of instability), and can often voluntarily reproduce their instability. Anterior and inferior multidirectional instability usually coexist. Isolated inferior instability is usually associated with deltoid and axillary nerve weakness. Concurrent anterior and posterior instabilities (without inferior instability) have been noted, usually with athletic performance or from iatrogenic causes.[18]

Case Study VIII

An 18-year-old high school athlete sustained a traumatic recurrent anterior instability and was unable to participate in sports. He underwent an anterior repair that resolved the anterior instability and resulted in a significant limitation of external rotation. Approximately 9 months postsurgery he became increasingly aware of symptoms associated with posterior instability, presumably induced by his initial injury and restricted motion following his anterior reconstruction. Following a course of soft tissue mobilization for his anterior contracture, which did not resolve the problem, he underwent a posterior reconstruction and continued a physical therapy approach to maintaining balanced shoulder function. His stability was improved, yet he continued to have difficulty throwing a baseball effectively. This difficulty caused him to change from his desired position of baseball catcher.

CONTROL

An individual with a voluntarily unstable shoulder is often able to demonstrate his or her instability either by arm positioning or selective muscle group activation. Generally, these shoulders are lax and may be at the minimally traumatic end of the spectrum. The symptoms are often surprisingly mild with the physical findings more impressive, and nonoperative care is often as successful as operative care.[19] A carefully supervised physical therapy rehabilitation program is an important first step in the treatment of voluntary instabilities.[20] Patients with involuntary instability who develop progressive laxity and muscle imbalance may gradually develop a voluntary component.

Case Study IX

A 16-year-old multi-sport woman fell on her abducted externally rotated left arm during a high jump performance. She sustained an anterior dislocation that could not be reduced at the site and required emergency room attention and significant medication to achieve reduction. During the next 4 months she experienced a progressive sequence of recurrent instability that became multidirectional, allowing her to demonstrate the instability on a voluntary basis (Fig. 11-5). She ultimately underwent a capsular shift procedure. The findings at surgery were a markedly atrophic subscapularis muscle and an attenuated capsule and ligaments, creating a capacious glenohumeral capsule.

The physician's judgment plays a role in the diagnosis of voluntary instability. Although individuals with voluntary instability can certainly have involuntary episodes, 10 to 15 percent of individuals who can voluntarily demonstrate their instability have a psychological basis for their presentation. These individuals may be difficult to identify, but the following findings are suggestive: (1) the "resistance to reduction sign" or the "hold out sign" (the examiner can actually observe the patient actively resisting any manual attempt to reduce the humeral head into the glenoid); (2) the patient finds it an enjoyable challenge to exhibit the maneuver and perceives it as a social trick. In addition, if the individual is an adolescent and the parents are present, abnormal dynamics may be noted as well as the sense that secondary gain is being achieved and realized from the "pathologic" situation. If these characteristics are observed, appropriate psychiatric consultation and testing may be helpful.[21]

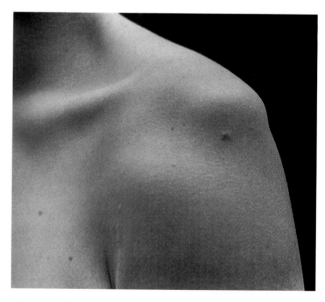

Figure 11-5 Sulcus sign associated with multidirectional voluntary instability.

DIAGNOSTIC PRINCIPLES

To formulate an appropriate and successful therapeutic plan, the characteristics of the instability must be determined. Diagnosis will be straightforward in patients who appear for treatment with an unreduced glenohumeral dislocation. The history, clinical evaluation, and radiographs of the glenohumeral joint will readily document the diagnosis. Patients with recurrent overt instability but with no prior radiographic documentation are more of a diagnostic challenge. Patients with lesser instabilities such as high performance or dynamic (e.g., fewer diagnostic signs; performance-related), who present with more subtle signs and symptoms are generally the most difficult to diagnose. The accurate diagnosis of unidirectional instability from multidirectional instability is critical.

A careful history and thorough physical examination is mandatory not only to determine shoulder instability and its direction(s), but also to rule out other possible causes of the patient's symptoms. Since there is a wide range of physiologic glenohumeral mobility, determining whether pathologic instability is present is often difficult. In such cases, the opposite shoulder can be used as a control. If the patient's symptoms can be reproduced in the other shoulder, it is generally a problem of abnormal tissue, that is, the patient has inherently lax ligamentous tissues, a smaller and looser labrum, and weakened stabilizing musculature. The patient should be examined in different positions for a complete evaluation of instability (see Ch. 10).

The traditional plain radiologic examination completes the initial acute incident evaluation: two views taken at 90 degrees to each other (a true AP view of the glenohumeral joint with the arm in as near-neutral rotation as possible; and either a true axillary or a true lateral scapular view are mandatory to rule out a dislocation). Although a patient's pain level should be recognized and considered, two views must be obtained so a posterior dislocation is not missed (see Case Study I). In the nonacute situation, a true AP view of the glenohumeral joint with the arm in neutral rotation, a true axillary view, and various supplemental projections (internal and external rotatory views of the proximal humerus and oblique views of the glenoid) may detect changes consistent with anatomic instability as well as lesions responsible for functional instability (Fig. 11-6). Unfortunately, in the acute injury setting, stress studies are difficult to obtain due to the positioning and discomfort level of the patient.

Supplemental radiologic image techniques may be helpful in the acute situation when it is uncertain if a dislocation with or without associated fracture(s) is present (Fig. 11-7). Glenohumeral computerized arthrotomography and MRI may be used to detect glenohumeral bony and soft tissue lesions and abnormalities

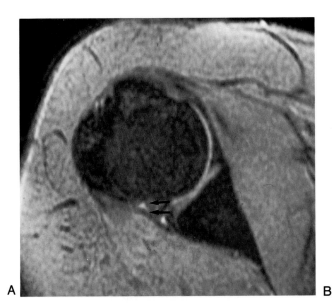 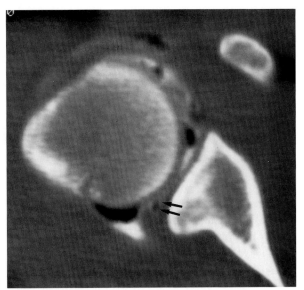

A   B

Figure 11-6 Eighteen-year-old male with posterior labral tear. Axial gradient echo scan (500/20 flip angle 20 degrees) with shoulder held in external rotation. **(A)** Linear midlevel signal intensity spans the midportion of the glenoid labrum posteriorly associated with small focus of extravasated joint fluid at the capsular margin *(arrows)*. **(B)** Axial image from CT/arthrogram shows extravasated contrast and air *(arrows)* correlating with posterior labral tear identified on MRI.

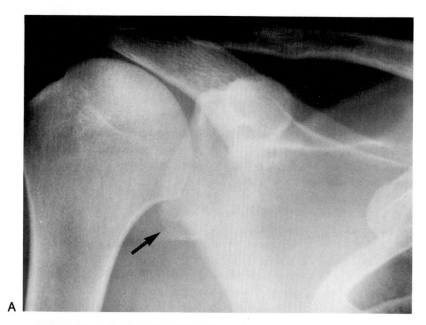

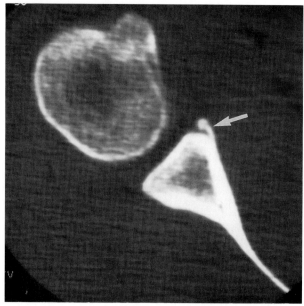

Figure 11-7 (A) Inferior glenoid ligamentous avulsion fracture resulting in recurrent dislocations. **(B)** CT scan demonstrating avulsion.

consistent with instability and, if present, to determine the direction(s) of that instability (see Ch. 1). There should be particular attention directed to the rotator cuff, which may be damaged or even disrupted in individuals with glenohumeral instability, especially in older patients[22] (see Ch. 13).

One must be careful not to overread image studies, as it is common to visualize changes that may not be related to an athlete's clinical problem. For example, most veteran overhead-activity athletes have labral and rotator cuff abnormalities. It is critical, therefore, to integrate clinical and ancillary test information prior to treatment. In fact, recent studies show a poor correla-

tion between MRI interpretation of the labral capsular anatomy and arthroscopic observations.[23,24] Considerable experience is necessary to recognize normal anatomic variants and to assign a relative clinical value to the different abnormalities that may be seen.

Other diagnostic studies include examination of the shoulder under anesthesia and glenohumeral arthroscopy. During an examination under anesthesia, the humeral head is manually directed anterior, posterior, and inferior relative to the glenoid with the arm in various positions of rotation and elevation. The examiner tries to detect pathologic instability either manually by palpating the humeral head or visually with the aid of fluoroscopy or plain radiographs. Specific attention should be directed to apparent anteroinferior instability and the decision to perform anteroinferior reconstruction. In some instances, there is a concurrent posteroinferior instability that is only discovered during an examination under anesthesia and this finding will obviously influence the surgical procedure. If the finding is not recognized, the patient will return with progressive symptoms of posterior instability, in part secondary to the unidirectional anterior surgery.

During a diagnostic arthroscopic procedure, an effort is made to actually visualize the instability, and the shoulder can be stressed at the same time it is examined intra-articularly. Although an arthroscopic examination may provide additional information, it will result in the athlete's nonparticipation in his or her sport for a period of time (see Ch. 12).

The major limitation with both examination of the shoulder under anesthesia and glenohumeral arthroscopy is the patient's inability to inform the physician whether a particular maneuver causes apprehension or duplicates the symptoms. Using the opposite shoulder as a control may be helpful, but under anesthesia shoulders are more mobile, making it even more difficult to differentiate lesser pathologic instability from physiologic mobility and ligamentous hyperlaxity. Since muscle control has been altered by anesthesia, these may not be finite tests, and although they may

provide information, they should not be the only determinants in the diagnosis.

Isokinetic testing should be considered in situations in which muscle weakness and imbalance are believed to be the underlying causes of instability (Fig. 11-8). Neurodiagnostic testing should be considered in situations where instability is thought to have a neurologic basis (e.g., axillary or suprascapular nerve injury) (see Chs. 3 and 4).

Finally, the most important component in the diagnosis is the physician's judgment and experience (i.e., the ability to assimilate all the information and laboratory data and to make a diagnosis). Often the final decision depends on a subjective experiential sense on the part of the physician, developed from observing and examining athletes and understanding the biomechanics and demands of athletic performance.

THERAPEUTIC PRINCIPLES

Nonoperative treatment will usually benefit individuals with symptomatic instability, individuals with muscle imbalance secondary to weakness and insufficient rehabilitation following injury, and individuals whose instability is due to lesser traumatic incidents and inherent soft tissue alterations. Patients are instructed to identify and avoid aggravating positions

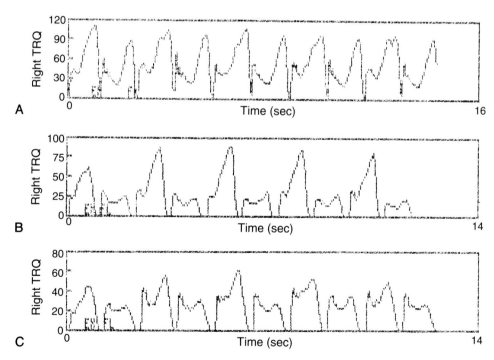

Figure 11-8 Isokinetic test patterns. **(A)** Normal. **(B)** Posterior shoulder weakness. **(C)** Internal derangement and torn anterosuperior labrum.

and activities while gradually increasing their level of activity as symptoms allow.

A monitored stretching program is indicated for individuals with glenohumeral and/or scapulothoracic motion limitation due to soft tissue contracture. An intensive muscle reeducation program is indicated in those with primary glenohumeral and/or scapulothoracic muscle weakness resulting in dynamic imbalance and impaired glenohumeral-scapulothoracic synchrony (see Ch. 16).

If an individual is thought to have an acute glenohumeral dislocation during athletic activity, one gentle attempt to reduce the dislocation is reasonable. This is often successful if performed before the onset of significant muscle spasm. Repeated forceful maneuvers are contraindicated at the site of the injury. Whether or not the reduction is considered successful, the arm is immobilized in a comfortable position and the patient is taken to an emergency room for comprehensive radiographic and neurovascular evaluation and care. Radiographs in two planes at 90 degrees to each other should be obtained to establish the diagnosis, confirm a successful reduction, and detect associated fractures. An anterior dislocation may be accompanied by a fracture of the greater tuberosity or the anteroinferior glenoid rim, while posterior dislocations are frequently associated with a fracture of the lesser tuberosity (Fig. 11-9).

A thorough neurologic and vascular examination should also be performed before and after the reduction to document any motor or sensory deficit. The axillary nerve is the structure most frequently involved — the overall incidence is 9 to 18 percent following acute anterior glenohumeral dislocations (see Case Study VI). Patients who have a neurologic basis for their muscle imbalance-instability are treated with strengthening of responsive muscle groups and if necessary, electric stimulation of impaired muscle groups while awaiting neurologic return (see Chs. 2 and 16 for a complete discussion on a program for gradual muscle strengthening and return to athletic activities). The likelihood of neural injury increases with the age of the patient (greater than 50 percent in patients over age 50), the duration of the dislocation, and the amount of trauma involved. Associated vascular injuries are also age-related, occurring primarily in the elderly; however, in younger athletes, the results can be catastrophic, requiring quick and aggressive care (see Ch. 5).

In the hospital setting, unreduced dislocations are managed with a closed reduction, with a variety of techniques described in the literature.[7,10,21] Regardless of the technique selected, it should be done as expeditiously and gently as possible, and when necessary, using intravenous sedation or occasionally general anesthesia. If an associated fracture remains in an unacceptable position following reduction of the dislocation, an open reduction is only necessary if there are fracture fragments or soft tissue interposition, an uncommon finding (see Ch. 15). Following reduction of an acute primary dislocation, the shoulder is immobilized for a variable period of time depending on the clinical situation. In individuals under the age of 40, who have sustained a significant traumatic acute dislo-

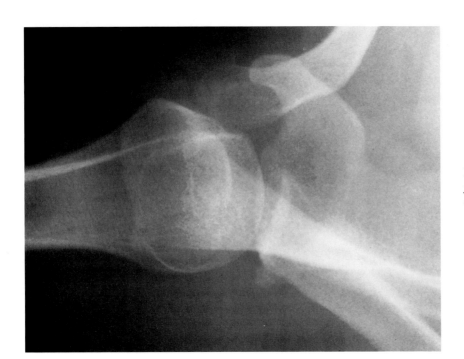

Figure 11-9 Posterior avulsion injury associated with posterior dislocation of glenohumeral joint.

cation for the first time, 4 to 6 weeks of immobilization is usually recommended. The therapeutic goal is primary healing of the damaged bony/soft tissue stabilizing structures to prevent recurrent instability. Immobilization other than for comfort is not necessary for those who have had previous episodes of instability, since other residual soft tissue problems versus acute damage is the primary pathology. These patients can progress with a gradual increase in functional use of the articulation as symptoms allow. If nonoperative modalities fail to provide adequate symptomatic relief and function (i.e., recurrent instability) corrective surgery (arthroscopic or open reconstructive procedures) should be considered. Patients over the age of 40 in whom the risk of adhesive capsulitis is far greater than that of recurrent instability are immobilized for 7 to 10 days for comfort (see Ch. 15). A sling and swathe bandage should be used for individuals who have sustained an anterior dislocation, while a shoulder spica or brace with the arm in 10 degrees of external rotation (described as a handshake position) should be used for those who have sustained a posterior dislocation (Fig. 11-10).

If the patient notes persistent severe pain, a thorough examination should be performed to rule out other sources of pathology. In particular, a rotator cuff tear may accompany anterior and inferior glenohumeral dislocations, the rate increasing with age: greater than 30 percent incidence in patients over the age of 40 and greater than 80 percent incidence in patients over age 60.[22]

After any period of immobilization, rehabilitation should be prescribed to initially regain shoulder range of motion followed by an aggressive strengthening program (see Chs. 2 and 16).

Arthroscopy can be used to remove intra-articular bony and soft tissue fragments responsible for intra-articular functional instability. Arthroscopy has also been used in recent years to repair some lesions responsible for dislocating and subluxating shoulders. Theoretically, arthroscopic techniques are ideal — the surgeon can identify and correct the pathology responsible for the instability while doing minimal damage to the surrounding soft tissue anatomy; thus, glenohumeral stability can be restored while mobility and function are preserved. Instability caused by detachment of the

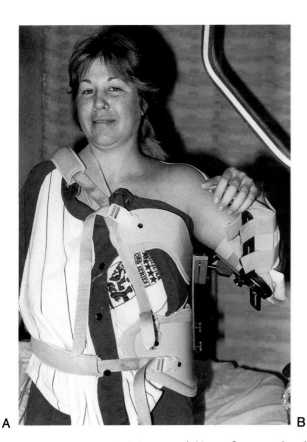 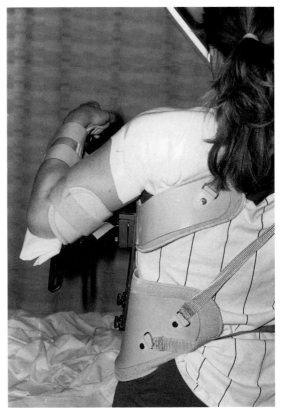

A B

Figure 11-10 (A & B) Commercial brace for control and immobilization of posterior dislocation postreduction or reconstruction.

labral-capsular-ligamentous complex from the glenoid is most amenable to arthroscopic techniques. Instabilities resulting from severe bony glenoid erosion, subscapularis damage, or capsular ligamentous laxity are not as effectively treated arthroscopically. In most instances, these arthroscopic techniques have a significantly higher failure rate compared to open reconstructive procedures due to tritissue etiology: glenoid ligamentous avulsion, midsubstance capsuloligamentous disruption, and subscapularis injury and atrophy (see Ch. 12).

Although restoration of stability and strength is fairly reliable (90 to 95 percent), open surgical procedures should be recommended with caution, since maintenance of full mobility is difficult. The patient should therefore understand the potential benefits and risks inherent in the surgery.

Case Study X

A 17-year-old high school multisport player sustained an acute dislocation of his shoulder while playing football. Following reduction and rehabilitation, he returned to activity in all his desired sports. However, his shoulder was symptomatic when he had to reach to catch a football or make a hard double play throw from his position at second base in baseball. He also experienced discomfort and apprehension when his arm was externally rotated and extended going after a basketball rebound. Radiographs confirmed a significant anteroinferior glenoid defect. An anteroinferior reconstruction was performed and his stability improved. The residual limitation of abduction external rotation extension interfered with his ability to throw a baseball effectively. The repair was considered successful, although the functional outcome limited his desired baseball skills.

Open reconstructive procedures should take the form of an *anatomic repair*—the pathology responsible for the instability is identified and a corrective procedure planned in an effort to restore stability while preserving mobility, flexibility, strength, and function. This is especially important in the athlete who requires maximum shoulder mobility as well as glenohumeral stability. The surgical techniques should reflect the selective needs for altering the involved anatomy: the capsule, ligaments, labrum, glenoid, and/or tendons.

Case Study XI

A 20-year-old man suffered twisting injuries to his right shoulder while wrestling. Thereafter, he experienced numerous episodes wherein the shoulder almost seemed to "come out of place." His shoulder was most uncomfortable and apprehensive when his arm was elevated above the horizontal, in the combined position of abduction, extension, and external rotation.

Despite advice to avoid aggravating shoulder positions and a rehabilitation program that focused on strengthening all of the glenohumeral muscle groups, the patient's symptoms persisted. Plain radiographs were normal. A computed arthrotomographic scan was obtained and demonstrated partial detachment of the anteroinferior glenoid labrum and an enlarged anterior capsular pouch (Fig. 11-11). Anterior subluxation of the humeral head could be demonstrated when stress was applied—changes consistent with anterior glenohumeral instability. An operative procedure was advised to restore stability. The findings during surgery included a patulous capsule, normal attachment of the ligaments to the glenoid, a moderate, midsubstance tear of the labrum, and intact tendons. The corrective procedure included excision of the damaged labrum and a plication capsulorrhaphy (Fig 11-12).

After a period of sling and swathe immobilization and a supervised formal rehabilitation program, the patient regained normal functional activity. Six months following the surgery, the patient was allowed to return to sports and continued a monitored rehabilitation program.

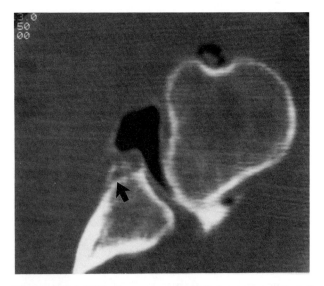

Figure 11-11 CT/arthrogram at the inferior aspect of the left glenohumeral joint of a 24-year-old man (with history of prior anterior dislocation and resultant anteroinferior instability) shows small Bankhart fracture and adjacent periostitis *(arrow)*. Capacious axillary recess on this and more caudal images (not shown) is evident.

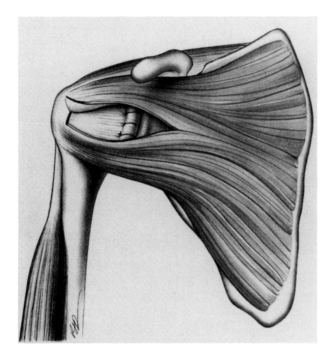

Figure 11-12 Capsulolabral reconstruction.

Unidirectional capsular ligamentous laxity, the most common pathology observed in recurrent subluxation instability, is corrected with a capsulorrhaphy. The type of surgical procedure is determined by the condition of the ligaments, labrum, and the capsule.[25] Specific attention should be paid to surgical details regarding induced contracture of the subscapularis.[26]

If the clinical findings are consistent with a recurrent dislocating shoulder, detachment of the capsular-labral-ligamentous complex in the region of the anteroinferior glenoid rim is the most common pathology. The damage to the labral-ligamentous complex is significant and variable. If the labrum and/or the ligaments are detached, a Bankhart procedure can be performed using traditional drill holes or self-anchoring sutures in the glenoid. If the labrum is loose, a capsulolabral reconstruction should be performed; if there is also a tear in the labrum, it should be debrided. The anatomic approach and surgical treatment of the subscapularis should be carefully planned and implemented to achieve the necessary repair to induce contracture and the desired functional result. Bone grafting should be considered if greater than one quarter of the anterior rim or one-third of the posterior rim is involved. A tricortical graft harvested from the iliac crest is favored since transfer of the adjacent coracoid process (the Bristow procedure) may significantly alter normal anatomy and is associated with a number of well-documented complications.[7] In addition, the use

and placement of metallic staples as part of a repair can result in problems (Fig. 11-13).

Case Study XII

A 24-year-old skier fell, sustaining a violent abduction, extension, and external rotational injury to his right shoulder. A clinical examination and subsequent AP and axillary radiographic views of the glenohumeral joint confirmed the presence of an anterior dislocation without fracture. Using intravenous sedation, a satisfactory reduction was achieved. Both the pre- and postreduction neurovascular examinations were within normal limits. Immobilization in a sling and swathe dressing was continued for a total of 4 weeks. The patient was then allowed to begin a progressive physical therapy program and to gradually increase the functional use of his shoulder as symptoms allowed.

Nine months later, while playing football, the patient sustained another glenohumeral dislocation. There was MRI evidence of complete detachment of the labral-capsular-ligamentous complex from the rim and neck and mild erosion of the bony glenoid. A Bankhart-type repair was performed to restore stability.

Immobilization in a sling and swathe bandage was continued for a total of 6 weeks. After 9 months, the patient was allowed to gradually return to athletics. Two years after his surgery, the patient has nearly a complete functional use of his shoulder with mild limitation of external ROM. No episodes of instability have occurred.

An inferior capsular shift is indicated if (1) the patient is multidirectionally unstable on evaluation; (2) the patient is found to have excessive inferior glenohumeral laxity on physical and radiologic examination (excessive inferior displacement of the humeral head on stress testing or an enlarged inferior capsular pouch seen on arthrography); and/or (3) the inferior pouch is found to be excessively capacious at the time of surgery (the inferior capsular pouch should not accommodate much more than one examining index finger). There is a dilemma with patients with multidirectional instability, since unidirectional repairs can cause increased instability or even symptomatic subluxation and dislocation of the humeral head to the opposite direction. The surgical approach and repair is performed on the region with the greater instability and includes an inferior capsular shift to eliminate inferior laxity and indirectly stabilize the opposite side of the articulation.[3,27,28] Patients who are equally unstable anteriorly and posteri-

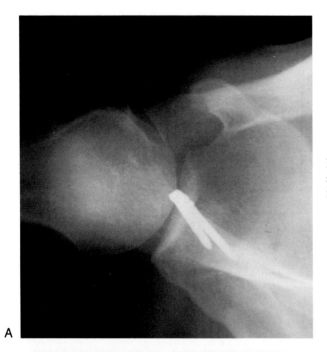

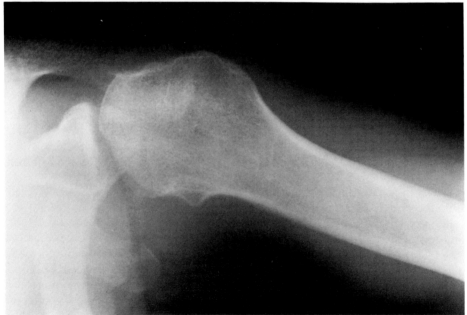

Figure 11-13 (A) Intra-articular position of staple following staple capsulorrhaphy. **(B)** Articular damage secondary to intra-articular staple.

orly should be repaired on both sides and should stop the inciting activity.

Case Study XIII

An 18-year-old female gymnast noticed gradually increasing left shoulder discomfort and a sensation of instability. In particular, she experienced discomfort when the shoulder was in the combined position of adduction, flexion, and internal rotation. She also began to sense that the shoulder "dropped down"

when she lifted heavy objects. Participation in gymnastics became increasingly difficult as glenohumeral instability worsened.

She could voluntarily posteriorly sublux the humeral head, and an inferior sulcus sign was readily demonstrable. Posterior and inferior subluxation of the humeral head could be produced on stress testing. Plain radiographs of the glenohumeral joint revealed increased distance between the acromioclavicular joint and humeral head. A computerized arthrotomographic scan demonstrated an extremely

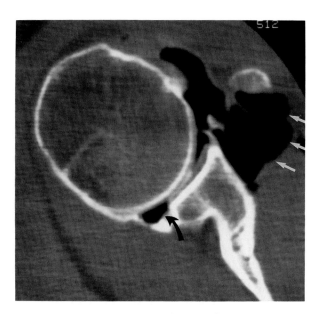

Figure 11-14 CT/arthrogram image of the midglenohumeral joint shows large volume, air-distended subscapularis recess *(straight arrows).* Posterior labral injury is also shown *(curved arrow).*

large posterior and inferior capsular pouch (Fig. 11-14), consistent with a posteroinferior multidirectionally unstable left shoulder. An intensive regularly monitored program of exercises designed to strengthen all shoulder muscle groups did not result

in improvement, and surgery was recommended. At surgery, a capacious posterior and inferior capsular pouch was present. A posteroinferior to anterosuperior capsular shift was designed and performed (Fig. 11-15).

Immobilization of the arm in an abduction splint with the shoulder in 10 degrees of external rotation was continued for a total of 6 weeks. Full functional use of the shoulder, including participation in gymnastics and other athletic activities was prohibited for 12 months. The patient has remained asymptomatic and returned to gymnastics at a competitive level.

Case Study XIV

A professional top draft choice right-handed hitting and throwing second baseman complained of left shoulder instability when hitting and going to his right to field. His symptoms were noted after a dive back to the base on an attempted pick-off play. During the ensuing 2 months his symptoms increased in frequency and his performance depreciated. His complaints were directed to the anteroinferior area, describing and demonstrating a motion while hitting. When initiating his back swing, he experienced left shoulder symptoms that improved once he started his power and follow-through components. His symptoms progressed to such a degree that he

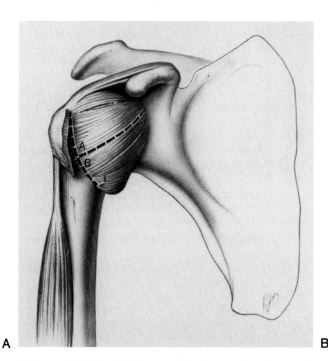

A

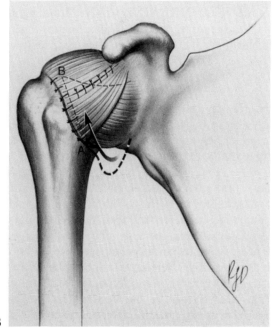

B

Figure 11-15 (A & B) Capsular shift procedure frequently used for multidirectional instability.

withdrew from competitive baseball and sought treatment.

His complaints were directed to the anteroinferior region, but his examination was more consistent with inferior and posterior findings. The question of multidirectional instability was considered. The image studies were not conclusive. An examination under anesthesia prior to an operative procedure was performed and indicated instability that was posterior and inferior. The shoulder was approached posteriorly and the musculotendon structures were normal; however, he presented with a patulous posterior capsule and a labrum that was detached from the glenoid — a posterior Bankhart lesion. The capsulolabral repair was performed using self-anchoring sutures to the posteroinferior glenoid and shift plication of the capsule was completed.

He was immobilized in a modified commercial brace that maintained his glenohumeral joint in 5-degree extension, 30-degree abduction, and 10-degree external rotation. He began a therapy program 3 weeks postsurgery, was brace-free 8 weeks postsurgery, and started light fielding and hitting at 12 weeks postsurgery. He returned to baseball without apparent impairment of function or loss of skills.

The postoperative rehabilitation program is tailored to the specific clinical situation and is directed to the restoration of flexibility, strength, maximal shoulder range of motion, and functional use. Individuals who undergo combined anterior and posterior repairs are immobilized in a shoulder spica or brace with the arm in neutral rotation. The postoperative immobilization device must prevent inferior displacement of the humeral head in patients who have undergone an inferior shift as part of their repair.

The optimal period of immobilization is both subjective and controversial, ranging from early-immediate motion to waiting 6 weeks to allow adequate soft tissue healing. A directed rehabilitation program is then prescribed and focuses initially on gradually regaining shoulder range of motion and strength (see Ch. 16).

Slower progress should characterize the rehabilitation program for individuals with multidirectional instability and/or inherent soft tissue laxity. Strengthening exercises are prescribed carefully, usually beginning with progressive isometrics postoperatively, and slowly increasing resistive exercises thereafter. These patients usually recover range of motion quite easily and may stretch repaired tissue beyond desired goal. Full functional use of the shoulder for demanding sports is often prohibited for 9 to 12 months and may require external protection.

The diagnosis and treatment of shoulder instability in the athlete is based on the practitioner's understanding of shoulder anatomy and function and the variables that define this specific entity. Determining the type of instability includes a thorough physical examination and history in addition to considering the specific anatomy and activity of the particular athlete. Treatment will depend on what characteristics and type of instability are present and the demands of the athlete's sport. Nonoperative treatment will be adequate with lesser instabilities while an "anatomic repair" (both open and arthroscopic approaches) will be the therapeutic option for athletes who require surgery. In these cases, concurrent stability and function cannot always be achieved.[29] Whether the treatment has involved surgery or not, rehabilitation will consist of muscle strengthening, range of motion, and functional performance needs. With appropriate treatment and rehabilitation, the long-term prognosis is optimistic. However, in certain sports, activity may need to be modified or limited.

REFERENCES

1. Hovelius L, Eriksson K, Fredin FH et al: Recurrences after initial dislocation of the shoulder. J Bone Joint Surg 65:343, 1983
2. Simonet WT, Cofield RH: Prognosis in anterior shoulder dislocation. Am J Sports Med 12:19, 1984
3. Bankhart ASB: The pathology and treatment of recurrent dislocation of the shoulder joint. Br J Surg 26:23, 1938
4. Bost FC, Inman VT: The pathological changes in recurrent dislocation of the shoulder. J Bone Joint Surg 24:595, 1942
5. Brostrom LA, Kronberg M, Nemeth G et al: The effect of shoulder muscle training in patients with recurrent shoulder dislocations. Scand J Rehabil Med 24:11, 1992
6. Hoelen MA, Burgers AMJ, Rozina PM: Prognosis of primary anterior shoulder dislocation in young adults. Arch Orth Trauma 110:51, 1990
7. Rockwood CA Jr, Matsen FA: The Shoulder. WB Saunders, Philadelphia, 1990
8. Cyprien JM, Vasey HM, Burdet A et al: Humeral retroversion and glenohumeral relationship in the normal shoulder and in recurrent anterior dislocations. Clin Orthop 175:8, 1983
9. Neer CS II: Shoulder Reconstruction. WB Saunders, Philadelphia, 1990
10. De Palma AF: Surgery of the Shoulder. JB Lippincott, Philadelphia, 1973
11. Rowe CR, Zarins B: Recurrent transient subluxations of the shoulder. J Bone Joint Surg [Am] 63:863, 1981
12. Protzman RR: Anterior instability of the shoulder. J Bone Joint Surg [Am] 62:909, 1980

13. Pappas AM, Goss TP, Kleinman PK: Symptomatic shoulder instability due to lesions of the glenoid labrum. Am J Sports Med 11:279, 1983
14. Ovesen J, Nielsen S: Anterior and posterior instability. Acta Orthop Scand 57:324, 1986
15. Fronek J, Warren RF, Bowen M: Posterior subluxation of the glenohumeral joint. J Bone Joint Surg [Am] 71:205, 1989
16. Wiley AM: Superior humeral dislocation. Clin Orthop 263:135, 1991
17. Weiner DS, McNab I: Superior migration of the humeral head. J Bone Joint Surg [Br] 52:524, 1970
18. Oveson J, Nielsen S: Posterior instability of the shoulder. Acta Orthop Scand 57:436, 1986
19. Burkhead WZ Jr, Rockwood CA Jr: Treatment of instability of the shoulder with an exercise program. J Bone Joint Surg [Am] 74:890, 1992
20. Aronen JG, Regan K: Decreasing the incidence of recurrence of first time anterior shoulder dislocators with rehabilitation. Am J Sports Med 12:283, 1984
21. Rowe CR: The Shoulder. Churchill Livingstone, New York, 1988
22. Johnson JR, Bayley JIL: Early complications of acute anterior dislocation of the shoulder in the middle-aged and elderly patient. Injury 13:431, 1982
23. Neuman CH, Petersen SA, Jahnke AH: MR imaging of the labral-capsular complex. Am J Radiol 157:1015, 1991
24. Garneau RA, Renfrew DL et al: Glenoid labrum: evaluation with MR imaging. Radiology 179:519, 1991
25. Jobe FW, Giangarra CE, Kivitner RS et al: Anterior capsulolabral reconstruction of the shoulder in athletes in overhead sports. Am J Sports Med 19:428, 1991
26. Symeonides DD: The significance of the subscapularis muscles in the pathogenesis of recurrent anterior dislocation of the shoulder. J Bone Joint Surg [Br] 54:476, 1972
27. Neer CS II, Foster CR: Inferior capsular shift for involuntary inferior and multidirection instability of the shoulder. J Bone Joint Surg [Am] 62:897, 1980
28. Altchek DW, Warren RF, Skyhar MJ et al: T-plasty modifications of the Bankhart procedure for multidirectional instability of the anterior and inferior types. J Bone Joint Surg [Am] 73:105, 1991
29. Matsen FA, Fu FH, Hawkins RJ: The Shoulder: A Balance of Mobility and Stability. American Academy of Orthopedic Surgeons, Rosemont, IL, 1993

12

Shoulder Arthroscopy

Dudley A. Ferrari
Arthur M. Pappas

Our knowledge of glenohumeral joint intra-articular anatomy and function has been significantly expanded with the technological advances of shoulder arthroscopy, computed tomography, and magnetic resonance imaging. This technology allows us to examine the entire joint through the range of motion without impact on normal and abnormal anatomy. As athletes mature, it is important to relate the effects of aging with changes of both normal and altered anatomy. Similarly, as we assimilate additional information on articular physiology and function, a further refinement of diagnosis and treatment will be achieved. While the clinical application of this information continues to evolve, these recent observations need to be integrated with existing knowledge of anatomy and function. Arthroscopy is an important tool in the treatment of athletic injuries. It serves both a diagnostic and therapeutic role.

ARTHROSCOPIC EXAMINATION

The arthroscopic examination of the shoulder should be performed in a sequential manner to assure a comprehensive recorded observation of the specific intra-articular structures. The shoulder joint is normally approached from the posterior vantage, and a specific pattern of views should be followed so that the entire joint is examined. The biceps tendon (Plate 12-1) is the initial landmark and should be seen through its entire intra-articular portion. Following the location and evaluation of the biceps tendon, the undersurface

of the rotator cuff should be identified, and the various components reviewed. The bare area (Plate 12-2) and posterior aspect of the humeral head should be evaluated, followed by the inferior recess and posterior labrum (Plate 12-3). The superior labrum and glenoid are viewed next (Plate 12-4). The arthroscope is then brought through the anterior triangle formed by the humeral head, glenoid and labrum, and biceps tendon (Plate 12-5). This position is used for the evaluation of the anterior structures, including the superior, middle, and inferior glenohumeral ligaments (Plates 12-6 and 12-7), the subscapularis tendon, the opening of the subscapularis bursa, and the anteroinferior and anterosuperior labrum.

Four determinations should be made when viewing all the segments. *First,* determine the presence or absence of the structures and whether there are anatomic variations within the anterior capsule. *Second,* determine whether there is evidence of injury to the capsule and ligaments. *Third,* observe the attachment of the ligaments to the labrum and glenoid, especially the insertion of the middle and inferior glenohumeral ligaments into the glenoid and labrum. Uhthoff and Piscopo[1] studied the anterior capsular insertion and noted that in 77 percent of the cases insertion was directly into the labrum, known as type I (Fig. 12-1), and in 23 percent of cases the capsule inserted directly into the glenoid neck, known as type II[1] (Fig. 12-2). *Fourth,* observe the labrum and its attachment, and determine whether there has been an injury; classify the injury as fibrillated (battered) or torn (flap or bucket handle)

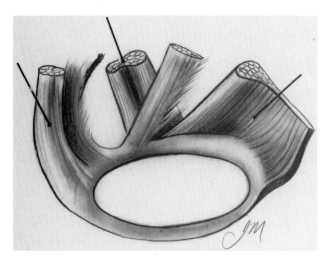

Figure 12-1 Type I insertion shows the middle ligament attaching directly into the labrum.

(Plate 12-8), also noting whether the labrum is attached, loosely attached, or detached (Plate 12-9).

The anterior capsule and its ligaments have been the subject of anatomic studies. Various classifications or groupings have been proposed. Many of the variations focus on the middle glenohumeral ligament. DePalma and colleagues[2] originally described six types of capsular arrangements. Rames and coworkers[13] recently proposed four groupings in which the middle glenohumeral ligament was separated and readily identifiable, confluent with the inferior ligament, cordlike, and attached superiorly on the glenoid or absent. Absence of the middle glenohumeral ligament has been noted in 8 to 18 percent[2-5] of cases (Plate 12-10); the higher number was based on a small number of specimens[2,4] while a combination of studies with a larger number of subjects suggests the incidence is closer to 8 percent.[2,3,5]

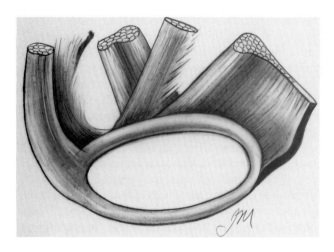

Figure 12-2 Type II insertion, the middle glenohumeral ligament, appears behind the anterosuperior labrum.

The appearance of the middle glenohumeral ligament is not only variable within the anterior capsule but also in itself. It can be described as thick or thin (Plate 12-11), and has been seen as split (Plate 12-12). The significance of the difference is not always apparent.

In one study twelve throwing athletes were observed to have an absent middle glenohumeral ligament (Ferrari, unpublished data). Their complaints indicate that pain usually occurs with ball release, occasionally in the cocking phase of throwing. Typically, the pain occurred over the anterior portion of the shoulder, specifically related to the biceps tendon. There was no apprehension in abduction external rotation and no evidence of impingement. One patient had a grade II rotator cuff tear and one had a grade I rotator cuff tear, but no other intra-articular pathology was noted. There were no lesions involving the anterosuperior or anteroinferior labrum nor were there any lesions involving the glenoid or the humeral head.

The observation that there were no lesions involving the anterosuperior labrum in these patients suggests that the middle glenohumeral ligament may be important in relation to the anterosuperior labrum. The consistent finding of biceps tenderness is most likely related to its function as a secondary restraint to external rotation and anterosuperior motion[6]; in these cases, it may have substituted for the absent middle glenohumeral ligament.

Labral injury has been the subject of a number of reports.[7-10] The success of pure labral debridement depends on the condition of the capsule, ligaments, muscle, and other restraints. The tears that are associated with significant capsular laxity are likely to cause symptoms consistent with instability. Examination under anesthesia will help determine the degree and area of instability. Arthroscopy and labral changes should corroborate the history and physical examination.

Labral changes that are noted must be classified and documented as lesions. In an attempt to classify the arthroscopic study of labral injuries, the glenoid and its capsular ligamentous attachments are divided into four segments: (1) the anterosuperior segment; (2) the superior segment, which includes the biceps attachment; (3) the anteroinferior segment; and (4) the posterior segment.

ANTERIOR LABRAL INJURIES

The labrum and attached capsule ligament complex provide the first line of defense to excessive motion to the humeral head. The capsular ligaments tighten and restrain in response to the rotation and the movement

Color Plates

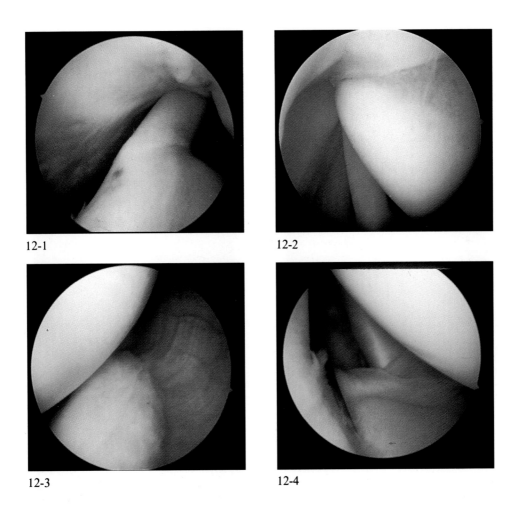

12-1

12-2

12-3

12-4

Plate 12-1 Biceps and biceps attachment overlying rotator cuff.

Plate 12-2 Overlying rotator cuff of humerus bare area seen at right.

Plate 12-3 Posterior labrum, posterior humeral head, and posterior capsule.

Plate 12-4 Superior labrum probe showing normal degrees of looseness.

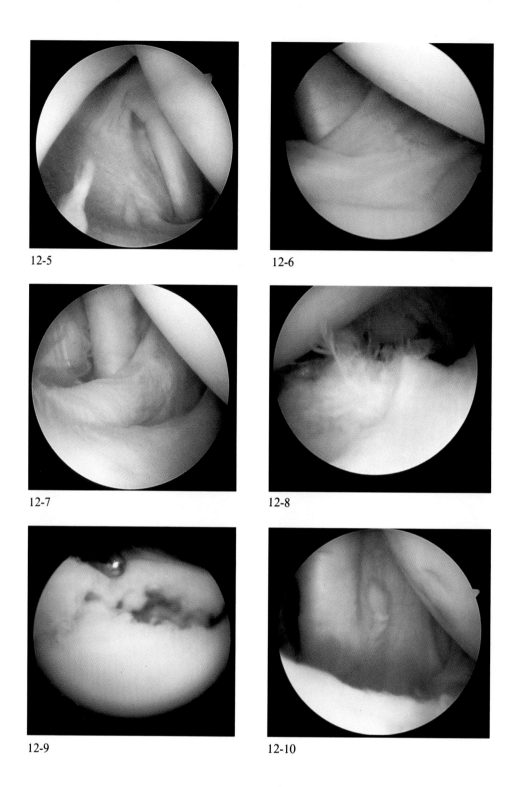

12-5

12-6

12-7

12-8

12-9

12-10

Plate 12-5 Through the triangle, the subscapularis tendon is identified as is the superior glenohumeral ligament.

Plate 12-6 Subscapularis muscle and middle and inferior ligament with a confluent appearance.

Plate 12-7 Subscapularis tendon and middle and inferior ligament are more easily identified because of the separation and recess below the middle glenohumeral ligament.

Plate 12-8 Battered appearance of anterior superior labrum of the left shoulder.

Plate 12-9 Loose but not detached anterior superior labrum with battered edges.

Plate 12-10 Absent middle glenohumeral ligament; large expansive subscapularis tendon and identifiable muscle.

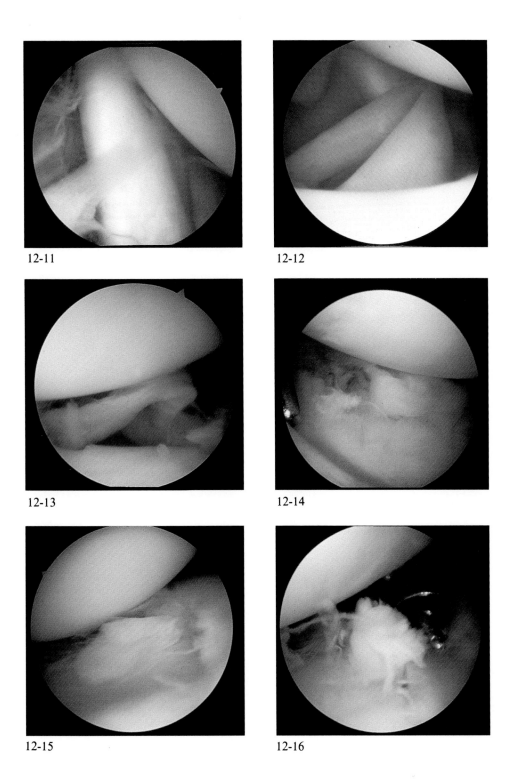

12-11

12-12

12-13

12-14

12-15

12-16

Plate 12-11 Thin middle glenohumeral ligament.

Plate 12-12 Split middle glenohumeral ligament.

Plate 12-13 Bucket handle tear of anterior superior labrum.

Plate 12-14 Probe is lifting superior labrum showing split at the junction of the superior and anterior superior labrum. Irritated middle glenohumeral ligament with an anterior flap present.

Plate 12-15 Anterior superior labral fibrillation (see text for details).

Plate 12-16 Loose chondral fragment from the glenoid at the junction of the superior and anterior superior labrum.

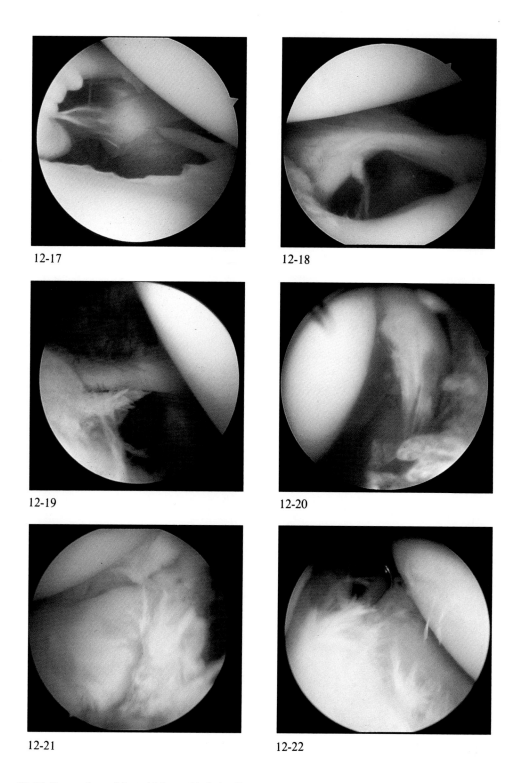

12-17

12-18

12-19

12-20

12-21

12-22

Plate 12-17 Separation of the middle and inferior ligaments, labrum not present, thin middle ligament attached superiorly, but break in the attachment between the middle and inferior ligaments is evident.

Plate 12-18 Looseness again noted by the anterior superior attachment of the middle glenohumeral ligament; however, separation between the middle and inferior ligaments has not taken place as it did in the other shoulder.

Plate 12-19 Middle glenohumeral ligament attached at the anterior superior labrum; some labral irregularities.

Plate 12-20 Indentation of the biceps tendon is appreciated along with some moderate irritation involving the rotator cuff from long-standing superior humeral head migration.

Plate 12-21 Torn anterior superior labrum, fibrillated superior labrum after acute injury.

Plate 12-22 Fibrillated type I superior labrum.

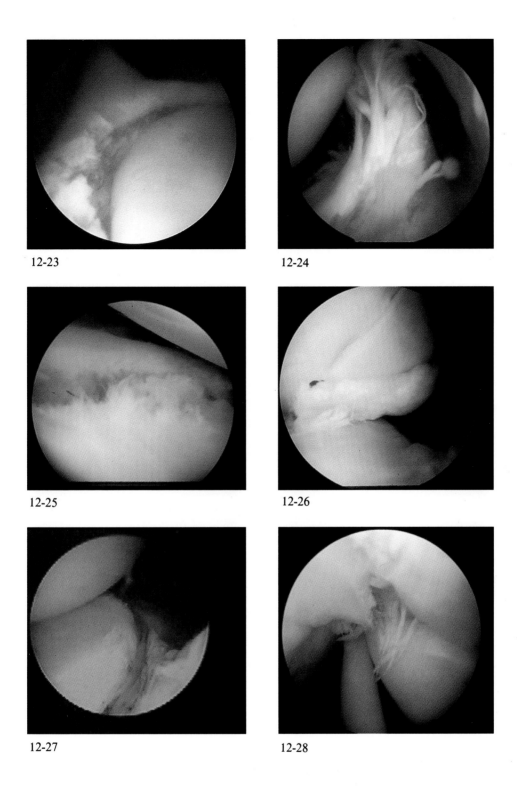

12-23

12-24

12-25

12-26

12-27

12-28

Plate 12-23 Loose type II superior labrum with synovitis in the area of the attachment.

Plate 12-24 Anterior split superior labrum extending into the biceps tendon.

Plate 12-25 Loose detached anterior inferior labrum.

Plate 12-26 Posterior labral tear.

Plate 12-27 Posterior labrum and capsular detachment.

Plate 12-28 Small rotator cuff tear undersurface.

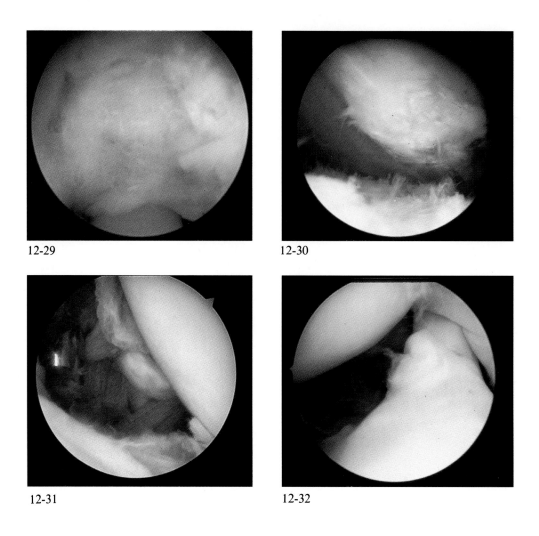

12-29

12-30

12-31

12-32

Plate 12-29 Larger grade II rotator cuff tear undersurface, not full thickness.

Plate 12-30 Stage III changes involving the coracoacromial ligament as well as the rotator cuff.

Plate 12-31 Injury to the subscapularis muscle and tendon surrounded by moderate irritation.

Plate 12-32 Biceps tendon injury.

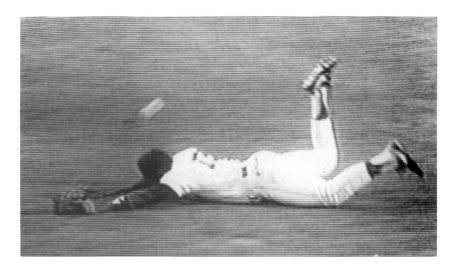

Figure 12-3 Outfielder falls on hand and externally rotated outstretched arm.

of the humeral head, and act as a buttress for anatomic constraint to excessive motion.

One violent episode or multiple less violent episodes may produce injury. The manifestation will be determined by the direction and magnitude of the force and strength of the structures. For example, a large force against a strong capsule and labrum may produce capsuloligamentous strain and stretch, while the same force against a smaller or weaker capsule and labrum may produce avulsion and dislocation. There are other manifestations between these two extremes. Motion of the head against a tight capsule and labrum may produce primary labral damages. A force that causes the head to move over the labrum and back may produce tears and fraying in the labrum. This repetitive force may loosen the capsule and labrum and initiate the process of performance functional instability.

Case Study I

A major league centerfielder fell on his flexed externally rotated arm while attempting to dive for a fly ball. He experienced immediate pain and limited ability to move his upper extremity. Radiographs were negative and magnetic resonance imaging revealed findings consistent with a torn labrum. Through arthroscopy, the finding was a bucket handle labral tear of the anterosuperior labrum (Fig. 12-3 and Plate 12-13). The capsular pattern was a stable capsular type II attachment. The position of the humeral head tore the labrum, but a stable capsular pattern kept the head from dislocating. The displaced bucket handle was removed arthroscopically. Following a carefully monitored rehabilitation program, the athlete returned to full-time major league baseball as a hitter 5 weeks postarthroscopy and as a centerfielder 6 weeks postsurgery.

This clinical example demonstrates a solitary disruption associated with a single episode of trauma with the capsular structures and ligaments appearing intact.[11] In this instance, the arthroscopic resection of the damaged labral area resulted in excellent results and the return of the athlete to a previously high level of athletic participation.

ANTEROSUPERIOR SEGMENT: THROWER'S LESIONS

The anterior superior labrum is difficult to evaluate because of the normal aging process that affects this area. DePalma and colleagues[2] noted that with each decade there is an increase in lifting of the anterosuperior labrum. A lesion associated with aging appears to be soft without surrounding erythema or injury to the other capsular ligamentous structures.

Injury to the anterosuperior labrum is often seen in the throwing athlete, with the anterior flap tear as one example (Fig. 12-4 and Plate 12-14). The lesion can be seen as an external rotation injury unrelated to sport. The flap tear is usually based at the area of the anterosuperior labrum, and the break occurs at the junction of the anterosuperior labrum and superior labrum and biceps attachment. This may occur because the middle glenohumeral ligament and attached labrum are under tension from the extreme external rotation. The superior migration of the humeral head is against the superior labrum and biceps. This lesion in the thrower can be accompanied by undersurface rotator cuff fraying and tears and is often associated with inflammation of the middle glenohumeral ligament.

The same motion (i.e., abduction external rotation) does not always produce flap tears. Movement of the

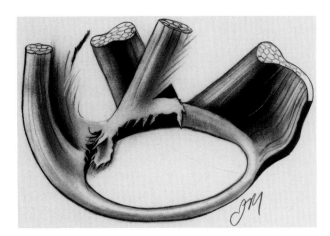

Figure 12-4 Anterosuperior flap lesion.

anterosuperior labrum and biceps attachment either over or along the glenoid rim may produce irritation or synovitis. Often thickened tissue and minor splits are seen under the labrum and biceps attachment. Debridement of these lesions and roughening the area on the glenoid rim followed by rehabilitation may return these athletes to overhead activities.

The biceps has been implicated in one study.[12] As of now, basic science has not demonstrated the forces, motions, or sequences that produce a variety of lesions at the anterosuperior and superior junction. When the arm is in maximal cocking position, the traction on the biceps labrum attachment may be under sufficient traction to create this lesion. Plate 12-15 shows an anterosuperior labral fibrillation, mostly reactive soft fibrous tissue hypertrophy beneath the labrum that was loose and not detached in a 27-year-old former minor league pitcher. Plate 12-16 shows a loose articular fragment from the glenoid in the same area.

Another lesion that occurs in the anterosuperior labrum is seen in both throwers and weight lifters. In these cases, it appears that the force of the humeral head is directed between the middle and inferior ligaments and that there may be some separation of these ligaments. The appearance is of a thin cordlike middle glenohumeral ligament usually attached superiorly in its segment. There may be flap tears of the anterosuperior labrum or the labrum may be absent.

Case Study II

A power weight lifter developed painful shoulders during the course of his activities. His shoulders became particularly painful with the benchpress. The examination revealed sensitivity over the biceps without apprehension in abduction external rotation. There was no clinical evidence of impingement. The findings at arthroscopy showed separation between the middle and inferior ligaments. In this case, both shoulders were arthroscoped—on one side there was separation between the two ligaments (Plate 12-17), and on the other side there was evidence that separation was occurring but was not complete (Plate 12-18).

Case Study III

A similar lesion was noted in a shortstop who successfully completed 4 years of Division I NCAA baseball. During his high-school career, he engaged in a course of power weight lifting. He developed a painful shoulder with benchpressing and was unable to throw. The lesion noted at arthroscopy was a thin cordlike middle (Plate 12-19) glenohumeral ligament with fibrillation of anterior superior labrum. He underwent debridement of the lesion and rehabilitation and successfully completed his college career.

This alteration of the middle glenohumeral ligament has been described as a normal variation in two studies.[3,13] Whether this appearance is developed or normal is debatable and whether produced by stress or traction or both is unknown. Irritations at the attachment may be a source of discomfort; however, reattachment is not necessary.

SUPERIOR SEGMENT

If the humeral head is forced into the superior direction, the superior labrum biceps attachment is subject to injury. The manifestations seen arthroscopically depend on whether the force is acute or chronic. In the fall on the oustretched arm, the humeral head may go over the labrum and come back, resulting in a torn labrum. If the force is sufficient, the humeral head may also injure the rotator cuff undersurface. The force may also split the biceps in addition to the superior labrum. If the movement of the humeral head superiorly is chronic due to loss of strength, fatigue, and inability of the supraspinatus to sufficiently centralize the humeral head during the abduction external rotation phase, the lesions may then appear different. In this case, the labrum may have a battered appearance or an indentation in the biceps tendon and possibly superior rotator cuff changes (Plate 12-20).

Case Study IV

A professional baseball shortstop slid back into first base on his abdomen and outstretched arm. The left nonthrowing arm struck the bag. The direction of the force appeared to be superior motion of the humeral head. The symptoms were pain and clicking in abduction. He had difficulty swinging a bat, but because of nondominance fielding was a minimal problem. The arthroscopic findings (Plate 12-21) were a superior labral tear, a loose superior labrum, and an undersurface rotator cuff tear. Following debridement of the rotator cuff and superior labrum and an off-season rehabilitation program, the patient returned to competitive major league baseball.

Snyder and associates[14] first reported on these lesions and termed them SLAP (superior labral anteroposterior) lesions. In 47 percent of the cases, the lesion appeared as an acute injury, usually from a fall onto the outstretched arm. The type I lesion consists of fraying and is often a chronic lesion (Plate 12-22). The type II separation of the labrum and biceps is difficult to evaluate due to a normal looseness at this attachment[15,16] (Plate 12-23). The bucket handle type III and the bucket handle that extends into the biceps tendon type IV are likely related to acute injuries (Plate 12-24). These injuries (as noted in the case report) may also produce rotator cuff injuries.

One cannot always separate anterosuperior and superior labral lesions. In some cases, the superior lesions may accompany an already loosened anterosuperior labrum. Often the anterior flap noted previously extends into the superior labrum. It is better to judge each segment separately and correlate them with the mechanism of the injury and the physical examination.

ANTEROINFERIOR SEGMENT

The anteroinferior labrum and the attached inferior glenohumeral ligament are strong buttresses to inferior and anteroinferior motion of the humeral head.[4,17] Force of the humeral head against this area in the abducted and externally rotated position may produce loosening of the capsule, disruption of the labrum, and dislocation of the humeral head. If the symptoms are of subluxation, there will be apprehension in abduction external rotation and other corroborating tests (see Ch. 10). The arthroscopic view is characteristic, revealing loosening and detachment of the anteroinferior labrum and capsule, and may also extend into other labral segments (Plate 12-25).

The treatment of anterior instability can be approached arthroscopically.[18-20] Open procedures, as noted in Ch. 11, have been tested and have a high degree of success. Arthroscopic procedures are newer and, subject to changes and modifications, have not been associated in all instances with the same degree of

success as open procedures.[18,21,22] As our understanding increases and techniques are improved, arthroscopic methods may become more successful.

POSTERIOR LABRAL INJURY

If the force is directed posteriorly, then the posterior capsule and labrum can sustain injury. The findings of a posterior labral injury (Plate 12-26) are frequently associated with posterior extra-articular ossification (Fig. 12-5). We have examined seven throwing athletes who have posterior ossifications and posterior labral lesions.[23] In each case, there was no anterior pathology. This lesion appeared consistent with Bennett's original description[24] in 1941. The pitchers had pain either in the cocking or follow-through phases of throwing. The etiologic force may have been an external rotational traction force on the posterior origin of the inferior glenohumeral ligament or the internal rotation adduction force of the humeral head after ball release. A physical examination demonstrated posterior tenderness in all cases, but other parts of the examination were varied. Although it can be viewed by radiographs, special views (e.g., Stryker notch views) are necessary to view the lesion. Arthro computerized axial tomography (CAT) scan and magnetic resonance imaging (MRI) may be helpful in finding the lesion earlier. Additionally, these studies may show intra-articular pathology. The ossification is not intra-articular. In each case, arthroscopy was performed to debride the posterior labral pathology and, in one case, a rotator cuff tear. The ossific lesion does not need to be surgically approached. Limited throwing and general conditioning should continue until the ossific lesion matures and there is no pain on palpation. In these specific cases, there was a high success rate in the return to throwing.[23] Isolated posterior labral injury without ossification may be produced by the same mechanism. Posterior labral ossification and posterior capsular injury may be found with posterior subluxation and dislocation.[25] Posterior lesions noted at arthroscopy should be correlated with the history and physical examination.

ANTERIOR AND POSTERIOR INJURIES

The humeral head may move excessively anterior and posterior producing problems in both segments. Symptoms may be those of anterior or posterior instability or a combination of both. Posterior lesions are occasionally associated with an anterior instability.[16]

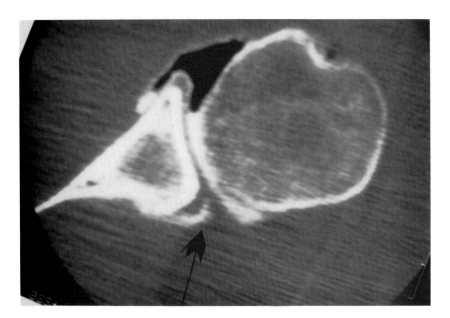

Figure 12-5 Posterior ossification noted. (Not seen arthroscopically.)

This should not be confused with multidirectional laxity, since generalized and inferior laxity are not present.

Case Study V

A large football interior lineman experienced pain with most shoulder motions. He had played both offense and defense, which required the frequent and forceful use of his arms and hands. He also pursued an extensive benchpressing and weight training program. The examination revealed clicking in abduction and external rotation and positive anterior and posterior apprehension tests as well as some crepitus posterior in the shoulder. The arthroscopic examination revealed anterior, superior, and inferior labral detachment in addition to a posterior labral injury with posterior detachment (Plate 12-27).

ACROMIOCLAVICULAR JOINT

The acromioclavicular joint responds to movement of the shoulder and stabilizes in rotation and elevation, as noted in Ch. 9. When stabilized in elevation, the ligaments tighten and pressure occurs across the joint. Excessive compressive pressure can occur with power weight lifting, resulting in osteolysis of the distal clavicle.[26] This injury responds to resection of the distal clavicle.[6]

Chronic acromioclavicular separation and the resulting laxity will cause degeneration and discomfort. The change seen anteriorly on the distal clavicle may be related to compressive pressure of the scapula across the joint during the acceleration phase of throwing.

Case Study VI

A 27-year-old major league pitcher complained of pain, weakness, and decreased velocity as he reached the acceleration phase of pitching. The examination revealed a tender acromioclavicular joint, and radiographic examination revealed osteolysis and an inferior spur fragment at the distal clavicle. The pitcher underwent resection of the distal clavicle where softening of the distal clavicle was noted. The area was approached from the superior position, as there was no evidence of undersurface or subacromial pathology on arthroscopic examination. The lesion was probably related to the throwing motion and the chronic protracted position of his scapula, producing compression across the acromioclavicular joint.

ROTATOR CUFF INJURY

Rotator cuff injuries must be mentioned in association with capsular labral injuries. They may be associated with superior migration of the humeral head, as reported in the SLAP lesion,[14] and may also be associated with a posterior ossification.[23] Rotator cuff injuries are seen in dislocations, power weight lifting, and repetitive overhead activity. The lesions in the throwers tend to be undersurface tears and not associated with subacromial changes (Plates 12-28 and 12-29).

Glenohumeral instability represents increased motion in a particular direction or directions. Weakened or atrophic rotator cuff musculature will contribute to instability and may result in rotator cuff damage in response to increased motion and shearing force. It cannot always be determined if the rotator cuff injury occurs at the same time as an initiating traumatic episode or is the result of increased motion after capsular labral injury. Likewise, labral injuries are seen with rotator cuff tears. These tears may result from altered mechanics produced by excessive and painful motion.

More recently, another mechanism has been demonstrated to cause rotator cuff injury.[27] This mechanism occurs in extreme abduction, which produces impingement of the rotator cuff between the humeral head and superior glenoid. This may have been associated with some of the other mechanisms, but it is not yet clear that it occurs at all times, and therefore this mechanism should be kept in mind when trying to understand the pathology noted at arthroscopy.

Isolated rotator cuff lesions in combination with other lesions may be approached athroscopically; smaller, undersurface lesions may be treated by arthroscopic debridement and have a high degree of success.[28,29] Open treatment of full-thickness tears may reduce pain, but may not return the throwing athlete to former levels of proficiency.[21] Arthroscopic treatment of full-thickness tears is changing, and newer techniques may permit a return to previous athletic performance status.

IMPINGEMENT

Classically, impingement is believed to be compression and abrasion of the bursa and rotator cuff tendons against the subacromial arc during the act of elevation.[30] In the throwing athlete, rotator cuff tears are often seen without any evidence of impingement pathology in the subacromial space. The impingement test may be positive. In these cases, the undersurface torn rotator cuff may abut the acromion, or the weakness of the rotator cuff, as a result of tearing and failure to centralize the humeral head, may be a cause of impingement symptoms. Weakness, which causes altered mechanics, can result in pain that produces the impingement sign. Lastly, weakness of scapular musculature may alter the motion of the scapula, resulting in impingement signs.

Arthroscopy is of value to view the subacromial space to see if changes are present (Plate 12-30). It is extremely rare to encounter subacromial changes in athletes under the age of 30. This suggests that the impingement is a secondary manifestation of some other cause, such as instability or weakness. Studies of acromioplasty in athletes and in younger patients[31,32] show excellent relief of pain but with lesser ability to return to sport.

Other intra-articular pathology may occur with sim-ilar history and examination to labral or capsular injuries. These lesions are also confusing in their appearance on diagnostic images; such examples are injuries of the subscapularis tendon and muscle, and the biceps tendon (Plates 12-31 and 12-32).

REFERENCES

1. Uhthoff HK, Piscopo M: Anterior capsular redundancy of the shoulder: congenital or traumatic? J Bone Joint [Br] 67:363, 1985
2. DePalma AF, Callery G, Bennett GA: Variational anatomy and degenerative lesions of the shoulder joint. AAOS Instr Course Lect 6:255, 1949
3. Rames RD, Morgan CD, Snyder SJ: Anatomical of the glenohumeral ligaments of the glenohumeral ligaments, abstracted. Arthroscopy 7:328, 1991
4. O'Brien SJ, Neves MC, Arnoczky SP et al: The anatomy and histology of the inferior glenohumeral ligament complex of the shoulder. Am J Sports Med 18:449, 1990
5. Ferrari DA: Capsular ligaments of the shoulder: anatomic developmental study of the anterior superior capsule. Am J Sports Med 18:20, 1990
6. Rodosky MW, Ruder MJ, Harner CH: The role of the biceps superior glenoid labrum complex in anterior stability of the shoulder, abstracted. Arthroscopy 6:160, 1990
7. Kohn D: The clinical relevance of glenoid labrum lesions. Arthroscopy 3:223, 1987
8. Payne LZ, Jokl P: The results of arthroscopic debridement of glenoid labral tears based on tear location. Arthrosc J Arthrosc Rel Surg 9:560, 1993
9. Altchek DW, Warren RF, Wickiewicz TL, Ortiz G: Arthroscopic labral debridement: a 3-year follow-up study. Am J Sports Med 20:702, 1992
10. Glasgow SG, Bruce RA, Yacobucci GN, Torg JS: Arthroscopic resection of glenoid labral tears in the athlete: a report of 29 cases. Arthroscopy 8:48, 1992
11. Pappas AM, Goss TP, Kleinman PK: Symptomatic shoulder instability due to lesions of the glenoid labrum. Am J Sports Med 11:279, 1983
12. Andrews JR, Carson WG Jr, McLeod WD: Glenoid labrum tears related to the long head of the biceps. Am J Sports Med 13:337, 1985
13. Snyder SJ, Buford D, Wuh HCK: The Buford complex: the loose anterior superior labrum-middle glenohumeral ligament complex: a normal variant. Presented at the Annual Meeting of the Arthroscopy Association of North America, Boston, MA 1992
14. Snyder SJ, Karzel RP, DelPizzo W et al: SLAP lesions of the shoulder. Arthroscopy 6:274, 1990
15. Cooper DE, Arnoczky S, O'Brien S et al: Anatomy, histology and vascularity of the glenoid labrum: an anatomical study. J Bone Joint Surg [Am] 74:46, 1992
16. Detrisac DA, Johnson LL: Arthroscopic shoulder anatomy. New Jersey, Slack, 1986
17. Turkel SJ et al: Stabilizing mechanisms preventing ante-

rior dislocation of the glenohumeral joint. J Bone Joint Surg [Am] 63:1208, 1981

18. Morgan CD, Bodenstab AB: Arthroscopic Bankart suture repair: technique and early results. Arthroscopy 3:111, 1987
19. Lane JG, Sachs RA, Riehl B: Arthroscopic staple capsulorrhaphy: a long-term follow-up. Arthroscopy 9:190, 1993
20. Benedetto KP, Glotzer W: Arthroscopic Bankart procedure by suture technique: indications, technique, and results. Arthroscopy 8:111, 1992
21. Tibone JE et al: Surgical treatment of tears of the rotator cuff in athletes. J Bone Joint Surg [Am] 68:887, 1986
22. Grana WA, Buckley PD, Yates CK: Arthroscopic Bankart suture repair. Am J Sports Med 21:348, 1993
23. Ferrari JD, Ferrari DA, Coumas J, Pappas AM: Posterior ossification of the shoulder the Bennett lesion: diagnosis and treatment. Am J Sports Med 22:171, 1994
24. Bennett GE: Shoulder and elbow lesions of the professional baseball pitcher. JAMA 117:51, 1941
25. Fronek J, Warren RF, Bowen MR: Posterior subluxation of the glenohumeral joint. J Bone Joint Surg [Am] 71:205, 1989
26. Cahill BR: Osteolysis of the distal part of the clavicle in male athletes. J Bone Joint Surg [Am] 64:1053, 1982
27. Walch G, Boileau P, Noel E, Donnell ST: Impingement of the deep surface of the supraspinatus tendon on the posterosuperior glenoid rim: an arthroscopic study. J Shoulder Elbow Surg 1:238, 1992
28. Andrews JR, Broussard TS, Carson WG: Arthroscopy of the shoulder in the management of partial tears of the rotator cuff: a preliminary report. Arthroscopy 1:117, 1989
29. Snyder SJ, Pachelli AF, Del Pizzo WD et al: Partial thickness rotator cuff tears: results of arthroscopic treatment. Arthroscopy 7:1, 1991
30. Neer CS II: Impingement lesions. Clin Orthop 173:70, 1983
31. Burns TP, Turba JE: Arthroscopic treatment of shoulder impingement in athletes. Am J Sports Med 20:13, 1992
32. Tibone JE, Jobe FW, Kerlan RF: Shoulder impingement syndrome in athletes treated by anterior acromioplasty. Clin Orthop 188:134, 1985

13

Musculotendinous Sport Injuries of the Shoulder

William B. Balcom
Arthur M. Pappas

Injuries to the musculotendinous structures surrounding the shoulder complex are common in the athlete, especially in sports requiring forceful and/or repetitive use of the upper extremity. Most injuries and clinical complaints of the shoulder area directly or indirectly involve the musculotendinous structures of the shoulder.[1] Some authors believe that 75 percent of these injuries are preventable.[2]

The muscles and tendons about an athlete's shoulder play a major role in maintaining stability of the glenohumeral and scapulothoracic articulations. The rotator cuff muscles, while weak movers of the glenohumeral joint, provide a balancing force and compressive containment for the joint, which has an important stabilizing effect, especially within the midrange of motion.[3] The scapular muscles control the thoracoscapular articulation and adjust the position of the scapula appropriate to the changing positions of the humerus. Because a stable thoracoscapulohumeral complex is a prerequisite for all satisfactory shoulder motion and function, loss of coordinated muscle action with resultant imbalance may cause both shoulder dysfunction and instability, with adverse effects on the athlete's performance.

Properly coordinated action of the muscles about an athlete's shoulder results in a multidimensional cohesive shoulder motion. This motion is a complex alternating sequence of concentric and eccentric contractions of the musculotendinous units, modulated by neuroproprioceptive mechanisms, and occurs with prerequisite flexibility and balanced strength. The end result should be a fluid and coordinated scapulothoracic and glenohumeral rhythm. If each unit does not interact in an integrated fashion, shoulder function will be compromised, resulting in injury and/or clinical complaints.

The muscles of the thoracoscapulohumeral articulation function both concentrically and eccentrically to accelerate and decelerate joint motion to stabilize these articulations.[4] Injury to a musculotendinous unit about the athlete's shoulder can result in an altered capacity to carry out these functions. Muscle injuries most often result from an eccentric muscle contraction or by application of an external stress that exceeds tissue tolerance.[5] Inadequate warm-up, lack of stretching, inflexibility, soft tissue contractures, weakness, imbalance, abnormal patterns of function, and fatigue are all factors associated with muscle injury. Muscles that cross several joints or that have been previously injured or incompletely rehabilitated are particularly susceptible.

Each musculotendinous unit consists of an origin, a muscle, a myotendinous junction, a tendon, and an insertion. Each component of the musculotendinous complex has a different gross and histologic appearance, with a resultant differentiation of function. The force generated by skeletal muscle is transmitted through the specialized myotendinous junction to the tendon and ultimately to the skeletal system. Although any component of the musculotendinous unit may be injured in a strain or eccentric-type injury, biomechanical studies and anecdotal observations have usually shown that the areas of the myotendinous junction and terminal few millimeters of muscle are the weak link and the site of most frequent failure. Because of their anatomic location, injuries to the biceps tendon and supraspinatus tendon are common exceptions to this general principle.

Injury prevention is critical in the athlete. Preparticipation physical examinations are an important facet of injury prevention in evaluating muscle strength and advanced and complete function. Properly performed strength and endurance training with appropriate warm-up and stretching prior to participation in athletic activities are also important. Correct warm-up and stretching increase the metabolic efficiency and the compliance of the muscle tissues. Strength and endurance training maximize the muscle's ability to absorb energy and minimize and delay fatigue. Whole-body conditioning, scheduled periods of rest, and an emphasis on proper sport-specific biomechanics are important for both injury prevention and during injury rehabilitation (see Ch. 16).

CONTUSION

A contusion is an injury to an anatomic structure (bony or soft tissue) caused by a directly applied force. Musculotendinous contusions in the shoulder area are common and are most often associated with collision sports (e.g., hockey). A clear inciting event is typically recalled by the individual. On physical examination, patients note pain to palpation directly over the involved structure and discomfort when the musculotendinous unit is either stressed or activated. Swelling and ecchymosis are often present. Radiographs usually demonstrate soft tissue swelling; magnetic resonance imaging (MRI) and ultrasound may more accurately define the extent of the injury. Treatment consists of rest, ice, and compression for 48 hours, followed by

moist heat, a well-structured rehabilitation program, and gradual return to sport (see Ch. 2).

STRAINS

A strain is an injury to a musculotendinous structure caused by an indirectly applied force. Muscle strains most often occur as the result of eccentric contraction or stretching of an activated muscle. The site of injury is influenced by the rate of loading, mechanism of injury, and local anatomic factors.[6] Lower rates of loading usually result in failure at the tendon-bone junction by bone avulsion or disruption at the insertion site, and higher rates of loading usually result in intratendinous injury or injury at the myotendinous junction.[7] This is an important distinction because bony avulsions and insertion site failures usually fare better than midsubstance disruptions. Direct trauma will most often produce injury within the muscle substance, while eccentric overload or other indirect injury will result in injury in the area of the distal muscle substance or myotendinous junction.[8] Excessive eccentric muscle activity may also result in injury within the muscle with the development of tender nodules early and a delayed muscle soreness occurring 24 to 48 hours after the inciting activity. The intra-articular path and impingement of the biceps, and poor vascularity and impingement of the supraspinatus are additional factors that predispose these structures to intratendinous injury.[6]

These musculotendinous injuries can be quantified in a clinical grading system. A grade I strain is a simple stretching of the soft tissue fibers. A grade II strain involves partial tearing of the musculotendinous unit. These two grades comprise the majority of musculotendinous strains. The clinical presentation in a grade I or II strain consists of pain and a limited ability to perform. Tenderness to palpation over the involved structure is noted, and discomfort is experienced when the musculotendinous unit is activated or stressed. Swelling of the tendons and ecchymosis are often present. The radiographs are negative. Ultrasound and MRI may help delineate the location and severity of the injury. Treatment is nonoperative and identical to that described for contusions. Prior to return to sport, the rehabilitation should emphasize flexibility and restoration of strength to decrease the incidence of reinjury.

Grade III strains are complete disruptions of the involved musculotendinous unit. Grade III strains are uncommon and are seen in athletes participating in sports where extreme forces are applied to the shoulder (weight lifting, wrestling). Other than disruptions of the rotator cuff or long head of the biceps tendon, complete disruptions of musculotendinous structures about the shoulder are rare in athletes. When grade III muscle injury does occur, the muscle elements are torn and a palpable defect may result. Diagnosis is based on the findings unique to disruptions, which include (1) presence of a palpable defect, (2) local sensitivity over the injured area, (3) significant decline in strength, and (4) development of atrophy with time. In recent years, computed tomography (CT) scan, ultrasound, and MRI have allowed objective visualization of these injuries. In the athlete, grade III injuries warrant consideration of acute surgical repair. Surgical repair can be difficult when injury occurs in the area of the muscle substance or myotendinous junction due to the problems of placing sutures directly into damaged and frayed muscle tissue. In instances where failure occurs within the bone substance (bony avulsion) or at the insertion site, surgical treatment consists of reattachment with staples, transosseous nonabsorbable sutures, screws with spiked washers, or suture anchors. Postoperatively, the arm should be immobilized in a position that protects the surgical repair. A progressive exercise program can then be implemented to optimize the athlete's rehabilitation efforts.

Specific musculotendinous injuries are discussed in the remainder of this chapter, with characteristics unique to the athletic population emphasized. Rotator cuff disease, longhead of the biceps tendon disorders, and impingement will be discussed together because they are clinically interrelated.

SPECIFIC MUSCULOTENDINOUS INJURIES

Deltoid

The deltoid is the most directly exposed muscle of the shoulder girdle. If there is irreversible injury to the deltoid muscle, shoulder function will likely be compromised. Grade I and grade II injuries are common, most often the result of a direct blow. Occasionally, in throwing athletes, the posterior deltoid may suffer eccentric injury during the deceleration phase of delivery. It is important to differentiate these grades I and II deltoid strains from the late muscle changes that occur secondary to axillary nerve or posterior cord injury, or to long-standing subdeltoid bursitis (see Chs. 4 and 11). Complete disruption of the deltoid in the athlete, however, is extremely rare, and if it does occur, it is the result of a significant load applied to a maximally contracted muscle. Physical findings vary depending on the site of injury. Loss of the normal convex shoulder

contour and weakness will be noted. The specific deficiency will depend on whether the anterior, middle, and/or posterior component of the deltoid is injured. If the injury is distal at or near its humeral attachment, the defect may be exaggerated by activation of the deltoid muscle.

Grades I and II strains of the deltoid can be treated with ice and compression acutely, followed by moist heat, a range of motion (ROM) regimen, stretching, and progressive strengthening with subsequent return to sport (see Ch. 2 for a complete discussion). In complete ruptures, if more than one-third of the deltoid is involved, prompt surgical exploration and primary repair are recommended, particularly in the athlete.[9]

Pectoralis Major

The vast majority of pectoralis major strains are grade I or grade II. Most often the pectoralis major is stretched while actively contracting (e.g., inability to complete the repetition during benchpressing). Grade III injuries are unusual, and when they do occur, they are usually seen in adult males under the age of 40. These severe injuries have been reported to occur at the muscle origin, within the muscle, at the musculotendinous junction, within the tendon, or at the bony insertion. Cases have been reported in weight lifters, wrestlers, and in athletes attempting to break a fall.[10] Wrestlers often injure the sternoclavicular portion. The injury results in sharp burning pain with accompanying swelling and ecchymosis. When the muscle is ruptured at its sternal or clavicular attachment, a bulge is noted within the anterior axilla. When the disruption is at or near the humeral attachment, a bulge appears over the chest wall. A visible or palpable defect is generally present. Resisted adduction and internal rotation are weak, elicit pain, and exaggerate the defect. Ultrasound and MRI will confirm the site of rupture but MRI will better quantify the extent of injury.

Grades I and II injuries respond to the nonoperative protocol previously outlined. The strengthening exercises should not be initiated until there is resolution of pain and restoration of full shoulder motion (see Ch. 2). Complete rupture demands early surgical treatment in the active athlete. Disruptions at the humeral attachment are repaired with heavy nonabsorbable sutures through drill holes or via suture anchors. Tendinous ruptures and musculotendinous junction tears are repaired end to end. A gentle range of motion program would begin with resolution of pain, but active motion should not begin for 6 to 8 weeks. Return to sport would be delayed until range of motion, strength, and coordination approximated that of the uninjured extremity.

Case Study I

A 36-year-old weight lifter heard a pop as he attempted to complete his final repetition during a benchpressing workout. He experienced significant pain and noted a defect in the anterior aspect of his right axilla. Over the ensuing days, a moderate area of ecchymosis developed. He sought consultation 8 weeks later because of the persistence of the defect and a perception of weakness (Fig. 13-1A). On physical examination, adduction and internal rotation were weak, and resisted adduction and internal rotation exaggerated the palpable defect. An MRI was obtained (Fig. 13-1B & C), which demonstrated complete detachment of the sternal head of the pectoralis major muscle from the humerus. The patient wished to continue weight training and desired treatment that would minimize the deformity and optimize his return of strength. At surgery, the detached sternal head was mobilized, the humeral surface denuded, and the sternal head reattached by three suture anchors. Pendulum motion was allowed 1 week postoperatively, and a more complete passive range of motion was begun at 4 weeks. Active range of motion was instituted at 6 weeks postoperatively, but a progressive return to weight training was not allowed until right shoulder motion, strength, and coordination approached that of the uninjured shoulder (4 months postoperatively).

Triceps

Most strains of the proximal triceps are grades I and II injuries located within the longhead of the triceps. These strains are especially common in throwing athletes and volleyball spikers and are caused by repetitive eccentric loads that occur with the deceleration of the upper extremity during the follow-through. These individuals present with deep, diffuse discomfort over the posteroinferior aspect of the glenohumeral joint and proximal arm. Ectopic calcification or bony spurring may be seen coincidentally on radiographs (Bennett's lesion).[11] Although this posteroinferior ossification is not related to the triceps attachment, its presence may prompt an investigation for concurrent intra-articular labral or posterior capsular pathology in patients with refractory symptoms.[12] The treatment of a triceps strain is nonoperative, consisting of symptomatic care followed by directed rehabilitation.

Case Study II

A 21-year-old college football player was involved in a pile-up in an attempt to recover a loose ball. His right arm was trapped underneath him with his right elbow maximally flexed when an opponent's helmet was driven into his triceps area. The patient felt a "tearing," which was accompanied by swelling and severe burning pain. The patient was referred for treatment with routine radiographs suggesting soft tissue swelling; an MRI demonstrated diffuse injury to the longhead of the triceps (Fig. 13-2). The injured triceps was iced intermittently for 48 hours, followed by periodic application of moist heat. The right arm was immobilized in a sling for 1 week, and then a stretching and progressive strengthening program was instituted. The patient returned to his sport 4 weeks from the time of his injury, at which time his right elbow and shoulder motions were full and pain-free, and triceps strength was equal to that of the uninjured extremity.

Serratus Anterior

Rupture of the serratus anterior is extremely uncommon. Winging of the scapula is more often the result of injury to the long thoracic nerve, which may be secondary to a traction neurapraxia, Parsonage-Turner syndrome, or a viral insult (e.g., mononucleosis) (see Ch. 4). The severity of pain can be helpful in differentiating chronic long thoracic nerve palsy from the more painful acute serratus anterior muscle disruption.[13] Serratus anterior atrophy occasionally may occur secondary to inflammation of the neighboring subcapsularis bursa. Regardless of the cause of serratus anterior insufficiency, the resultant scapular winging and altered scapular orientation may result in secondary rotator cuff injury, glenohumeral instability, or impingement, emphasizing the importance of the serratus anterior for normal shoulder function. In the case of a serratus anterior injury, recovery depends on the proper diagnosis and then the initiation of a directed rehabilitation program. Surgery may be considered in cases of chronic serratus anterior insufficiency and winging of the scapula. In most instances, however, the postsurgical impairments are greater than the original problem.

Coracobrachialis

Rupture of the coracobrachialis is also extremely uncommon. The reported cases in the literature were significantly improved by surgery.[14] The limited antici-

pated functional disability may make observation a reasonable treatment alternative. Musculocutaneous nerve function and biceps innervation must be specifically documented.

Subscapularis

Partial ruptures, especially of the lower one-fourth are frequently associated with anterior dislocation of the glenohumeral joint.[15,16] Eccentric injury may also occur during the late cocking or early acceleration phase of the throwing motion as the maximally stretched subscapularis contracts. These muscle injuries are treated with immobilization of the affected shoulder in internal rotation, followed by a flexibility and strengthening rehabilitation program. Reports of complete traumatic ruptures of the subcapsularis are uncommon, but those reported in the literature have been successfully treated with primary repair.[17] An incompletely rehabilitated subscapularis injury may predispose the athlete to recurrent anterior glenohumeral instability.

Case Study III

On a cold, wet night in May, a 26-year-old major league pitcher was in the ninth inning of a one-run difference game. In an attempt to strike out a batter, he describes reaching back for a "little extra" (i.e., increasing his shoulder extension external rotation sequence, which placed additional stress on the front of his shoulder). He felt discomfort with the pitch but was able to complete it and then was removed from the game due to the pain. On the following day, examination demonstrated discomfort with attempted abduction and external rotation, but there was no evidence of swelling or focal sensitivity.

His discomfort persisted, and he was placed on the disabled list. Approximately 4 weeks later he felt he could return to major league baseball. He pitched three innings but again experienced discomfort with maximum external rotation, and requested to be removed from the game. An MRI was performed and the findings were consistent with changes in the subscapularis muscle (Fig. 13-3A). He was maintained on a limited activity program and again attempted to return approximately 6 weeks later and experienced a recurrence of his symptomatology. Another MRI was performed that demonstrated progressive change in the subscapularis area (Fig. 13-3B). There was a question of these changes being tumorous rather than an acute injury. For additional consulta-

tion the MRI was reviewed and the findings were thought to be consistent with injury and repair and not a tumor. Accordingly, he was placed on a nonthrowing rehabilitation program to maintain maximum function of his subscapularis, minimizing contracture and maximizing strength.

The pitcher continued with his rehabilitation program and an MRI in November revealed some improvement. His program was increased, which included some resistance exercises and some gradual overhead athletic functions but without maximum output. A final evaluation and MRI performed in January, 8 months after his initial injury (Fig. 13-3C) and 4 months after the most recent injury, demonstrated continued improvement in the healing of the subscapularis muscle. He was able to return to his position as a starting major league pitcher in the following season and has continued to perform as a major league pitcher for an additional 5 years at this time.

The injury of the subscapularis muscle occurred in a maximum cocking phase when there was an additional eccentric force that resulted in the internal disruption. Attempts to return too soon postinjury resulted in recurrent injury and a delay in improvement. The interval between the recurrent injury and his returning to throw effectively was monitored, and more than 4 months were required for adequate repair and rehabilitation of the injured subscapularis muscle prior to the pitcher returning to his sport.

Infraspinatus and Teres Minor

Grades I and II injuries of the infraspinatus and teres minor are common in the overhead athlete. They are usually the result of eccentric injury during the follow-through phase in an attempt to decelerate the forward flexion and internal rotation of the affected arm. On examination, patients note pain to palpation over the distal muscle and myotendinous junction. Tender nodules are typically noted at the time of initial presentation. Treatment is as previously discussed. Firm cruciform or friction massage techniques may be of benefit if palpable nodules are present. The strengthening component of care should utilize techniques emphasizing eccentric muscle contractions. Infraspinatus dysfunction and atrophy may occur secondary to a traction neuropathy of the suprascapular nerve as it courses around the spinoglenoid process, and this may need to be specifically ruled out (see Chs. 4 and 11). Grade III injuries are extremely rare.

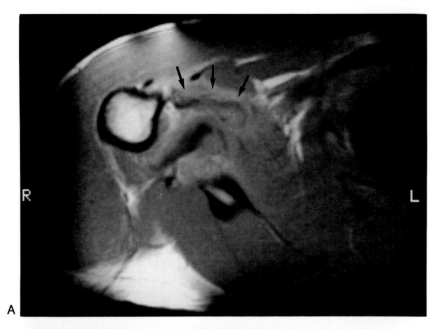

A

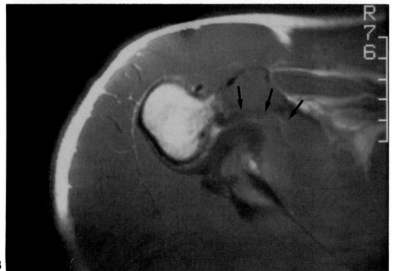

B

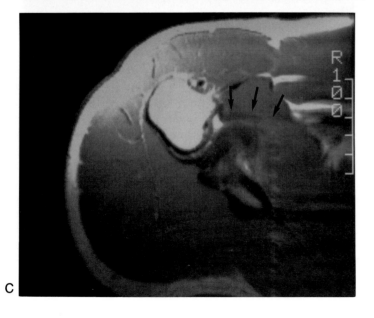

C

Figure 13-3 (A) Sequential T1-weighted axial image through the inferior glenohumeral joint, demonstrating an abnormal bulbous configuration to the distal myotendinous junction of the inferior component of the subscapularis with moderate redundancy of the tendon *(arrows).* Concurrent midlevel signal intensity within the distal muscles substance is consistent with geographic infiltration of inflammatory fluids. **(B)** MRI image a few months after the first demonstrates interval reduction in mass effect with persistent thickening of the tendon *(arrows).* **(C)** Image 2 months later shows resolution of the mass effect *(arrows)* with some persistent post-traumatic degenerative change of the inferior aspect of the subscapularis tendon.

Case Study IV

A 26-year-old major league catcher did not have any complaints about his shoulder. He was participating in a game when a base runner attempted to steal from first to second base. As he was about to release the ball, he experienced some discomfort in the back of his shoulder and was unable to control the direction and velocity of the ball. He denied the pain as being a sharp pain, but it continued whenever he attempted to throw the ball any distance at any velocity. He was removed from the game, and the sensitivity in the back part of his shoulder was reviewed. Radiographs were negative. An MRI revealed changes in the area of the teres minor and there was a question as to whether this was a disruption that required surgery.

Careful examination of his shoulder revealed a functional and intact infraspinatus, but there was definite sensitivity in the region of the teres minor, both to palpation and on attempted eccentric activity. The muscle was boggy; however, a major deficit was not palpated. All nerve conduction studies were within normal limits and the only abnormality on needle electromyography was the evidence of major fasciculation in the teres minor. On the basis of the history, physical examination, and lack of major neurodiagnostic indications of damage, it was recommended that a surgical procedure be delayed and that a rehabilitation program be instituted with continued observation.

He was maintained on a program for control of shoulder function and gradual strengthening and utilization of the infraspinatus, teres minor complex. Approximately 4 weeks later he was prepared to return to all of his required activities as a major league catcher. Three seasons have passed since the injury, and he remains on an active program for flexibility and strengthening of his shoulder muscles with no problems.

Case Study V

A 24-year-old major league relief pitcher complained of discomfort with pitching during the acceleration phase. He was unable to recall a specific pitch when this was first noticed and continued to pitch, yet the next day he experienced soreness in the back of his shoulder.

On examination, he had definite fullness and sensitivity over both the infraspinatus and teres minor musculotendinous areas in an attempt to bring his arm across his chest in a flexed and adducted position, while stabilizing his scapula. He experienced

acute sensitivity with palpation of the infraspinatus and teres minor muscles. Acute strain and inflammation in the musculotendinous junction of the infraspinatus and teres minor was diagnosed. He began a course of restricted activity, ice packs, massage and then gradual rehabilitation. He was not allowed to return to pitching until he had a full pain-free active and passive range of motion without evidence of contracture. A rehabilitation program of 4 months was necessary prior to his return to participation.

Rhomboid and Trapezius Muscles

The rhomboids and the horizontal component of the midtrapezius, like the infraspinatus and teres minor, may suffer eccentric injury in their attempt to decelerate protraction of the scapula during the follow-through phase of the pitcher's delivery. Tender palpable nodules are often present and these typically respond to firm cruciform massage techniques. The trapezius and rhomboid muscles need to be specifically addressed in the conditioning or rehabilitation program of any overhead athlete. The trapezius may also be injured by a direct blow in collision sports. The injuries are usually grade I or grade II in severity.

Case Study VI

The day after each starting role, a successful major league pitcher presents for evaluation and treatment of his trapezius and rhomboid musculature. The sensitive nodules within these muscles are present after each pitching occasion, and massage therapy is necessary for treatment of what could be considered either eccentric sprains, eccentric injury, or metabolic fatigue nodules. The importance of the identification, treatment, and rehabilitation focus on these muscles is critical to the maintenance of a sound shoulder throwing mechanism. Continuous care of his shoulder is a critical part of his in-season as well as out-of-season program. Particular attention has been directed toward his posterior shoulder and scapula muscles.

Impingement

The impingement space is defined by the undersurface of the anterior one-third of the acromion, distal clavicle, and acromioclavicular joint superiorly, the proximal humerus inferiorly, and the coracoacromial ligament anteriorly. Impingement refers to the compression of the rotator cuff, biceps tendon, and/or accompanying bursa between one or more of these confining structures.

Pure impingement in the young athletic population is rare. It is most often a manifestation of underlying subtle superior, anterosuperior, or posterosuperior glenohumeral instability. It may be secondary to a number of other causes as well: thoracoscapular weakness and instability; rotator cuff or longhead of biceps dysfunction; displaced acromioclavicular joint disruptions and other double disruptions of the superior suspensory complex of the shoulder; lesions of the acromion (congenital or posttraumatic) or distal clavicle, including undersurface bony spurs; loss of lower extremity strength or faulty biomechanics, transferring increased stress to the shoulder; iatrogenic following anterior or posterior shoulder reconstruction; and other less common etiologies. In a small number of veteran athletes (usually over the age of 35) primary impingement will occur with overhead activity. In this subgroup of athletes, years of repetitive overhead activity cause an overgrowth on the undersurface of the acromion or acromioclavicular articulation or a thickening and/or ossification of the acromioclavicular ligament with resultant narrowing of the impingement space.[18] The characteristic signs and symptoms include discomfort over the anterior and anterolateral aspect of the shoulder; discomfort to palpation over the impingement interval; maximal pain when the arm is elevated from 60 to 120 degrees (the so-called painful arc), increased within the internal rotation and decreased with external rotation of the arm; pain with forward flexion of the humerus as the acromion is manually depressed (impingement sign); and transient relief of discomfort when the impingement interval is injected with xylocaine (impingement test). In patients with concurrent rotator cuff tears or instability, the superior migration of the humeral head may make the impingement symptoms worse.

Case Study VII

A major league pitcher began experiencing discomfort in his shoulder, and, despite rest and rehabilitative treatment over the next few weeks, he became less effective as a pitcher. The highlights of his examination were pain with pitching motion, definite limitations of motion with stabilization of his scapula and weakness of his supraspinatus, infraspinatus, trapezius, and rhomboid muscles. His scapula was positionally displaced, protracted, and depressed demonstrating (1) limited motion, (2) muscle imbalance, and (3) an image study of irregular labral and cuff pathology. An arthroscopic procedure was performed and noted was a definite poste-

rior labral tear that extended from the superior to near-inferior area with irritation of the superior and superoposterior cuff. His ligaments were intact. After the involved areas had been debrided, he started an intensive physical therapy program in preparation for the next year's baseball season. The highlights of the program were directed toward reestablishing normal scapulothoracic and scapulohumeral motions and synchrony of motion. It was recommended that he not attempt any throwing of a ball for approximately 4 months postarthroscopic procedure. He progressed slowly through the postarthroscopic rehabilitation program, working on form pitching until he was ready to return to baseball training in the spring.

He continued his therapy program and progressed from the spring season to Triple A level and within 3 months was back at a major league level. He has remained at a major league level as an effective starting pitcher for 7 years.

This is an example of proceeding from labral tear and rotator cuff irritation to progressive alteration of normal biomechanic pitching with an effective loss of his pitching skill and progressive discomfort. The arthroscopic debridement helped with the posterior labral and undersurface of the cuff lesion, which were probably secondary to the dynamic change in his scapulothoracic glenohumeral function. He also had some mild instability noted on examination and clunking of his labral tear. He continues with his prescribed rehabilitation program. Surgery is helpful, but a continued commitment to rehabilitation is critical.

Case Study VIII

A 46-year-old recreational tennis player presented with a complaint of progressive left shoulder pain. Her shoulder pain with overhead motion had progressed to the point where she was incapable of serving the ball. On initial examination, she had pain with elevation of the arm in the scapular plane beyond 70 degrees. She received 8 weeks of relief after a subacromial injection of an anesthetic and corticosteroid suspension and a rotator cuff rehabilitation program. However, with the return of shoulder pain, she received only 2 weeks of relief following a second subacromial injection. An MRI and a CT arthrogram were obtained and the glenohumeral joint and the synovial surface of the rotator cuff were normal. A bursogram, however, clearly demonstrated bursal side injury to the supraspinatus tendon (Figs. 13-4). An arthroscopic subacromial decompression and a debridement of the partial thickness

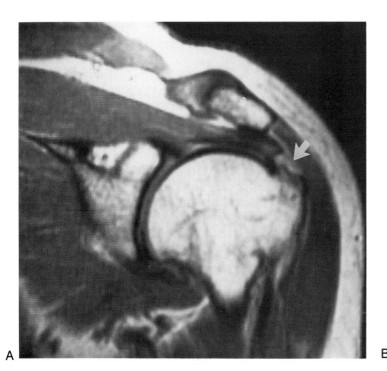

A

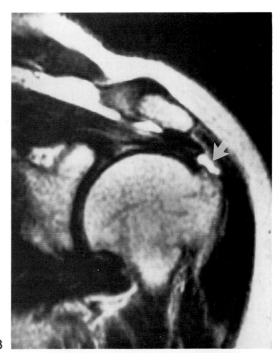

B

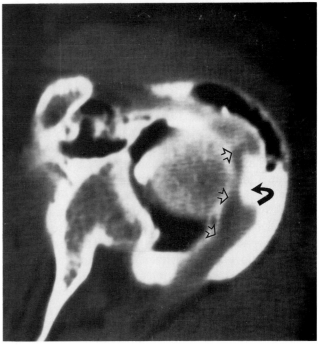

C

Figure 13-4 **(A)** Oblique coronal spin density image at the level of the midglenohumeral joint shows a focus of abnormal midlevel signal intensity interrupting the superficial fibers of the distal supraspinatus tendon. **(B)** This area markedly increases in signal intensity on the T2-weighted scan. No through-and-through discontinuity of the supraspinatus tendon is demonstrated. **(C)** Axial image of CT arthrogram and bursogram performed at the superior aspect of the glenohumeral joint demonstrates an intact synovial surface *(open arrows)* but notchlike defect of the bursal surface *(curved arrow)* of the supraspinatus tendon.

bursal side rotator cuff tear was undertaken. Her left arm was placed in a sling for 1 week. A program to rehabilitate her rotator cuff musculature was then initiated. At 8 weeks, she had painless synchronous left shoulder motion and successfully returned to playing tennis without recurrence of shoulder symptoms.

Biceps Pathology

The biceps tendon originates off the supraglenoid tubercle and/or posterior superior labrum. It courses intra-articularly toward the intertrochlear groove where it is stabilized by the shoulder capsule, coracohumeral ligament, and opposing edges of the supraspinatus and subscapularis tendons.[19] The biceps tendon functions at the shoulder as a dynamic and static depressor of the humeral head, especially with an externally rotated arm, which positions the tendon directly over the humeral head (see Fig. 9-8). It also functions as a secondary restraint to excessive anteroposterior motion of the humeral head.[20]

The past decade has brought forth a better appreciation of the association of glenohumeral instability, impingement, and rotator cuff pathology with bicipital disorders. Due to its location within the impingement interval, if a diagnosis of biceps tendon pathology is considered, a diagnosis of impingement of the rotator cuff should also be considered (see Fig. 9-10).

In the athlete, injury to the biceps tendon can result from a single violent injury or from repeated microtrauma. A fall on a flexed and abducted arm (head-first slide) may result in a compressive load on the superior joint surface with injury to the biceps and the superior labral tissues. If the proximally directed force continues, a rotator cuff tear can occur as well. Indirect injury is also seen in overhead athletes. In throwing activities, for example, the longhead of the biceps tendon decelerates the elbow extension and forearm pronation during the follow-through and may be injured by repetitive eccentric overload. In the extreme external rotation, abduction, and extension characterizing the late cocking phase, a contracted biceps may elevate a part or all of the superior labrum off the underlying glenoid producing the so-called SLAP lesion (see Ch. 12).

Impingement, whether primary or secondary, may cause bicipital tendon injury or instability. Repeated trauma of the biceps, rotator cuff, coracohumeral ligament, and accompanying shoulder capsule against the undersurface of the acromion may result in direct injury to the biceps tendon and to the soft tissues that stabilize the tendon within its groove. In these patients, the biceps pathology is directly related to the fact that it lies within the impingement space. Impingement is probably the most common cause of both bicipital tendonitis and subluxation of the biceps tendon in overhead athletes.[21]

An accurate history and physical examination are important in attempting to differentiate bicipital tendonitis, bicipital instability, and impingement syndrome. Patients with bicipital tendonitis usually have persistent anterior shoulder pain. Typically, the patient has a history of repetitive overhead action, such as is seen in golf, tennis, swimming, and throwing sports. In all of these activities, the rotation of the arm above the horizontal presents the tuberosities, biceps tendon, and rotator cuff to the undersurface of the anterior acromion and coracoacromial ligament. Patients with

biceps tendon instability have a similar pain pattern, but shoulder motion is often accompanied by a palpable snap or audible pop.

On physical examination, point tenderness in the biceps groove is best localized with the arm in 10 degrees of internal rotation. The locus of the tenderness should move with rotation of the arm but may disappear as the groove rotates medially under the conjoined tendon. The tenderness associated with impingement is usually less localized and should not resolve with rotation.[22]

Several tests have historically been used to support the diagnosis of biceps tendonitis or biceps tendon instability. Pain referred to the bicipital groove upon resisted supination with a flexed elbow[23] or upon resisted shoulder flexion with an extended elbow[24] are suggestive of bicipital tendonitis. In turn, when bringing the arm from a fully abducted and externally rotated position down to one's side and an audible and palpable click is produced, biceps tendon instability is considered likely.[25] Although these clinical signs may suggest biceps tendon pathology, they contribute little to determining the cause of the pathology or ruling out other contributing or associated disorders. In addition to impingement, glenohumeral instability, labral tears, coracoid impingement,[26] thoracic outlet syndrome, peripheral nerve entrapment, and brachial neuritis must all be ruled out. Selective injection of a local anesthetic with elimination of pain is an important part of the examination. Routine radiographs are typically normal. Special views, including bicipital groove view[27] and outlet view,[28] may help differentiate impingement syndrome from bicipital tendonitis or instability. Ultrasound, CT arthrography, MRI, and arthroscopy may be helpful as well. The usefulness of ultrasound depends on the experience of the examiner and interpreter. Visualization of the bicipital tendon within the groove on CT arthrography may be limited when a rotator cuff tear is present. With MRI, the biceps and rotator cuff can be adequately visualized through most of their course and, as technologies improve, its role will continue to expand. Arthroscopy can often detect the subtle patterns of abnormal anatomy that result in impingement or bicipital damage (e.g., partial tears, SLAP, etc.) or dysfunction, which may not have been appreciated in other investigative studies (see Ch. 12).

Although biceps tendon pathology is not uncommon, complete disruption of the biceps tendon proximally is rare in the younger athlete. It may occur in athletes involved in overhead activities or weight lifters, where a sudden significant load results in failure of the biceps tendon origin or musculotendinous junction. Complete disruptions within the muscle substance have been reported in parachutists where an ill-placed strap tightens across the contracted biceps muscle. Musculocutaneous nerve injury can occur concurrently.[29] Regardless of the specific site of failure, a tearing or popping sensation in the arm often accompanies the injury, followed by severe pain, swelling, and loss of strength. Depending upon the site of failure, a visible and palpable defect may be present. Plain radiographs generally are not helpful, but MRI and ultrasound will provide information on the site of rupture and will determine the state of the rotator cuff. For the athlete with a complete disruption of the biceps within the muscle substance or at the myotendinous junction who wishes to continue athletic activities, treatment should consist of control of the hematoma if possible with immobilization in acute flexion[29] or acute surgical repair and appropriate immobilization. In cases of failure within the proximal biceps tendon, reattachment of the tendon to the supraglenoid tubercle should be attempted. Tenodesis is indicated only if severe attritional wear of the tendon is present. These treatment regimens will optimize a return of muscle power and resistance to fatigue in the athletic population.

Case Study IX

A 42-year-old active right-handed recreational weight lifter presented with a complaint of right shoulder discomfort. His history was significant, since he had a Bristow reconstruction of his right shoulder 20 years before and had progressive anterior shoulder pain over the previous 2 years. Two weeks prior to seeking consultation, he experienced a tearing sensation in his right shoulder while performing pull-downs on a resistance-style exercise machine. He described the pain as a burning discomfort. He had a second episode of significant pain 1 week later when he tossed a heavy rock underhand with an extended elbow. On initial examination, he had moderate tenderness over the bicipital groove and the locus of discomfort did move with rotation of the arm. There was an asymmetry in the contour of the biceps when compared to the opposite extremity (Fig. 13-5A). Radiographs of the right shoulder including anteroposterior, axillary, lateral, and outlet views, were normal. An arthrogram did not visualize the normal intra-articular course of the biceps (Fig. 13-5B). (An MRI was not obtained because of a retained screw in the right shoulder.) A CT scan suggested attenuation of the biceps within its groove (Figs. 13-5C & D). Over the next 8 weeks, the patient's burning sensation persisted; he was dissatisfied with the discomfort and perceived weakness of

elbow flexion and the readily apparent clinical deformity. The patient was brought to the operating room where a nearly complete disruption of the biceps tendon within its groove was noted. The proximal intra-articular biceps was excised, and the residual stump of tendon was tenodesed into the denuded bicipital groove. The patient's right arm was immobilized in a sling and swathe postoperatively for 2 weeks, and then pendulum exercises were begun. At 4 weeks, active-assisted exercises were begun and at 8 weeks a progressive strengthening program was instituted. The patient has returned to his weight training exercise without difficulties.

Although biceps tendon instability is most often a consequence of traumatic degeneration of the cuff, acute dislocations have been reported. The tendon dislocation is usually the result of a direct blow to the shoulder or a fall on an outstretched upper extremity. Dislocation of the biceps tendon is more common in softball pitchers because of the forceful supinator strain that occurs with delivery of the ball toward the plate.[22] Patients with bicipital tendon instability are best treated with open reduction of the tendon, reconstruction of the fibrous roof, and acromioplasty. Tenodesis is indicated only in the context of severe attritional wear of the tendon or an unreconstructable roof.

Case Study X

A 29-year-old competitive racquet ball player presented with a 3-month history of pain and "snapping" in the right shoulder. This pain worsened when she extended and externally rotated her right arm in preparation for a forehand shot. On physical examination, her tenderness was located over the bicipital groove. From a maximally elevated position, bringing her right arm to her side elicited a painful snap in the anterior shoulder area. A CT scan was obtained which demonstrated the medial dislocation of her biceps tendon with passive external rotation of her arm (Fig. 13-6).

The racquet ball player wanted to continue tournament play so an open reduction reconstruction of the coracohumeral ligament and supporting capsular structures and acromioplasty was performed. She was placed in a sling for 1 week and then pendulum motion was initiated. At 3 weeks, active-assisted shoulder motion was instituted. At 6 weeks, her range of motion was full and a comprehensive strengthening program was begun. At 10 weeks, she returned to full play and competed in her first tournament postsurgery 4 weeks later without recurrence of symptoms.

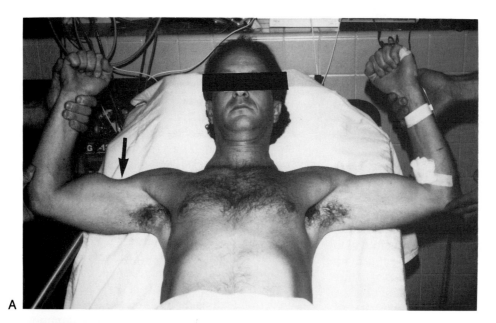

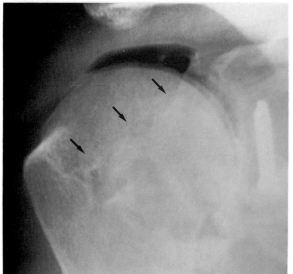

Figure 13-5 **(A)** Note asymmetry in the contour of the biceps muscles and loss of the normal fullness proximally on the right. **(B)** AP view held in external rotation following double contrast arthrography fails to delineate the intra-articular course of the proximal longhead of the biceps *(arrows)* delineate expected course. **(C)** Double-contrast CT arthrogram at the level of the inferior glenoid demonstrates dystrophic mineralization around the expected course of the transverse ligament anterior to the bicipital groove with poor delineation of the tendon secondary to lack of air or iodinated contrast within the bicipital sheath *(arrow)*. Note degenerative changes about the bicipital groove and hardware within the anterior glenoid from prior Bristow procedure. **(D)** More caudal image shows the distal portion of the bicipital groove with normal-appearing tendon delineated by air.

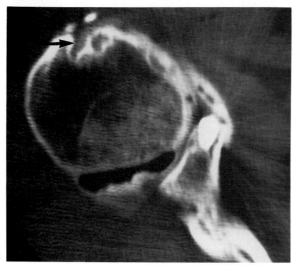

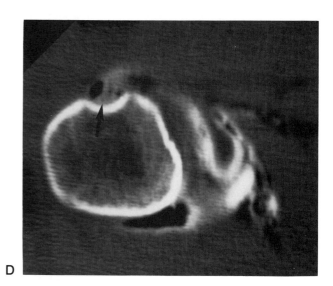

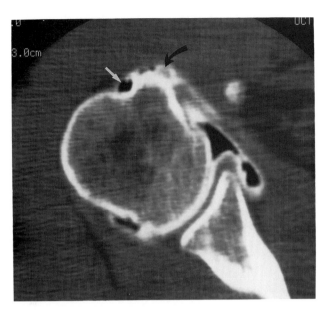

Figure 13-6 Axial CT arthrographic image of the mid- to inferior glenohumeral joint demonstrates an "empty" air distended sheath within the bicipital groove *(white arrow)*. Rounded filling defect projecting just medial to the lesser tuberosity reflects intact but dislocated longhead of biceps tendon *(curved arrow)*.

ROTATOR CUFF PATHOLOGY

As with impingement, rotator cuff pathology in the athlete is often a manifestation of underlying glenohumeral instability. Other less common causes of secondary rotator cuff injury include developmental variations in the coracoacromial arch, scapulothoracic or scapulohumeral dysfunction, and capsular contracture. Primary rotator cuff injury can and does occur. It may result from a single violent injury, or, more often, as a consequence of repeated microtrauma, particularly in athletes using overhead motion. The injury should be classified as a partial- (specifying depth) or full-thickness injury and whether the injury is on the bursal or synovial side of the tendon. The dimensions of the injured area should be determined as well (CT arthrogram, MRI, arthroscopy). The supraspinatus tendon is the component of the rotator cuff that is most frequently affected. In these overhead athletes, repetitive eccentric tensile loading of the articular side of the rotator cuff in an area where the blood supply is variable may result in partial-thickness undersurface tears, most often just proximal to the supraspinatus insertion, with resultant dysfunction.[30]

Case Study XI

A 35-year-old major league pitcher was seen for shoulder pain. The initial incident of discomfort started 4 months earlier when he experienced shoulder pain after a very irregular pitch. He was coming forward to plant his contralateral leg on a wet ground surface and slipped. As he came forward, he describes his arm going into hyperabduction, in addition to the usual extension and external rotation. Because of the sensitivity following that incident, he did not pitch for 3 weeks. A progressive rehabilitation program and return to pitching as a relief pitcher carried him through the major league season, league championships, and the World Series.

In the final stages of the playoff schedule he noted progressive discomfort in his shoulder, and after the final game he was seen for additional evaluation. An MRI and CT arthrogram were performed and the findings included evidence of disruption in the tendinous portion of the supraspinatus (Fig. 13-7). This was interpreted to be an incomplete tear of the rotator cuff. It was noted there was some irregularity of his anterior labrum; however, his symptomatology was directed to the rotator cuff area. Due to the incomplete nature of the disruption it was determined that he would follow a course of nonsurgery with intense rehabilitation goals. The plan was to repeat an MRI in 1 month and then reevaluate treatment.

The repeat MRI demonstrated a decrease in the overall intensity and amount of fluid identified in the rotator cuff, suggesting a progressive improvement in the injury and probably progression of the healing process. He continued rehabilitation and progressed with his throwing activity, returning to his position as a premier relief pitcher. He also continued with recommended conditioning both on- and off-season. He has since completed 4 additional years as a major league pitcher, including winning the Cy Young and Most Valuable Player awards.

Supraspinatus weakness will also allow mild superior humeral head subluxations with secondary impingement.[31] These athletes present with pain over the supraspinatus insertion, motion limitation, muscle spasm, and atrophy. Dynamic stabilization of the glenohumeral joint may be compromised, resulting in excessive excursion of the humeral head and incremental attenuation and elongation of the glenohumeral ligaments and capsule. Instability may thus result secondarily (see Ch. 11).

It can be difficult to differentiate rotator cuff pathology, impingement, and glenohumeral subluxation in this group of patients. The apprehension sign and relo-

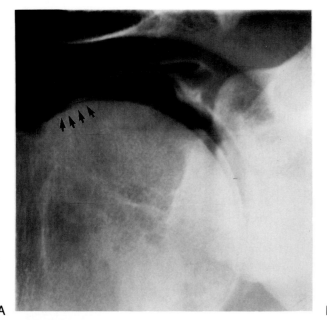

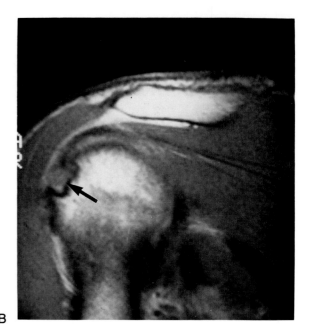

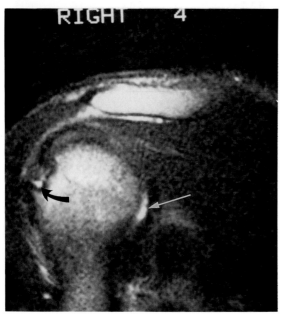

Figure 13-7 (A) Plain films double-contrast arthrogram shows partial defect involving the synovial surface with local intravasation of contrast at the distal supraspinatus tendon *(arrows)*. No extravasation to the subacromial-subdeltoid bursal plane is seen. **(B)** Oblique coronal spin density scan shows an abnormal focus of midlevel signal intensity at the synovial side of the supraspinatus at the level of its attachment to the greater tuberosity *(arrow)*. **(C)** This area shows abnormal increased signal intensity *(black arrow)* on the T2-weighted image, which is isointense with joint fluid *(white arrow)*.

cation test can be helpful (see Ch. 11). CT arthrogram, MRI, and arthroscopy may all have a diagnostic role. Arthroscopic examination can directly evaluate both the articular and bursal surfaces of the rotator cuffs, and can detect other lesions that might affect treatment. For young active patients in whom primary instability and impingement are ruled out, restoration of rotator cuff function will correct the secondary instability and impingement. A successful rehabilitative effort, though it may take many months, will interrupt the self-perpetuating cycle of rotator cuff dysfunction, instability, and impingement.

NONOPERATIVE TREATMENT

In the athletic population, most impingement, rotator cuff, and biceps tendon difficulties can be successfully managed nonoperatively. In the athlete with evidence of inflammation of the rotator cuff, longhead of the biceps tendon, or subacromial bursa, treatment initially consists of rest, use of nonsteroidal anti-inflammatory drugs (NSAIDs), and rehabilitation. Treatment is potentially more effective if this process is detected early and aggressively managed before imbalance, altered function, and irreversible damage to the periarticular soft tissues occur (see the section, *Dynamic Instability* in Ch. 11).

For acute symptoms, resting the shoulder articulation and irritated soft tissues should be emphasized; however, long-term immobilization, which can lead to adhesive capsulitis, especially in the older athlete, should be avoided. The athlete should move the shoulder through as full a range of motion as possible several times each day, active-assisted passively. As acute symptoms subside, the formal rehabilitation program should be initiated and serves both a therapeutic and a prophylactic function. Shoulder range of motion, flexibility, and strength must be regained before the athlete begins a gradual return to sports. When pain hinders the rehabilitative effort, injection of an anesthetic and corticosteroid suspension may provide relief.[32] The injection should be extratendinous, with a maximum of three injections spaced a minimum of 6 weeks apart. Strengthening activities should be avoided for 1 to 3 days after each injection, with the rehabilitative program resumed in a progressive fashion. When the range of motion is full and painless and strength is adequate, the athlete may return to his or her sport. The program is prolonged but important, since surgery is not a desirable option for most athletes.

The initial emphasis of the rehabilitative program is to regain full shoulder range of motion and flexibility, with tight contracted soft tissues identified and targeted (see Ch. 16 for a complete discussion). A strengthening program is then begun. As flexibility, range of motion, and strength return to normal, the patient is placed on a gradual return to sports program and instruction on proper shoulder mechanics is provided.

SURGICAL TREATMENT

Nonoperative treatment for most impingement, rotator cuff, and biceps tendon disorders is successful in returning the athlete to his or her sport. However, the following situations merit surgical treatment. In athletes with anterosuperior glenohumeral instability (i.e., deficiency or disruptions of the labral-capsular-ligamentous complex) resulting in impingement or rotator cuff dysfunction and unresponsive to an extended supervised course of nonoperative treatment, surgery is warranted (see Ch. 11). In athletes with impingement not related to anterosuperior instability and unresponsive to a long and supervised course of nonoperative treatment, a surgical decompression to enlarge the impingement space should be considered. In athletes with significant full-thickness tears of the rotator cuff or an acute rupture of the longhead of the biceps tendon,

surgical repair and decompression may be warranted to alleviate acute symptoms and prevent long-term deterioration of shoulder function and pain. In cases of double disruptions of the superior shoulder suspensory complex, resulting in an anteroinferior tilt of the scapula/anterior acromion (e.g., an old type III disruption of the acromioclavicular joint), surgical correction may be necessary. The particular corrective procedure in this situation is dictated by the nature of the double disruption.

Arthroscopic surgical techniques may be appropriate: (1) in cases where correction of anterior glenohumeral instability resulting from deficiency or disruption of the labral-capsular-ligamentous structures is indicated (see Chs. 11 and 12) (although controversial, arthroscopic stabilization may best be reserved for noncontact athletes because of the higher redislocation rate associated with arthroscopic stabilization as compared to open techniques); (2) in patients where decompression or enlargement of the impingement spaces is elected; and (3) in circumstances in which subacromial decompression and repair or debridement of small full-thickness rotator cuff tears is appropriate. For larger rotator cuff tears, arthroscopic subacromial decompression and rotator cuff mobilization can be combined with a miniarthrotomy for definitive cuff repair. The arthroscopic techniques, however, remain technically demanding, and the incidence of surgical failure presently still exceeds that which is seen when open techniques are utilized (see Chs. 11 and 12 for a complete discussion). Because arthroscopy offers the potential for repair of pathology with minimal damage to the surrounding normal anatomy (thus providing the athlete the opportunity for a quicker and full recovery), it will continue to have a role in the surgical management of shoulder disorders in athletes.

Injuries to the musculotendinous structures about the shoulder are common in certain sports and can produce considerable disability to the injured athlete. Most contusions and grades I and II strains will respond satisfactorily to early symptomatic care followed by a directed flexibility and strengthening program and a gradual return to sports program. In grade III strains, consideration should be given to early direct repair followed by a structured rehabilitation. Most impingement, biceps tendon, and rotator cuff disorders can be managed with rest, use of NSAIDs, and implementation of a directed and closely supervised rehabilitation program. Surgery is reserved for cases unresponsive to nonoperative regimens. For all musculotendinous shoulder injuries, a successful rehabilitation will not only optimize return of function to the injured part but will avoid the secondary disorders that commonly occur and are often more difficult to treat.

REFERENCES

1. Jobe FW, Tibone JE, Perry DR et al: An EMG analysis of the shoulder in throwing and pitching: a preliminary report. Am J Sports Med 11:3, 1983
2. Ekstrand J, Gillquist J, Liljedahl SO: Prevention of soccer injuries: supervision by doctor and physiotherapist. Am J Sports Med 11:116, 1983
3. Vanderhoff E, Lippitt S, Harris S et al: Glenohumeral stability for concavity-compression: a quantitative analysis. Orthop Trans 16:774, 1992
4. Lephart S, Kocher M: The role of exercise in the prevention of shoulder disorders. p. 601. In Matsen FA, Fu FH, Hawkins RJ (eds): The Shoulder: a Balance of Mobility and Stability. American Academy of Orthopedic Surgeons, 1993
5. Zarins B, Ciullo JV: Acute muscle and tendon injuries in athletes. Clin Sports Med 2:167, 1983
6. Caughey M, Welsh P: Muscle ruptures affecting the shoulder girdle. p. 863. In Rockwood CA, Matsen FA (eds): The Shoulder. WB Saunders, Philadelphia; 1990
7. Welsh, RP, MacNab I, Riley V: Biomechanical studies of rabbit tendon. Clin Orthop 81:171, 1971
8. McEntire JE, Hess WE, Coleman S: Rupture of the pectoralis major muscle. J Bone Joint Surg [Am] 43:81, 1961
9. Caughey M, Welsh P: Muscle ruptures affecting the shoulder girdle. p. 867. In Rockwood CA, Matsen K (eds): The Shoulder. WB Saunders, Philadelphia, 1990
10. Zeman SC, Rosenfeld, RT, Lipscomb PR: Tears of the pectoralis major muscle. Am J Sports Med 7:343, 1979
11. Bennett GE: Shoulder and elbow lesions of the professional baseball pitcher. JAMA 117:510, 1941
12. Ferrari JD, Ferrari DA, Coumas J, Pappas AM: Posterior ossification of the shoulder—the Bennett lesion: etiology, diagnosis, and treatment. Am J Sports Med 22:171, 1994
13. Overpeck DO, Ghormley RK: Paralysis of the serratus magnus muscle. JAMA 114:1994, 1940
14. Tobin WJ, Cohen LS, Vandover JT: Parachute injuries. JAMA 117:1318, 1941
15. DePalma AF, Cooke AJ, Prabhaker M: The role of the subscapularis in recurrent anterior dislocations of the shoulder. Clin Orthop 54:35, 1967
16. Symeonides PP: The significance of the subscapularis muscle in the pathogenesis of recurrent anterior dislocation of the shoulder. J Bone Joint Surg [Br] 54:476, 1972
17. McAuliffe TB, David GS: Avulsion of the subscapularis tendon: a case report. J Bone Joint Surg [Am] 69:1454, 1987
18. Jobe F, Tibone J, Jobe C, Kvitne R: The shoulder in sports. In Rockwood CA, Matsen FA (eds): The Shoulder. WB Saunders, Philadelphia, 1990:965
19. Meyer AW: Spontaneous dislocation of the tendon of the long head of the biceps brachii. Arch Surg 13:109, 1926
20. Rockwood CA, Matsen FA: Biceps Tendon. p. 807. In Rockwood CA, Matsen K (eds): The Shoulder. WB Saunders, Philadelphia, 1990
21. O'Donahue D: Subluxating biceps tendon in the athlete. Clin Orthop 164:26, 1982
22. Burkhead W Jr: The biceps tendon. p. 810. In Rockwood CA, Matsen FA (eds): The Shoulder. WB Saunders, Philadelphia, 1990
23. Yergason RM: Rupture of the biceps. J Bone Joint Surg 131:160, 1931
24. Gilcrest EL, Albi P: Unusual lesions of muscles and tendons of the shoulder girdle and upper arm. Surg Gynecol Obstet 68:903, 1939
25. Abbott LC, Saunders LB de CM: Acute traumatic dislocation of the tendon of the long head of biceps brachii: report of 6 cases with operative findings. Surgery 6:817, 1939
26. Warren RF: Lesions of the long head of the biceps tendon. AAOS Instr Course Lect 34:204, 1985
27. Cone RO, Danzig L, Resnick D, Goldman AB: The bicipital groove: radiographic anatomic and pathologic study. AJR 41:781, 1983
28. Neer SC II, Poppen NK: Supraspinatus outlet. Orthop Trans J Bone J Surg 11:234, 1987
29. Heckman JD, Levine MI: Traumatic closed transection of biceps brachii in the military parachutist. J Bone Joint Surg [Am] 60:369, 1978
30. Lohr JF, Unthoff HK: The microvascular pattern of the supraspinatus tendon. Clin Orthop 254:35, 1990
31. Jobe FW, Kvitne RS: Shoulder pain in the overhand or throwing athlete: the relationship of anterior instability and rotator cuff impingement. Orthop Rev 18:963, 1989
32. Cyriar J, Trosier O: Hydrocortisone and soft tissue lesions. Br Med J 2:966, 1953

14

Ligamentous Disruptions of the Shoulder Complex

Thomas P. Goss
Arthur M. Pappas

The shoulder complex includes three diarthrodial joints: glenohumeral, acromioclavicular, and sternoclavicular. Each of these articulations may become symptomatically unstable if the periarticular soft tissue stabilizing structures (particularly the ligaments) are traumatized. Injuries involving the glenohumeral joint are discussed in Chapter 11. Acute injuries and chronic problems involving the acromioclavicular and sternoclavicular joints are discussed in this chapter, as are a group of related injuries termed "double disruptions of the superior shoulder suspensory complex."

DISRUPTIONS OF THE ACROMIOCLAVICULAR JOINT

A discussion of the anatomy and function of the acromioclavicular joint is presented in Chapter 9. Figure 14-1 shows the ligamentous structures that provide stability to the articulation. Injuries to the acromioclavicular joint are common in all sports but occur most frequently in those involving high-impact collisions between the participants (football, rugby, hockey, wrestling), and those in which the participant may strike a fixed object with considerable force (motor

vehicle racing, equestrian events, skiing). In most instances, the mechanism of injury is a direct blow applied over the superolateral aspect of the acromial process. Less common mechanisms include a direct anterior or posterior blow to the shoulder, a fall onto the outstretched hand or elbow, or an indirect downward pull applied to the upper extremity. The severity of the injury is determined by the magnitude and direction of the applied force and the resultant damage to the acromioclavicular ligaments, the coracoclavicular ligaments (occasionally the coracoid process may be fractured), the intra-articular meniscus, and the deltoid-trapezius sling. In general, the more severe the force and damage to the soft tissue stabilizing structures, the greater the acromioclavicular discontinuity and likelihood of post-traumatic, symptomatic acromioclavicular instability.[1-14]

Clinical Evaluation

Evaluation of acute injuries to the acromioclavicular joint begins with a history from the athlete. One should try to determine the mechanism of injury, an estimate of the severity of the force, the degree of pain and functional limitation, and the length of time from injury to

239

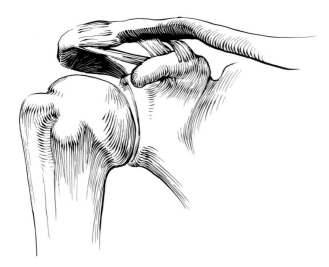

Figure 14-1 Shoulder region with particular attention to the bony and ligamentous anatomy of the acromioclavicular joint.

presentation. The physical examination should begin with a visual inspection of the shoulder complex, noting any deformity of the acromioclavicular articulation. The involved area is gently palpated to determine if local sensitivity is present. The examiner should manually depress the distal end of the clavicle to determine the extent of discomfort and whether abnormal motion is present between the distal clavicle and the acromial process. The athlete is then requested to actively put his or her shoulder through a limited range of motion while the examiner notes local crepitus, the degree of associated discomfort and any change in the appearance of the acromioclavicular deformity (if present). An overall examination of the surrounding soft tissues, including the muscles and a neurovascular assessment, is always included.

Radiographic Examination

The radiographic examination should include true anteroposterior (AP) and axillary projections of the glenohumeral joint. An AP-view radiograph should be obtained with both acromioclavicular joints on one film and 10-lb weights hung from both wrists (Fig. 14-2). It is important that the patient not hold these weights with the hands, since this may cause isometric contraction of the shoulder musculature with resultant reduction of any acromioclavicular separation that may be present. The position of the distal clavicle rela-

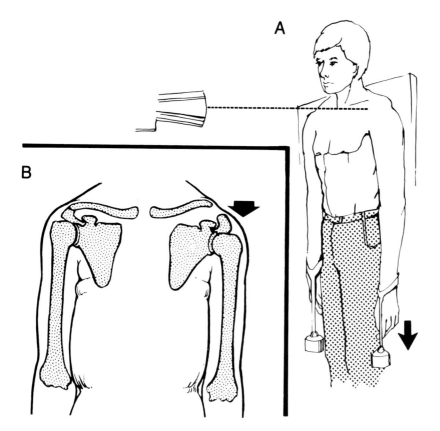

Figure 14-2 Weightbearing AP radiographic view of the acromioclavicular joint. **(A)** Patient standing for the AP-view radiograph with 10-lb weights attached to both wrists *(arrow)*. **(B)** AP-view radiograph including both shoulders showing a type III or type V disruption of the left acromioclavicular joint *(arrow)* (the acromion is significantly displaced relative to the distal end of the clavicle).

tive to the acromion may help to determine the mechanism of injury. A "high-riding" clavicle is generally associated with a downward force applied over the superior aspect of the acromion, which then displaces inferiorly due to ligamentous damage and the weight of the arm. Conversely, acromioclavicular disruptions caused by a fall onto the elbow or an outstretched hand initially present with the acromion displaced superiorly relative to the distal clavicle. Supplemental radiographs that may be beneficial include the Zanca view[15] and the Alexander view.[16] These projections often provide valuable information regarding the intra-articular acromioclavicular relationships and may detect adjacent fractures (Fig. 14-3). Occasionally, for complex injuries, computed tomography (CT) scans, arthro-

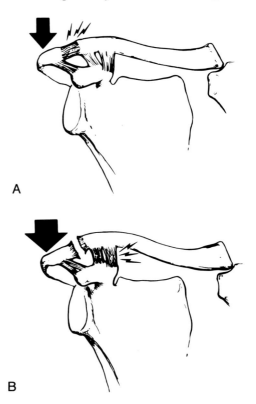

A

B

Figure 14-4 Ligamentous injuries of the acromioclavicular joint. (**A**) Type I disruption, stretched acromioclavicular ligaments. (**B**) Type II disruption, torn acromioclavicular ligaments and stretched coracoclavicular ligaments allowing partial displacement of the acromioclavicular joint.

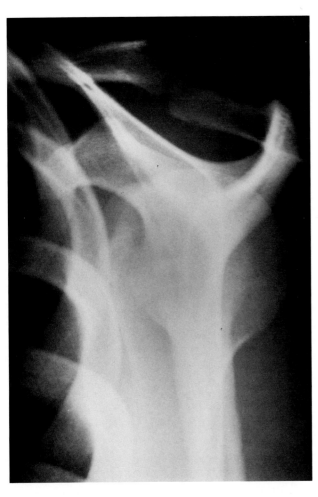

Figure 14-3 An Alexander or scapulolateral radiographic view of the acromioclavicular joint: The distal clavicle is superiorly displaced and overlapped with the acromion—findings consistent with a ligamentous disruption of the acromioclavicular joint.

graphic CT scanning, and/or magnetic resonance imaging may be indicated to evaluate possible damage to adjacent bony, articular, and soft tissue structures as well as to determine the true position of the distal clavicle relative to the acromion.

Classification

Rockwood's classification includes six types of acromioclavicular disruptions, reflecting increasing degrees of damage to the soft tissues that secure the clavicle to the acromion and scapula as a whole.[12,13] The type I injury is equivalent to a grade I or II sprain of the acromioclavicular ligaments (Fig. 14-4) and a possible grade I sprain of the coracoclavicular ligaments. Clinical characteristics include minimal (if any) visible deformity over the acromioclavicular joint, mild to moderate sensitivity to palpation over the articulation, full or nearly full range of motion of the shoulder complex with mild to moderate discomfort, and no radiographic displacement at the acromioclavicular articulation, even on distraction views (see Ch. 16 for a complete discussion of grades I to III sprains).

In the type II injury, a grade III sprain of the acromioclavicular ligaments is present, as well as a grade I or a grade II sprain of the coracoclavicular ligaments (Fig. 14-4). Clinically, there is often a visible deformity indicating a disruption of the acromioclavicular relationship, discomfort localized over the acromioclavicular joint, and restriction of shoulder range of motion secondary to pain. A standard AP-view radiograph supplemented by distraction radiographs as well as other views (Zanca or Alexander) will reveal the altered relationships. The inferior border of the distal clavicle lies above the inferior border but below the superior border of the acromion, and the coracoclavicular distance is widened.

The type III acromioclavicular separation is a grade III sprain of the acromioclavicular and coracoclavicular ligaments (occasionally the coracoid process is fractured or there is an avulsion fracture at the point where the coracoclavicular ligaments attach to the clavicle or coracoid process). In addition, there is damage to the intra-articular meniscus and the deltoid-trapezius sling of varying degree (Fig. 14-5). Rarely, an intra-articular fracture is identified (see Ch. 15 for a complete discussion). There is an obvious deformity in the area with the acromion resting inferior to the distal clavicle due to the loss of ligamentous support and the weight of the arm. Standard AP-view radiographs, distraction views, and supplemental Zanca or Alexander projections document the inferior displacement of the acromion relative to the distal clavicle such that the inferior border of the clavicle lies above the superior border of the acromion. In addition, the coracoclavicular distance is significantly widened as compared to the opposite shoulder unless the coracoid process is fractured, in which case displacement at the fracture site is noted.

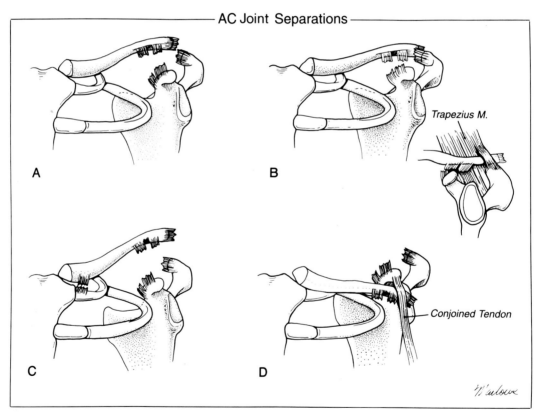

AC Joint Separations

Figure 14-5 Acromioclavicular joint disruptions. **(A)** Type III, torn acromioclavicular and coracoclavicular ligaments allowing complete displacement of the acromioclavicular joint. **(B)** Type IV, torn acromioclavicular and coracoclavicular ligaments allowing posterior displacement of the distal clavicle into and through the trapezius muscle. **(C)** Type V, extensive disruption of the clavicular soft tissue support structures allowing severe dissociation of the acromioclavicular joint. **(D)** Type VI, torn acromioclavicular and coracoclavicular ligaments associated with dislocation of the distal clavicle inferior to the coracoid process and posterior to the conjoined tendon.

Type I, II, and III acromioclavicular joint disruptions account for most of the acromioclavicular injuries seen in athletes. Occasionally, more violent forces result in type IV, V, and VI disruptions. The type IV injury is characterized by disrupted acromioclavicular and coracoclavicular ligaments, a torn deltoid-trapezius sling, and displacement of the distal end of the clavicle posteriorly through and locked within the fibers of the trapezius muscle (Fig. 14-5). Oblique- and axillary-view radiographs are needed to diagnose this variant. The type V injury is an extensive acromioclavicular joint dissociation in which all of the soft tissues joining the clavicle to the acromion and scapula are disrupted. The deltoid and trapezius muscles are detached from the distal *half* of the clavicle. In addition, the medial clavicular support structures, including the costoclavicular ligaments, may be disrupted, allowing extreme instability of the clavicle, not only at the acromioclavicular joint but throughout its length. Weight distraction radiographs reveal severe displacement of the acromion relative to the clavicle (Fig. 14-5). In the type VI injury, the acromioclavicular and coracoclavicular ligaments are disrupted as well as the deltoid-trapezius sling, and the clavicle is dislocated either inferior to the acromion or inferior to the coracoid process, posterior to the conjoined tendon. This variant is readily diagnosed on the standard AP-view radiograph (Fig. 14-5).

Treatment

Treatment for type I and II injuries is nonoperative, including rest and protection of the upper extremity, local application of ice followed by moist heat, and appropriate analgesic medications (see Ch. 2). Use of a sling minimizes motion, thereby alleviating pain and preventing additional soft tissue damage. The individual is allowed to return to athletic activities when he or she is asymptomatic and shoulder range of motion and strength are normal and consistent with the demands and risks of anticipated events (approximately 2 to 6 weeks).

Treatment of type III acromioclavicular disruptions has changed significantly in the last 20 years.[17-20] When surveyed in the 1970s, 90 percent of orthopedic surgeons recommended some form of open management. A similar study in 1992, however, revealed that 86 percent of sports physicians and 72 percent of orthopedic department chairmen recommended closed treatment.[21] This change most likely relates to studies that have reported equal or better outcomes associated with closed management. These "successful" results, however, may be short-term, with increasing discomfort and disability occurring later, resulting in compromised athletic performance.

For nonoperative treatment, there are a variety of shoulder taping methods and harnesses designed to reduce the acromioclavicular disruption. These methods, however, have the disadvantages of requiring close follow-up as well as optimal patient compliance and are associated with a significant incidence of skin pressure breakdown and recurrence of acromioclavicular displacement. Consequently, most orthopedists recommend simple symptomatic care, including protection of the arm in a sling for comfort and gradual increase in functional use of the shoulder as symptoms allow. A progressive rehabilitation program is prescribed, with the individual allowed to return to athletic activities any time after 12 weeks (approximately) when asymptomatic and shoulder function is satisfactory for anticipated demands. For those sports that include hard physical contact, a longer time interval should be considered to minimize the risk of additional injury.

Patients with type III injuries who do not undergo surgery should be advised that a visible prominence will remain in the acromioclavicular joint area, and there may be a 5 to 10 percent loss of shoulder strength. Surgical treatment should be considered in high-demand athletes who require maximal shoulder function. Surgical principles and techniques are well described in the literature and include debridement and stabilization of the acromioclavicular joint, repair of the acromioclavicular and coracoclavicular ligaments, and repair of the deltoid-trapezius sling (Fig. 14-6).

Type IV and type VI injuries require general anesthesia to reduce the posteriorly or inferiorly displaced clavicle, respectively. If a closed reduction is successful, additional treatment is dependent upon whether a type III or a type V dissociation results. If an open reduction of the displaced clavicle is needed, surgical restoration of the normal clavicle-scapula relationship is performed. For the type V injuries (including the type IV and type VI disruptions, which assume a type V dissociation following reduction of the displaced clavicle), surgical reconstruction of the articulation is necessary to restore satisfactory shoulder function (Fig. 14-7).

Adverse Late Sequelae

There is a surprisingly significant incidence of adverse late sequelae associated with type I and type II acromioclavicular disruptions—36 percent with the type I injuries and 48 percent with the type II injuries.[22] Patients may begin to experience chronic discomfort and crepitus, especially with repetitive overhead activ-

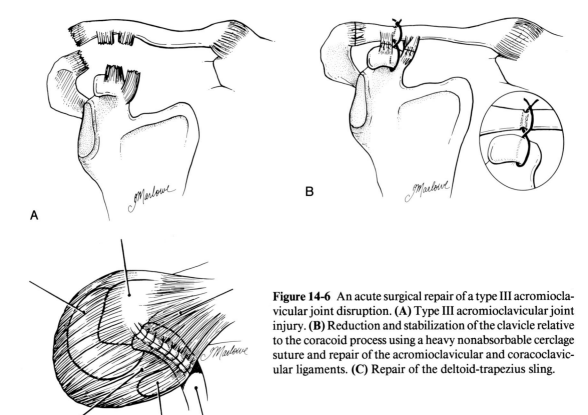

Figure 14-6 An acute surgical repair of a type III acromioclavicular joint disruption. (**A**) Type III acromioclavicular joint injury. (**B**) Reduction and stabilization of the clavicle relative to the coracoid process using a heavy nonabsorbable cerclage suture and repair of the acromioclavicular and coracoclavicular ligaments. (**C**) Repair of the deltoid-trapezius sling.

ity due to a torn intra-articular meniscus, degenerative joint disease, or osteolysis of the distal clavicle.[23] If nonoperative therapeutic modalities are ineffective, resection of the distal 1.5 to 2 cm of the clavicle[24] will generally provide excellent pain relief and reliably allow the individual to return to athletic competition in approximately 3 to 4 months (Fig. 14-8). Data obtained by Cooke and Tibone[25] reveal good to normal return of strength.

Type III acromioclavicular injuries (as well as types IV to VI disruptions) represent a double disruption of the superior shoulder suspensory complex,[26] since both the acromioclavicular and coracoclavicular ligaments are completely torn (see the next section). Although generally managed nonoperatively, type III injuries represent an anatomically unstable situation, which can result in subacromial impingement, neurovascular compromise, and decreased strength as well as muscle fatigue discomfort. If these adverse late sequelae develop and are sufficiently symptomatic, a reconstruction of the acromioclavicular linkage must be considered[27,28] (Fig. 14-9).

Case Study I

Injury, Initial Evaluation, and Management

An 18-year-old male experienced a driving board check during a hockey game, the area of impact centered over the superolateral aspect of his shoulder. Localized pain and swelling were present over the acromioclavicular joint, and the distal clavicle appeared prominent superiorly. The acromioclavicular joint was exquisitely tender to palpation and painful on attempted range of motion. Radiographs of the shoulder were obtained in two planes as well as a distraction view of the shoulder complex. No fractures were seen, but the inferior margin of the distal clavicle was noted to lie above the superior border of the acromion (Fig. 14-10A). The patient had sustained a grade III disruption of his acromioclavicular joint. Nonoperative symptomatic management was chosen. The patient was provided a sling and swathe immobilizer and instructed to gradually increase the

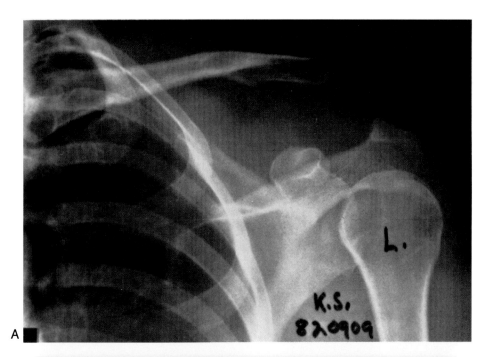

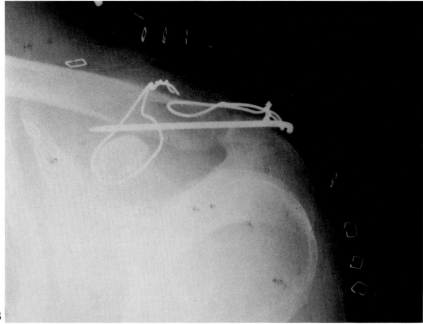

Figure 14-7 An individual who sustained a type V acromioclavicular joint separation. **(A)** Preoperative AP radiographic view showing severe displacement of the distal clavicle relative to the acromion. **(B)** Postoperative AP radiographic view showing anatomic reduction of the clavicle relative to the acromion using a cerclage wire passed around the coracoid process and through a drill hole in the clavicle as well as a K-wire passed across the acromioclavicular joint.

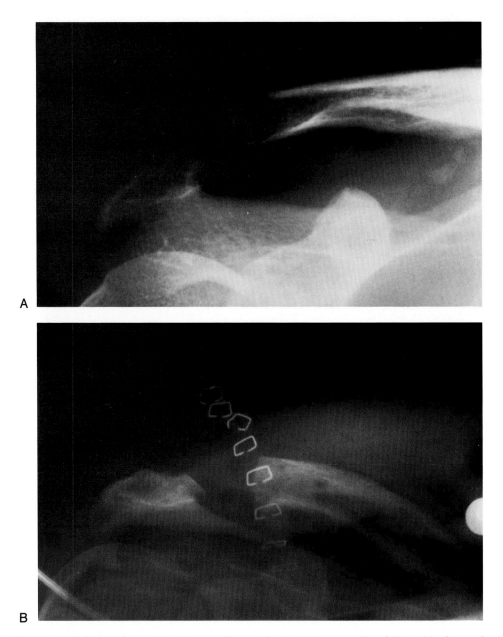

A

B

Figure 14-8 An individual who sustained a type II acromioclavicular separation followed by increasing local discomfort. **(A)** Initial AP radiographic view showing partial displacement of the clavicle relative to the acromion. **(B)** Postoperative AP radiographic view showing the acromioclavicular joint with the distal 2 cm of the clavicle resected.

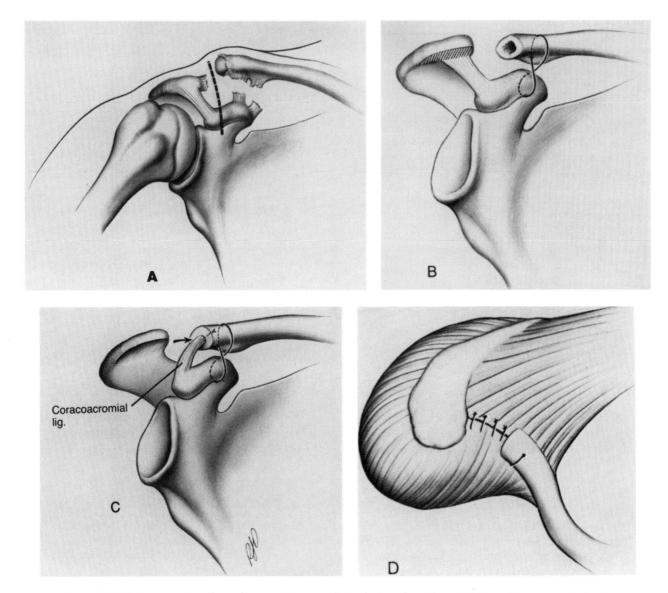

Figure 14-9 Late reconstruction of a type III acromioclavicular disruption. (**A**) Type III acromioclavicular disruption. (**B**) Resection of the distal clavicle, debridement of the acromioclavicular interval, and reduction/stabilization of the coracoclavicular interval using a heavy nonabsorbable cerclage suture. (**C**) Transposition of the coracoacromial ligament into the intramedullary canal of the clavicle to serve as a coracoclavicular ligament substitute. (**D**) Repair of the deltoid-trapezius sling.

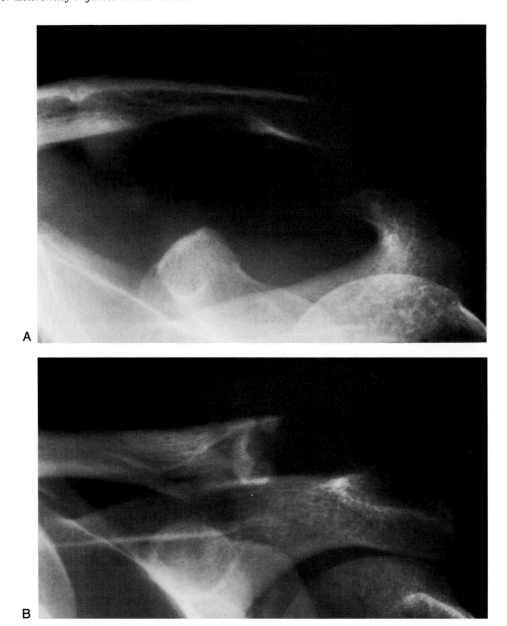

Figure 14-10 "Late" surgical management of an 18-year-old man who sustained a type III acromioclavicular joint disruption. **(A)** Initial weight-bearing AP radiographic view showing complete displacement of the distal clavicle relative to the acromion. **(B)** Postoperative radiograph showing removal of the distal 2 cm of the clavicle and reduction/stabilization of the remaining clavicle relative to the coracoid process.

use of his upper extremity as symptoms allowed, while avoiding aggravating positions and activities.

Six weeks after the injury, the patient's shoulder discomfort had resolved and full range of motion had returned. By 16 weeks postinjury, he had returned to competitive hockey. However, 3 years later, the patient began to experience impingement symptoms: discomfort over the anterolateral aspect of the shoulder, pain to palpation over the impingement interval, and maximal pain when the arm was actively elevated from 60 to 120 degrees (increased with

internal rotation of the arm). Nonoperative therapeutic modalities were ineffective. Surgery to reconstruct the acromioclavicular articulation was recommended.

Operative Management

The distal 2 cm of the clavicle was removed, and the degenerated acromioclavicular meniscus was excised (Fig. 14-10B). The acromioclavicular and coracoclavicular ligaments could not be identified for repair. The clavicle was reduced relative to the acromion and coracoid, and stabilized using heavy nonabsorbable sutures passed beneath the coracoid process and through a drill hole in the clavicle. The coracoacromial ligament was exposed—its acromial end was detached and reattached to the distal end of the clavicle. The deltoid-trapezius sling was reconstructed.

Postoperative Management

Postoperatively, the patient's arm remained immobilized in a sling and swathe bandage. At 6 weeks postoperatively, external immobilization was discontinued and a rehabilitation program was initiated, focusing on regaining shoulder range of motion and flexibility. At 12 weeks postoperatively, strength exercises were added. At 18 weeks postoperatively, the patient was asymptomatic, the shoulder had full range of motion, and strength was subjectively normal. The patient was placed on a carefully monitored program designed for his sport (hockey). At 24 weeks following surgery, unrestricted competition was allowed.

There are athletes who develop symptomatic degenerative disease or altered function of the acromioclavicular joint without historical evidence of a specific single incident of trauma.[23] These athletes perform forceful repetitive motions that result in intense compressive and rotational forces across the acromioclavicular joint. In many instances, these forces are enhanced by altered biomechanical shoulder function,

usually associated with poor scapulothoracic control: a persistent protraction of the scapula and an anterior adduction position of the shoulder, resulting in additional compression across the acromioclavicular articulation. The continued repetitive functional performance contributes to various presentations of degenerative joint disease—narrower articular space subchondral cyst formations, spur formations, and distal clavicle osteophytes. Osteophytes on the bursal side of the acromioclavicular articulation can irritate the bursal side of the rotator cuff. This irritation causes an inflammation (tendonitis) that contributes to pain, secondary weakness, and altered function and performance (Fig. 14-11).

Case Study II

A 25-year-old man presented with the chief complaint of acromioclavicular joint pain. He had been a competitive pairs figure skater for 15 years, achieving national championship and U.S. Olympic team status. His pain was reproduced with motions of upper-extremity adduction and internal rotation—a position he frequently repeated when lowering his partner from an overhead figure skating maneuver. The two most notable features of his physical examination were the lateral positions of scapula on his thorax and weakness of the muscles controlling his scapula and scapular humeral motions. The pain was reproduced with compression of the acromioclavicular joint and the position of shoulder adduction internal rotation (Fig. 14-12).

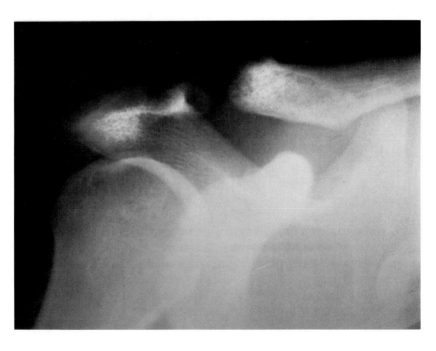

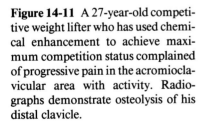

Figure 14-11 A 27-year-old competitive weight lifter who has used chemical enhancement to achieve maximum competition status complained of progressive pain in the acromioclavicular area with activity. Radiographs demonstrate osteolysis of his distal clavicle.

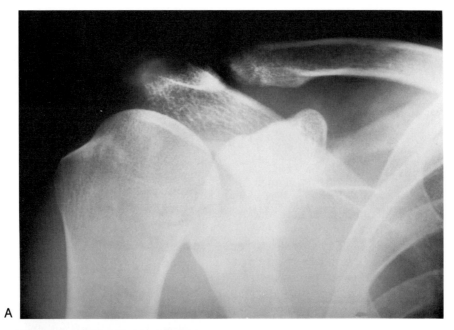

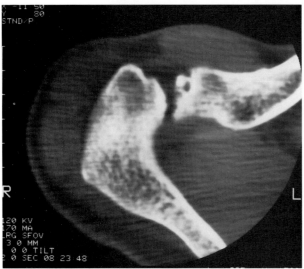

Figure 14-12 **(A)** Radiograph and **(B)** CT scan of the acromioclavicular joint demonstrate the articular and subchondral changes consistent with an acquired degenerative joint.

A treatment program was instituted with an initial program of rest, nonsteroidal anti-inflammatory medications, and appropriate nonresistive postural and scapula positioning physical therapy. The later stages of rehabilitation included a program for strength and proper mechanics of integrated shoulder complex motions (e.g., proper scapula and humeral coordinated patterns of function). The final stages of rehabilitation and return to competitive figure skating were the floor practice sessions with his partner, emphasizing proper lifting positioning of his scapula and avoidance of compression of his acromioclavicular joint. This process was enhanced by video recording to reinforce the desired mechanics

and compared with previous videotapes of improper techniques that contributed to the problem (i.e., protracted lowering of the scapula in front of the trunk and across the body). When these stages of rehabilitation were achieved, and he was pain-free (approximately 3 months from onset), he returned to practice on ice with his partner and later to exhibitions and performances.

The clinical significance of these examples underscores the importance of preventive exercise programs to ensure balanced kinesiologic and articular functions as well as periodic physical examinations and performance observations.

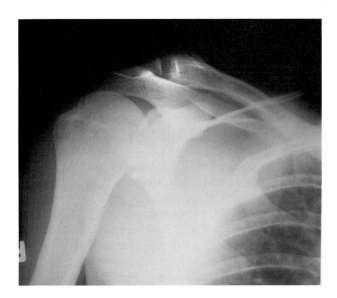

Figure 14-13 Radiograph showing subchondral changes of the acromioclavicular joint in a 29-year-old major league pitcher. There is evident enlargement of the acromioclavicular joint area. However, he presented full range of motion, well-balanced total shoulder muscle groups, and has pitched more than 200 innings for each of the past seven years without symptoms related to his acromioclavicular joint.

In certain cases of radiographic change indicating acromioclavicular degeneration, the etiology may have been a prior collision sport injury. Various image studies may be performed for nonacromioclavicular-related problems, with significant acromioclavicular

changes considered incidental findings. The variable physical and/or psychological interpretation of pain and the motivation level may be factors in the lack of acknowledgment of the injury. However, these findings in athletes may be associated with significant functional impairment and an indication for therapeutic intervention (Fig. 14-13). This raises questions for discussion concerning the clinical significance of radiographic findings, individual pain interpretation and tolerance, and motivational factors related to athletic and nonathletic activities.

DOUBLE DISRUPTIONS OF THE SUPERIOR SHOULDER SUSPENSORY COMPLEX

Several of the injuries described in this chapter and Chapter 15 have been termed "double disruptions of the superior shoulder suspensory complex."[26] The superior shoulder suspensory complex is a bony-soft tissue ring at the end of a superior and an inferior bony strut (Fig. 14-14). The ring is composed of the glenoid process, the coracoid process, the coracoclavicular ligaments, the distal clavicle, the acromioclavicular joint, and the acromial process. The superior strut is the clavicle, and the inferior strut is the lateral scapular body/spine. Each of the individual components has its own specific function(s). As a whole, the complex (1) maintains a normal stable relationship between the scapula-upper extremity and the axial skeleton; (2) allows mo-

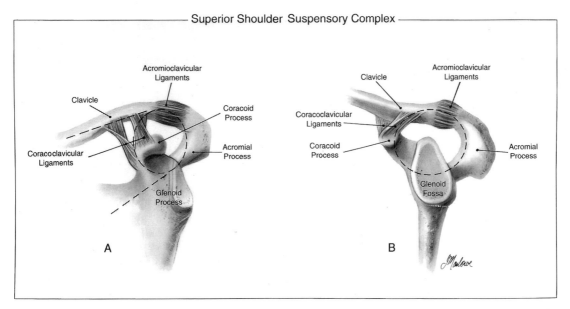

Figure 14-14 Superior shoulder suspensory complex. **(A)** AP view of the bony/soft tissue ring and the superior and inferior bony struts. **(B)** Lateral view of the bony/soft tissue ring.

tion to occur through the acromioclavicular joint and the coracoclavicular ligaments; and (3) provides a firm attachment point for various soft tissue structures.

Traumatic disruptions of one of the components of the superior shoulder suspensory complex (type I distal clavicle fractures and type II disruptions of the acromioclavicular joint) are common. They tend to be minor injuries, however, since these single disruptions do not significantly compromise the overall integrity of the complex. Displacement is minimal, and nonoperative treatment is sufficient. However, if the traumatic force is sufficiently severe or adversely directed, the suspensory complex may fail in two or more places (Fig. 14-15). In these situations, significant displacement at both the individual sites and of the suspensory complex in general often occurs. This, in turn, can lead to significant adverse healing and long-term functional consequences—delayed union, nonunion, malunion; impingement; decreased strength and muscle fatigue discomfort; neurovascular compromise; and degenerative joint disease—depending upon the particular injury. This double disruption principle unites and allows one to understand several well-described, but difficult to treat, shoulder injuries, including (1) type III to VI acromioclavicular joint disruptions (see p. 260); (2) type II and V distal clavicle fractures (see Ch. 15, p. 261); (3) type III glenoid fossa fractures with an associated superior shoulder suspensory complex disruption (see Ch. 15, p. 263); and (4) glenoid neck fractures with an associated suspensory complex disruption (see Ch. 15, p. 266) (Fig. 14-16).[26] Other unusual combinations include an acromial fracture with an associated suspensory complex disruption; a coracoid process fracture with an associated suspensory complex disruption; and fractures of the acromial and coracoid processes in the same individual (see Ch. 15, p. 270) (Fig. 14-17).

Injuries to the superior shoulder suspensory complex should be carefully evaluated for a double disruption (CT scanning with reconstructions is often necessary due to the complex bony anatomy in the region). If present and displacement is unacceptable, surgical reduction and stabilization of one or more of the injury sites is necessary to restore a stable shoulder complex and avoid the adverse sequelae described earlier. Often surgical reduction and stabilization of one of the injury sites will indirectly reduce and stabilize the accompanying injury adequately.

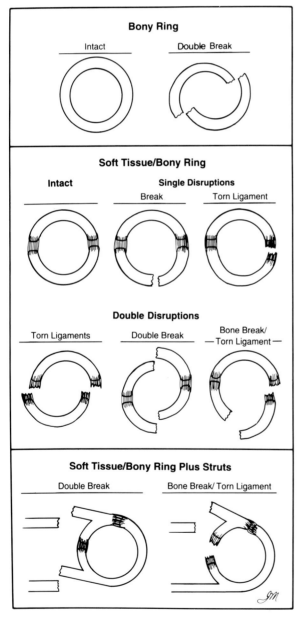

Figure 14-15 Traumatic ring/strut disruptions.

DISRUPTIONS OF THE STERNOCLAVICULAR JOINT

Disruptions of the sternoclavicular joint are uncommon injuries resulting from strong and unusually directed forces applied to the stabilizing ligaments.[1,3,4,6-8,10,11-14] Three grades may occur, reflecting increasing degrees of damage to the soft tissues (the sternoclavicular ligaments and the costoclavicular ligament) that secure the clavicle to the sternum and first rib.

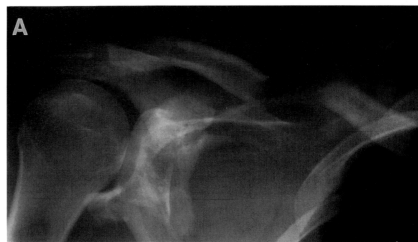

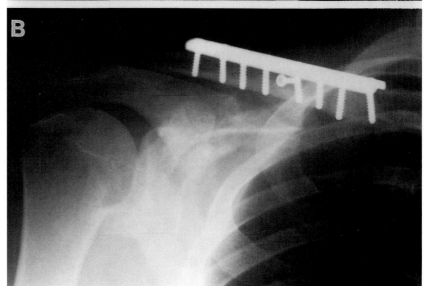

Figure 14-16 An individual who sustained a double disruption of the superior shoulder suspensory complex —fractures of the midclavicle and glenoid neck. **(A)** Initial AP-view radiograph showing the two fractures (note the severe separation at the clavicle fracture site and the medial translation of the glenoid fragment). **(B)** Postoperative AP-view radiograph showing the clavicle fracture reduced and securely fixed with a dynamic compression plate (the glenoid neck fracture was treated nonoperatively).

Grade I and Grade II (Subluxation) Sprains of the Sternoclavicular Joint

A grade I sprain represents a stretching or partial tear of the sternoclavicular ligaments, while a grade II sprain (subluxation) represents a complete tear of the sternoclavicular ligaments and a stretching-partial tear of the costoclavicular ligament (Fig. 14-18). Both injuries present with pain (especially with shoulder motion), tenderness, and swelling over the articulation. Treatment is symptomatic: sling or figure-of-eight splintage is prescribed (as necessary) for comfort, followed by increase in functional use of the extremity as symptoms allow. Ice is applied to the involved area during the first 48 hours, followed by local moist heat. Analgesic medications may be needed. Return to athletic activities is allowed when the patient is asymptomatic and shoulder range of motion and strength are normal.

Grade III Sprain (Dislocation) of the Sternoclavicular Joint

In a grade III sprain, the costoclavicular ligament as well as the sternoclavicular ligaments are completely torn, allowing the articulation to dislocate either anteriorly or posteriorly[29] (Fig. 14-18). Severe pain and tenderness are present over the sternoclavicular joint. Any movement of the shoulder causes increased discomfort. There is maximum pain when the patient is supine, so the patient prefers to be in the sitting position supporting the arm on the injured side.

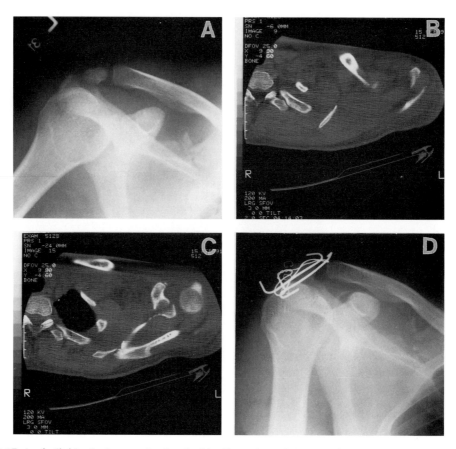

Figure 14-17 An individual who sustained a double disruption of the superior shoulder suspensory complex —fractures of the acromial and coracoid processes. **(A)** AP-view radiograph of the involved shoulder. **(B)** Axial CT image showing significant displacement at the acromial fracture site. **(C)** Axial CT image showing the coracoid process fracture. **(D)** Postoperative AP-view radiograph showing reduction and stabilization of the acromial fracture using a dorsal tension band technique (the coracoid fracture was treated nonoperatively).

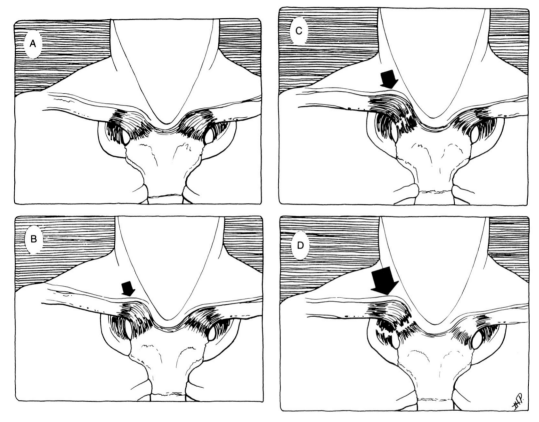

Figure 14-18 Grades I, II, and III sprains of the sternoclavicular joint. **(A)** Normal sternoclavicular joint with intact sternoclavicular and costoclavicular ligaments. **(B)** Grade I sprain with stretched sternoclavicular ligaments *(arrow)*. **(C)** Grade II sprain with torn sternoclavicular ligaments and a stretched costoclavicular ligament *(arrow)* allowing partial displacement of the sternoclavicular joint. **(D)** Grade III sprain of the sternoclavicular joint with torn costoclavicular and sternoclavicular ligaments *(arrow)* allowing the articulation to dislocate.

Anterior Dislocation

The anteriorly displaced medial end of the clavicle is generally quite visible (Fig. 14-19). At least one attempt at a closed reduction is reasonable. Intravenous sedation is usually adequate, but occasionally general anesthesia is necessary. The patient is positioned supine at the edge of a table with a sandbag under the scapula. The injured arm is abducted 90 degrees and extended to the point of resistance (about 15 degrees). While traction is applied to the injured extremity, the medial end of the clavicle is manipulated posteriorly. Reduction is usually achieved but is frequently unstable. If stable, a figure-of-eight bandage is worn for 6 weeks. If unstable, a sling is provided for comfort for 7 to 10 days followed by a gradual increase in functional use of the arm as symptoms allow. Patients may return to athletic activities any time after 8 weeks when they are asymptomatic and shoulder range of motion and strength are normal. Satisfactory painless function usually results. In patients who develop symptomatic degenerative

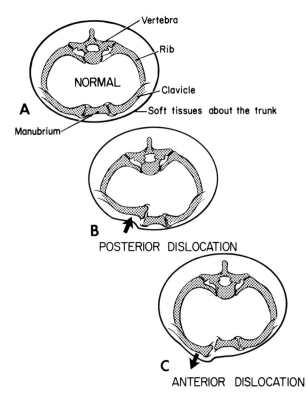

Figure 14-19 Grade III sprains of the sternoclavicular joint as seen in the axillary plane. **(A)** Normal sternoclavicular joint. **(B)** Posterior dislocation of the sternoclavicular joint —the proximal end of the clavicle is displaced posteriorly relative to the sternum *(arrow).* **(C)** Anterior dislocation of the sternoclavicular joint—the proximal end of the clavicle is displaced anteriorly relative to the sternum *(arrow).*

disease of the sternoclavicular joint unresponsive to nonoperative treatment, resection of the medial 2.0 cm of the clavicle combined with a ligamentous reconstruction is a consideration.

Case Study III

Injury and Initial Evaluation

A 20-year-old college football running back was tackled by a 260-lb defensive lineman who landed on top of him, driving the lateral aspect of his left shoulder against a hard artificial surface. Acute severe and persistent pain was noted along the entire length of his left clavicle. On physical examination, he was exquisitely tender over both the sternoclavicular and acromioclavicular articulations. In addition, the proximal end of the clavicle was visibly prominent anteriorly, the distal end of the clavicle seemed to be displaced posterosuperiorly to palpation, and the clavicle as a whole was abnormally mobile. AP and axillary views of the left shoulder showed the distal end of the clavicle to be displaced posteriorly relative to the acromion. Anteroposterior and oblique radiographic views of the sternoclavicular joint were difficult to interpret. A CT scan revealed an anterior dislocation of the sternoclavicular joint and a type IV disruption of the acromioclavicular joint (Fig. 14-20A).

Operative Treatment

The patient was taken to the operating room to improve the overall stability of the sternal-clavicular-acromial linkage by reducing and stabilizing the sternoclavicular and acromioclavicular disruptions.

The distal clavicle was found to be "buttonholed" through the trapezius muscle. It was gradually mobilized and reduced relative to the acromion. (The acromioclavicular meniscus within the acromioclavicular articulation was removed). A smooth Kirschner-wires were passed across the acromioclavicular joint and down the intramedullary canal of the clavicle. The coracoclavicular and acromioclavicular ligaments, along with the rent in the trapezius muscle, were repaired. Reduction of the anterior sternoclavicular dislocation was easily achieved but was extremely unstable and could not be maintained. The shoulder complex and upper extremity were immobilized in a sling and swathe dressing (Fig. 14-20B).

After 6 weeks, all protection was discontinued, the transfixing K-wires were removed, and the patient was instructed to gradually increase the functional use of his shoulder as symptoms allowed, while

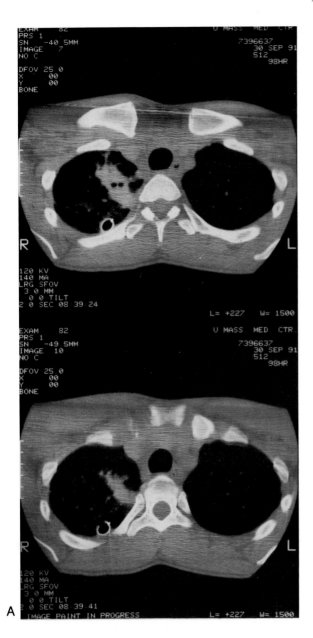

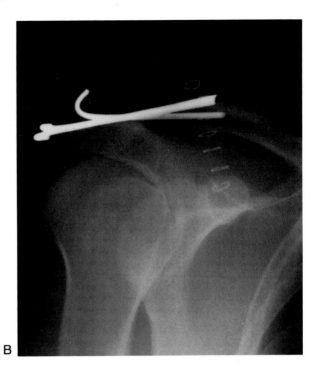

Figure 14-20 A 20-year-old man who sustained a panclavicular dislocation. (A) Preoperative axial CT image showing the proximal end of the clavicle to be dislocated anteriorly and superiorly relative to the sternum. (B) Postoperative radiograph showing reduction/stabilization of the distal end of the clavicle relative to the acromion using transfixing K-wires.

avoiding aggravating positions and activities. A closely supervised physical therapy program was prescribed. At 12 weeks postoperatively, the patient was begun on a carefully monitored return to sports program. By 16 weeks postoperatively, the patient was asymptomatic, had regained nearly full shoulder range of motion and strength, and had returned to competitive athletics.

Posterior Dislocation

The usually prominent medial end of the clavicle is not visible or palpable due to its posterior displacement[30,31] (Fig. 14-19). Posterior dislocation of the ster-

noclavicular joint may cause pressure on the great vessels, the trachea, or the esophagus. Either the dislocation itself or associated injuries to the chest wall may result in a pneumothorax. Radiographic assessment is necessary to confirm the presence of a posterior sternoclavicular dislocation. Oblique projections are quite helpful, since the standard AP view is often difficult to interpret. Due to the complex bony anatomy in the area, however, a CT scan is generally necessary to establish the diagnosis.[32] When pressure on the great vessels or the trachea is posing a threat to life, reduction of the dislocation becomes an emergency. Unless the patient is in extremis, general anesthesia or intravenous sedation should be used. The patient is positioned supine at the edge of a table with a sandbag beneath the scapula. The arm is abducted 90 degrees and extended to the point of resistance (approximately 15 degrees). As traction is applied to the extremity, reduction of the dislocation may occur. However, it may be necessary to pull the medial end of the clavicle outward, either manually or with a towel clip. Reduction of all posterior sternoclavicular joint dislocations must be achieved, and operative intervention may be necessary. Once obtained, the reduction is generally quite stable. A figure-of-eight bandage is then applied and maintained for 6 weeks, with strenuous activities prohibited for an additional 2 weeks. The patient may return to athletic activities when asymptomatic and shoulder range of motion and strength are normal. If recurrent subluxation or dislocation of the sternoclavicular joint articulation occurs, a reconstructive procedure using fascia lata, the semitendinosis tendon or the toe extensor tendons passed between the clavicle, the first rib, and the manubrium may be considered. In patients who develop symptomatic degenerative disease of the sternoclavicular joint that is unresponsive to nonoperative treatment, resection of the medial 2.0 cm of the clavicle, combined with a ligamentous reconstruction, is a consideration.

REFERENCES

1. Allman FL: Fracture and ligamentous injuries of clavicle and its articulations. J Bone Joint Surg [Am] 49:774, 1967
2. Bach BR, Van Fleet TA, Novak PJ: Acromioclavicular injuries. Phys Sports Med 20:87, 1992
3. Bateman JE: The Shoulder and Neck. 2nd Ed. WB Saunders, Philadelphia, 1978
4. DePalma AF: Surgery of the Shoulder. 3rd Ed. JB Lippincott, Philadelphia, 1983
5. Heppenstall RB: Fractures and dislocation of the distal clavicle. Orthop Clin North Am 6:477, 1975
6. Hoyt WA: Etiology of shoulder injuries in athletes. J Bone Joint Surg [Am] 49: 755, 1967
7. Neer CS II: Shoulder Reconstruction. 1st Ed. WB Saunders, Philadelphia, 1990
8. Nevaiser JS: Injuries of the clavicle and its articulations. Orthop Clin North Am 11:233, 1980
9. Nevaiser RJ: Injuries to the clavicle and acromioclavicular joint. Orthop Clin North Am 18:433, 1987
10. Post M: The Shoulder. 2nd Ed. Lea & Febiger, Philadelphia, 1988
11. Quigley TB: Injuries to the acromioclavicular and sternoclavicular joints sustained in athletics. Surg Clin North Am 43:1551–1554, 1963
12. Rockwood CA Jr, Green DP: Fractures in Adults. 2nd Ed. JB Lippincott, Philadelphia, 1984
13. Rockwood CA, Matsen FA: The Shoulder. 1st Ed. WB Saunders, Philadelphia, 1990
14. Rowe CR: The Shoulder. 1st Ed. Churchill Livingstone, New York, 1988
15. Zanca P: Shoulder pain: involvement of the acromioclavicular separation. Am J Radiol 112:493, 1971
16. Alexander OM: Radiography of A-C joint. Med Radiogr Photogr 30:34, 1954
17. Bjerneld H, Hovelius L, Thorling J: Acromioclavicular separations treated conservatively: a 5-year follow-up study. Acta Orthop Scand 54:743, 1983
18. Imatani RJ, Hanlon JJ, Cady GW: Acute, complete acromioclavicular separation. J Bone Joint Surg [Am] 57:328, 1975
19. Larsen E, Bjerg-Nielsen A, Christensen P: Conservative or surgical treatment of acromioclavicular dislocation: a prospective, controlled randomized study. J Bone Joint Surg [Am] 68:552, 1986
20. Powers JA, Bach PJ: Acromioclavicular separation closed or open treatment? Clin Orthop 204:213, 1974
21. Cox JS: Current method of treatment of acromioclavicular joint dislocations. Orthopedics 15:1041, 1992
22. Cox JS: The fate of the acromioclavicular joint in athletic injuries. Am J Sports Med 9:50, 1981
23. Cahill BR: Osteolysis of the distal part of the clavicle in male athletes. J Bone Joint Surg [Am] 64:1053, 1982
24. Mumford EB: Acromioclavicular dislocation: a new operative treatment. J Bone Joint Surg 23:799, 1941
25. Cook FF, Tibone JE: The Mumford procedure in athletes: an objective analysis of function. Am J Sports Med 16:97, 1988
26. Goss TP: Double disruptions of the superior shoulder suspensory complex. J Orthop Trauma 7:99, 1993
27. Bosworth BM: Acromioclavicular dislocation: end-results of screw suspension treatment. Ann Surg 127:98, 1948
28. Weaver JL, Dunn HK: Treatment of acromioclavicular injuries. J Bone Joint Surg [Am]54:1187, 1972
29. Heppenstall RB: Sternoclavicular Dislocations. p. 417. In: Fracture Treatment and Healing. WB Saunders, Philadelphia, 1980
30. Heinig CF: Retrosternal dislocation of the clavicle: early recognition, x-ray diagnosis, and management. J Bone Joint Surg [Am] 50:830, 1968
31. Selesnick FH, Jablon M, Frank C, Post M: Retrosternal dislocation of the clavicle: report of four cases. J Bone Joint Surg [Am] 66:287, 1984
32. Levinsohn EM, Bunnell WP, Yuan HA: computed tomography in the diagnosis of dislocations of the sternoclavicular joint. Clin Orthop 140:12, 1979

Fractures of the Shoulder Complex

Thomas P. Goss

Shoulder fractures in athletes are typically seen in sports in which the shoulder is subjected to high-energy direct trauma or in which significant indirect loading, levering, or twisting stresses are applied to the shoulder complex. Evaluation and treatment of shoulder fractures in the athlete follow the same principles as those developed for the general population. However, for the high-performance athlete, restoration of range of motion, flexibility, strength, and overall functional use are especially important, particularly for those in whom upper extremity function is critical (throwing athletes, gymnasts, weight lifters). Thus, treatment of the fracture followed by rehabilitation should be provided with these needs in mind.

In general, fractures are considered functionally healed, and protection can be discontinued when (1) the average healing time for that particular fracture has been reached; (2) the patient is nontender to palpation over the fracture site and no abnormal motion is detected; (3) movement of the extremity does not cause pain at the fracture site; and (4) hard bridging mature callus is radiographically visible. Rehabilitation focuses initially on regaining shoulder range of motion followed by strengthening exercises. As the individual progresses, a gradual return to athletics program specific to the patient's particular sport is initiated. Return to competitive sports is prolonged for those activities in which severe forces are applied to the shoulder (foot-

ball) and in those that require high degrees of motion, flexibility, and indirect stress (tennis, pitching). Supervised follow-up and sportwise judgment on the part of the physician and the therapist are critical to an optimal result (see Ch. 2).

FRACTURES OF THE CLAVICLE

Fractures of the clavicle make up approximately 10 percent of all fractures, with approximately 85 percent occurring through the middle one-third; 10 percent through the distal one-third; and 5 percent through the proximal one-third.[1-10] Of the three bones in the shoulder complex, the clavicle is the one most often fractured. Since it is the only bony link between the upper extremity and the axial skeleton, direct and indirect forces (inherent in many sports) tend to be concentrated over its course. Most fractures can be managed nonoperatively, but surgical intervention is occasionally required.

Fractures of the Middle Third of the Clavicle

Fractures of the middle third are the most frequently seen clavicular disruption in athletes. The mechanism of injury may either be a directly applied force (com-

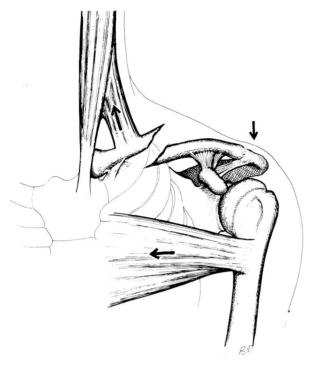

Figure 15-1 Fracture of the middle third of the clavicle. Note the superior displacement of the proximal segment and the inferior displacement of the distal segment.

mon in collision sports such as football) or an indirectly applied force (a blow to the shoulder region or a fall onto an outstretched arm) seen in those sports where the individual impacts the ground, a wall, and so on

with significant violence (e.g., a fall while skiing on icy terrain). The medial or proximal fragment is usually displaced superiorly by the pull of the sternocleido-mastoid muscle, while the lateral or distal fragment is drawn inferiorly by the weight of the arm (Fig. 15-1). Although anatomic reduction of the fracture fragments is seldom obtained, these fractures generally heal with full restoration of shoulder function and an acceptable cosmetic deformity. Complications include nonunion (reported incidence of 0.9 to 4.0 percent), malunion (patients with more than 15 mm of overriding have been noted to have significantly more discomfort), and neurovascular sequelae (following both united and un-united fractures) (Fig. 15-2). Surgical open reduction internal fixation is rarely necessary and neurovascular injury is uncommon.

The figure-of-eight bandage is the traditional method of treatment. Its intent is to reduce overriding and decrease motion at the fracture site, thereby lessening the patient's discomfort. The figure-of-eight bandage should be worn snugly but not so tight as to cause excessive discomfort, skin breakdown, and/or neurovascular compromise. It should be adjusted frequently to prevent secondary spasm and looseness and worn constantly (it may be removed to wash) for a period of at least 6 weeks (4 weeks in preadolescents). During the first 2 weeks after the injury, a sling may be added to support the weight of the arm and provide further pain relief. Evidence of early bony union is usually present before 6 weeks. The figure-of-eight bandage can be removed when adequate callus is visible on radiographic

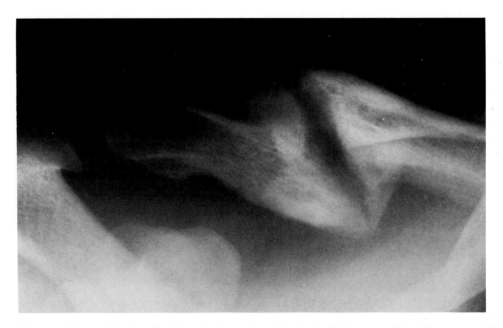

Figure 15-2 AP radiographic view of a delayed union of a midshaft clavicle fracture. The injury eventually went on to union.

examination, and the patient can fully move the arm without discomfort. After removal, the patient is encouraged to gradually increase the functional use of the affected extremity while working on regaining range of motion and strength. Collision sports and sports requiring strenuous use of the shoulder girdle should be avoided for a minimum of an additional 6 weeks.

Fractures of the Distal Third of the Clavicle

In the athlete, fractures of the distal third of the clavicle are considerably less common than those of the middle third.[7,11-13] They are generally caused by forces similar to those that disrupt the acromioclavicular joint: a blow to the superior or (less frequently) the anterior or posterior aspects of the shoulder or a fall onto the outstretched arm. Consequently, these fractures are most often seen in collision sports (e.g., rugby) and sports in which the individual's shoulder may impact hard, immobile surfaces with considerable force (e.g., hockey with its frequent "board checks").

Type I fractures (those in which the coracoclavicular ligaments remain attached to the medial segment [Fig. 15-3]) comprise 80 percent of all distal third injuries.

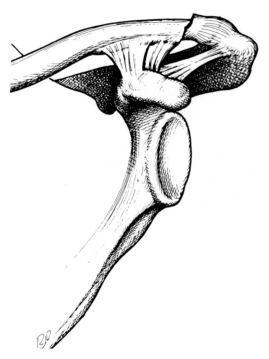

Figure 15-3 Type I fracture of the distal clavicle. Note the coracoclavicular ligaments remain attached to the proximal segment preventing significant displacement at the fracture site.

These are managed in the same manner as fractures of the middle third of the clavicle.

In type II and type V distal clavicle fractures, the coracoclavicular ligaments are detached from the medial segment (Fig. 15-4), creating a double disruption of the superior shoulder suspensory complex[14] (see Ch. 14). The lateral segment-scapula-upper extremity are drawn anteriorly, inferiorly, and medially by the weight of the arm and the pull of the pectoralis major, pectoralis minor, latissimus dorsi, and teres major muscles. The pull of the trapezius and sternocleidomastoid muscles draws the medial segment superiorly and posteriorly. This often creates a large gap at the fracture site, posing a significant risk for a delayed union or even a symptomatic nonunion.

Case Study I

Injury, Initial Evaluation, and Operative Management

A 25-year-old soccer player collided with another player and landed heavily on the superolateral aspect of his right shoulder. Initial AP-view films revealed a comminuted fracture of the distal third of the clavicle. Supplemental views revealed significant inferior displacement of the lateral portion of the clavicle relative to the medial segment. (A type II separation of the acromioclavicular joint was also present.) A type V fracture of his distal clavicle was diagnosed (i.e., a fracture had occurred through the distal third of the clavicle and the coracoclavicular ligaments were totally detached from both the medial and lateral segments remaining attached to a small inferior fragment) (Fig. 15-5A). Surgical management was advised and performed (Fig. 15-5B).

Postoperative Management

Postoperatively, the patient's arm was immobilized in a sling and swathe bandage; however, limited use out of the sling and gentle passive range of motion exercises were permitted. At 6 weeks after surgery, the transfixing pin was removed, and all immobilization was discontinued. The patient was instructed to gradually increase the functional use of his shoulder as symptoms allowed. An intensive physiotherapy program was prescribed to help him regain shoulder range of motion, flexibility, and strength. At 16 weeks following his injury, the patient was asymptomatic, shoulder range of motion had improved steadily (forward flexion 160 degrees, abduction 90 degrees, extension 60 degrees, internal rotation to the high lumbar area, and external rotation 45 degrees) and strength was subjectively nor-

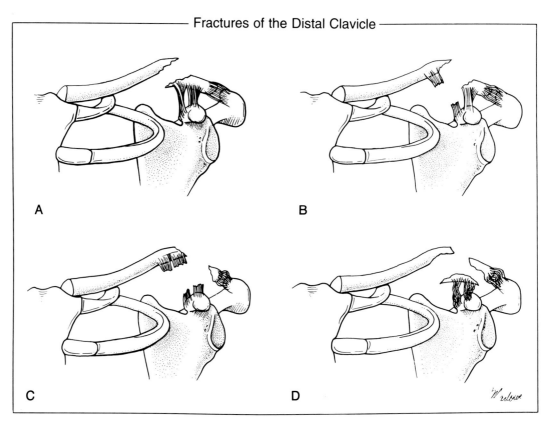

Fractures of the Distal Clavicle

Figure 15-4 Type II and type V distal clavicle fractures. **(A–C)** Three type II variants: in each the coracoclavicular ligaments are detached from the proximal segment allowing significant displacement to occur at the fracture site. **(D)** Type V: the coracoclavicular ligaments are attached to a small inferior clavicular fragment but detached from the proximal clavicular segment allowing significant displacement to occur at the fracture site.

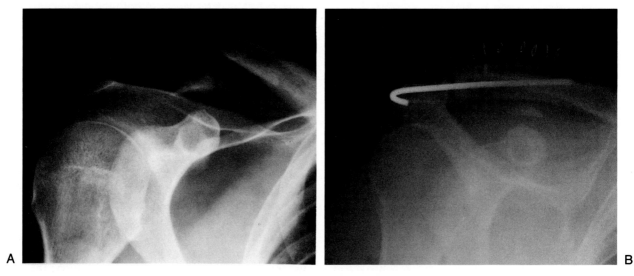

Figure 15-5 A 25-year-old soccer player who sustained a type V fracture of the distal clavicle. **(A)** Weightbearing AP-view radiograph showing significant inferior displacement of the distal clavicular segment relative to the proximal segment and a small inferior fragment to which the coracoclavicular ligaments were attached. **(B)** Postoperative AP-view radiograph showing the fracture to be reduced and stabilized with an intramedullary K wire.

mal. He was begun on a carefully monitored gradual return to soccer program. By 24 weeks postoperatively, he had returned to unrestricted competition.

The potentially serious nature of these fractures needs to be recognized. For all disruptions of the distal third of the clavicle, an AP-view radiograph should be obtained of both shoulders on one film with the patient standing and a 10-lb weight attached to each wrist. If the coracoid process-medial clavicle distance is significantly increased compared to the normal side, one can assume that the coracoclavicular ligaments are detached. Since much of the displacement is in the AP plane, however, two additional radiographs are worthwhile: anterior and posterior 45 degree oblique views with the patient erect and the injured shoulder against the radiographic film. These projections will demonstrate the extent of separation between the two fragments. Computed tomography (CT) scanning of the area can also be considered.

If displacement is unacceptable, the clavicular fracture site should be anatomically reduced and internally fixed. A variety of fixation techniques are available, but one of the most effective is a smooth Steinmann pin passed across the fracture site and bent at its lateral end to prevent medial migration. Generally, this will indirectly restore the normal anatomic relationships among the medial clavicle, the coracoclavicular ligaments, and the coracoid process. The arm is then placed in a sling and swathe dressing for 6 weeks, at which time all metallic implants are removed, immobilization is discontinued, and rehabilitation to regain normal function is begun.

Type III distal clavicle fractures are those in which the articular surface of the distal clavicle is involved. These fractures may be subtle and easily confused with a type I acromioclavicular joint injury. Special radiographic views (oblique projections and even CT scanning) may be required to visualize the fracture. Treatment is usually nonoperative. Open reduction internal fixation is indicated if a single large fragment is present and associated with a significant articular step-off. If post-traumatic symptomatic degenerative joint disease occurs, resection of the distal 1.5 cm of the clavicle must be considered (Fig. 15-6).

A clinical entity commonly referred to as "weight lifter's shoulder" is a symptomatic pathologic process that involves the distal articular end of the clavicle and is caused by chronic trauma. Individuals who subject the acromioclavicular joint to significant repetitive compressive stresses (weight lifters, throwing athletes) frequently develop pain over the region. Athletes who use chemical enhancers to increase their strength often stress the soft tissues and cartilage to excess, thereby making the acromioclavicular joint and other areas more susceptible to injury. Although plain radiographs may be negative, in severe cases, resorption (osteolysis) of the distal clavicle may be seen and is thought to be due to increased vascularity secondary to microtrauma or microfractures (Fig. 15-7). Treatment initially consists of rest and avoidance of aggravating activities. Anti-inflammatory medications as well as a local injection of cortisone may be of value. If unacceptable discomfort persists, resection of the distal 1.5 cm of the clavicle is the surgical procedure of choice. Although there is usually some loss of maximum benchpress strength and possible residual weakness of shoulder flexion and extension, the athlete subjectively feels stronger due to pain relief and is generally able to return to competitive sports.

Fractures of the Proximal Third of the Clavicle

Fractures of the proximal one-third are quite uncommon, since this portion of the clavicle is not as exposed and is relatively protected by the surrounding anatomy. Fractures through the proximal epiphysis occur before age 25 and must be differentiated from an injury to the sternoclavicular joint. These fractures are caused by the same forces that can disrupt the adjacent sternoclavicular joint (Fig. 15-8), and treatment is identical to that described for the corresponding sternoclavicular injury (see Ch. 14). Mechanisms of injury include a direct blow or a force of considerable violence applied over the outer aspect of the shoulder complex as occur in such high-velocity sports as motorcycle or auto racing. Due to the severe forces involved, injuries to adjacent structures are common and may be life-threatening.

FRACTURES OF THE SCAPULA

Fractures of the scapula are uncommon in athletes. The scapula is well-protected by surrounding osseus and soft tissue structures, and its mobility allows dissipation of traumatic forces. These fractures make up only 1 percent of all fractures and 5 percent of all shoulder fractures. Approximately 45 percent involve the body, 25 percent the glenoid neck, 10 percent the glenoid cavity, and 20 percent the acromian, the coracoid process, and the scapular spine combined (Fig. 15-9). These fractures are seen in the most violent sports, generally when the shoulder impacts a hard immobile surface (being driven against the artificial turf in

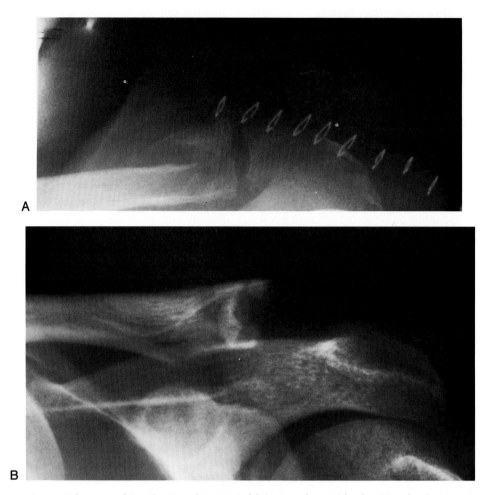

Figure 15-6 Type III fracture of the distal clavicle. **(A)** Initial AP radiographic view showing involvement of the articular surface and a significant articular step-off. **(B)** Postoperative AP radiographic view showing the clavicle with its distal end resected.

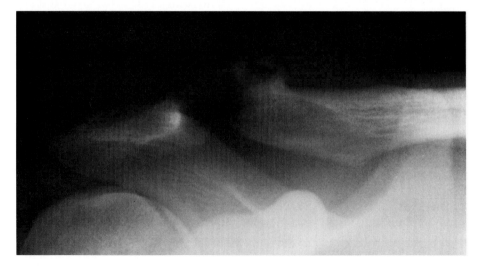

Figure 15-7 AP-view radiograph of a weight lifter's shoulder showing severe resorption of the distal articular end of the clavicle, resulting in painful degenerative disease of the acromioclavicular joint.

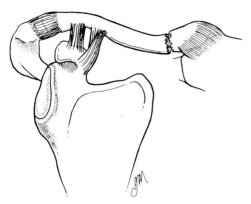

Figure 15-8 Fracture of the proximal third of the clavicle. Displacement is usually acceptable due to strong soft tissue support structures.

football, striking the pavement in motor racing, etc.). Consequently, there is a significant incidence (80–95 percent) of associated bone and soft tissue injuries that can be multiple, major, and even life-threatening. The radiologic evaluation is critical and, due to the complex anatomy in the area, CT scanning with reconstructions is almost always necessary in addition to routine plain radiographs. Most scapular fractures can be managed nonoperatively with surgical treatment rarely indicated.[2–4,8–10,15]

Fractures of the Body and Spine

Injuries to the body and spine are caused by severe forces applied directly over the scapular body and spine. The large surrounding soft tissue mass usually makes displacement minimal (significant displacement is rare) and uncomplicated union is the norm. Symptomatic nonoperative care consisting of initial immobilization for comfort followed by early and progressive range of motion and functional use generally yields good to excellent results. Union usually occurs within 6 weeks.

Fractures of the Glenoid Neck

Fractures of the glenoid neck are the second most common scapular fracture.[16] They are caused by direct trauma, a fall onto the point of the shoulder, or a fall onto an outstretched arm. The articular surface of the glenoid cavity is intact, as the fracture usually runs from the lateral margin of the scapula through the spinoglenoid interval and out the superior border of the scapula, or up the inferior glenoid neck along the scapular spine and out the medial border of scapula (Fig. 15-10). Generally, displacement is acceptable (type I fractures) and nonoperative treatment is sufficient (6 weeks is required for bony union). If the traumatic force is particularly violent, however, and especially if the coracoid process, the coracoclavicular ligaments, the acromioclavicular joint, the acromion, or most commonly, the clavicle is also disrupted (i.e., a double disruption of the superior shoulder suspensory complex[14]), significant displacement of the glenoid fragment may occur. Translational displacement (antero-

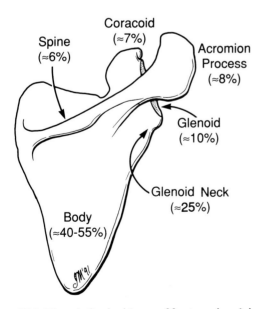

Figure 15-9 The relative incidence of fractures involving the various segments of a scapula.

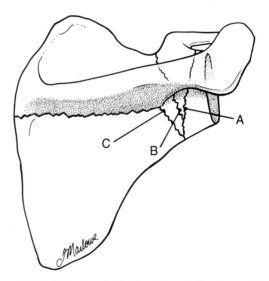

Figure 15-10 The three basic glenoid neck fracture patterns: *A*, fracture through the anatomic neck; *B*, fracture through the surgical neck; *C*, fracture of the inferior glenoid neck coursing across the scapular body, and exiting out the medial scapular border.

Type I

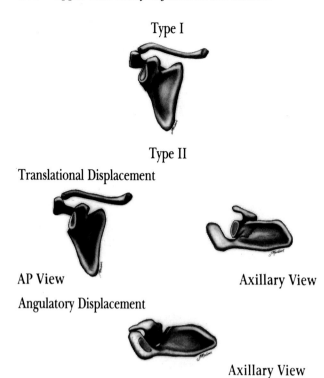

Type II

Translational Displacement

AP View

Axillary View

Angulatory Displacement

Axillary View

Figure 15-11 Glenoid neck fracture classification scheme: type I (minimal displacement); type II (significant translational displacement); type II (significant angular displacement).

medial is most common) of 1 cm or more or angulatory displacement of 40 degrees or more in the transverse or coronal plane (type II fractures) are indications for surgical open reduction internal fixation (Fig. 15-11).

Fractures of the Glenoid Cavity

Although fractures of the glenoid cavity are rare, they are intra-articular injuries that can result in instability and/or degenerative joint disease.[17-19] These fractures are seen in motor sports, equestrian events, and other "hard-hitting" activities. Around 90 percent of cases are minimally displaced and are managed nonoperatively with sling and swathe protection for comfort and early progressive range of motion and use out of the sling as symptoms allow. Usually, 6 weeks is required for union, and the prognosis is excellent. However, 10 percent of these fractures are significantly displaced, and surgical treatment should be considered to avoid post-traumatic glenohumeral instability and/or degenerative joint disease.

Glenoid cavity fractures are divided into two categories: fractures of the glenoid rim and fractures of the glenoid fossa (Fig. 15-12). Glenoid rim fractures occur when a laterally applied force drives the humeral head

directly against the glenoid margin (Fig. 15-13). These injuries are distinct from the smaller avulsion fractures that occasionally occur when a dislocating humeral head impacts the periarticular soft tissues. The type Ia variant is a fracture of the anterior rim, and the type Ib variant is a fracture of the posterior rim. Glenoid fossa fractures (types II to VI) occur when a violent force is applied laterally over the humeral head, which in turn is driven directly into the glenoid cavity. A transverse fracture across the fossa occurs, which then propagates in one of several directions, depending upon the exact direction of the traumatic force (Fig. 15-14).

If a glenoid cavity fracture is noted or suspected on the basis of the patient's history, physical examination, and/or admission chest radiograph, the standard radiographic evaluation includes true AP and axillary views of the glenohumeral joint. Transthoracic lateral and lateral scapular views may be of value. If a fracture is present but further delineation is needed, tomography in the AP plane, a CT scan with axial images and coronal reconstructions, or even a three-dimensional CT scan can be performed.

If significant displacement at the fracture site is present, surgical management must be considered. The glenoid may be approached anteriorly, posteriorly, or superiorly, depending upon the clinical situation. If necessary, these approaches can be combined to allow optimal exposure of the glenoid. Four regions of thick, solid bone are available for internal fixation: (1) the glenoid neck, (2) the coracoid process, (3) the base of the scapular spine, and (4) the lateral margin of the scapular body (Fig. 15-15). There are several possible internal fixation devices that can be considered, but the 3.5-mm cannulated interfragmentary compression screw is the most useful (Fig. 15-16). The final choice depends upon the available bone stock and the surgeon's preference.

Case Study II

Injury, Initial Evaluation, and Operative Management

A 25-year-old motorcycle racer lost control and was thrown off his bike, striking the lateral aspect of his left shoulder against the pavement. In the emergency room, he complained of pain only over the shoulder region and resisted any attempt to move his arm. Diffuse swelling and exquisite tenderness to palpation were noted over the anterior and posterior aspects of the glenohumeral joint. His neurovascular examination was normal.

Radiographs of the shoulder were obtained in two planes at 90 degrees to each other—a true AP projection of the glenohumeral joint with the arm in as

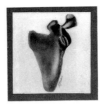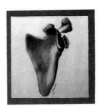

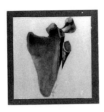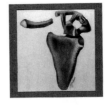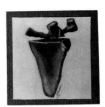

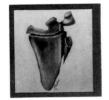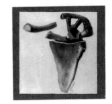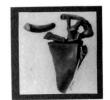

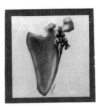

Figure 15-12 Glenoid cavity fracture classification scheme: type Ia and b fractures involve the glenoid rim; types II to Vc fractures involve the glenoid fossa; type VI fractures include all comminuted injuries.

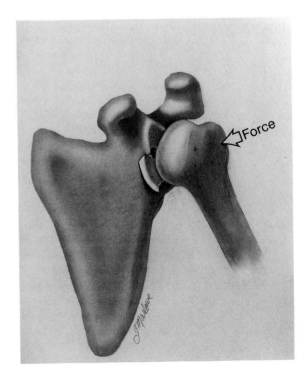

Figure 15-13 Mechanism of injury associated with fractures of the glenoid rim: a laterally applied *force* drives the humeral head against the glenoid rim creating a type Ia fracture.

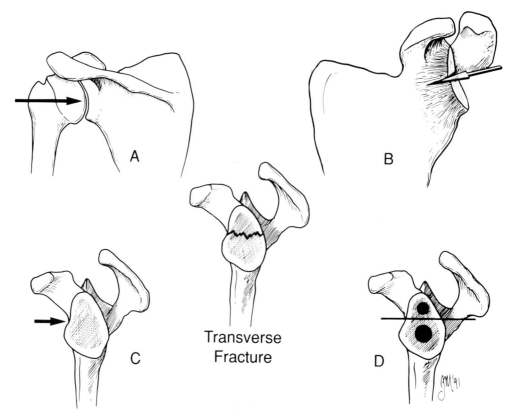

Figure 15-14 Possible reasons why glenoid fossa fractures begin as a transverse disruption. **(A)** The force of the humeral head is concentrated across the apex of the glenoid concavity. **(B)** Fracture lines tend to follow the transversely oriented subchondral trabeculae. **(C)** The abrupt change in contour along the anterior glenoid rim creates a stress riser at which point fractures are likely to originate. **(D)** The glenoid cavity is formed from two ossification centers which leaves a "weak" fusion area centrally.

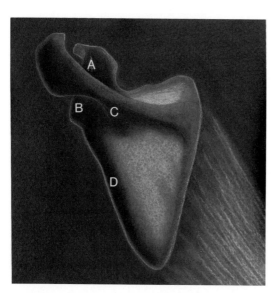

Figure 15-15 The four areas of substantial scapular bone stock available for internal fixation: *A*, the glenoid neck; *B*, the coracoid process; *C*, the base of the scapular spine and *D*, the lateral scapular border.

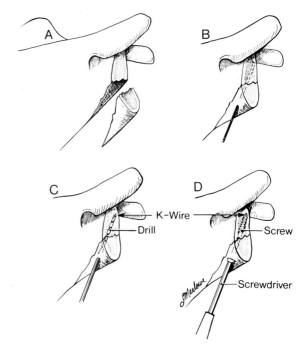

Figure 15-16 Reduction and stabilization of a displaced glenoid fragment using a 3.5-mm cannulated interfragmentary compression screw.

near neutral rotation as possible and a true axillary view. The AP-view radiograph revealed a type II fracture of the glenoid fossa with significant displacement of the inferior glenoid fragment (Fig. 15-17A). Surgical management of the glenoid fracture was advised and performed (Fig. 15-17B).

Postoperative Care

Since rigid fixation was achieved, a physiotherapy program was begun immediately. Two weeks postoperatively, the patient began gentle but progressive passive and active-assisted range-of-motion exer-

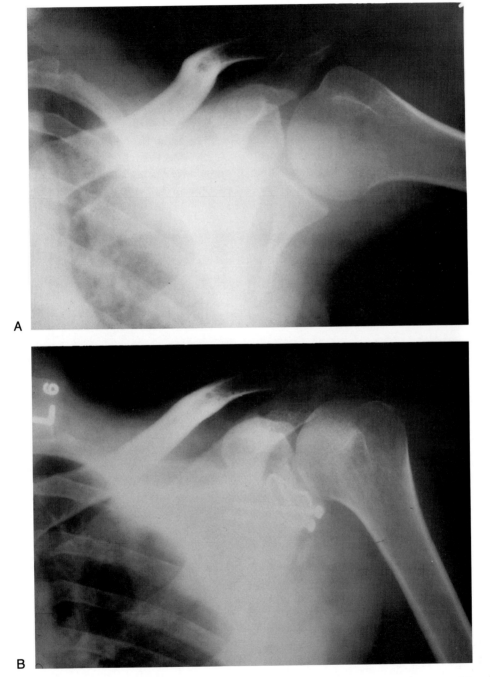

Figure 15-17 A 25-year-old individual who sustained a significantly displaced type II fracture of the glenoid fossa. **(A)** Initial AP-view radiograph showing a large displaced inferior glenoid fragment and a significant articular step-off. **(B)** Postoperative AP-view radiograph showing reduction of the glenoid fragment and stabilization using two cancellous screws and a cerclage wire.

cises in all directions. In addition, he was allowed to use his arm for gentle activities out of the sling (see Ch. 2).

Six weeks postoperatively, the fracture was sufficiently healed to allow discontinuation of external immobilization. The patient was instructed to gradually increase the use of his shoulder as symptoms allowed while avoiding aggravating positions and activities.

Strengthening exercises were slowly added. As overall shoulder function improved, the patient was allowed to gradually return to sports and he was able to resume competitive motorcycle racing 6 months following his injury. One year after surgery, the patient was pain-free and his shoulder strength was subjectively normal.

For type VI (comminuted) fossa fractures, surgical open reduction internal fixation is not an option due to the extensive comminution present. Treatment con-

sists of immobilization for comfort combined with early progressive range of motion, with the hope that movement of the humeral head will mold the fracture fragments into a more congruous position. Bony union occurs within 6 weeks. However, even with optimal care, type VI glenoid fossa fractures pose the greatest risk of late symptomatic glenohumeral degenerative joint disease.

Isolated Fractures of the Coracoid and Acromial Processes

Isolated fractures of the coracoid process are occasionally seen in the athletic population.[20-22] Fractures at the base are the most common — often secondary to a direct blow to the area as seen in the more violent "stick" sports such as lacrosse. Fatigue or stress fractures have been associated with very specific athletic activities (high-impact rifle shooting), while avulsion

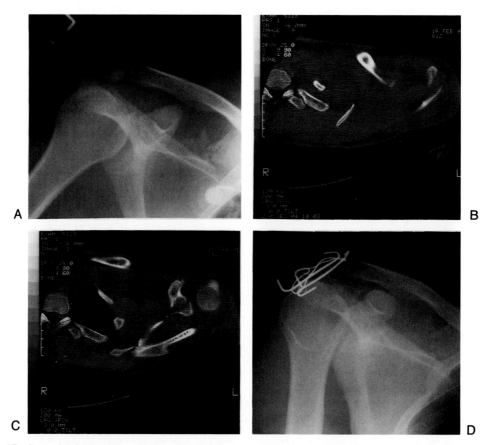

Figure 15-18 An individual who sustained a double disruption of the superior shoulder suspensory complex-fractures of both the acromial and coracoid processes. **(A)** AP-view radiograph of the involved shoulder. **(B)** Axial CT image showing significant displacement at the acromial fracture site. **(C)** Axial CT image showing the coracoid process fracture. **(D)** Postoperative AP-view radiograph showing reduction and stabilization of the acromial fracture using a dorsal tension band technique (the coracoid fracture was treated nonoperatively).

injuries of the coracoid tip due to the pull of the biceps, coracobrachialis, and/or pectoralis minor muscles or a direct blow from a dislocating humeral head have been described. Radiographic visualization is difficult and generally requires one of the following views: (1) an AP 35- to 60-degree cephalic tilt view, (2) a Stryker notch view, or (3) a posterior oblique 20-degree cephalic tilt view. Accessory ossification centers and epiphyseal lines may complicate the evaluation.

Isolated coracoid fractures are generally minimally displaced, treated nonoperatively, and sufficiently healed in 6 weeks. Occasionally, a fibrous union occurs, but these are rarely symptomatic. Symptomatic nonunions of the coracoid tip may be treated with excision of the bony fragment and reattachment of the conjoined tendon to the remaining coracoid. Isolated fractures of the acromial process (which must be distinguished from a developmental os acromiale) are usually minimally displaced and progress to uncomplicated union in 6 weeks with symptomatic care.

In situations in which the traumatic forces are particularly violent, fractures of the coracoid and acromial processes may be associated with another disruption of the superior shoulder suspensory complex (Fig. 15-18) (see Ch. 14). Displacement at one or both sites is frequently unacceptable, and, if so, surgical open reduction internal fixation must be considered.

FRACTURES OF THE PROXIMAL HUMERUS

Proximal humeral fractures make up 4 to 5 percent of the fractures in the general population.[2-4,8-10,15,23-26] Approximately 80 percent of these injuries can be managed nonoperatively, while 20 percent are significantly displaced and pose challenging problems for the orthopedic surgeon.

Neer's four-segment classification[25,26] is well described in standard orthopedic texts. It allows one to understand these fractures, provides a guide to treatment, and facilitates early prognostic judgments (Figs. 15-19 and 15-20). The radiologic assessment is critical to fitting the individual case into the classification scheme and ultimately determining appropriate treatment. Standard radiographic views include true AP (in neutral rotation) and lateral views of the glenohumeral joint, a true axillary view, and a true transthoracic lateral view. In particularly difficult cases, CT scanning of the area with reconstructions can be especially useful.

In the athletic population, these injuries are seen in sports where severe direct forces are applied to the proximal humerus (collision sports where the athletes

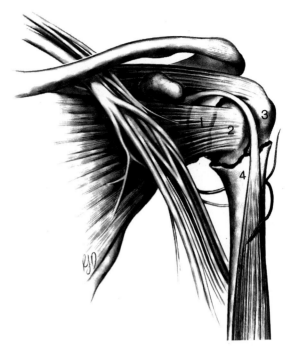

Figure 15-19 The four segments of the proximal humerus: *1*, the articular segment; *2*, the lesser tuberosity; *3*, the greater tuberosity; and *4*, the humeral shaft.

strike each other or hard surfaces). These fractures also result when significant indirect forces are applied to the upper extremity (sports associated with falls and those in which the upper extremity is grasped and twisted by another individual, e.g., wrestling, barroom arm wrestling).

Fracture-dislocations are caused by extreme forces and are therefore seen in the most violent sports. In addition to the fracture, the humeral head is levered or twisted out of the glenoid cavity so indirect forces applied to the upper extremity are always involved to some degree. Two-part fractures involving the anatomic neck, three- and four-part fractures, and fractures of the articular surface are not discussed here, since they are rarely seen in the athletic population and are well described in most orthopedic texts.

One-Part Fractures/Fractures with Minimal Displacement

One-part fractures make up approximately 80 percent of all proximal humeral fractures and include those in which none of the major segments is displaced 1 cm or more nor rotated 45 degrees or more. Treatment consists of immobilization of the arm in a sling and swathe dressing until the entire humerus moves as a unit (approximately 2 weeks), followed by progressive

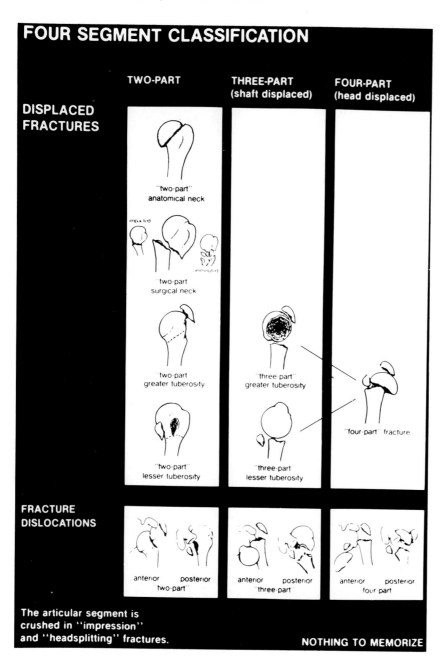

FOUR SEGMENT CLASSIFICATION

| | TWO-PART | THREE-PART (shaft displaced) | FOUR-PART (head displaced) |

DISPLACED FRACTURES

"two-part" anatomical neck

"two-part" surgical neck

two-part greater tuberosity

"two-part" lesser tuberosity

"three-part" greater tuberosity

"three-part" lesser tuberosity

"four-part" fracture

FRACTURE DISLOCATIONS

anterior   posterior
"two-part"

anterior   posterior
"three-part"

anterior   posterior
"four-part"

The articular segment is crushed in "impression" and "headsplitting" fractures.

NOTHING TO MEMORIZE

Figure 15-20 Neer's four-segment proximal humeral fracture classification scheme.

range of motion exercises during the subsequent 4 weeks (dependent circular and pendulum range of motion exercises as well as external rotation to neutral during weeks 3 and 4, and more aggressive range of motion exercises in all directions during weeks 5 and 6). At the 6-week point, bony healing is usually clinically solid and active use can be allowed. Physiotherapy continues until full range of motion and strength are obtained or until the patient reaches a plateau. In addition, the patient is carefully guided through a "gradual return to sports" program. The prognosis for these fractures is generally very good.

Two-Part Fractures

Greater and Lesser Tuberosities

If the greater tuberosity is involved (Fig. 15-21), a full-thickness rotator cuff tear is present by definition. In addition, posterior displacement of the greater tuberosity can result in limitation of external rotation, while superior displacement can lead to impingement difficulties and limitation of abduction. In rare instances, a symptomatic nonunion may occur. Surgical treatment is necessary and involves an anatomic re-

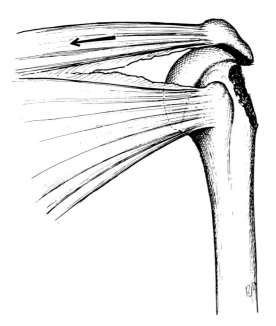

Figure 15-21 A two-part (greater tuberosity) proximal humeral fracture.

duction and internal fixation of the displaced tuberosity as well as repair of the rotator cuff tear. Isolated displaced fractures of the lesser tuberosity are rare and associated with some damage to the subscapularis tendon (Fig. 15-22). They may result in some loss of internal rotation, and, theoretically, a nonunion may occur. In general, however, these fractures are not of functional importance and require only symptomatic care.

If widely displaced, surgical open reduction internal fixation and repair of the rotator cuff must be considered.

Surgical Neck

Severely angulated (≥45 degrees) and/or rotated fractures at this level may go on to union but with significant limitation of glenohumeral motion in one or more directions (Fig. 15-23). Also, the greater the separation between the segments, the greater the risk of a nonunion. Nonsurgical treatment involves a closed reduction to correct the angulation-rotation, impaction of the fracture surfaces, and immobilization of the arm in a sling and swathe dressing or a shoulder splint, brace, or spica designed to relax the deforming pull of the surrounding soft tissues. Absolute immobilization continues until the entire humerus moves as a unit (approximately 2 weeks), followed by progressive passive range of motion exercises during the subsequent 4 weeks. At the 6-week point, bony healing is usually sufficient, and active use can be allowed. Physiotherapy continues until range of motion and strength are maximized. Percutaneous pinning of the fracture following the closed reduction can also be considered, especially if the fracture is unstable. Overhead olecranon pin traction may be of use in patients with multiple injuries and those with extensive comminution in the region of the surgical neck (seen in the most violent sports, such as auto racing). If despite all attempts the fracture remains in an unacceptable position, surgical open reduction internal fixation must be considered.

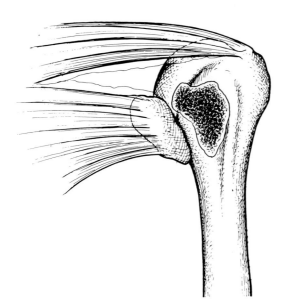

Figure 15-22 A two-part (lesser tuberosity) proximal humeral fracture.

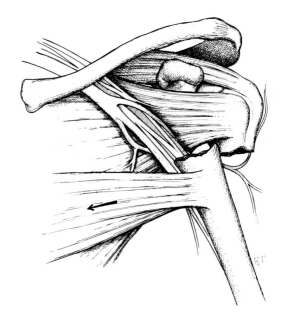

Figure 15-23 A two-part (surgical neck) proximal humeral fracture.

Fracture-Dislocations of the Glenohumeral Joint

Any proximal humeral fracture can be associated with a glenohumeral dislocation (anterior, posterior, or inferior) and vice versa. Well-described combinations include an anterior dislocation with a fracture of the greater tuberosity, a posterior dislocation with a fracture of the lesser tuberosity, and a dislocation with an impression fracture of the humeral head. The dislocation must be reduced first, and one closed attempt is reasonable. The accompanying fracture(s) may make closed attempts impossible, however (particularly if the articular-tuberosity segment is dissociated from the shaft), in which case an open surgical reduction must be performed. Additional treatment is then dictated by the nature of the associated fracture(s).

Case Study III

Injury, Initial Evaluation, and Operative Management

A 35-year-old skier fell while trying to negotiate an icy mogul field, sustaining a severe twisting injury to his shoulder. The initial evaluation revealed his arm

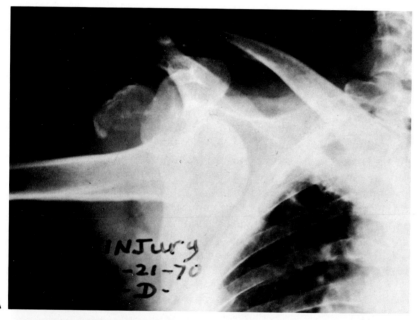

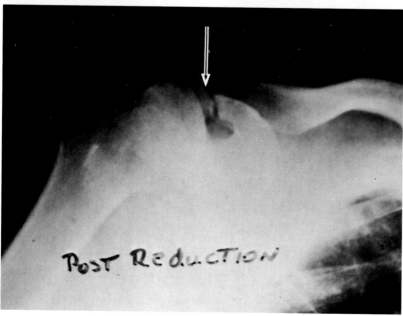

Figure 15-24 A 35-year-old skier who sustained a two-part (greater tuberosity) anterior fracture dislocation of the proximal humerus. **(A)** Initial AP radiographic view showing the humeral head anteriorly dislocated relative to the glenoid fossa and the greater tuberosity significantly displaced relative to the proximal humerus. **(B)** Postreduction AP radiographic view of the shoulder showing the humeral head relocated within the glenoid fossa but the greater tuberosity significantly displaced superiorly, lying within the subacromial space. *(Figure continues.)*

to be held close to his body, slightly abducted, and internally rotated. The shoulder appeared flattened laterally and unusually prominent anteriorly. Radiographs of the shoulder were obtained in two planes: an AP view with the arm in as near-neutral rotation as possible and a lateral scapular view (an axillary projection could not be obtained because the patient could not tolerate shoulder abduction). These radiographs confirmed the presence of a two-part anterior fracture-dislocation (the humeral head was dislocated anteriorly, and the greater tuberosity was fractured and displaced) (Fig. 15-24A).

Treatment

Using appropriate intravenous sedation, the dislocation was reduced gently and promptly; however, the greater tuberosity remained significantly displaced (Fig. 15-24B). Consequently, the patient was taken to the operating room for an open reduction internal fixation of the greater tuberosity fragment and repair of the rotator cuff tear (Fig. 15-24C).

Postoperative Care

Due to the secure nature of the fixation achieved, the patient was begun on a physiotherapy program 48 hours following his surgery when pain had diminished (see Chs. 2 and 16 for a full discussion).

Six weeks postoperatively, the fracture dislocation

was judged fully healed and in a good position. All protection was discontinued and progressive active functional use of the shoulder within the patient's limits of comfort was encouraged. Physiotherapy continued on a daily basis until range of motion and strength were maximized. Six months postoperatively, the patient was asymptomatic, had achieved nearly full shoulder range of motion (external rotation was limited to 60 degrees as opposed to 90 degrees on the normal side), and had regained full shoulder strength. The patient was allowed to gradually return to athletic activities following a carefully monitored program.

EPIPHYSEAL INJURIES OF THE PROXIMAL HUMERUS

For a discussion of epiphyseal injuries of the proximal humerus, see Chapter 8.

REFERENCES

1. Allman FL: Fracture and ligamentous injuries of clavicle and its articulations. J Bone Joint Surg [Am] 49:774, 1967
2. Bateman JE: The Shoulder and Neck. 2nd Ed. WB Saunders, Philadelphia, 1978
3. DePalma AF: Surgery of the Shoulder. 3rd Ed. JB Lippincott, Philadelphia, 1983
4. Neer CS II: Shoulder Reconstruction. 1st Ed. WB Saunders, Philadelphia, 1990
5. Nevaiser JS: Injuries of the clavicle and its articulations. Orthop Clin North Am 11:233, 1980
6. Nevaiser RJ: Injuries to the clavicle and acromioclavicular joint. Orthop Clin North Am 18:433, 1987
7. Parkes JC, Deland JD: A three-part distal clavicle fracture. J Trauma 23:437, 1983
8. Post M: The Shoulder. 2nd Ed. Lea & Febiger, Philadelphia, 1988
9. Rockwood CA Jr, Green DP: Fractures in Adults. 2nd Ed. JB Lippincott, Philadelphia, 1984
10. Rowe CR: The Shoulder. 1st Ed. Churchill Livingstone, New York, 1988
11. Heppenstall RB: Fractures and dislocations of the distal clavicle. Orthop Clin North Am 6:477, 1975
12. Neer CS II: Fractures of the distal third of the clavicle. Clin Orthop 58:43, 1968
13. Rockwood CA: Fractures of the outer clavicle in children and adults. J Bone Joint Surg [Br] 64:642, 1982
14. Goss TP: Double disruptions of the superior shoulder suspensory complex. J Orthop Trauma 7:99, 1993
15. Rockwood CA, Matsen FA: The Shoulder. 1st Ed. WB Saunders, Philadelphia, 1990

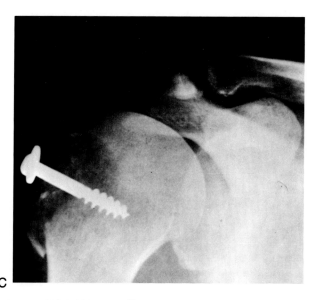

C

Figure 15-24 *(Continued)* **(C)** Postoperative AP radiographic view of the shoulder showing the humeral head relocated within the glenoid fossa and the greater tuberosity reduced and internally fixed relative to the proximal humerus (fixation using heavy nonabsorpable sutures would have been another option).

16. Goss TP: Fractures of the glenoid neck. J Shoulder Elbow Surg 3:42, 1994

17. Goss TP: Fractures of the glenoid cavity. J Bone Joint Surg [Am] 74:299, 1992

18. Goss TP: Fractures of the glenoid cavity (operative principles and techniques). Techn Orthop 8:199, 1994

19. Ideberg R: Fractures of the scapula involving the glenoid fossa. p. 63. In Bateman JE, Walsh RP (eds): Surgery of the Shoulder. BC Deck, Philadelphia, 1984

20. Boyer DW: Trap shooter's shoulder: stress fracture of the coracoid process. J Bone Joint Surg [Am] 57:862, 1975

21. Froimson AL: Fracture of the coracoid process of the scapula. J Bone Joint Surg [Am] 60:710, 1978

22. Mariani PP: Isolated fracture of the coracoid process in an athlete. Am J Sports Med 8:129, 1980

23. Cofield RH: Comminuted fractures of the proximal humerus. Clin Orthop 230:49, 1988

24. Heppenstall RB: Fractures of the proximal humerus. Orthop Clin North Am 6:467, 1975

25. Neer CS: Displaced proximal humeral fractures. Part I. Classification and evaluation. J Bone Joint Surg [Am] 52:1077, 1970

26. Neer CS: Displaced proximal humeral fractures. Part II. Treatment of three-part and four-part displacement. J Bone Joint Surg [Am] 52:1090, 1970

16

Care and Rehabilitation of the Throwing Shoulder

Arthur M. Pappas

Claire F. McCarthy

Richard M. Zawacki

Conditioning, competitive-season care, and rehabilitation programs for athletes have common goals: the prevention of injury and achievement of optimal performance. In sports that place high stress on the shoulder complex (e.g., baseball pitching, swimming, tennis), the main focus of these programs is on maintaining normal articular biomechanics, flexibility, and muscle balance. Baseball pitching is described as one of the most demanding and highly dynamic skills in all sports. Accordingly, this chapter uses the pitching shoulder as the example to describe a comprehensive shoulder conditioning program, aspects of competitive-season care, and a rehabilitation program. Principles and concepts described for the pitching shoulder can serve as a basis for developing programs and addressing shoulder problems in other sports and other postoperative programs.

The success of any program requires an understanding by health professionals of how total shoulder movement occurs and how that movement can be disturbed by a pathologic process (see Ch. 9). The pitching mechanism requires and combines flexibility, balanced strength, endurance, and a high level of neuromuscular coordination of the upper extremities, trunk and pelvis, and lower extremities. An interruption of any one of these integrated movement patterns places additional stress on the shoulder and its surrounding soft tissue structures. A biomechanically unsound shoulder generally develops secondary to one of the following: abnormal pitching biomechanics, weakness of some of the shoulder complex musculature, laxity or contracture of the surrounding capsular and ligamentous structures causing an alteration or decrease in glenohumeral motion, and intra-articular disruptions. As a result, altered or decreased performance demonstrated by loss of velocity, accuracy of ball location or placement, or general consistency may be experienced.

Throwing is a sequential pattern of movement. The timing and execution of each contributing segment of the body is critical to ball velocity and overall effectiveness of the throw. One segment's motion must follow the preceding segment's motion while the latter is increasing in speed, preferably at its peak of velocity and acceleration. The greater the desired speed, the more segments needed to increase the body's momentum. To throw a pitch at 90+ mph requires a highly coordinated and maximum effort. Eight dimensions are noted in a throwing motion:

1. Ipsilateral total lower extremity thrust (toe and ankle plantar flexion/knee extension)
2. Pelvic flexion and rotation
3. Stride and thrust from the pitching plate
4. Trunk extension, rotation, and flexion
5. Vertebroscapular and scapulothoracic action
6. Glenohumeral function
7. Elbow function
8. Wrist and hand function

Movements that facilitate a smooth uninterrupted pathway for the center of gravity are important for proper shoulder mechanics. Disruptive movements are caused by tight hamstrings, thereby limiting forward flexion, or an adductor strain which will limit stride, result in additional muscle stress at the shoulder. Pelvic motion, lumbar extension, and thoracic rotation occur in the early moments of the throwing mechanism. Trunk extension and rotation, particularly thoracic extension and rotation in conjunction with glenohumeral and scapulothoracic motion, increase the body's axial rotation and thus increase the excursion and distance through which force may be applied to the ball prior to release.

A comprehensive approach to conditioning and competitive-season care will maximize performance and minimize the risk of injury and the debilitative effect of the season. A conditioning program prepares the pitcher for the baseball season; competitive-season care addresses competitive-season physical challenges, particularly the postgame effects of pitching; and rehabilitative care provides an injured pitcher with directed treatment and guidance through the recovery process, strategies for return to sport participation, and a directed preventative program specific for the injured area.

CONDITIONING

All high-use shoulder athletes, whether competitive or recreational, require a conditioning program that addresses cardiorespiratory fitness, flexibility, balanced muscle function and strength (though not necessarily power), endurance, and skill practice. The realization that conditioning is a continuous process throughout the year is helpful for both the athlete and trainer. For athletes with a defined season, such as the baseball pitcher, the year can be broken down into seasonal components (Table 16-1). Each season will have its specific objectives and requirements. A thorough conditioning program for a pitcher should include both general and specific types of exercises to ensure the athlete is optimally fit to withstand the general stresses of pitching on the entire body, as well as to meet the special demands and skills specifically required of the shoulder complex. It should be noted that at the end of the competitive season most pitchers have weakness of the supraspinatus (and sometimes infraspinatus) secondary to repetitive function, as well as tightness of the glenohumeral capsule. Therefore, it is recommended that the concepts in Phases II and III of the Rehabilitation section be referred to in conjunction with the following conditioning information.

Flexibility

Flexibility should be a part of every conditioning program since it is the key to injury prevention and fluidity of motion. Good flexibility allows for complete motion and control through maximal allowable ranges. As a result, stresses on ligaments, muscles, and tendons at individual joints are reduced and greater freedom of movement is allowed.

Proper technique is essential when doing flexibility exercises. The flexibility component of a conditioning program should follow an initial warm-up (e.g., a slow 5-minute jog). Part or all of the flexibility exercises can be repeated at the end of the conditioning program. Various books are available with good diagrams devoted to stretching programs (see Suggested Readings, Anderson). Incorrect technique can be counterproductive and may be unsafe. A flexibility program can be designed as a self-program or one with the assistance of a partner, and a towel or tube can be used. In either a self- or assisted format, a stretch should always be done smoothly and in a comfortable range. It is important not to be too vigorous with passive stretching, since stretch beyond a desired range results in acquired laxity. The athlete should not experience sharp pain, but the perception of stretch or tension should be felt in the desired area, such as the hamstring or calf muscle. The position should be held for a brief period, followed by a period of relaxation or further stretch.

General stretching exercises should involve the entire body with the aim of achieving full range of motion at each joint as well as for each muscle group, particularly muscles that cross two joints. These exercises should include allowable motions at the toes, ankles, knees, hips, trunk, fingers, wrists, elbows, shoulders, and neck. Because pitching involves the whole body, general flexibility is important in the pitcher. A limitation in any area of the body can cause an alteration in timing or the pitching motion itself. A truly effective stretching program should be regularly performed throughout the year to improve musculotendinous flexibility and joint suppleness. Activities such as aerobics, yoga, ballet, and karate offer excellent flexibility exercises.

Table 16-1 Annual Monthly Conditioning Schedule[a]

	Conditioning Schedule by Months			
	1 & 2 (Off season)	3+ (Preseason)	4–10 (Competitive)	11–12 (Postseason)
Aerobic	XXX	XXXX	XXXX	X
Flexibility	XX	XXXX	XXXX	XX
Muscle strength	XXXX	XXX	XXX	XX
Endurance	XXX	XXXX	XXXX	X
Skill	XX	XXXX	XXXX	X

[a] A conditioning program can be projected according to the individual's sport schedule. Expected levels of achievement by certain dates or times are helpful.

A specific flexibility program for a pitcher is designed to obtain and maintain normal glenohumeral, scapulothoracic, and vertebrothoracic motion. If a pitcher is to be effective, achieving normal shoulder motion is an absolute necessity before strengthening programs are initiated. With normal glenohumeral motion, the glenohumeral-scapulothoracic musculature can interact and coordinate the forces that impact on all surrounding soft tissue structures of the shoulder. Without adequate flexibility, poorly supervised strength enhancement programs will contribute to abnormal movement patterns. To achieve and maintain true glenohumeral flexibility, scapular motion on the thorax must be complete and synchronous.

In the throwing shoulder, there should be a focus on two patterns of glenohumeral motion: horizontal flexion in neutral rotation and combined abduction to 150 degrees. Pitchers who have inherent tightness can attain flexibility effectively through the use of a proprioceptive neuromuscular facilitation, of which rotation is an important component. The one technique most frequently used to achieve joint range, known as "contract-relax," involves an isotonic contraction of the antagonist, followed by a period of relaxation and passive stretch of the antagonist. It is particularly effective in conditions where muscle tissue is the limiting factor. (See later discussion on flexibility).

Because of the innate instability of the shoulder complex, attention to appropriate stabilization and technique is required to prevent unwanted joint accommodations or adjustments. Stretching with an experienced partner who is specifically instructed on the individual pitcher's program is strongly recommended.

Strength Training and Muscle Care

Strength training for pitchers can be divided into specific anatomic regions: lower body, trunk, and upper body. Each anatomic region has unique contributions to the art of pitching and is addressed at various time periods of the baseball conditioning schedule. The use of machines and mechanical resistance can be included, but with caution.

A strength training program should be performed three times per week. Three sets of 20 repetitions per set of each exercise are sufficient. The amount of weight lifted in each set should progressively increase. The initial set is low to allow for an initial warm-up period. The last set comprises the maximum amount of weight that can be properly lifted through 20 repetitions. Each repetition should be performed with good form in a controlled manner, both raising and lowering the weight through a complete range of motion.

Lower Body

Leg strength and endurance are critical for proper pitching mechanics and endurance throughout a game. A program that addresses the strength and endurance of all lower extremity musculature is essential. The slide board is an excellent apparatus for pitchers because it provides concentric and eccentric challenges to knee flexors and extensors and for hip adductors, abductors, flexors, extensors, and rotators. In addition, a variety of weight-training machines are available.

Endurance training, related to but not synonymous with aerobic conditioning, is a key factor in injury prevention. A conditioned athlete can sustain an activity for a longer period of time while a fatigued athlete has diminished reaction time and is less able to respond to an unexpected stress or demand (such as slipping from a wet mound or dodging a batted ball). For a pitcher, leg muscle endurance, including aerobic conditioning, is a prerequisite for effective pitching. Thus, an aerobic and endurance program for the lower extremity should be combined. Endurance-type activities are in those that utilize large muscle mass, such as running, swimming, cycling, and rowing, or by using generally available exercise equipment.

Trunk

The trunk plays a critical role in the pitching mechanism. Force generated from the wind-up and initial push-off is transferred through the trunk to the pitching extremity. In addition, the trunk through axial rotation contributes to those forces and the resultant acceleration. A conditioning program for the trunk needs to concentrate on the abdominals, back extensors, and trunk rotators. Partial, traditional, and rotation sit-ups can be used for the abdominals and intercostals while trunk extension from a prone position can be used for the back extensors. Trunk rotation exercises can be performed either by incorporating trunk rotation into the partial sit-ups or by using weight-training equipment designed to provide resistance. Upper trunk rotation with extension should also be included, and trunk exercises using medicine balls should be included in each workout.

The training and development of shoulder musculature is not exclusive to the pitching motion or open-loop activities. Scapular stabilization and control in closed-loop activities is important as a protective mechanism in falls or in response to oncoming batted balls. Push-ups performed against the wall, in hand-knee position, or in full prone position, can be used selectively to develop the upper body. Scapula position

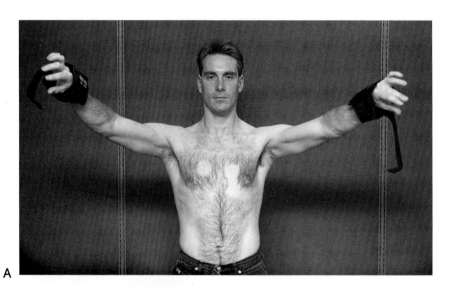

A

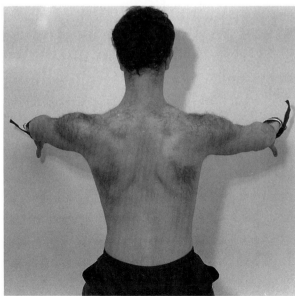

B

Figure 16-1

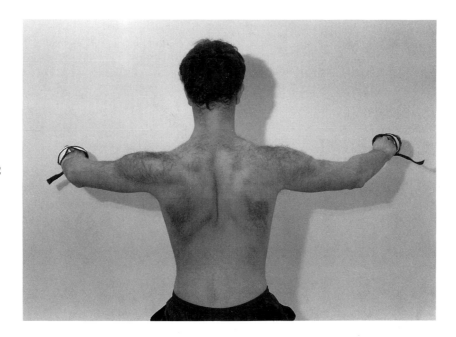

Figure 16-2

on the thorax as well as full excursion in retraction and protraction are essential to any effective push-up sequence. Seated push-ups are also included to facilitate depression of the scapula on the thorax.

Both proprioceptive neuromuscular facilitations and plyometric-type motions can also be considered as an advanced form of exercise. The latter designed to utilize the stretch or elastic component of muscle; an eccentric contraction is followed by a quick or explosive concentric contraction. For a pitcher, this is represented in the cocking phase with an eccentric contraction of the biceps, pectorals, and subscapularis, followed by concentric contractions and powerful acceleration. These techniques can be gradually introduced using surgical tubing, Thera-Band or pulleys, and progression to two-handed catching and throwing of a large ball. Progression to unilateral use of weighted balls is not recommended.

Upper Body

The use of many popular power weight exercise programs, either through free weights or exercise equipment for the upper body, is discouraged for baseball pitchers. Success in benchpressing is not related to how effective an individual will be as a pitcher. In our experience, power lifting generally results in greater strength in the larger muscles of the anterior shoulder and a relative imbalance in the smaller rotator cuff muscles and scapular control muscles, which are very important in allowing the shoulder to function properly while throwing. Pitching is a neuromuscular skill activity and not a strength power activity. Most pitching coaches recognize the need for balanced strength; however, emphasis on power strength training is perceived to decrease arm speed and balanced throwing. In addition, improper lifting, particularly in the benchpress, may lead to intra-articular damage (i.e., anterior labral fragmentation and capsular hyperlaxity). The larger muscles may be conditioned by using any of the popular weight-training machines or free weights; it is important, however, to use less weight and more repetitions. For the rotator cuff muscles and other smaller shoulder muscles, a lightweight, high repetition exercise program (i.e., maximum weight of 5 lb and 3 sets of 10 repetitions, held for a count of 5) is recommended. This program should be performed five times a week during the off-season, decreasing to three times a week during the season.

Recommended Exercise Program

These four exercises are performed in a standing position with good posture and starting with arms at the sides:

1. Slowly raise arms approximately 30 degrees in front of body to shoulder level with thumbs pointed down (Fig. 16-1: supraspinatus and anterior deltoid).
2. Slowly raise arms directly in front of body with palms down (Fig. 16-2: supraspinatus and anterior deltoid).
3. Slowly raise arms to slightly above shoulder level, turning palms toward ceiling as arms are being elevated (Fig. 16-3: supraspinatus and anterior and middle deltoid).
4. Slowly raise arms to or slightly above shoulder level, flex elbows to 90 degrees, externally rotate shoulders and then horizontally extend upper arms and retract (adduct) scap-

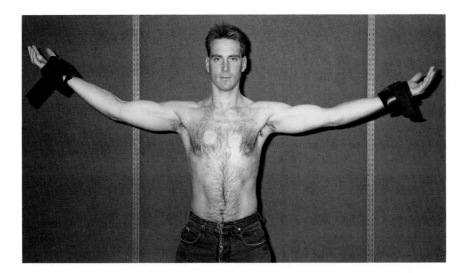

Figure 16-3

ulae. It is important to keep elbow higher than shoulder in the horizontal plane (Fig. 16-4: posterior deltoid, infraspinatus, teres minor, trapezius, and rhomboids).

The next three exercises are performed on a table in a prone position:

5. With arms hanging over the end of table, raise arms to 90° abduction, horizontally extend and then externally rotate shoulders and retract (adduct) scapulae. It is important to keep hand higher than elbow in the horizontal plane (Fig. 16-5: posterior deltoid, infraspinatus, teres minor, trapezius and rhomboids).
6. With throwing arm hanging over side of table, raise externally rotated arm as a unit with thumb pointing toward ceiling (Fig. 16-6: same muscles as Fig. 16-5).

7. With head and chest on table, keeping arms close to head, raise both arms up off table (Fig. 16-7A: upper and middle trapezius and rhomboids; Fig. 16-7B: lower trapezius and latissimus dorsi).

This exercise should be performed in a standing position facing a wall:

8. Standing approximately 3 ft away from a wall, place hands against wall, hand turned in, and extend arms. Elbows extended, alternately adduct (retract) and abduct (protract) scapula. Do one set of 25 wall push-ups (Fig. 16-8: serratus anterior).

Tubing Exercises

Use of surgical tubing, Thera-Band, or pulley weight system can be used as a progression with the small muscles of the shoulder as well as in the more extensive full patterns of movement. What is most important is that appropriate posture, stabilization, and technique are not compromised. Tubing exercises can be part of a home program. The pattern should be completed in a smooth, coordinated, synchronous manner, to condition both concentric and eccentric patterns. The choice of resistance, color Thera-Band, size of tubing, amount of pulley weight, and progression should depend on the execution of the movement and the related goal within the program.

The following patterns of function should be performed a minimum of once daily, (twice a day if time permits), 20 repetitions, 5 to 6 days per week. Thera-Band can be anchored to a wall bracket or doorframe.

1. Sitting or standing position, tubing anchored below waist level, shoulder at 90 degrees of abduction, extend upper arm, back, and externally rotate shoulder (Fig. 16-9).

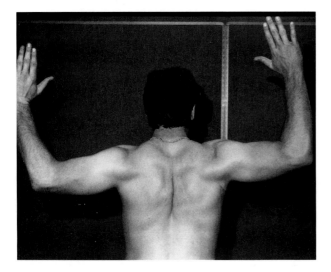

Figure 16-4

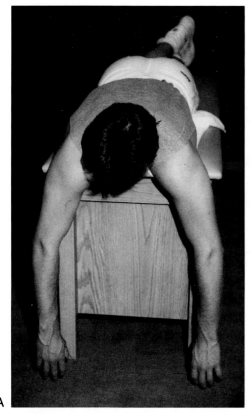
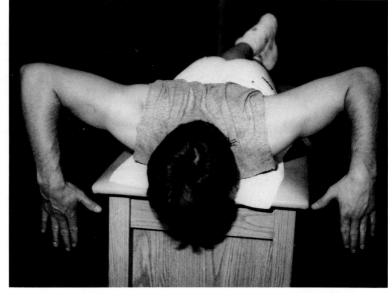

Figure 16-5

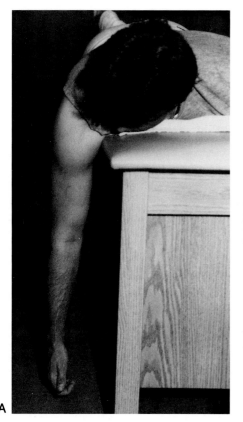
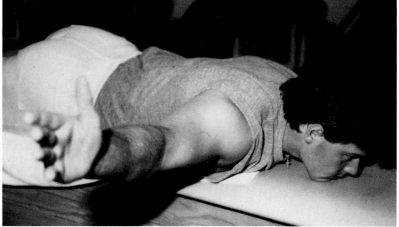

Figure 16-6

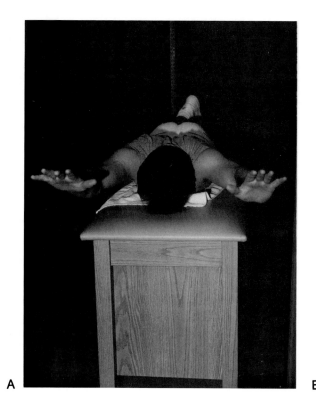 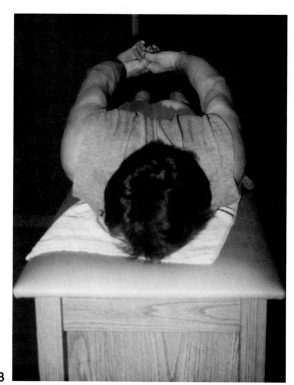

A   B

Figure 16-7

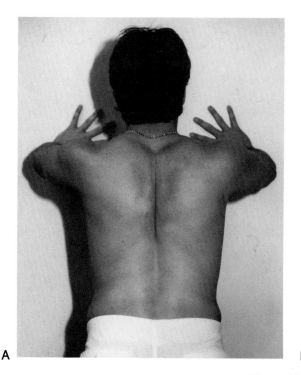 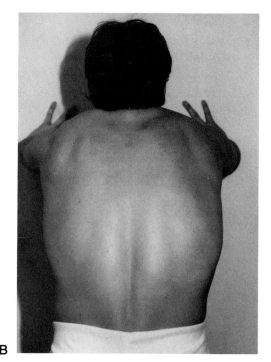

A   B

Figure 16-8

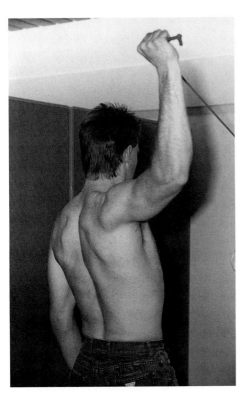

Figure 16-9

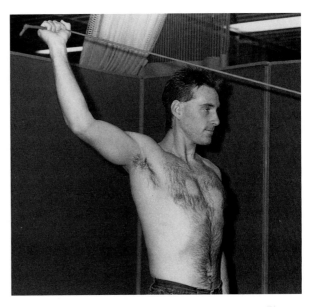

Figure 16-10

fully considered. For example, running will provide a better coordinated and combined program for the pitcher's lower extremity than swimming, biking, or rowing. Running requires total lower extremity in-

2. Sitting or standing position, tubing anchored below waist level, raise arm diagonally upward into cocking position (Fig. 16-10).
3. Sitting or standing position, tubing anchored above shoulder level, extend arm diagonally downward (Fig. 16-11).
4. Standing position, arm at side, tubing at elbow level, externally rotate shoulder (Fig. 16-12).
5. Standing position, tubing at elbow level, internally rotate shoulder (Fig. 16-13).

Aerobic Conditioning

Aerobic conditioning is reflected in improved cardiovascular efficiency and demonstrated by an athlete's ability to perform a task for progressively longer periods of time. Since throwing requires total body participation, aerobic conditioning is critical for the pitcher. An aerobic exercise program should consist of a 5- to 10-minute warm-up, a minimum period of 20 minutes, which is performed at 60 to 75 percent of maximum heart rate, and a 5- to 10-minute cooldown period. The program should be performed 3 to 5 times per week.

The endurance and cross-training benefits of the activity selected for aerobic conditioning should be care-

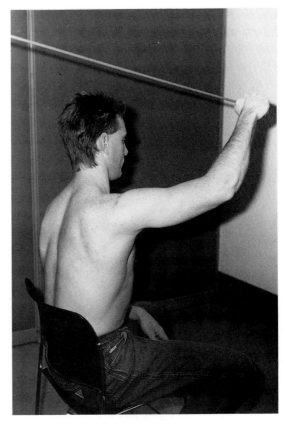

Figure 16-11

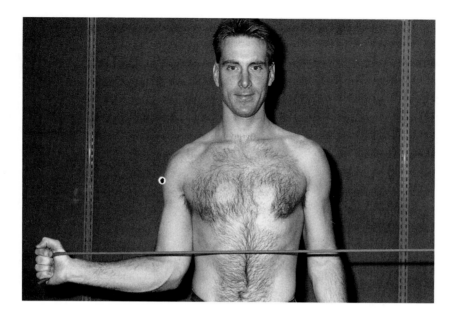

Figure 16-12

volvement, foot and ankle push-off motion as well as hip and knee activity, with the weight of the athlete as the resistance force. Swimming and rowing provide better cross-training benefits for the pitcher's upper extremity. The activity selected as part of the aerobic conditioning program should be considered as part of the strength training program. A well-designed aerobic program combined with a weight-training and flexibility program will condition both the cardiorespiratory and neuromuscular systems.

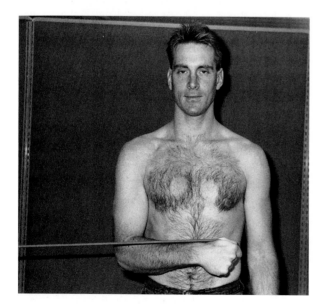

Figure 16-13

Throwing Skill Practice

Skill practice is an integral component of a general conditioning program. After the postseason rest period of 4 weeks, off-season skill practice is initiated at a low level of intensity. Long-toss throwing should begin on a 3 times per week basis, for a period of 10 to 15 minutes per session. Since timing and sequence of muscle actions are critical in pitching and can be improved with practice, proper throwing mechanics should be used even when playing catch. There should be a focus on the complete cocking phase to throw the ball versus pushing the ball. Weight shifts, trunk rotation, arm pattern, eye-hand-target coordination and follow-through should all be present. Progression in skill conditioning occurs through changes in distance, number of throws, velocity, types of pitches, and delivery location.

About 6 to 8 weeks before the spring practice reporting date, throwing off a mound 2 to 3 times per week for 10 minutes should begin. In the first few days that a pitcher throws off the mound, the focus should be on proper mechanics and not velocity or the ability to pitch breaking balls. There should be a progressive build-up of skill and endurance. About 2 weeks prior to preseason reporting, velocity should be increased and breaking balls can be thrown, but on a limited basis, for example, 10 to 15 breaking balls per session.

Conditioning and training is a continuous process throughout the year. Similar schedules can be extrapolated for other high-use shoulder athletes. Table 16-2 outlines a postseason schedule for a baseball pitcher.

Table 16-2 Postseason Conditioning Schedule for the Professional Pitcher

October	Rest
	Care of shoulder, if necessary
Nov.–Dec.	(Rehabilitation of any specific problems) Care continued
	Maintenance of general flexibility
	Maintenance of shoulder flexibility
	Strength: 3 times per week; progress in all areas to maximum weight by end of December
	Aerobic training: 3 times per wk for 20 to 30 minutes, choice of activity
	Skills: light throwing
Jan.–Feb.	Flexibility: full body achieved
	Flexibility: shoulder achieved
	Strength: 3 times per week, no increase weight
	Aerobic training: continue
	Skills: throwing: progress to off-the-mound 2-3×/week, 10 minutes; gradual increase in velocity; progress to 10 to 15 breaking balls per session
Preseason (training camp)	
Feb.–March	Flexibility: full body and shoulder daily
	Strength: maintenance 3 times per week
	Aerobic training: continue as above
	Skills: under the tutelage of pitching coach
	Shoulder care, as needed

COMPETITIVE-SEASON CARE AND CONDITIONING

This section describes the competitive-season conditioning schedule of both starting and relief pitchers and introduces the concept of competitive-season care, which includes monitoring and therapeutic intervention for the cumulative effects of pitching over the competitive season.

The repetitive high-velocity nature of throwing generates such stresses that postgame specialized care is accepted practice. Therapeutic modalities such as ice, massage, nonsteroidal anti-inflammatory drugs (NSAIDs) and electric stimulation, and interventions such as rest, massage, and therapeutic exercise are selectively utilized and serve to facilitate readiness of the shoulder for the next game. Deep massage is effective in eliminating the muscular nodules throwers occasionally acquire after stressful throwing. Although modalities may provide symptomatic relief, the underlying defects need to be addressed. Pitchers are individualis-

tic in their choice of postgame care. Pitchers vary in style and technique, games vary in number and type of pitches thrown each inning and in total, and environments, including weather, vary. A comprehensive competitive season program, carefully monitored, can help minimize the individual's potential for injury and the cumulative effects of game stress and microtrauma over the competitive season. Subtle changes in range of shoulder motions, additional use of modalities, or increases in degrees of postgame soreness are important to document and review. (If gradual changes are observed, preplanning a miss or delay in the pitching rotation may be a reasonable therapeutic strategy.)

To assure maintenance of full shoulder joint range of motion required for effective pitching, flexibility exercises performed with an experienced qualified professional are recommended. Physical therapy techniques such as proprioceptive neuromuscular facilitation are preferred to active or passive uniplanar motions. All treatment should be directed to maintenance of the functional composite patterns of pitching.

Pitchers are usually classified as either starting or relief pitchers. Starting pitchers know in advance when they will pitch. Relief pitchers must be available on a daily basis, and because of their varied time schedules, structured competitive-season care is not possible.

Relief Pitcher Care

Most relief pitchers will ice their shoulders after they pitch (which reduces edema and acts as an analgesic), believing that this will assist in a speedier recuperation and thus prepare them for the next day. On occasion, they will request a posterior shoulder massage. To maintain shoulder strength, relief pitchers will plan to exercise at least three times a week during the season. The time of exercise during the day varies; certain pitchers will exercise 5 to 6 hours prior to the game, while others wait to exercise after the game if they have not pitched. Assisted shoulder flexibility to maintain full range of motion is important at least three times per week. A short, low repetition, self-administered flexibility program performed daily is helpful.

Due to their lower number of pitches per game (as compared to starters), relief pitchers generally do not experience excessive soreness around their shoulders. A conditioning program, however, should address the need of relief pitchers to warm up in a short time prior to game participation. The number, velocity, and type of pitches should be considered. In addition, the likelihood of daily warm-ups without game participation should be considered. Care should be taken to address the residual responses of the shoulder to the stresses described above.

Starting Pitcher Care

Starting pitchers usually pitch every fifth day. The following list represents a typical 5-day period (Table 16-3):

Day 1: This is the pitching day. General stretching exercises for the entire body are important. Prior to the game, assisted flexibility of the throwing shoulder is carried out. Pitchers may apply hydrocollator packs to "warm up" their throwing shoulders prior to stretching. Some pitchers

Table 16-3 Starting Pitcher's Competitive-Season Conditioning and Care

Day 1 (pitching day)
  Pregame warm-up
    General stretching exercises for entire body
    Assisted flexibility of the throwing shoulder with or without
      previous use of an hydrocollator pack
    Optional: set of active shoulder exercises
    Optional: massage
  Game warm-up
    Long ball toss for 5 minutes
    50 to 60 throws from the mound
  Between innings: Warm-up
  Start of each inning: Warm-up, 8 pitches
  Postgame care
    Application of ice to shoulder and/or elbow (15 to 20 minutes)
Day 2 (first day postpitching)
  Run with other pitchers
  Massage
  Full shoulder exercise program at 100% resistance level
  Assisted flexibility program
  Light catch for 5 to 10 minutes
Day 3 (second day postpitching)
  General body aerobic and leg conditioning program
  Assisted flexibility
  Supervised pitching from the mound; time is variable
  Application of ice if requested
Day 4 (third day postpitching)
  General body aerobic and leg conditioning program
  Normal exercise program
  Light massage
  Easy catch
Day 5 (fourth day postpitching)
  Total rest
  Assisted flexibility exercises
  Limited exercise program
  "Game face"/mental preparation

do one set of each of their shoulder exercises without resistance to warm up. They may also want to have a massage on the posterior aspect of their shoulder or apply a liniment or analgesic balm to their throwing arms; these actions not only serve as a warm-up, but dilate the blood vessels, which enhances flexibility. Most pitchers usually begin warm-ups 20 to 25 minutes prior to the game, for example, 5 minutes of long toss, and then progress to the mound for pregame warm-ups, the duration of which varies from pitcher to pitcher (the usual warm-up range is 50 to 60 pitches).

After the game, most pitchers ice their shoulders and/or elbows because they believe it reduces the amount of soreness experienced the next day (i.e., periarticular stress and eccentric muscle contractions). Since icing reduces edema and acts as an analgesic, it should be encouraged for any pitcher who has been experiencing mild discomfort while throwing and for pitchers who are returning to competition following an extended period of inactivity because of shoulder and/or elbow problems.

Day 2: All pitchers experience muscle soreness about their shoulders, as well as in their low back and forearm musculature. Some pitchers prefer a deep massage to all affected areas to reduce the soreness. The purpose of the massage is to (1) enhance blood flow, (2) decompress muscular nodules in the posterior shoulder, which frequently appear after pitching, and (3) desensitize any muscular trigger points. It is recommended that pitchers complete their entire shoulder exercise program with usual weight resistance. Assisted flexibility will maintain normal glenohumeral motion. They will play light catch (i.e., 5 to 10 minutes before the game) and do some type of aerobic activity (e.g., run with the other pitchers).

Day 3: The pitcher will throw off the mound under the tutelage of the pitching coach. Duration of throwing (i.e., number of pitches) will vary depending on how many pitches were thrown in the outing 2 days previously. Assisted flexibility is imperative (see section on Flexibility in Phase II of Rehabilitation). Ice, if requested, is applied after throwing. Although there is no specific exercise for the shoulder, the normal aerobic and leg endurance program should be followed.

Day 4: The normal shoulder exercise program is performed. Light massage is provided to promote flexibility and reduce muscle soreness. Easy catch during batting practice occurs as does the normal aerobic and leg endurance routine.

Day 5: A day of relative rest; assisted flexibility exercises and a limited exercise program are recommended. The day before he pitches, the pitcher will watch this day's game and chart each pitch and location of the pitcher. This record provides an opportunity for peer involvement and prepares the pitcher mentally for pitching the next day—what some pitchers refer to as preparing their "game face."

Day 6: Pitch again.

REHABILITATION OF THE PITCHING SHOULDER

A rehabilitation program becomes necessary when a pitcher is unable to pitch or pitch effectively over a period of time due to an acute injury from a single pitch or through gradual failure of the shoulder complex to withstand the repeated physiologic demands of pitching. The injuries incurred may be intra-articular, capsular, tendinous, muscular, neural, and vascular in nature. Pain, muscle stiffness, weakness, and fatigue may be present and certain daily activities may be affected. The athlete's primary concern, however, is losing the ability to pitch and the amount of time required away from the game for rehabilitation. Whether the approach to the injury or problem is nonoperative or operative, the desired outcome is the same: the return of the pitcher to his prior level of performance as safely and as quickly as possible. It should be remembered that a rehabilitation program is not something "done" to an athlete, but a program that is followed in partnership with health professionals and trainers to meet agreed-upon goals.

Inherent in the achievement of the rehabilitation goals is the education of the athlete. Understanding the nature of the injury and the progressive stages of the rehabilitative process will facilitate active participation by the athlete, commitment to the program, and acceptance of responsibility. With shoulder injuries in particular, an understanding of shoulder anatomy, the mechanism of injury, and the principles on which the rehabilitation program is based can be most beneficial. Education of the athlete should be continuous throughout the program, ultimately directed toward strategies to prevent a recurrence or a secondary injury. Education of the clinical team on the mechanics of pitching, particularly applied to the athlete referred for rehabilitation, is helpful.

A pitcher is often able to describe the process of deterioration of his pitching mechanics and perhaps identify the phase of pitching that is the most troublesome. Correlation of the athelete's report with clinical findings will serve to direct the rehabilitation program. Any injury can lead to a disruption of the fluidity of the throwing motion that may predispose to further injury or stress on the shoulder.

If a pitcher is able to throw without excessive discomfort, observation and filming of his throwing motion without a shirt is valuable. Four components of his motion should be observed: (1) the mechanics of his entire body during the throw, (2) the height to which he elevates his arm, (3) the amount of posterior excursion of the humerus during the cocking phase, and (4) the

humerus-shoulder girdle-trunk relationship. A comparison with films prior to injury is beneficial to familiarize both the clinician and the pitcher with the specifics of the pitcher's motion during effective pitching.

Pain has a secondary effect of inhibiting muscle action and causes a cycle to develop eventually leading to disuse, weakness, and atrophy (see Fig. 2-5). Chronic discomfort of recurrent shoulder pain are the more frequent complaints among baseball pitchers, and offer the greatest challenge to a clinical team. In these instances, pain may not be the primary symptom, but a secondary one caused by repeated minimal injuries to the shoulder. Our approach to chronic shoulder pain is to address it through resolution of limitations in range of motion, muscle imbalances, and asynchronous movement patterns. The use of modalities and NSAIDs are often a component of an initial strategy, but are usually considered adjunctive.

Occasionally, individuals with acute or chronic shoulder problems will require arthroscopic intervention either to define the pathology more clearly or to provide definitive treatment of involved structures and intra-articular damage. Knowledge of arthroscopic technique and the details of the specific procedure by the involved clinicians is critical to an effective rehabilitation program (see Ch. 12). All team members, including the athlete, must understand that operative shoulder arthroscopic intervention will delay the return to sport a minimum of 8 weeks. This is the time period required for the necessary healing processes. For a pitcher, throwing off the mound can be anticipated at 8 to 12 weeks and competitive pitching between 12 and 24 weeks postarthroscopic surgery. For hitters and other position players who comparatively place lower amounts of stress across the shoulder, progress toward sport participation may be at an accelerated rate— anticipated at 8 to 12 weeks.

If an open surgical repair becomes necessary (e.g., cuff reconstruction, open repair of instability), the specifics of the rehabilitation program need to be carefully and thoroughly reviewed with the athlete. The outline of a plan, beginning with the surgical anatomy involved and specific details of the surgical procedure, desired position of the shoulder, and postoperative care, should be discussed. Time parameters are of particular importance, for example, period of immobilization, period of restricted motion, and anticipated time to begin throwing. For pitchers and other athletes involved in repetitive overhead activities, the rehabilitation process is intense and return to competitive sports can extend to 12 months or longer. The physician is the best member of the health care team to have this discussion with the athlete, with other members of the team (physical therapist, trainer, coach, and involved family members) informed of the plan. Consistent and appropriate communication between team members, including the athlete, is central to the success of the total program.

The goal of a postarthroscopic or postsurgical rehabilitation program is the same as a nonoperative program: to return the athlete to athletic participation safely and as quickly as possible. The program is progressive and sequential in design. The timing, however, is guided by the specifics of the injury or surgical procedure and the healing processes of the involved tissues and structures. The key to postoperative management is communication between the physician and the physical therapist. Details of the operative procedure, precautions, and any specific contraindications should be known and discussed.

A rehabilitation program should be specifically designed for the individual athlete, based on findings from a comprehensive and thorough examination, ancillary tests, and the resultant clinical diagnosis. Whether the program addresses an acute or chronic shoulder problem, or is part of postsurgical management, there are some guiding common principles:

1. Pain should not result from any physical therapeutic strategy. An increase in or unexpected experience of pain would indicate unwarranted stress. Therapeutic techniques and progression of exercise parameters should be reviewed.
2. The plane of the scapula is the preferred position for exercise and testing. In the plane of the scapula, the glenohumeral joint is in a comfortable and biomechanically advantageous position for the muscles of the rotator cuff. The axis of the glenohumeral joint coincides with the common axis of the periarticular muscles of the shoulder; there is maximum congruency of the glenohumeral joint, thus greater stability.
3. Scapula control is a major component of the program for scapulothoracic stabilization and position of the glenohumeral joint. The glenoid of the scapula must follow the movement of the humeral head to maintain glenohumeral joint congruency. Static and dynamic control of the scapula is required to maintain a stable foundation upon which the freedom of the upper extremity relies.
4. Correct postural and joint alignment should be addressed throughout the program. Appropriate resting position of the scapula on the thorax is necessary for the full excursion of scapula motion available for tracking the humeral head. Glenohumeral congruency and scapulohumeral alignment will minimize tendencies toward unwanted anterior or posterior translation of the humeral head and stress on rotator musculature.
5. Education of the athlete is a core component. An understanding of the pathology and some specifics of the rehabilitation process fosters long-term carryover and preventive practices on the part of the athlete.

6. Acceptance of responsibility for participation and compliance with the program by the athlete.

The sequential goals of a rehabilitation program for the pitcher's shoulder are to (1) eliminate pain, (2) return to normal passive and active range of motion and reestablish synchrony of motion, (3) increase strength and endurance in integrated muscle actions, (4) progressively return to pitching, and (5) return to sport (game) participation. These goals are outlined in five specific phases:

Phase I/acute rehabilitation: Control pain and inflammation and protect the injured or postsurgical area. Limited function is determined by the severity of the injury and tissue involvement. The goal of this phase is not to aggravate the injury or surgical anatomy.

Phase II/initial rehabilitation: Normal passive and active range of motion and reestablishment of synchrony and articular patterns of motion.

Phase III/progressive rehabilitation: Increase motion and initiate strength and endurance in integrated muscle action, joint mobilization and neuroproprioceptive techniques. Begin skill performance.

Phase IV/integrated functions: Continue with Phase III skills and progressively return to maximal skill performance and simulated performance. Determine need for medication and protection.

Phase V/ return to sport: Monitor reentry to competitive level at this point; maintenance of motion, strength, performance.

The time necessary to progress through these phases will vary depending on the underlying pathologic process to be rehabilitated. The complexity of the injury or operative intervention and the recovery healing period for specific tissues will guide the rate of the rehabilitation program (i.e., bone, ligament, muscle, tendon, articular surface). Nonoperative or conservative management is the preferred approach to recurrent shoulder pain or chronic shoulder discomfort. It is also the choice in acute pain, unless the need for surgical intervention is obvious. Although the goals of a rehabilitation program are sequential, they are often interrelated and addressed simultaneously in the development and implementation of intervention strategies.

Phase I: Acute Rehabilitation

The goals of the acute phase are elimination of pain and control of edema and swelling. Pain is often the major presenting symptom. The use of modalities alone or in conjunction with NSAIDs can be effective.

An early period of nonactivity, cryotherapy, and gentle exercises should be implemented. Subjective evaluation and measurement of pain should be part of the initial examination and periodically assessed throughout the rehabilitation process. Measures of the sensation of pain are often done; emotional pain is not measured, but should also be considered and should occur away from peers. The latter is of value with competitive and team athletes, particularly when involved in a long-term rehabilitation program. How an athlete "feels" about not pitching or not contributing to the team can be a significant psychological concern throughout the rehabilitation program.

Unless pain is resolved, a secondary effect, inhibiting muscle action, can occur with the development of a cycle leading to disuse, weakness, and atrophy. Attempting to pitch through such acute episodes can often lead to the chronic or recurrent painful shoulder. As the level of pain diminishes, attention to a question such as "How can I prevent a recurrence?" as well as to analyses of pitching mechanics is most important.

The immediate postarthroscopic period is directed toward decreasing pain and inflammation and achieving full and pain-free range of motion. Modalities such as ice, ultrasound, electric stimulation and NSAIDs can be considered and used selectively in conjunction with assisted and active exercise. Motion is the critical intervention. Pendulum exercises may be introduced immediately and done frequently throughout the day. In the supine position, self-assisted exercises with the use of a lightweight bar can be initiated within a day or two. Flexion is the most comfortable movement to initiate. Changes in elbow position, hand distances, and hand grip on a bar can be used as elements for progression. All motions should ultimately be attempted but kept within a comfortable range. No increase in pain should be experienced. When the use of modalities and NSAIDs are no longer necessary, and good consistent isometric contractions of the rotator cuff musculature are achieved, progression to active exercise can begin (see the sections, *Phase II* and *Phase III*).

Similarly, the immediate postoperative period for open procedures is focused on pain control, positioning and the initiation of muscular contractions and selectively guided motion, and wound care. There should be a discussion between the athlete and the physical therapist on how the brace, sling, or other supportive device is to fit and be used.

The transition from the acute phase requires knowledge and assessment of the extent of injury or impairment and tissue healing. Careful clinical observation to ensure incremental motions and muscle contractions are performed without pain and active muscle substi-

tutions. If pain is associated with any motion, there will be a postural change that affects the positions of the scapula and control of the glenohumeral joint. The education of the athlete to the importance of these factors is critical to the success of rehabilitation. Frequently the athlete will prefer a program that includes resistance exercises, only to delay the ultimate return to skill rehabilitation.

Phase II: Initial Rehabilitation

Achievement of full range of motion with progressive muscle function and synchrony of motion are addressed in this phase. Prior to the initiation of a strengthening program, discrete muscular problems must be solved. Muscle conditioning should be a priority if muscles are found to have either minimal contractions or limiting contractures. Progressive range of motion without pain should occur. The plane of the scapula is the preferred position for exercise and testing. Scapular control is a major component of the program to achieve scapulothoracic stabilization for control of the glenohumeral joint. Unless all muscles surrounding the shoulder are able to be actively controlled, abnormal movement patterns will be aggravated in any exercise program that requires multiple sequential contractions.

Prior to the initiation of a muscle training or strengthening program, discrete muscular problems must be solved; shortened muscles need to be lengthened and weakened or atrophied muscles should be conditioned and strengthened. As pain/discomfort is resolving and joint range of motion is normalized, isometric exercises, particularly for scapular positioning and the rotator cuff musculature, are begun (determined by the details of the open procedure). These exercises can be done independently or with a partner. Encouragement is also given to move within pain-free ranges. The rehabilitation program will focus on the correction of muscle imbalances at the glenohumeral joint and scapulothoracic articulation. Muscle control throughout a full range of motion is the major goal. The initial evaluation will have identified the presenting problem areas. Exercises to address these problems are designed and activities selected and implemented; some exercises are to stretch certain muscles, others are to strengthen certain muscles. In this phase of the rehabilitation program, the importance of precise execution of an exercise or activity cannot be overstated. This is true both in those performed with a therapist and those that are part of a home program, independently or with a partner. Repeated assessments during treatment sessions will monitor progress and help reset direction and priorities.

Active motion is an important aspect in achieving and maintaining joint range of motion. Use of the arm in biomechanically appropriate exercises and selected activities is recommended. As additional joint range is achieved through any of the mentioned techniques, the ability to move into, through, and maintain position in the new ranges of motion is essential. It is a requirement for achieving muscle balance and synchrony of motion.

In pitching, the rotator cuff muscles are particularly stressed. Frequently, the supraspinatus and infraspinatus are weak and atrophied. Occasionally, a pitcher may be unable to elicit any contraction in the supraspinatus during abduction. Such a finding is critical; a proper functioning supraspinatus is a prerequisite for accurate centralization of the humeral head within the glenoid during the phases of throwing.

Pitchers with supraspinatus difficulty will frequently shrug their shoulders to initiate and complete abduction. As they abduct, they may describe discomfort in the superior aspect of their shoulder, suggesting a proximal decentralizing elevation of the humeral head within the glenoid due to absence of supraspinatus action, creating impingement. It is imperative that a strong supraspinatus contraction be present in the early range of abduction before major strengthening exercises begin.

If difficulties with supraspinatus action are noted, the pitcher should concentrate on initiation of supraspinatus contraction during the first 30 degrees of abduction. This can be achieved by having the pitcher sit upright and abduct his shoulder against slight resistance provided by the clinician. The exercise can be reinforced at home by doing a similar isometric set while sitting in an armchair facing a mirror. The pitcher should concentrate on "setting" his shoulder just prior to initiating abduction. The initial abduction motion should not be initiated with a total shoulder elevation. The pitcher only needs to abduct to 30 to 45 degrees to initiate supraspinatus action. This can also be reinforced by practice by doing a few selected daily activities. The athlete may need to continue to "set" the supraspinatus when skill practice is initiated. Once supraspinatus contraction is present in the early range of abduction, further active abduction to 90 degrees may be performed. It is crucial that the supraspinatus contracts throughout the entire range of abduction in order for synchronous and rhythmic abduction to occur. If unable to locate supraspinatus contraction, the use of electric stimulation may assist in the achievement of the goal.

The infraspinatus is also frequently weak and atrophied in the pitching shoulder with chronic problems. In conjunction with infraspinatus weakness, the entire posterior shoulder girdle musculature may have diminished strength. Weakness of the posterior shoulder musculature compromises (1) the horizontal extension necessary at the beginning of the cocking phase, (2) the fixation of the shoulder girdle during the acceleration phase, and (3) the proper eccentric contractions necessary for a smooth deceleration during the follow-through phase, for control of scapular protraction and glenohumeral internal rotation and adduction.

As with the supraspinatus, it is important that the pitcher can contract both his infraspinatus and teres minor before further strengthening exercises for the posterior shoulder musculature can begin. To isolate the infraspinatus and teres minor, the pitcher should be on his affected side with his arm hanging over the edge of the table, and instructed to externally rotate his arm. Palpation will reveal the extent of contraction. If difficulties in contraction are evident, this position should be used until the pitcher is able to consistently contract these muscles. Assisted flexibility exercises, with proprioceptive neuromuscular facilitation if necessary, should be initiated. There are some successful pitchers who have permanent incomplete infraspinatus function. The specific conditioning of the remaining posterior shoulder muscles is critical for them to continue pitching.

Lack of scapular fixation and control is also a common finding. The resting position of the scapula is frequently in a protracted position. The rhomboids, middle and lower trapezius, and levator scapulae are weaker or fatigue earlier with repetitive scapula retraction and the serratus anterior may fail to control motion of the scapula to the thorax (i.e., clinical "winging" of the scapula). As a result, the glenoid turns anteriorly and inferiorly during arm movements leading to glenohumeral joint incongruency.

If specific muscles are not responding or require additional therapy, electric stimulation or specific therapeutic exercises may be used.

Full range of motion at the glenohumeral joint and scapulothoracic articulation without joint compensatory adjustment is critical and serves as the major criterion for progression to muscle strengthening and endurance program components. Once the early stages of individual muscle actions are achieved, the use of 1-lb hand weights can be used through the range of motion that is normal.

An injury to the capsule usually results in the formation of scar tissue limiting motion; a tear of the capsule or a ligament inappropriately increases joint motion.

Table 16-4 Proprioceptive Neuromuscular Facilitation

Contract-relax
   This technique is based on the concept of reflex activation and inhibition; a maximum contraction of a muscle results in maximum relaxation of the same muscle
Reciprocal relaxation
   This technique is based on reciprocal inhibition; an isometric contraction against resistance results in reciprocal relaxation of the antagonist

Overhead athletes and pitchers in particular frequently present with capsular tightness, reflected in limitation of internal rotation, horizontal adduction, and combined abduction. Muscles and tendons that cross the joint, if shortened, will also limit motion. There is rarely a primary restriction in the scapulothoracic articulation, but occasionally a slight restriction or weakness in scapular retraction (adduction) is found, the scapula positioned in protraction (abduction).

A shoulder flexibility program will consist of a combination of stretching exercises, joint mobilization, and active exercise. Active and passive static stretching and proprioceptive neuromuscular facilitation (Table 16-4) are the stretching techniques of choice. It should be noted that only an experienced therapist should perform posterior capsule stretching.

The technique of active and passive static stretching consists of:

Static Stretch
   Passive: The arm is moved into maximum comfortable range, then moved further so that a slight tension or slow stretch is felt, held for 15 to 30 seconds and released. Return to starting position. Repeat.

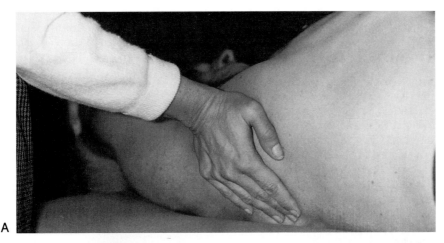

A

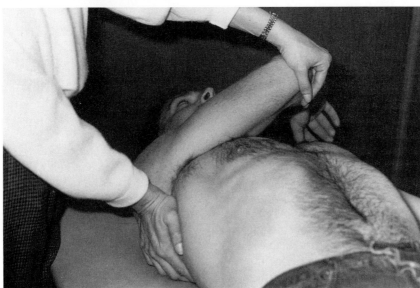

B

Figure 16-14

Active: Arm is moved into position as above. Slowly contract the antagonist muscle to gain further motion, hold and slowly release. Return to starting position. Repeat.

Assisted Stretch

  To achieve flexibility in horizontal flexion, the athlete should be supine. The physical therapist stabilizes the scapula behind the thorax by firmly holding the scapula from above and along the lateral thoracic wall (Fig. 16-14A). A slow, sustained stretch is applied as the humerus is brought across the chest wall to gain glenohumeral horizontal flexion and adduction to either 45 degrees or within the limits allowed by the chest wall (Fig. 16-14B).

  To achieve an increased excursion of the combined flexion/abduction pattern, the athlete should be supine and the scapula should be stabilized at the edge of the thoracic wall. A slow and gentle sustained passive stretch alone or in combination with the use of active neuromuscular facilitation techniques is applied to the externally rotated arm in a downward direction toward the table (Fig. 16-15).

  External rotation at full abduction: The patient should be in the supine position. The arm should be brought into full abduction. The arm should be stretched into external rotation by positioning one hand at lateral elbow for stabilization and the other hand at dorsum of wrist to provide stretching force into external rotation. Hold 20 seconds. Stretch inferior capsule.

  Posterior glide of humerus: The patient should be in the supine position with the arm close to edge of table. The arm is placed in 90 degrees of flexion with slight horizontal adduction and elbow flexion. Force is applied through the elbow pushing the humerus posteriorly. Hold 20 seconds. Stretch posterior capsule and subscapularis tendon.

Movement beyond the horizontal may cause the anterior capsule of the shoulder to be stretched too far, precipitating a local inflammatory response and increasing joint laxity, possibly leading to anterior instability, associated bicipital tendinitis, and an anterior labral injury (see Ch. 9 for information on glenoid position and articular effect).

Proprioceptive neuromuscular facilitation patterns performed with a therapist directed toward stabilization of the scapula are most effective (Table 16-4). In addition, exercises for the muscles that control and stabilize the scapula can be part of a home program. Recommended positions are described in manual muscle testing. Pitchers should be instructed in postural correction and encouraged to do frequent repetitions of scapula retraction independent of arm movement. This position is the first-stage correction to develop the proprioceptive phase of cocking. A number of these repetitions can be done hourly during other activities. When the athlete is comfortable with scapular retraction, added demand can occur by progression to wall push-ups. Fixation of the scapula in the shortened position followed by a full excursion of protraction and retraction is necessary. If a wall mirror is available, the push-up should be performed into the mirror; the visual feedback on shoulder position can be very helpful (as described in the section *Conditioning* above).

Joint mobilization is a specialized form of passive motion which utilizes distraction and translatory gliding motions with varying degrees of intensity.

The specific techniques of joint mobilization are described in the literature. Use of joint mobilization techniques for the pitcher's glenohumeral joint would be indicated when lack of extensibility in periarticular structures limits caudal movement of the humeral head during abduction or posterior movement during horizontal adduction. Resolution of such restrictions would facilitate restoration of normal joint mechanics and muscle function.

When flexibility, individual muscle action, and syn-

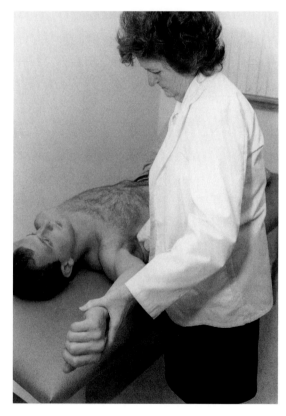

Figure 16-15 (Photograph courtesy of James Koepfler.)

chronous movements have been attained, the functional patterns of pitching should be instituted with an observant health professional present. Flexibility and range of motion gained through proprioceptive neuromuscular facilitation techniques require a pattern, which in the initial stages of a rehabilitation program are applied by a physical therapist.

Active motion is an important aspect in achieving and maintaining joint range of motion. Use of the arm in biomechanically appropriate exercises and selected activities is recommended. As additional joint range is achieved through any of the above-mentioned techniques, the ability to move into, move through, and maintain position in the new ranges of motion is essential. It is a requirement for achievement of muscle balance and synchrony of motion.

Progression to synchronous movement patterns occurs as muscle imbalances are corrected. In the plane of the scapula, the following sequence can be used to note progress toward scapuloglenohumeral rhythm: abduction to 90 degrees, external rotation, reach toward the ceiling, hold and check position, return to each position slowly. Scapular stabilization and coordinated muscle control should be repeatedly checked. Eccentric control is usually the most difficult for the athlete recovering from an injury. The challenge to clinicians is to incorporate movement components into a variety of complex movement patterns, with a preference given to those related to specific sport activity. Synchrony of scapulothoracic and glenohumeral motion is the end product of this phase of rehabilitation.

Synchrony of Motion

A proper pattern of muscle action is an important prerequisite to a healthy pitching shoulder. A sequence of shoulder abduction, horizontal extension with scapular adduction, and external rotation occurs during the cocking phase. A pitcher must be able to perform this sequence in an upright position, symmetrically, and with no indication of weakness or abnormal scapular motion. Symmetrical scapulothoracic synchrony cannot be accomplished by a pitcher with marked shoulder weakness, especially of the supraspinatus. The pattern of active abduction, horizontal extension, scapular adduction, and external rotation exercises is the primary component of skill practice. Initially, this sequence should be performed without additional resistance (Fig. 16-16).

Pitchers should practice this pattern at least four times per day, 25 repetitions each. The focus should be on scapular control and bilateral symmetrical motion.

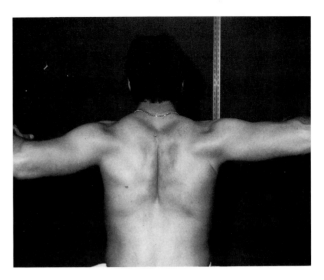

Figure 16-16 Skill practice sequence.

As flexibility, strength, and scapular control improve, lateral scapular migration will decrease. Proper attention to this functional pattern of muscle action will ensure a stable shoulder during the entire pitching sequence and serve as the singular criterion for progression to the next phase of rehabilitation.

For the postarthroscopic athlete, motions in the plane of the scapula are recommended to minimize unnecessary stress within the glenohumeral joint. Centralization of the humeral head in the glenoid and coordinated scapula participation should be observed and emphasized. There can be gradual progression in strengthening exercises. A simple change from an elbow bent to elbow straight position can substantially increase force requirements. Progression can be reflected in the number of repetitions, sets, and sessions utilized. Pain or loss of full joint mobility and range should not be a by-product of any exercise strategy. Both should be carefully monitored; regression in either would be of concern and require immediate attention. A physical therapist may choose to begin proprioceptive neuromuscular facilitation patterns to facilitate neuromuscular coordination.

At approximately 3 to 4 weeks postarthroscopic surgery, steady progress in performance and good control over the shoulder musculature should be exhibited. A weight of 1 to 2 lb is routinely used in exercise and the extremity is used in common daily activities without pain (patterns as described). Progression to a dynamic strengthening program can be specifically outlined, and activities such as low-stress swimming and limited short distance basketball shooting can begin.

Phase III: Progressive Rehabilitation

Strengthening Program

Once an individual is able to actively contract and control synchrony of all glenohumeral and scapulothoracic musculature and has demonstrated complete flexibility, and has full range of motion, a specific strengthening program may begin. This strengthening program should be followed in conjunction with the conditioning exercises previously outlined (see the section *Conditioning* above). Initially, the exercises should be completed throughout the ranges and functional patterns without any weight, with a progression of 1- to 2-lb increments once the exercises can be completed without muscle fatigue or fasciculation. This phase is designed to address the functional requirements of the athlete. For the pitcher, sequences of high-velocity concentric and eccentric movements are required and will need to be specifically addressed.

The use of free hand-held or wrist weights is probably the most compatible method with the throwing shoulder. The gradual use of free weights can place progressive demands on the shoulder musculature in a variety of movement patterns. Concentric and eccentric control can be addressed, changes in position and speed easily altered, and maintenance of postural alignment observed and corrected, if necessary. The exercises are performed in a concentric-eccentric manner with a slow concentric contraction followed by a slow eccentric contraction to the starting position. Eccentric contractions are important, for the deceleration of the arm in the follow-through phase requires eccentric contraction. Frequent repetition, with progressive weight resistance (5 lb maximum) exercises are recommended. Weights heavier than 5 lb are not recommended, since they will cause abnormal movement patterns and use of larger muscles, precipitating a loss of muscular balance around the throwing shoulder. For each exercise, the goal should be three sets of 10 to 12 repetitions. Substitution patterns reflected in shoulder adjustments or body realignments should be noted and analyzed in relation to pitching for future consideration in the transition to a preventative maintenance program.

Use of surgical tubing, Thera-Band, or pulley weight system can be used as a progression with the muscles of the shoulder as well as in the more extensive full patterns of movement. What is most important is that appropriate posture, stabilization, and technique are not compromised. The choice of resistance, color Thera-Band, size of tubing, amount of pulley weight, and progression should depend on the execution of the movement and the related goal within the program.

The use of machines and mechanical resistance can be included, but with caution. Development of the larger musculature must be done in conjunction with the development of the smaller musculature to maintain a balanced shoulder and to minimize the potential for substitution patterns. If synchronous movements are disrupted or substitution of muscle action is evident, the weight resistance must be decreased.

Introduction to isokinetic exercise can occur when good control of the shoulder complex is observed. A comprehensive isokinetic evaluation should be done as early as is feasible; positioning of the extremity in the plane of the scapular is strongly recommended for all testing. The various isokinetic instruments are now able to perform both concentric and eccentric testing and also accommodate patterns of movement. The isokinetic equipment should be positioned so that the athlete can perform a modified flexion-extension pattern (similar to throwing pattern) while seated (Fig. 16-17). The same instrument should be used in repeated testing as data are not interchangeable. Data, particularly with rotation, are also position-specific. Therefore, for monitoring progress, comparison with the opposite extremity is preferred.

Pitching is a high-speed, high-velocity activity requiring fluidity of training movement. Strength and endurance are better achieved at the high speeds. Speed ranging from 300 degrees per second down to 210 degrees per second in 30 increments are used with 15 repetitions per set. After an initial warm-up, a typical workout would be 15 repetitions at each of the following degrees: 300, 270, 240, 210, 210, 240, 270 degrees per second. Slower speeds than 210 degrees per second are not recommended for athletes in the rehabilitation phases.

Again, as in the use of regular exercise machines, isokinetic exercise should be used in conjunction with a flexibility and lightweight exercise program. If available, isokinetic training is recommended three times a week. As muscle performance improves, the pitcher will also begin to throw and progress, as indicated in skill practice.

At 6 to 8 weeks postarthroscopic surgery, exercising with a 3-lb weight is anticipated. Exercises are performed throughout a full range and without pain. Synchrony of scapular glenohumeral motion is also easily observed. It is at this point that a comprehensive review of general physical fitness and conditioning should occur. Identified needs can be gradually incorporated into the rehabilitation program and represent the beginning of the transition period to general conditioning and training. If all criteria are satisfied, the progressive throwing program can be initiated.

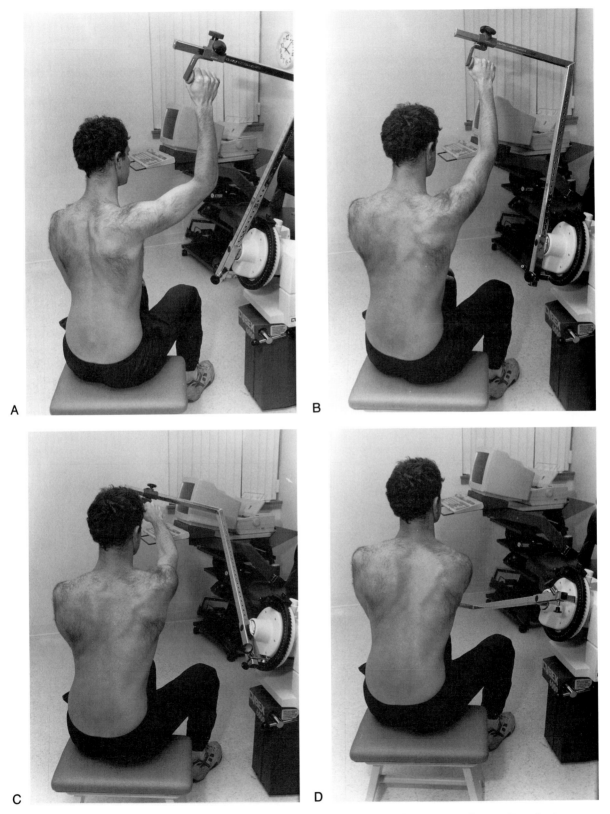

Figure 16-17 (A – D) Modified flexion-extension pattern. (Photographs courtesy of James Koepfler.)

Skill Practice

Skill Motion

The pitcher with chronic shoulder discomfort has often not thrown with his normal motion for at least half a season (usually longer). When flexibility has been restored, muscle integration attained, and clear control of the shoulder during the patterns of the pitching motion achieved, practice of the pitching motion with a weighted ball (1 lb) in the throwing hand can be initiated. The pitcher is instructed to use his normal pitching motion in front of a mirror and take note of each phase, particularly the exaggeration of the horizontal extension and external rotation scapular adduction of the cocking phase (Fig. 16-18A). By performing the act slowly, each muscle is conditioned in three specific activities: (1) the posterior excursion of the throwing arm, (2) fixation of the shoulder girdle necessary to provide an eccentric resistance so that the shoulder might rotate about a fixed point, and (3) the smooth follow-through so that the stress of deceleration and eccentric contractions might be distributed among all soft tissue structures. This deceleration awareness exercise is an excellent method of conditioning the posterior shoulder musculature in the eccentric contractions necessary for the large deceleration forces of the follow-through (Fig. 16-18B).

Short-Distance Throwing

When shoulder function patterns and mirror throwing demonstrate satisfactory muscle function and integration, the pitcher may begin to throw a ball for short distances of 30 to 50 ft and progress from an initial period of 2 to 5 minutes daily. The purpose of short distance throwing is to regain the throwing motion in a coordinated fashion, using the sequential aspects of total body motion. At this stage, it is critical to initiate proper throwing mechanics to avoid poor habits that create additional stress on the shoulder. Velocity is not a concern at this point. Fluidity of motion and accuracy are emphasized, with close observation to assure a proper synchronous pattern.

Phase IV: Integrated Functions: Muscle Action/Strength-Endurance and Progressive Return to Pitching

Once a pitcher has demonstrated complete flexibility and synchronous control of his shoulder girdle during exercise, the pitcher may increase throwing and also

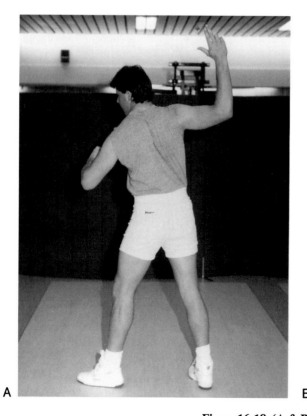 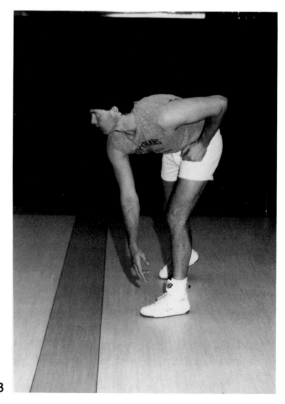

Figure 16-18 (A & B) Skill practice.

use resistance tubing or isokinetic exercise equipment as a rehabilitation tool. The various types of isokinetic exercise equipment allow maximum resistance throughout the entire range of motion.

Skills Practice

Skills practice is an important component of all rehabilitation programs. For a pitcher, skill practice represents the sequential return to throwing and progression to pitching and game participation. During this program, the pitcher should expect some mild, generalized soreness to occur; however, sharp pains are not normal. If pain arises at any step in the program, the program should be reviewed by a physical therapist and trainer, and the pitcher should stop and rest a day or two, and apply ice regularly. If pain does not resolve with ice and rest, a medical consultation is recommended. While working on the return to throwing program, the pitcher should continue with stretching and strengthening exercises as instructed.

When the pitcher is able to throw short distances on an arc with appropriate patterns of function for 10 minutes comfortably, longer distance throwing can begin. Again, the focus is fluid motion and accuracy. Distances should gradually increase up to 150 ft, determined by monitored observation by a baseball coach. At this point, velocity is still not a concern. The throw should be delivered to a partner on an arc. The pitcher should concentrate on proper mechanics and use total body motion while throwing. Long-distance throwing should be done every other day for periods ranging from 5 minutes initially, up to 15 minutes.

A review and analysis with the pitcher of a video taken of him prior to injury can be helpful. This can also facilitate communication between all team members and represent a period of transition in the rehabilitation process to specific sport activity.

Form Pitching

Once a pitcher is able to throw comfortably over short and long distances, he may begin to throw off a mound, initially 6 to 8 minutes, progressing to 12 to 15 minutes. For a pitcher with a history of chronic shoulder discomfort, this period may require at least 6 to 8 weeks after the start of a conditioning program. Attention is given to the proper mechanics of throwing, and velocity is progressively increased. Initially, a pitcher should only throw fast balls.

For the postsurgical pitcher, progress is essentially dictated by the pitcher's response to the stresses of throwing. This is achieved by increasing distance and velocity and changing the types of pitches thrown.

Throughout this period, there should be careful monitoring of the healing process of tissue and external demands. Changes in joint range and/or signs of discomfort should be noted. Any effect on the specific site of the surgery is of particular importance. When the pitcher has reached the milestone of throwing from the mound with reasonable velocity, an isokinetic test is recommended; first, as an indicator for readiness to pitch a simulated game or batting practice, and second, to use for comparison in follow-up tests. When batting practice velocity of the fast ball is reached, breaking balls may be gradually introduced into the throwing regime.

Throughout the progressive throwing phases, individuals should remain on their prescribed exercise programs. In fact, even when they return to competition, the exercises should be done a minimum of three times per week.

Advanced Skill Practice

Progression to this level occurs when the pitcher's velocity approaches 70 to 75 percent effort without any discomfort. This should be done under the tutelage of the pitching coach in addition to members of the clinical team.

Batting Practice

Batting practice is another step in the progression to game participation. Although eye-hand-target is a component of any skills practice, pitching batting practice clearly focuses the pitcher's attention to location and control. Batting practice provides an opportunity for feedback from the catcher and batters.

Simulated Game

The simulated game consists of the pitcher throwing a series of pitches at maximum velocity, pausing for a period similar to the time between innings, then repeating another series of pitches. The session should begin with the usual number of warm-up pitches, followed by warm-up pitches off the mound. The session should end with a few pitches of low velocity. A week's schedule should be planned in advance with simulated game days and rest days identified. Also included is the anticipated progression, that is, altering intensity by the number of pitches thrown per series plus the number of series scheduled, increasing velocity and increasing the type and frequency of pitches thrown. Only one parameter should be altered at a time so that the cause of any discomfort or changes in range of motion can be identified.

Phase V: Return to Sports

In this phase, the reentry to competitive sports should be monitored by the professional health care team. In the first outing with any pitcher, the coach and health care team should focus on the pitch count (specific to the pitcher's time away from participation) and biomechanic control, location, and velocity. A post-pitching physical examination 24 and 48 hours after this first outing should be directed to muscle action and synchrony and any potential muscle nodules and trigger points.

The time required for a return to pitching will depend on the complexity of the presenting diagnosis. In general, lesser degrees of pathology will make for a speedier return. The individual with an acute inflammatory tendonitis will progress rapidly through a sequence of rehabilitative steps and may be ready within 2 to 3 weeks with a course of rest and anti-inflammatory medication and appropriate therapeutic modalities and exercises. An individual with a more complex series of problems (e.g., tight capsule, muscle imbalance, and altered biomechanics) may require 4 to 6 months of different rehabilitative considerations. Return to competitive pitching is generally expected to occur 3 to 6 months postarthroscopic surgery. A program designed to maintain full joint range of motion, integrated muscle action and dynamic strength should become a routine component of the pitcher's ongoing conditioning program. Continued improvement in shoulder strength and biomechanical adjustments are expected for at least 1 year postsurgery, and a maintenance program should continue throughout the pitcher's competitive years.

It is not possible to present a single program for all shoulders that require rehabilitation. The principles of rehabilitation have been presented in five phases. The return to competition phase must be individually defined. The observations of performance are invaluable. The following is a generic program that can be used for baseball pitchers or other overhead athletes who are returning from a tissue or inflammatory injury.

Return to throwing program I

Step I (week 1)
Throw on an arc 40 to 60 ft.
Begin with 5 minutes on day 1. Progress gradually in duration to 15 minutes by day 5. Throw 5 days in a row, then rest 2 days
Work on proper mechanics and form, no velocity

Step II (week 2)
Throw on an arc 90 to 120 ft.
Throw up to 15 minutes each day for maximum of 5 continuous days, then rest 2 days
Work on proper mechanics and form, no velocity

Step III (week 3)
Throw 90 to 120 ft progressing from "arc" throwing to line throwing
Increase velocity gradually and as tolerated
Throw up to 15 minutes maximum for 5 days, rest 2 days

Step IV (week 4)*
Begin throwing off of the pitcher's mound 5-10 minutes, alternate days
Begin with easy throws and increase velocity, as tolerated
When close to full velocity with line pitches, breaking pitches can begin

SUGGESTED READINGS

Anderson B: Stretching. Shelter Publications, Bolinas, California, 1980

Andrews JR, Harrellson GH: Physical Rehabilitation of the Injured Athlete. WB Saunders, Philadelphia, 1991

Basmajian JV, DeLuca CJ: Muscles Alive: Their Functions Revealed by Electromyography. 5th Ed. Williams & Wilkins, Baltimore, 1985

Braatz JH, Gogia PP: The mechanics of pitching. J Orthop Sports Phys Ther 9:56, 1987

Cookson JC, Kant BE: Orthopedic manual therapy-an overview. Part I: The extremities. Phys Ther 59:136, 1987

Dillman CJ, Fleisig GS, Andrews JR: Biomechanics of pitching with emphasis upon shoulder kinematics. J. Orthop Sports Phys Ther 18:402, 1993

Donatelli R: Physical Therapy of the Shoulder. 2nd Ed. Churchill Livingstone, New York, 1991

Greenfield B, Donatelli R, Wooden M et al: Isokinetic evaluation of shoulder rotational strength between the plane of the scapula and the frontal plane. Am J Sports Med 18:32, 1990

Jobe FW, Tibone JE, Perry J et al: An EMG analysis of the shoulder in throwing and pitching. Am J Sports Med 11:3, 1983

Kaltenborn FM: Mobilization of the Extremity Joints: Examination and Basic Treatment Techniques. Ola Noris, Oslo, 1980

Luttgens K, Wells, K: Kinesiology: Scientific Basis of Human Motion. 7th Ed. WB Saunders, Philadelphia, 1982

Maitland GD: Treatment of the glenohumeral joint by passive movement. Physiotherapy 69:3, 1983

Meeusen R, Lievens P: The use of cryotherapy in sports injuries. Sports Med 3:398, 1986

Michlovitz SL: Thermal Agents in Rehabilitation. 2nd Ed. FA Davis, Philadelphia, 1990

Newham DJ, Mills KR, Quigley BM, Edwards RHT: Pain and fatigue after eccentric and concentric contraction. Clin Sci 64:55, 1983

---

* For pitchers only. Others can progress with gradual increases in number of throws, distance or velocity, as tolerated. Progression in one dimension is recommended on a given day to assess the effect.

Pappas AM, Zawacki RM, McCarthy CF: Rehabilitation of the pitching shoulder. Am J Sports Med 13:4, 1985

Pappas AM, Zawacki RM, Sullivan TJ: Biomechanics of baseball pitching. Am J Sports Med 13:216, 1985

Paris SV: Extremity Dysfunction and Mobilization. Institute Press, Atlanta, GA, 1980

Pearl ML, Perry J, Torburn L, Gordon LH: An electromyographic analysis of the shoulder during cones and planes or arm motion. Clin Orthop 284:116, 1992

Seaver T: The Art of Pitching. Hearst Books, New York, 1984

Smith CA: The warm-up procedure: to stretch or not to stretch—a brief review. J Orthop Sports Phys Ther 19:12, 1994

Soderberg GJ, Blaschak MJ: Shoulder internal and external rotation peak torque productions through a velocity spectrum in differing positions. J Orthop Sports Phys Ther 8:518, 1987

Stokes M, Young A: The contribution of reflex inhibition to arthrogenous muscle weakness. Clin Sci 67:7, 1984

Tata GE, Ng L, Kramer JF: Shoulder antagonistic strength ratios during concentric and eccentric muscle action in the scapular plane. J Orthop Sports Phys Ther 18:654, 1993

Voss DE, Ionta MK, Meyers BJ: Proprioceptive Neuromuscular Facilitation: Patterns and Techniques. 3rd Ed. Harper & Row, Philadelphia, 1985

Whitney SL: Physical agents: head and cold modalities. p. 844. In Scully RM, Barnes MR (eds): Physical Therapy. JB Lippincott, Philadelphia, 1989

Wilk KE, Voigth ML, Keirns MA, Cambetta V et al: Stretch-shortening skills for upper extremities: theory and clinical application. J Orthop Sports Phys Ther 17:225, 1993

Zachazewski JE: Improving flexibility. p. 698. In Scully RM, Barnes MR (eds): Physical Therapy. JB Lippincott, Philadelphia, 1989

17

Elbow Anatomy and Function

Arthur M. Pappas
John Vitolo

The elbow is an intricate link in all upper extremity function, transfer of force, and skill movements. This chapter presents elbow anatomy, correlating the functional aspects of the anatomic structures with the known biomechanic requirements of specific athletic skills (e.g., baseball pitch). The functional anatomy and biomechanic interactions of the elbow must be understood for the evaluation, treatment, and rehabilitation of sport-related injuries and dysfunction.

TOPICAL ANATOMY

With the forearm supinated, the contours of the cubital fossa outline the topical anatomy of the anterior elbow. The landmarks of the triangular fossa consist of the pronator teres medially, the brachioradialis laterally, and the base, a line between the two humeral epicondyles. The anatomic structures within the cubital fossa from lateral to medial are the biceps tendon,

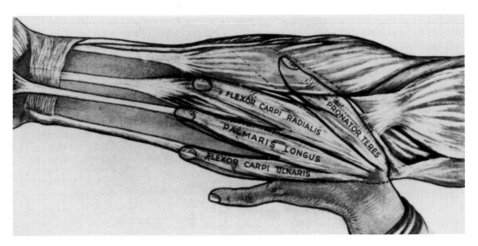

Figure 17-1 Muscles that arise from the medial epicondyle can be reviewed topographically by placing the opposite hand over the muscle mass with the thenar eminence located over the epicondyle, as presented by Henry.

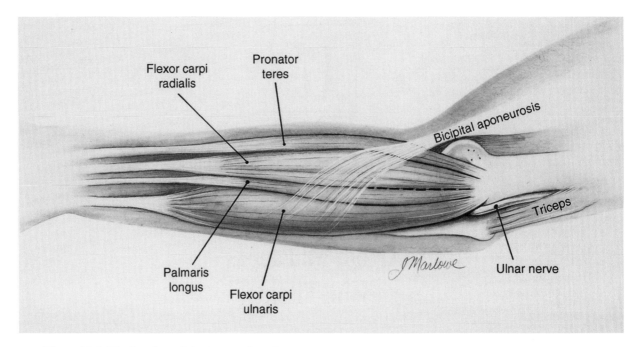

Figure 17-2 The location of the lacertus fibrosis, the aponeurotic extension from the biceps tendon that covers the muscles of the medial forearm.

brachial artery, median nerve, and musculocutaneous nerve. The medial muscle group includes the muscles that have a primary origin from the medial epicondyle, from central to medial: the pronator teres, flexor carpi radialis, palmaris longus, flexor digitorum superficialis, and flexor carpi ulnaris[1] (Fig. 17-1). The bicipital aponeurosis (lacertus fibrosis) overlies the medial muscle group (Fig. 17-2). The medial epicondyle is the origin for the medial (ulnar) collateral ligament, and the ulnar nerve is palpable as it passes behind the medial epicondyle within the cubital tunnel.

The lateral muscle group, described by Henry[1] as the "mobile wad," includes from central to lateral, the brachioradialis, extensor carpi radialis longus and brevis, extensor digitorum communis and minimis, extensor carpi ulnaris, and anconeus (Fig. 17-3). The posterior vantage views the tip of the olecranon with the insertion of the triceps tendon and the medial and lateral epicondyles. When the elbow is fully extended, the relationship of the olecranon and lateral and medial epicondyles forms a straight line. In maximum flexion, the relationship between these three bone landmarks is an equilateral triangle (Fig. 17-4). When the elbow is flexed 90°, the relationship forms an isosceles triangle. These topical areas serve as landmarks for evaluation, aspiration of effusions, and arthroscopy reference points.

ELBOW OSTEOLOGY AND ARTICULATIONS

The distal humerus is comprised of the bony medial and lateral epicondyles, the trochlea and capitellum which articulate with the sigmoid fossa of the proximal ulna, and the head of the radius, respectively (Figs. 17-5 and 17-6). These articulations form the three joints of the elbow: the radiocapitellar, the ulnotrochlear, and the radioulnar. The distal humerus forms an angle of approximately 6 degrees of valgus when viewed in the AP plane and approximately 30 degrees of anterior inclination when viewed from the lateral plane. There is a 3- to 5-degree internal rotation of the proximal humerus in relationship to the intercondylar line (Fig. 17-7). The articular surface of the trochlea presents an arc of approximately 330 degrees and the capitellar articular surface is nearly hemispherical and makes an arc of approximately 180 degrees.[2]

The proximal ulna forms the greater sigmoid fossa, which posteriorly forms the olecranon and anteriorly forms the coronoid process and the radial notch. The proximal ulna makes a 4-degree valgus angle with the ulnar shaft. In addition, the articular surface of the proximal ulna is rotated approximately 30 degrees posteriorly when viewing from the lateral plane (Fig. 17-8). The posterior rotation of the ulna matches the anterior

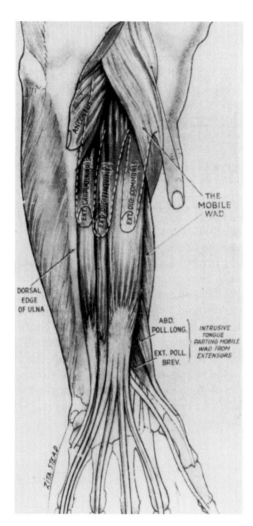

Figure 17-3 The topographic contour of the muscles on the lateral or extensor surface. The thumb of the opposite hand overlies the lateral epicondyle along the course of the anconeus, index, long, and ring fingers running parallel, overlying the extensor muscles of the "mobile wad."

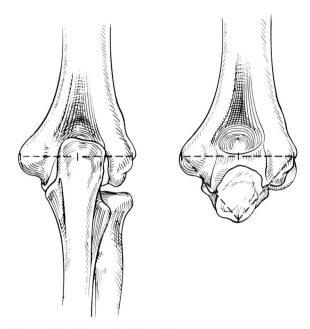

Figure 17-4 When the elbow is fully extended the relationship of the olecranon, lateral and medial epicondyles forms a straight line. When the elbow is flexed to 90 degrees, the relationship of the olecranon to the two epicondyles is an isosceles triangle.

rotation of the distal humerus. The greater sigmoid notch of the proximal ulna and the increased trochlea articular surface allows for articular contact through a greater range of motion. The congruous articulation between the proximal ulna and the trochlea is responsible for much of the elbow joint's inherent stability. The valgus angle of the distal humerus, along with the valgus at the proximal ulna, determines the carrying angle.

The radial head presents a cylindrical shape with a depressed midportion and articulates with the capitellum. The depressed cylindrical radial head articulation and the domed spherical capitellum provide mobility for wide ranges of supination and pronation in varying degrees of elbow flexion and extension. The radius

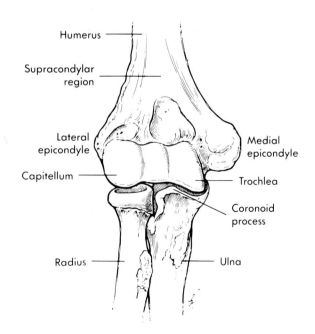

Figure 17-5 Osteology of the elbow from the anterior view with the forearm in supination.

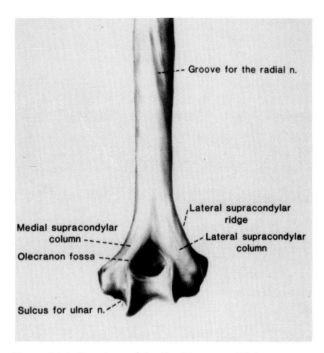

Figure 17-6 Osteology of the distal humerus (R) from a posterior view.

maintains its rotatory articulations with the radial ulnar notch by the annular ligament (Fig. 17-9). The integrity and stability of this ligament are crucial to elbow function and forearm rotation (e.g., effect of a radial neck fracture or Monteggia fracture) and the congruity of radiocapitellar and radioulnar articulations. Distal to the radial head, the radial tuberosity serves as the bone attachment for the biceps tendon, the anchor for elbow flexion and forearm supination. This proximal portion of the radius makes a direction of approximately 15 degrees with the shaft of the radius, influencing capitellum forces in pronation and supination.

The articular geometry of the three elbow joints contributes remarkable mobility and stability. The tongue and groove configuration of the humeral ulnar joint, along with supportive ligaments and musculotendon structures, creates stability primarily in flexion and extension and secondarily in varus and valgus. The varus and valgus stresses of overhead athletic performance create extraordinary traction-tension forces on the medial and lateral articular areas. In addition, the rotatory forces on the radiocapitellar articulation are frequently coupled with the valgus and varus forces and together contribute to articular cartilage shearing and injury.

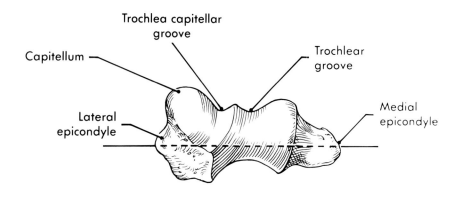

Figure 17-7 There is a 3- to 5-degree internal rotation of the humerus (L) in relationship to the epicondyles and a projected intercondylar line.

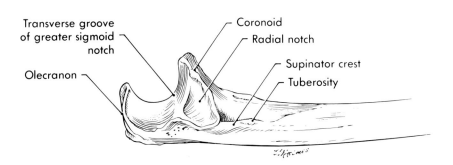

Figure 17-8 A lateral view of the proximal ulna with the relationships of the olecranon, greater sigmoid notch, and radial notch. The greater sigmoid notch with its extension to the coronoid provides an effacement, which minimizes the potential for dislocation unless there is excessive extension.

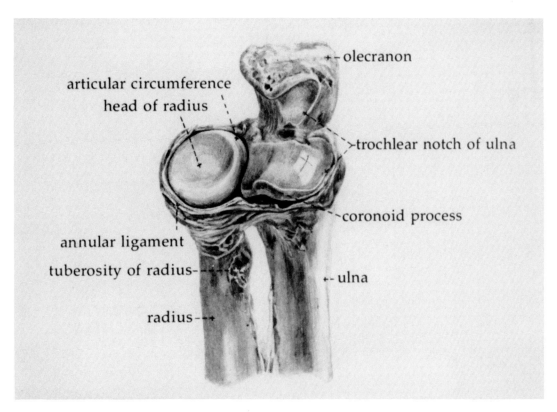

Figure 17-9 The articular surface of the radial head as well as the trochlear notch provide an extensive arc of hyaline cartilage. Approximately 240 degrees of the radial head is covered with hyaline cartilage. Its articulation in the radial notch of the ulna is supported by the annular ligament. This accounts for the containment and rotation of the radius in pronation and supination of the forearm.

Joint Capsule

The anterior capsule attaches to the margin of the coronoid on the medial aspect and the annular ligament on the lateral aspect. Some stability is provided by the oblique and transverse bands. The anterior capsule is taut in extension and loose in flexion. Posteriorly, the capsule attaches just above the olecranon fossa, along the supracondylar ridges and along the margins of the posterior trochlea. The noninflamed anterior capsule is a transparent opaque structure that permits a view of the prominent articular condyles. The synovial lining follows the configuration of the joint capsule, especially significant in relation to radioulnar articulation and evaluation of motion and injury.

Elbow Ligaments

The collateral ligaments are identifiable thickenings of the elbow capsule medially and laterally. The medial (ulnar) collateral ligament consists of three separate bundles: the anterior, posterior, and transverse por-

tions of the ligament. The anterior bundle is the most discrete and appears to be functionally the most important. The posterior bundle is a thickening in the posterior capsule and is well defined only when the elbow is at 90 degrees of flexion. The transverse ligament is not considered a major contributor to elbow joint stability but gives medial support to the greater sigmoid notch (Fig. 17-10).

The origin of the medial collateral ligament is from the anteroinferior surface of the medial epicondyle. The anterior portion originates just posterior to the axis of the rotation of the elbow joint and inserts on the medial aspect of the coronoid process.[3] The anterior component is approximately 27 mm long and the posterior segment is 24 mm long. The width of the anterior segment is approximately 5 mm. The anterior portion seems to tighten as the elbow approaches 20 to 30 degrees of flexion.

The posterior portion originates inferior and posterior to the axis of the rotation. The posterior bundle inserts into the middle of the margin of the semilunar notch. The posterior segment is approximately 5 mm wide at the midportion. The posterior position is lax to

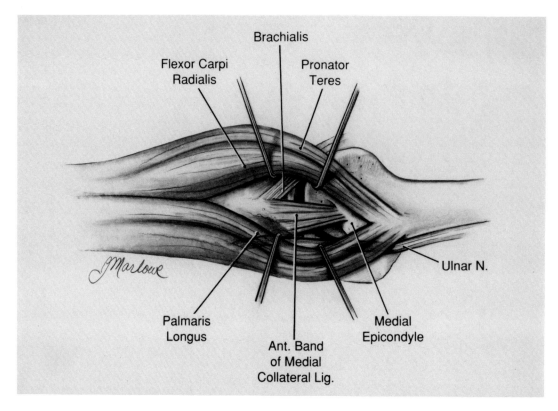

Figure 17-10 The anterior bundle of the medial collateral ligament provides the greatest resistance to the valgus force of overhead pitching activity.

about 60 degrees of flexion and then becomes tightest at 90 degrees. This so-called "cam effect" occurs due to the relationship of the origin of the ligaments to the axis of rotation.[2] These anatomic relationships of the ligaments are critical when planning and performing medial collateral ligament reconstruction.[4]

The lateral (radial) ligament complex of the elbow is often less consistent than the pattern of the medial ligament complex. There are four separate components[2]: (1) the radial collateral ligament, (2) the lateral ulnar collateral ligament, (3) the accessory lateral collateral ligament, and (4) the annular ligament (Fig. 17-11).

The lateral (radial) collateral ligament originates from the lateral epicondyle, terminates by blending with the fibers of the annular ligament, and is not as well defined as the anterior band of the medial collateral ligament. This portion of ligament is uniformly taut throughout the range of flexion and extension, indicating that the origin is very near the axis of rotation. The lateral ulnar collateral ligament extends from the lateral epicondyle to the supinator crest of the ulna and is present in approximately 90 percent of elbow studies. It has been suggested that the function of this portion of the lateral complex is to stabilize the elbow

against varus stress.[5] The annular ligament is a strong band of tissue originating on the anterior ulna and inserting on the anterior and posterior margins of the radial notch of the ulna, and provides stability for the radial head articulation with the ulna (Fig. 17-12). The anterior insertion tightens with supination, and the posterior insertion becomes taut in extremes of pronation.

Musculotendon Structures

This section does not cover all the anatomic details of the musculotendon units around the elbow, but instead presents information of clinical relevance in the evaluation and treatment of an athletic injury or complaint. The sequence begins with the medial epicondyle origin of the pronator flexor group. Figure 17-1 illustrates the relationship of the flexor pronator muscles.

The pronator teres usually has two heads of origin, the primary arising from the medial epicondyle and the second from the coronoid process of the ulna. These two origins provide an arch through which the median nerve passes to the forearm—at times, the source of neural compression either related to an injury or overdevelopment of the pronator muscle (see Ch. 3). The

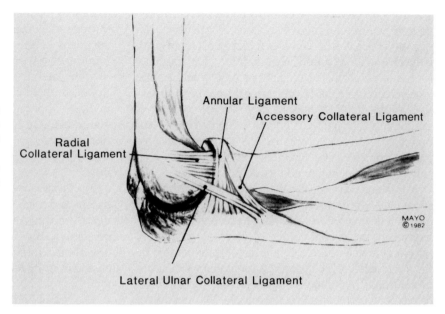

Figure 17-11 The components of the lateral collateral ligament, which are of lesser significance on varus valgus stability are demonstrated. However, the annular component is very significant in controlling the maximum arc of pronation supination.

pronator teres proceeds radially and distally under the brachioradialis, inserting at the junction of the proximal middle third of the radius. It is a strong pronator of the forearm as well as a weak flexor of the elbow. The pronator is frequently a source of discomfort for baseball pitchers, secondary to eccentric contracture associated with certain pitches. The flexor carpi radialis originates just inferior to the origin of the pronator teres at the anterior inferior aspect of the medial epicondyle. It passes distally and radially where it inserts into the base of the second and sometimes third metacarpal. It functions as a wrist flexor and is important for forceful

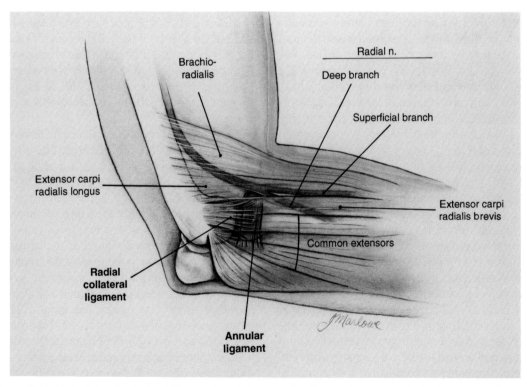

Figure 17-12 The lateral collateral ligament and the annular ligament are presented with the overlay of the extensor muscles.

wrist flexion activities (e.g., bowling, archery). It may be a source of tendonitis secondary to repetitive motion, and thus with certain sports the use of a rigid glove is recommended to limit wrist motion. The palmaris longus arises from the medial epicondyle and inserts into and becomes continuous with the palmar aponeurosis of the hand. It may be absent in 10 percent of individuals. The palmaris longus is often an important biologic transfer structure, used as a donor source for tendon transfers and ligament reconstruction, especially the medial collateral ligament.

The flexor carpi ulnaris is the most posterior of the superficial common flexor tendons, one head originating from the medial epicondyle. The second head originates from the medial border of the coronoid and the proximal medial aspect of the ulna. It is innervated by the ulnar nerve, which passes between the two heads of origin imparting branches either just before or after it passes between the heads of the muscle. The location of the ulnar nerve branches to the flexor carpi ulnaris is critical when surgery for ulnar nerve transposition or flexor carpi ulnaris transfer is performed. The muscle travels distally to insert into the pisiform, serving as a flexor and ulnar deviator of the wrist, important motions for both bat and racquet control and the spin motion of curveballs. Deep to these muscles lies the flexor digitorum superficialis and flexor digitorum profundus. The flexor digitorum superficialis has a complex origin. Medially it arises from the medial epicondyle via the common flexor tendon and the medial aspect of the coronoid. The lateral head is smaller and arises from the proximal two-thirds of the radius. The unique origin of the muscle forms a fibrous margin under which the median nerve and the ulnar artery emerge as they exit from the cubital fossa. The flexor digitorum profundus originates from the proximal medial ulna as well as the medial coronoid process and interosseus membrane. It is deep to the median nerve as the nerve crosses distally to the wrist (Fig. 17-1) (see Chs. 3 and 4). The relationship of flexor digitorum muscles with the neurovascular structures of the forearm is important to consider in the evaluation of nerve compression and/or vascular impairment of compartment compromise syndrome.

The predominant muscle in the posterior aspect of the elbow is the triceps. The function of the triceps is to extend the elbow by concentric contraction and decelerate elbow flexion by eccentric contraction. The radial nerve innervates the triceps and is shielded by the triceps as it passes around the humerus into the spiral groove and lateral toward the lateral epicondyle see Ch. 3). The medial and lateral heads of the triceps are innervated prior to the spiral groove, except for one

branch to the medial that enters proximally and passes through the head, terminating and innervating the anconeus (Fig. 17-13). This is an important anatomic feature when considering surgical approaches to the lateral elbow such as those by Kocher, Bryan, and Boyd. The incisional internervous plane in these approaches lies between the anconeus (radial nerve) and the extensor carpi ulnaris (posterior interosseous nerve). The anconeus covers the lateral portion of the annular ligament and the radial head.

The ulnar nerve passes along the medial border of the triceps and medial to the olecranon before it enters the ulnar groove (cubital tunnel) posterior to the medial epicondyle and passes toward the flexor carpi ulnaris. The clinical implications of the neuroanatomy are discussed in more detail later in this chapter and in Chapter 19.

The biceps and brachioradialis muscles are predominant anterior muscles and are the primary flexors of the elbow joint (Fig. 17-14). The biceps covers the brachialis in the distal arm and passes into the cubital fossa as the biceps tendon. The tendon attaches to the posterior aspect of the radius and the bicipital aponeurosis (lacertus fibrosis) is a broad band of tissue that is a continuation of the anterior medial and distal muscle fascia, runs obliquely superficial to the median nerve and brachial artery, and inserts into the deep fascia of the forearm. When the elbow is flexed to 80 degrees the medial margin of the aponeurosis is readily palpable on the medial aspect of the cubital fossa. The biceps and brachialis are major flexors of the elbow, with concentric contraction and deceleration of elbow extension by eccentric contraction. When the forearm is in the pronated position, the biceps serves as a strong supinator.

The brachialis muscle originates from and covers the anterior distal half of the humerus. The muscle crosses the anterior elbow capsule and inserts along the base of the coronoid and into the tuberosity of the ulna. The biceps and brachialis are innervated by the musculocutaneous nerve. Approximately 95 percent of the cross-sectional area of the brachialis is muscle tissue anterior to the elbow joint, thus explaining the high incidence of trauma to the muscle, secondary to elbow hyperextension and dislocation. Laterally, the brachialis covers the radial nerve after it spirals around the humerus away from under the triceps. The median nerve and brachial artery travel superficial to the brachialis and deep to the biceps in the cubital fossa. The brachioradialis originates on the lateral supracondylar bony ridge of the humerus and lies between the lateral head of the triceps and the brachialis muscle.

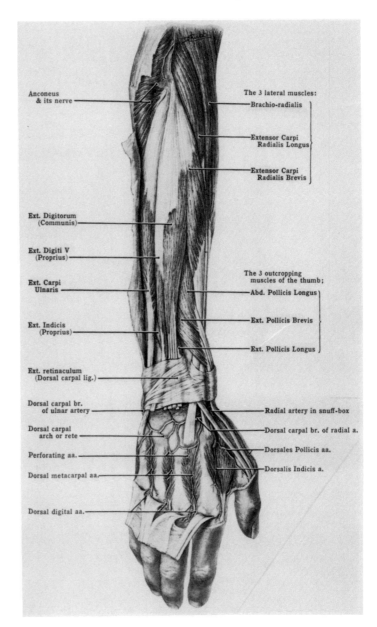

Figure 17-13 The posterolateral elbow demonstrating the course of the radial nerve and its distributions to the triceps as well as the muscles of the lateral epicondyle origin.

This muscle crosses the elbow joint covering the proximal origin and extensor carpi radialis and forms the lateral border of the cubital fossa, and extends along the course of the radius and inserts into the base of the radial styloid. The muscle is superficial to the radial nerve and is innervated by it as it emerges from the spiral groove. The extensor carpi radialis longus originates from the supracondylar ridge just below the origin of the brachioradialis. It inserts to the dorsal base of the second metacarpal. It lies deep to the brachioradialis and superficial to the extensor carpi radialis brevis. The extensor carpi radialis brevis originates from the

lateral inferior aspect of the lateral epicondyle. The extensor carpi radialis brevis inserts into the base of the third metacarpal and functions as a wrist extensor (Fig. 17-15). The major function of these muscles is wrist extension and radial deviation. The extensor digitorum communis originates from the common extensor tendon, and is just medial or ulnar to the extensor carpi radialis brevis. In the proximal forearm, the muscle fibers of the extensor carpi radialis longus and the extensor digitorum communis are indistinguishable from those of the extensor carpi radialis brevis. All of the extensor muscles are innervated by the radial nerve.

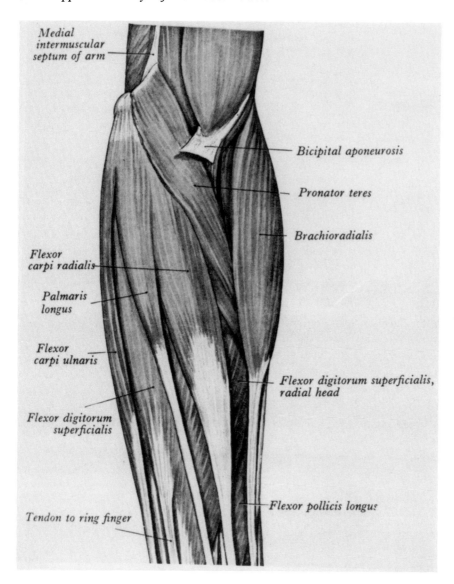

Figure 17-14 The muscles of the anterior elbow, the biceps and brachioradialis, and the relationship to the brachial artery and median nerve.

The extensor carpi ulnaris originates from two heads. The humeral origin is the most medial of the common extensor group. The ulnar attachment is along the aponeuroses of the anconeus and the superior border of this muscle. It inserts on the dorsal base of the 5th metacarpal. The clinical significance of these lateral muscles in the etiology of lateral epicondylitis are discussed in other chapters.

The supinator is a flat muscle with a complex origin and insertion. It originates from the lateral anterior aspect of the lateral epicondyle, the lateral collateral ligament, and the proximal anterior crest of the ulna. The muscle is rhomboidal in shape and runs distally and obliquely to wrap around the proximal radius. The radial nerve bifurcates above or passes through the supinator on its way to the distal forearm to become the superficial sensory radial nerve and the deeper poste-

rior interosseous nerve, important in surgical observations during surgery of the proximal radius (Fig. 17-16). The sensory branch is frequently compressed by tight wrist straps and gloves, in sports such as baseball and golf causing numbness and distal paresthesias.

Bursae

Several bursae have been identified around the elbow joint. The most frequent clinical bursal problem on the posterior aspect of the elbow is the superficial olecranon bursa between the olecranon process and the subcutaneous tissue. A deep intertendinous bursa may be present in the substance of the distal triceps tendon, and an occasional deep subtendinous bursa is noted between the tendon and the tip of the olecranon. The

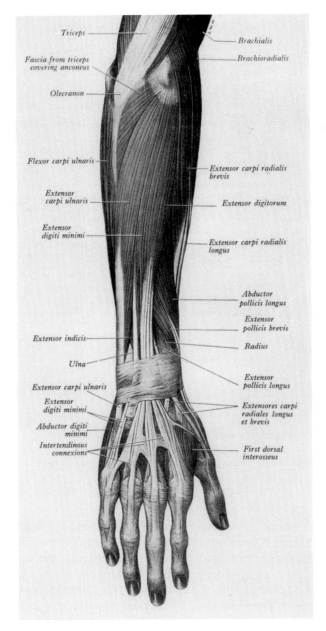

Figure 17-15 The lateral muscles arising from the distal humerus and the lateral epicondyle as well as the radial nerve innervations.

subcutaneous medial epicondylar and lateral epicondylar bursae and the radiohumeral bursa deep to the common extensor tendon superficial to the radiohumeral joint capsule have been recorded, with the latter implicated in the etiology of lateral epicondylitis (Fig. 17-17). The bicipital radial bursa exists between the biceps tendon from the tuberosity of the radius. Another bursa has been observed between the ulnar nerve and the medial epicondyle, and the margin of the triceps muscle. These bursae must be considered in the

evaluation of possible sources of elbow pain associated with athletic injury or overuse.

VASCULAR ANATOMY

The brachial artery, a continuation of the axillary artery, enters the cubital fossa running on the lateral side of the median nerve and lying superficial to the brachialis. The brachial artery continues distally at the medial margin of the biceps muscle and enters the antecubital space medial to the biceps tendon and lateral to the median nerve. It crosses under the bicipital aponeurosis and at the level of the radial head extends its terminal branches, the ulnar and radial arteries, which continue into the forearm (Fig. 17-18) (see Chs. 3 to 5). The brachial artery is usually accompanied by medial and lateral brachial veins. The continuation of the brachial artery, the radial artery, emerges from the antecubital fossa between the brachioradialis and the pronator teres and continues down the forearm under the brachioradialis muscle. The ulnar artery is the larger of the two terminal branches of the brachial artery, and at the level of the radial head usually passes distally, traversing the pronator teres between its two heads and continues deep to the flexor digitorum superficialis muscle.

A rich collateral arterial network of anastomoses exists around the elbow. These collateral arteries on both the radial and ulnar aspects of the elbow become significant if there is any injury either directly or indirectly to the cubital fossa or the brachial artery.

NERVE ANATOMY

The complete anatomy of the upper extremity peripheral nerves is presented in Chapter 3. This section details the anatomic and functional aspects of the neurologic complaints presented by athletes with elbow problems. It must be restated that pain can be focused about the elbow and more distally, yet the etiology may be an alteration that occurred more proximally (e.g., cervical disc, cervical rib, thoracic outlet syndrome, congenital anomaly) that causes compressive neuropathy. In addition, nerves are not static conduction lines. External pressures and excessive and repetitive motions are capable of altering nerve function and cause clinical symptoms at the site of impact or referred to other areas. The ulnar, median, radial, and musculocutaneous nerves will be the focus of this section on elbow anatomy and function.

The ulnar nerve passes from the anterior compartment to the posterior compartment approximately

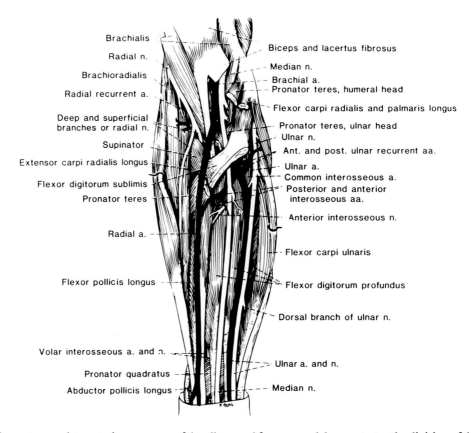

Brachialis
Radial n.
Brachioradialis
Radial recurrent a.
Deep and superficial branches or radial n.
Supinator
Extensor carpi radialis longus
Flexor digitorum sublimis
Pronator teres
Radial a.
Flexor pollicis longus
Volar interosseous a. and n.
Pronator quadratus
Abductor pollicis longus

Biceps and lacertus fibrosus
Median n.
Brachial a.
Pronator teres, humeral head
Flexor carpi radialis and palmaris longus
Pronator teres, ulnar head
Ulnar n.
Ant. and post. ulnar recurrent aa.
Ulnar a.
Common interosseous a.
Posterior and anterior interosseous aa.
Anterior interosseous n.
Flexor carpi ulnaris
Flexor digitorum profundus
Dorsal branch of ulnar n.
Ulnar a. and n.
Median n.

Figure 17-16 Presents complete anterior exposure of the elbow and forearm and demonstrates the division of the radial nerve proximal to the supinator.

10 cm above the medial epicondyle and through a dense, fibrous arcade of Struthers, a potential site of compressive entrapment. The nerve passes along the medial border of the triceps toward the posterior aspect of the medial epicondyle. Another occasional source of entrapment proximal to the epicondyle is an anomalous portion of the triceps inserting into the epicondyle. The nerve passes within the cubital tunnel, which is between the posterior epicondyle and the olecranon and is covered by the cubital retinaculum. The region of the cubital tunnel is a common site for ulnar nerve compressive entrapment neuropathies. There may be a deficient or absent posterior epicondylar groove, permitting medial subluxation of the nerve with flexion, extension, and valgus stress. The etiology can be an anatomic variant or abnormal functional stress, and at times a combination of the two. The ulnar nerve passes through the cubital tunnel and inferior to the epicondyle, where it is adjacent to the medial collateral ligament and under the arcuate ligament before passing between the two heads of the flexor carpi ulnaris, a

source of nerve irritation secondary to medial (ulnar) collateral ligament instability. The motor branches to the flexor carpi ulnaris, and an elbow articular branch, are the first to emerge from the ulnar nerve, at varying locations distal to the epicondyle. This area demands meticulous intraoperative surgical attention and technique. The anatomic sites most frequently associated with sports-related ulnar nerve symptoms are the arcade of Struthers, an aberrant band of triceps, the cubital tunnel (depth of groove and containment of retinaculum), the integrity of the medial collateral ligament and medial elbow capsule, the arcuate ligament, and the flexor carpi ulnaris muscle (see Chs. 3 and 19).

The median nerve enters the arm anterior to the brachial artery and crosses the intermuscular system to become medial to the biceps tendon and the brachial artery in the antecubital fossa. The median nerve lies on the surface of the brachialis muscle and beneath the bicipital aponeurosis (lacertus fibrosis) as it crosses the elbow. The median nerve provides some articular

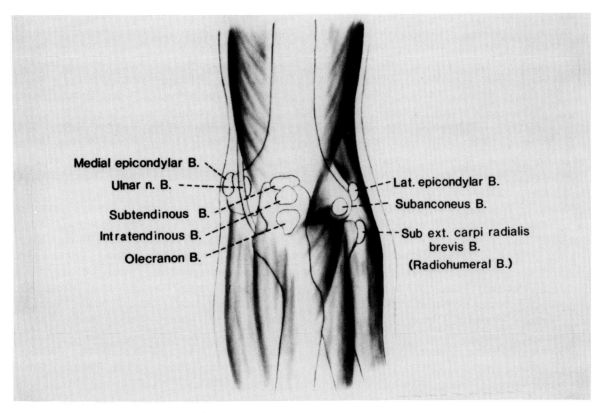

Figure 17-17 The posterior view of the elbow demonstrating the various bursae present about the elbow joint.

Figure 17-18 Diagrammed details of the rich arterial anastomoses about the elbow.

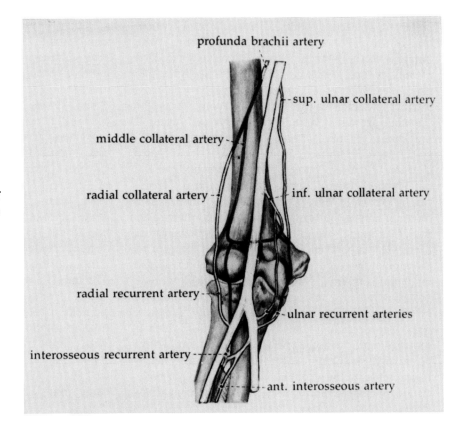

branches to the anterior elbow, and then passes between and supplies the motor branches of the humeral and ulnar heads of the pronator teres. Within a short distance, additional motor branches (all in a medial direction) are directed to the flexor carpi radialis, palmaris longus, and the flexor digitorum superficialis. The median nerve passes deep to the flexor superficialis and along the anterior interosseous membrane, becoming the anterior interosseous nerve, and providing branches to the flexor pollicis longus and a portion of the flexor digitorum profundus.

The anatomic site most associated with sport-related median nerve problems is the supracondylar area of the humerus secondary to fracture, direct contusion, hyperextension, and posterior dislocation of the elbow. Conditions most associated with sport-related median nerve problems include: 1) potential compression under the lacertus fibrosis secondary to biceps overdevelopment, 2) pronator teres syndrome secondary to overdevelopment or eccentric injury and swelling of the pronator teres, and 3) compression or injury at the arch of the flexor digitorum superficialis, that is, impending compartment syndrome.

The radial nerve, a continuation of the brachial plexus posterior cord, enters the arm in the posterior compartment where it provides branches for heads of the triceps. At approximately the midlevel of the humerus, it passes around the bone in the spiral radial groove, and enters the lateral compartment, approximately 10 cm above the lateral epicondyle. The location of the radial nerve around and adjacent to the humerus accounts for the associated neurologic deficits of trauma and surgery (see Ch. 3, Case Study I). The nerve lies under the brachioradialis and brachialis muscles and anterior to the lateral epicondyle. Motor branches are directed to the anconeus and terminal branches to the medial triceps, brachioradialis, and extensor carpi radialis longus. As the radial nerve passes over the lateral epicondyle and in the regions of the radiocapitellar articulations, it divides into the posterior interosseous and superficial radial nerves. The motor branch to the extensor carpi radialis brevis either is a direct branch from the radial or superficial radial nerve. The superficial radial nerve passes anterior to the supinator muscle and deep along the course of the brachioradialis to the distal forearm and hand. The posterior interosseous nerve (recurrent radial nerve) travels around the posterolateral aspect of the radius, passing through or under the supinator for which it provides motor branches. When it comes from within or under the supinator, it provides motor branches to the extensors of the wrist and hand and abductor pollicis longus. The posterior interosseous nerve, as it ap-

proaches the supinator muscle, passes under a fibrous arch, the arcade of Froshe, a common area for entrapment or compression (e.g., posterior interosseous nerve syndrome and some resistant tennis elbow symptoms). In addition, its relative location to the posterolateral radius is a site for potential injury associated with fractures of the proximal radius. Common sites of injury are around the spinal groove of the humerus, the arcade of Frohse, the posterior interosseous nerve along the radius, and the sensory nerve branch.

The musculocutaneous nerve is a mixed motor and sensory nerve that arises from the lateral cord of the brachial plexus. It pierces and innervates the coracobrachialis muscle, emerging below the coracoid, and travels distally between the biceps and brachialis muscles where it supplies innervation to each muscle. The sensory component then continues laterally to the biceps and becomes superficial anterolaterally as it penetrates the deep brachial fascia above the elbow. At this point, it becomes the lateral cutaneous nerve of the forearm. Athletic injuries of the anteroinferior area of the shoulder and medial brachium are the most common sites of musculocutaneous nerve damage (see Ch. 3, Case Study II).

ELBOW JOINT FUNCTION

The elbow is an integral link in the kinematics of all athletic activities that require upper extremity function. Stability of the elbow is essential for the transmission of activity from the shoulder to the wrist and the hand. Clinical problems that affect the shoulder will potentially affect the elbow. For example, a restriction of shoulder motion will increase the demand for forces that will be transmitted to the elbow, resulting in altered stress. Likewise, any injury to the radiocarpal or distal radius ulnar joint will potentially alter rotational strength and motion, thus altering the normal function of the elbow joint.

The elbow should not be thought of as purely a hinged joint of the humeral ulnar articulation. In addition to the flexion extension hinge motion, there are degrees of axial and angular change. The radiocapitellar joint is the most complex of the three elbow joints. The intricate relationship of the proximal radius and congruity of the depressed radial head on the spherical capitellum contributes to the multiple composite motions of rotation, flexion extension, and varus valgus. This complexity of motion is accommodated by the slight rotational effacement in the distal humerus as well as the angulated normal valgus alignment of the elbow joint. The proximal radioulnar joint is critical for both the rotational control of pronation and supination and the direction of radial head to the capitellum throughout the extreme ranges of radiocapitellar motion.

If any of these motions become excessive, most likely secondary to a fracture or congenital variant, an acute soft tissue injury, or associated with incremental ligamentous and muscular pathology, there will be an impact on athletic performance (i.e., radial head and neck fractures, capitellar fractures, coronoid fractures, medial collateral laxity, chronic medial or lateral epicondylitis, posteromedial traction osteophytes, and intra-articular cartilage damage).

The significant effect of ligament injury or disruption to elbow stability cannot be overemphasized. An acute disruption or progressive attenuation with secondary laxity of the medial collateral ligament, lateral collateral ligament, annular ligament will alter all degrees of potential motion, resulting in abnormal excessive motion causing a progressive alteration of athletic performance[4] (see Ch. 19).

The musculotendon effect on elbow function is more significant as a source of discomfort and secondary instability in conjunction with ligamentous alteration. Chronic musculotendon inflammatory conditions and unbalanced forces (e.g., medial elbow eccentric forces of pitching, lateral eccentric forces and inflammation of the tennis elbow, bicipital tendinitis of weight lifters) are examples of the inflammatory problems of musculotendon structures that cause imbalance, discomfort, and altered athletic performance.

This section focuses on the functional aspects of elbow motion and the baseball pitch. The athletic example is used to integrate the various anatomic aspects of the elbow articulation, stability, and total function. The stages of the baseball pitch (see Ch. 9) consist of the wind-up, cocking, acceleration, and deceleration stages. Similar stages have been defined for other athletic activities, (e.g., tennis, swimming, golf).

The coordinated motions of the shoulder and elbow are closely related in a timed sequence. Most of the stressful changes occur in the final stages of cocking through acceleration and ball release with lesser changes during the period of deceleration. When the pitcher has achieved the maximum cocking stage, the elbow is flexed to approximately 90 degrees, the early stage of valgus stress on the medial elbow. In the transitional moment from maximum cocking to initial acceleration, there is an additional 20 to 30 degrees of elbow flexion, an additional stress on the medial elbow. Some pitchers will refer to this as their moment of explosion or the initiation of arm speed. If all anatomic components are not integrated and synchronized, pain or instability will occur at this moment, and the remainder of the pitch will probably be biomechanically abnormal. The maximal stress on the medial elbow, as observed and calculated from 200 frames per second synchronized high-speed cinematography and computer-assisted analysis, is at the end of the cocking phase and the early acceleration phase, approximately 40 to 60 ms before ball release. As the shoulder initiates the acceleration phase of explosive internal rotation

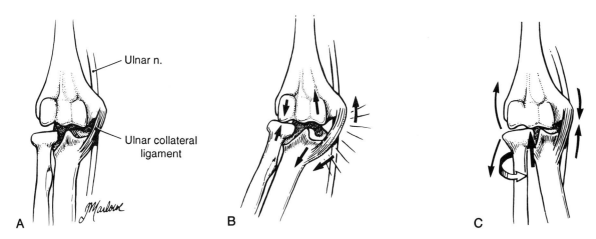

Figure 17-19 (A) Neutral position. (B) Forces on elbow at time of maximal cocking to early acceleration. The valgus force stresses all medial structures: medial collateral ligament, ulnar nerve, posterior medial insertion of triceps, and pronator flexor muscles originating from medial epicondyle. The varus compression force across radiocapitellar articulation, with elbow flexed and supinated. During this phase, the forearm is supinated. (C) After ball release, late acceleration to deceleration, the valgus force is directed to lateral elbow (much less than earlier medial valgus force and the radial head pronates and impacts on the inferomedial capitellum.

from a position of 150 degrees external rotation, elbow flexion increases to approximately 110 degrees, and the forearm is in near-full supination. This combination of forces concentrates on the medial elbow and challenges all of the anatomic structures with the combined axial and rotatory valgus force.[7] The forces at this time are valgus and eccentric contraction on the medial elbow and a varus compression, supination, and lateral muscle concentric contraction on the lateral elbow, concentric contraction of the biceps and brachialis muscles, and eccentric contraction of the triceps.

During these forces, the most clinically significant forces are on the medial and lateral sides of the elbow. On the medial elbow, the major stability that is challenged is that of the anterior band of the medial collateral ligament, with eccentric force on the pronator flexor muscle origins (Fig. 17-19). There is the potential for limited excursion of the ulnar nerve secondary to the shoulder external rotation, valgus force through the elbow, and wrist extension and supination. O'Driscoll and colleagues[6] have observed that with elbow flexion, there is compression and a decrease in size of the cubital tunnel which flattens the ulnar nerve (Fig.

17-20), and in extension, a recovery to maximal space/volume of the cubital tunnel.[6] The medial valgus traction force of overhead athletic activity, (e.g., baseball pitching) creates significant potential impact on ulnar nerve excursion. This valgus force is more significant if there is weakness or disruptions of the medial collateral ligament and/or chronic epicondylitis. The ultimate effect of elbow and wrist flexion, extension, and varying degrees of valgus is to increase the compression on the nerve and limit the excursion of the ulnar nerve, which produces neurologic symptoms.

The passage of the ulnar nerve between the two heads of the flexor carpi ulnaris is another site of potential nerve compressions. The two most common sport-related etiologies are overdevelopment of the flexor carpi ulnaris secondary to resistance weight training (heavy forearm curls) and spasticity of the flexor carpi ulnaris in crutch-using athletes, particularly individuals with cerebral palsy.

As the pitcher's elbow moves through the stage of acceleration, the forces are similar to the forces recorded at the shoulder in these stages—the elbow rapidly extends within a period of 20 ms from more

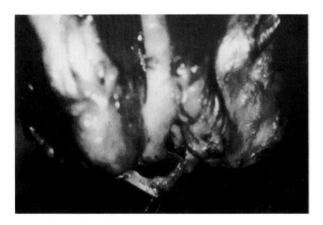
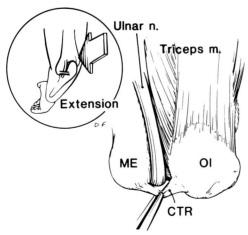

Figure 17-20 (A) Laxity of the retinaculum when the elbow is extended. **(B)** Compression of the retinaculum when the elbow is flexed acting as a compressive and constricting force along the ulnar nerve. (*Figure continues.*)

A

than 100 degrees of flexion to approximately 10 degrees of flexion. During this time, the velocity peaks at approximately 5,000 degrees per second[7] (Fig. 17-21). These changes appear to be occurring at a time that is virtually concurrent to the changes of position and velocity within the shoulder (see Ch. 9). While these forces and anatomic positions are changing, the medial valgus force subsides and there will be lateral radiocapitellar compression.

The articular forces change in the final stages of pitching—as the elbow extends, there is progressive pronation, resulting in a changing anatomic relationship of the radial head to the capitellum. In addition to the rotation, there is an axial force when the radial head impacts on the capitellum. During the final stages of pronation, the axial rotational shearing force is focused on the inferior and medial aspect of the capitellum. This is the force that causes some fibrillation and injury to the articular surface, and is generally the position and sequence noted at the termination of a baseball pitch. This compressive shearing force frequently results in articular changes that are the genesis of intra-articular cartilaginous fraying and the development of

osteocartilaginous fragments. In many instances the osteocartilaginous "loose bodies" are the result of fragments of cartilage undergoing metaplasia and growth within the synovial fluid medium.[8] The biceps is converting from a concentric to an eccentric contraction and the triceps is converting from an eccentric to a concentric contraction. The ability to facilitate these sudden changes in neuromuscle function is an important training consideration. If the conversion from eccentric to concentric and concentric to eccentric is not well coordinated, there will be additional stress on the ligaments and articulations of the elbow, especially the posterior olecranon impaction.

The pronation supination motion is directed by the radioulnar joint, which, if normally developed, is a stable articulation because of the annular ligament (see Ch. 8). The motion is also associated with minor degrees of varus valgus motion and some axial motion. It is these motions that are most significant when considering the negative effect of wrist pathology on elbow function. Any dysfunction of the distal radial ulnar joint or radiocarpal mechanism can cause pain and altered proximal radioulnar joint function. Any signif-

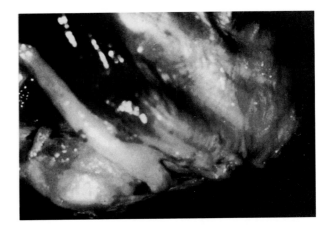

Figure 17-20 *(Continued)*

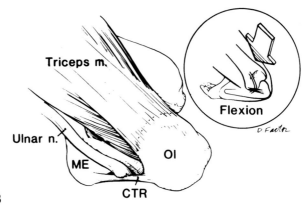

B

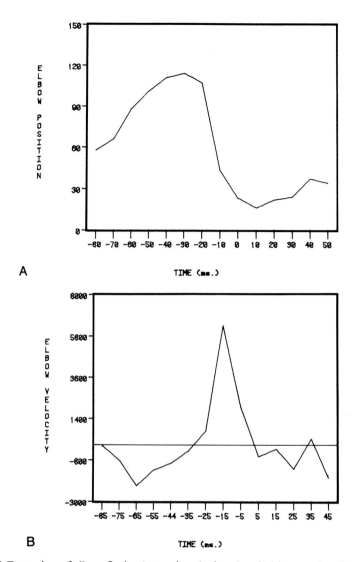

Figure 17-21 (A) Excursion of elbow flexion/extension during the pitching acceleration phase. Positive values are external rotation. Ball release occurred at zero on the time scale. (B) Velocity of elbow-extension during the pitching acceleration phase. The velocities shown are an average 10-ms time spans.

icant damage to the annular ligament will result in radioulnar and radiocapitellar instability and altered function associated with subluxation or frank dislocation of the radial head. In addition, deformities or injuries of the radial head will cause wrist discomfort and altered motion.

The final stages of the pitch from ball release through deceleration creates lesser forces medially and laterally. These forces are not nearly so significant as the early medial valgus and lateral compression. The final phase of the pitch is most involved with the concentric and eccentric changes in muscle function, most notably the deceleration of elbow flexion associated with biceps and brachialis eccentric contraction and triceps con-

centric contraction. If the forces are not closely integrated, the olecranon may impact on the posterior humerus, resulting in focal irritation and osteophytic impingement. The posterior elbow joint has different periods of impact during the baseball pitch — the early posteromedial valgus tension/traction and the final triceps extension traction and late pitching phase olecranon posterior humerus impaction.

When considering the osteology of the shoulder and elbow, both acceleration and deceleration within the elbow are potentially more stressful than to shoulder osteology. The bony constraints of the elbow limit the potential for mobility whereas the shoulder has more soft tissue constraints, allowing a longer deceleration moment and the potential for additional deceleration or eccentric injury of the soft tissues. The changes that occur from tennis and golf motion are not as stressful to the articulations when compared to the ligaments and musculotendon components.

REFERENCES

1. Henry, AK: Extensile Exposure. 2nd Ed. Williams & Wilkins, Baltimore, 1966
2. Morrey BF: In: The Elbow and Its Disorders. 2nd Ed. WB Saunders, Philadelphia, 1993
3. O'Driscoll SW et al: Anatomy of the attachment of the medial ulnar collateral ligament. J Hand Surg 17:154, 1992
4. Jobe F, Stark H, Lombardo SJ: Reconstruction of the ulnar collateral ligament in athletes. J Bone Joint Surg [AM] 68:1158, 1986
5. Morrey BF, Tanaha S, An KV: Valgus stability of the elbow. Clin Orthop 265:187, 1991
6. O'Driscoll SW et al: The cubital tunnel and ulnar neuropathy. J Bone Joint Surg [Br] 73:613, 1991
7. Pappas AM, Zawacki RM, Sullivan TJ: Biomechanics of baseball pitching: a preliminary report. Am J Sports Med 13:216, 1985
8. Milgram JW: The development of loose bodies in human joints. Clin Orthop 124:292, 1977

18

History and Examination of the Elbow

R. Maxwell Alley

Arthur M. Pappas

Proper treatment of the clinical problems and injuries of the athlete's elbow requires a clear and systematic diagnostic approach. Through a detailed history, the etiology, severity, and frequency of the injury can usually be determined. In conjunction with a careful physical examination, this will provide much of the information necessary for treating most athletes with elbow problems.

HISTORY

Standardized questionnaires (Figs. 18-1 and 18-2) streamline the interview component of the examination. Data are given by the patient without the potential distractions and anxiety associated with the examination room. The level of pain and disability of an injury is subjectively ranked by the patient. This offers a quick estimate of the severity of the injury and will help direct the course of the interview and examination. Moreover, this initial documentation is helpful when gauging the progress of rehabilitation.

An understanding of the mechanism of injury is critical for the diagnosis of any sports injury. It is essential to discern whether the injury is a result of a single,

violent force or the sum of repetitive stresses across the elbow. In the former injury, termed *macrotrauma,* a single force transmitted across the joint exceeds the yield point of the bone-ligament-tendon complex. A spectrum of injury severity does exist, depending on the energy of the force. Conversely, a *microtrauma* is the sum of repetitive lesser forces (each of which individually falls below a threshold for diagnosis of clinical injury), which eventually may produce a bone-ligament-tendon chronic attenuation and/or disruption. Thus, the injury patterns sustained while tackling a runner in football or falling during an alpine ski race differ from those incurred during repetitive activities, such as baseball pitching or hitting a backhand in tennis. Physically challenged athletes using wheelchairs are also subjected to repetitive stresses about the shoulder, elbow, and wrist. If the joint is required to assume weightbearing loads, as in Olympic style weight lifters or gymnasts, osteochondral fractures and osteoarthrosis are more common due to these increased compression and shearing forces.

The onset and frequency of the injury should then be considered. Is the onset of injury acute, with the athlete performing to his or her normal potential until the injury? If so, the injury was generally caused by a spe-

Name:_____

Date: _____ MR#: _____

PATIENT SCREEN (PREVISIT):

Completed by patient:

Sport(s): _____

               Competitive   Recreational

                  R   L

Hand used in eating/writing: _____   _____

Hand used in throwing: _____   _____

Hand used in batting: _____   _____

Describe (injury, condition, problem); be specific:

    Initial problem:

    How:

    When:

    Major problems:

    Major limitations:

Pain (with activity): _____Yes _____ No. If yes, complete below:

    Location (pain and activity):

    _____

    _____

Acute Pain Management Guideline Panel

0	1	2	3	4	5	6
None	Annoying	Uncomfortable	Dreadful	Horrible	Agonizing	

Pain (without activity): _____Yes _____ No. If yes, complete below:

    Location: Level

                               0   6

    _____   0   6

Pain on touch/pressure: _____Yes _____ No. If yes, complete below:

    Location: Level

                               0   6

    _____   0   6

Changes in sensation (numbness, dullness, etc.): _____Yes _____ No.

    If yes, describe (location, type, level):

    _____

    _____

Impact on/interference with athletic participation:

    _____Yes _____ No

                                                         (Continues)

Figure 18-1 Sample questionnaire to be filled out by the patient before being examined.

If yes, describe (amount of time, intensity level, ability to perform, etc.):

_____

_____

_____

On the scale below, rate how you "feel" about your injury.

      0 _____ 10

     (Best)   (Worst)

Medications taken: _____ Yes   _____ No

     If yes,   _____ Prescription   _____ Nonprescription

                 _____ Name   _____ Name

                 _____ Dosage   _____ Dosage

                 _____ Frequency   _____ Frequency

     Side effects: _____ Yes _____ No

         If yes, describe:

     Impact on performance: _____ Yes _____ No

         If yes, describe:

Daily activities affected in order of rank (worst/most painful = 1):

     _____ Putting on shirt, jacket, blouse

     _____ Taking off shirt, jacket, blouse

     _____ Putting on overhead sweater/shirt

     _____ Taking off overhead sweater/shirt

     _____ Eating/drinking

     _____ Driving

     _____ Removing milk jug from refrigerator

     _____ Carrying a suitcase

     _____ Tying shoes

     _____ Combing hair

     _____ Brushing teeth

     _____ Pulling off bed sheets/spreads

     _____ Rectal cleaning

     _____ Opening doors

     _____ Pushing doors/objects

     _____ Reaching for objects overhead

     _____ Other, describe

Assistive equipment used: _____ Yes _____ No

     If yes, describe (type, frequency/duration of use, affect):

Other concerns:

Figure 18-1 *(Continued)*

Name:_____
Date:_____ MR#: _____

ELBOW ASSESSMENT SCREEN

Presenting problems:
_____
_____

Associated problems:
_____
_____

Pre-examination observations:
  Difficulty with general activity: _____Yes _____ No
    If yes, describe:
  Arm symmetry when walking: _____Yes _____ No
    If no, describe:
  Pain or discomfort in evidence: _____Yes _____ No
    If yes, describe:

Physical examination—positive findings:
  Observations:
    Posture (head, shoulders, carrying angle, hand):
    Asymmetries:
    Areas of concern:
  Palpation:
    Pain/discomfort: _____Yes _____ No   Location: _____
    Joint/muscle/tendons: _____Yes _____ No   Location: _____
  Active motion (range and asymmetries):
    Movement patterns:

	Right		Left	
	Active	Passive	Active	Passive
Flexion:				
Extension:				
Pronation:				
Supination:				

    Quality of endpoint: _____ Firm   _____ Soft
    Crepitus: _____Yes _____ No

	Strength	Pain
Muscle performance:		
Flexion:		
Extension:		
Pronation:		
Supination:		
Selected movements related to sport:		

  Provocative tests:
    Varus/valgus stability:
    Extension overload:
    Pivot shift:
  Sensation:
    Reflexes:
  Ancillary tests:
  Other comments:
Impression: _____
_____

Other tests considered:
    _____
    _____
    _____

                                    _____   _____
                                    Signature   Date

Figure 18-2 Sample questionnaire used by the physician before and during the examination.

cific incident (e.g., a triceps rupture in the previously asymptomatic weight lifter or osteocartilaginous fragments in a gymnast).

A recurrent injury is one in which the athlete sustains the injury, appears to improve and is able to perform to his or her usual level, and then a reinjury occurs (e.g., recurrent lateral epicondylitis in the mature recreational tennis player or triceps tendinitis in the body builder or weight lifter). These athletes seem to experience periods when they are performing to their usual level, but then resuming repetitive training activities results in a decreased level of performance.

Chronic injuries are those that create a cycle of decreased performance or an inability to perform the particular sport (e.g., chronic medial collateral ligament instability or ulnar nerve irritation in the professional or collegiate baseball pitcher). These are sometimes the most difficult elbow problems to diagnose and treat, since the symptoms have occurred and recurred for a prolonged period of time. In the skeletally immature pitcher, medial epicondylitis is an example of a chronic injury (see Ch. 8).

The severity of the injury should then be considered, since this will affect the athlete's ability to perform. A grade I sprain of the ulnar collateral ligament complex sustained by a football tackle is a separate and much less debilitating injury than an incompetent ulnar collateral ligament from repetitive indirect trauma in the javelin thrower. Also, an injury such as a biceps tendon rupture or a dislocation of the elbow with accompanying risk of heterotopic bone formation is more severe than a triceps or biceps tendinitis where the athlete can perform (though at a decreased level). Associated symptoms such as numbness or paresthesias should also be noted. Are there any complaints of popping, locking, or clicking? When a sudden loss of motion occurs without injury, one should suspect an intra-articular loose body.

When no obvious causal incident is offered by the patient, the examiner must search for any changes in the athlete's equipment and training performance regimen. A change of equipment (e.g., composite tennis racquet, longer golf clubs) may be the etiology of the injury or reduction in performance. Any increase in the intensity or duration of workouts should be noted. Has the weight lifter been increasing his maximum weight or the baseball player taking extra batting practice? Has the baseball pitcher been learning a new pitch (i.e., slider or curve ball?)

It should always be remembered that injury of anatomically distant areas may alter mechanics and place new demands on the athlete's elbow. Any related factors such as injuries to the neck, shoulder, wrist, or hand should be reviewed. For example, a relatively minor shoulder injury in a football quarterback may

place the elbow at risk of injury. Injuries to the cervical spine or the shoulder are often referred to the elbow, while injuries to the hand and wrist can be proximally referred.

Other related information includes the age and development of the athlete. Certain injuries to the elbow of a skeletally immature pitcher will be different from those sustained by a collegiate athlete or an adult recreational athlete. The injuries in the adolescent population are more likely to be medial epicondylar or capitellar-type problems, whereas those in the mature athlete are more likely to be ligamentous or degenerative in nature, such as ulnar collateral ligaments, spurs, or osteophytic processes in the joint. Once these historical facts are obtained, the clinician can proceed with a careful physical examination and evaluation of the injured athlete.

The transition to the physical examination should be made with the clinical examiner present. In a somewhat distracted setting, one can gain valuable observations of the patient's elbow function during activities of daily living. The examiner should observe upper extremity contribution while the patient rises from a chair or removes outer garments. Expressions of discomfort and an impression of overall function should be noted before a structured, thoughtful physical examination.

PHYSICAL EXAMINATION

Physical examination of the athlete's elbow begins with an unobstructed exposure of both upper extremities and the full torso. The elbow must be viewed as a link in a kinetic chain of several joints. Function in the athlete must follow from the lower extremity of the axial skeleton to the upper extremity. This continuity of function demands that one rule out any related or referred problems when diagnosing an upper extremity injury. Examination of these anatomically distant though functionally related areas is usually performed first. This order provides several benefits. The patient is given an opportunity to relax, as this aspect of the examination is seldom painful, but more important, it ensures that this significant part of the examination will not be inadvertently omitted. Careful attention must be paid to the cervical spine where neuropathy may simulate elbow disease. In a similar manner, a complete examination of the shoulder, the wrist, and the hand must be undertaken to eliminate these areas as possible causes of elbow pain.

The majority of the formal elbow component of the examination may be performed with the patient seated and should follow a standard planned sequence. Comparison is always made with the contralateral uninjured extremity. This is especially helpful in athletes with generalized joint laxity to prevent overdiagnosis.

Our preferred order of the examination is as follows:

1. inspection;
2. palpation;
3. active motion;
4. passive motion;
5. individual muscle examinations;
6. sensation tests;
7. reflex tests;
8. provocative tests.

Depending on the findings of the examination, further tests (plain or stress radiographs, arthrograms, magnetic resonance imaging, electromyograms) may be obtained.

Inspection

The trained examiner can obtain much information from visual inspection of the elbow. Since much of the joint is subcutaneous, alterations in musculoskeletal anatomy are often detectable. Usually soft tissue swelling, joint effusion, or muscle atrophy can be visualized. In addition, areas of contusion or ecchymosis, indicating a traumatic superficial or deep injury, may be observed. The topographic location of such ecchymosis will suggest certain injuries. For example, if the examiner observes swelling and bruising proximally in the cubital fossa, a biceps tendon rupture should be suspected. Observation of the carrying angle, when compared to the nondominant side, may suggest prior trauma or growth disturbance. Determining the carrying angle is usually accomplished by holding the hand supinated and the elbow in full extension. Throwing athletes will often have a combined deformity of flex-

ion and valgus on the dominant arm. At times this may be difficult to diagnose due to the frequent flexion deformity in those that are long-standing throwers; such a contracture may mask a significant humeroulnar malalignment. Observation of fullness about the recess inferior to the lateral condyle may suggest synovitis with increased joint fluid or radial head pathology. The prominent subcutaneous olecranon bursa is readily observed posteriorly when it is distended, and this may indicate some type of traumatic, infectious, or inflammatory effusion or olecranon bursitis.

Palpation

Medial

Careful palpation of bony landmarks is performed in a stepwise fashion. Beginning at the medial epicondyle, discomfort associated with compression of the medial epicondyle suggests either acute or chronic tendon avulsion. Palpation begins with the flexor pronator muscle origins and their attachment to bone. (Fig. 18-3) This is the area where developmental problems can exist for the skeletally immature. The examiner searches for a defect, tenderness, or nodules in the muscles of the pronator, flexor carpi radialis, palmaris longus, and flexor carpi ulnaris. The examiner must also palpate and percuss along the course of the ulnar nerve and cubital tunnel to determine if there is any ulnar nerve tenderness, soft tissue masses, or bony protrusion. A positive Tinel's sign demonstrates irritability of the ulnar nerve. Hypermobility of the nerve may be seen with attempts to manually sublux it from the cubital tunnel. Palpation along the medial joint line may reveal any osteophytes or spurring of the olecranon or medial epicondyle. Finally, palpating along the course

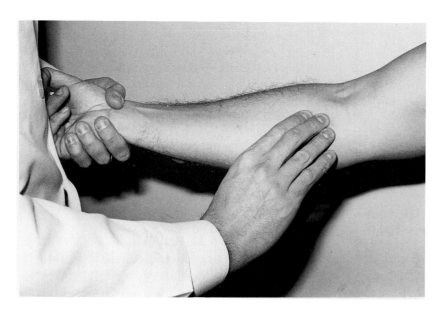

Figure 18-3 Palpation of the medial elbow should include the flexor/pronator muscle mass as well as the medial epicondyle.

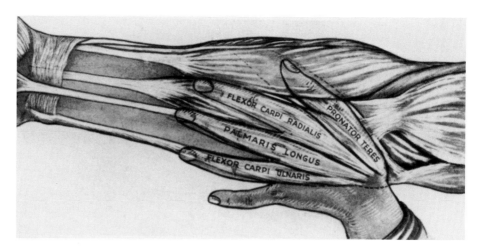

Figure 18-4 Anatomy of the medial elbow.

of medial collateral ligament may reveal injury to this structure at its origin, insertion, or intrasubstance (Fig. 18-4).

Lateral

Lateral palpation begins along the lateral epicondyle and lateral supracondylar ridge. Palpation of the mobile wad of the three muscles, the brachioradialis, the extensor carpi radialis longus, and the extensor carpi radialis brevis, is then undertaken, with any defects or areas of tenderness noted (Fig. 18-5). The radial head and the radial capitellar articulation may then be palpated for crepitus or osteophytic spurs. This should be performed while gently pronating and supinating the forearm in varying degrees of elbow flexion, allowing the examiner to feel the entire radial head as well as its articulation with the capitellum. At all degrees of elbow flexion, the radial head should have a constant, firm articulation with the capitellum. An increased prominence or discomfort during pronation and supination of the radial head should suggest fracture, arthrosis, or dislocation.

Posterior

The important relationship of the epicondyle and the olecranon can also be appreciated with the elbow in flexion. The medial and lateral epicondyles and the tip of the olecranon form an equilateral triangle while in flexion. This relationship usually becomes a straight line when the elbow is held in full extension (Figs. 18-6). When this normal relationship is observed, it allows the examiner to rule out a fracture or dislocation of the elbow. Deep pressure allows the examiner to appreciate the tip of the olecranon. Generally, this is done with the arm held in approximately 15 degrees of flexion to release tension on the triceps tendon. The posterior, medial, and lateral aspects of the olecranon

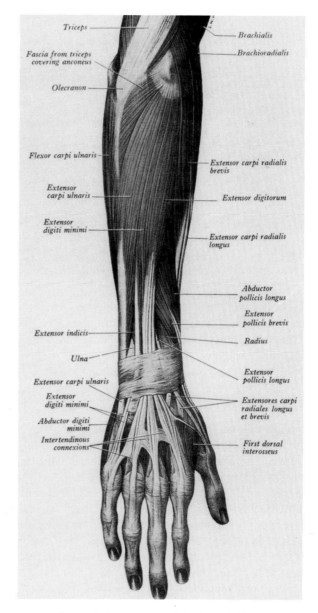

Figure 18-5 Anatomy of the lateral elbow.

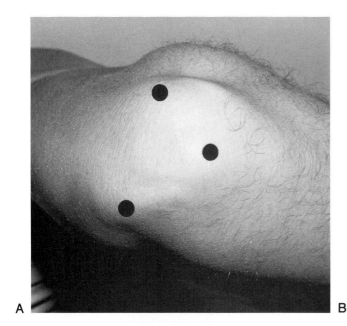
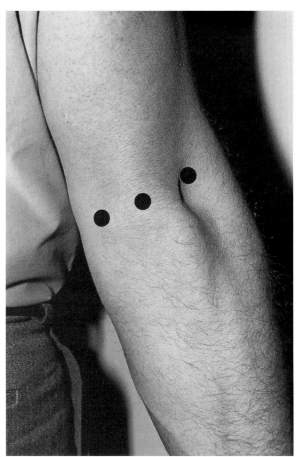

Figure 18-6 The lateral epicondyle, medial epicondyle, and olecranon form **(A)** an equilateral triangle when in flexion and **(B)** a straight line when in extension.

are palpated for evidence of osteophytes, crepitus, or loose bodies. The olecranon bursa is examined for tenderness, since inflammation often arises after direct contact in sports such as football, hockey, or lacrosse, especially when played on artificial turf. The integrity of the triceps tendon may be assessed as well.

Anterior

The cubital fossa is bound laterally by the brachioradialis and medially by the pronator teres. Structures in this area include the bicipital tendon, the lacertus fibrosis, brachial artery, median nerve, the terminal portion of the musculocutaneous nerve, and the lateral antebrachial cutaneous nerve. The deep structure overlying the anterior capsule, the brachialis muscle, can be found in the floor of the antecubital fossa (Fig. 18-7). In this area, the examiner can palpate the brachial artery pulse and tenderness along the course of the median nerve. Soft tissue masses, such as lipomas, may exert compressive effects in this area. In addition, the

examiner can palpate the biceps tendon to detect swelling, tenderness, or rupture.

Range of Motion: Active and Passive

Elbow joint motion occurs about two axes, flexion-extension and pronation-supination. Normally, a few degrees of varus-valgus motion should exist. When nonphysiologic varus-valgus motion exists, ligament incompetence and/or bony deficiency is present. Arcs should be measured and recorded both actively and passively, with a comparison to the contralateral elbow noted. Normal flexion-extension is from 0 to 140 degrees, while supination-pronation is 90 degrees, respectively.[1] Any discrepancy between active and passive arcs can usually be attributed to pain. When a deficit does exist, the quality of the end point should be characterized.

Firm end points are often due to bony blocks, arising from joint incongruity, osteochondral loose bodies, or

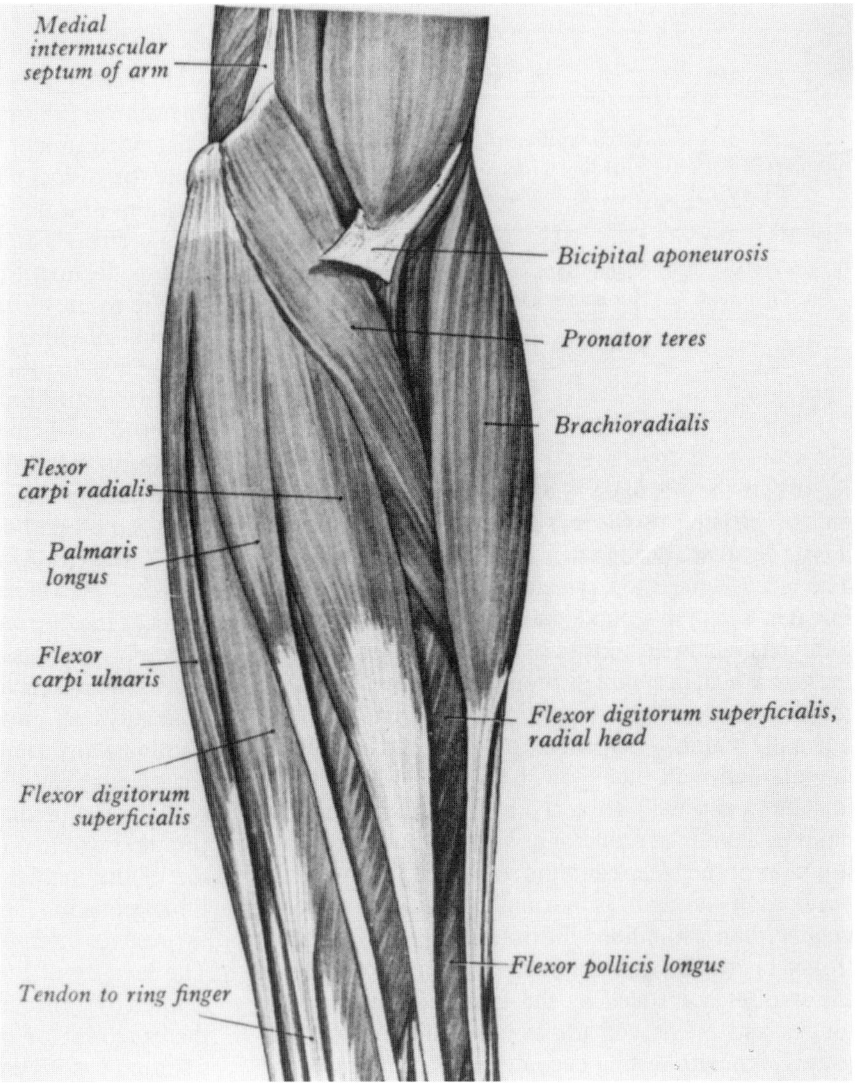
Medial intermuscular septum of arm
Bicipital aponeurosis
Pronator teres
Brachioradialis
Flexor carpi radialis
Palmaris longus
Flexor carpi ulnaris
Flexor digitorum superficialis, radial head
Flexor digitorum superficialis
Flexor pollicis longus
Tendon to ring finger

Figure 18-7 Anatomy of the anterior elbow.

congenital or acquired synostoses. When assessing a loss of pronation or supination, the entire length of the forearm must be examined, since distal radioulnar incongruity may be the cause. When pronation-supination is limited, wrist symptoms often evolve as more demands for motion are placed on it.

Soft, rubbery end points are more often caused by soft tissue contractures. Flexion contractures are commonly encountered in throwing athletes and weight lifters, presumably caused by recurrent anterior capsular sprains, brachialis injury, or forearm flexor strain. Pathology of the radial head or capitellum may result in flexion contracture and in a decreased pronation-supination arc. Gymnasts have been found to exhibit a statistically significant increase in elbow supination (although not in elbow extension) when compared with age-matched controls.[2]

Strength Testing and Muscle Examination

Strength testing should be included in the physical examination. Although the grading of muscle strength is a subjective examination, it is the basis for assigning a comparative normative grade (see Ch. 10 for more information on muscle testing). A numerical scale (Table 18-1) is most commonly used. Interobserver differences are often due to variations in examination technique. Many muscles have more than one function, and most movements are controlled by more than a single muscle. Thus, the use of different starting points may affect perceived muscle strength.[3]

Flexion and extension strength testing are conducted against resistance with the forearm in neutral rotation and the elbow at 90 degrees of flexion. The major elbow

Table 18-1   Grading of Muscle Strength

Grade	Observation
0/0	No contraction
I/TR	Twitch
II/Poor	Joint movement with gravity eliminated
III/Fair	Joint movement against gravity
IV/Good	Slightly damaged strength
V/Normal	Normal strength

flexors are the brachialis, the biceps, and the brachioradialis. The latter two flexors cross two joints; therefore, it is understandable that they both have several actions. The biceps appear to have increased activity when the forearm is held in complete supination, and the brachioradialis seems to increase its activity of flexion when the arm is held in complete pronation. The triceps is the major extender of the elbow joint. Extension strength is normally about 70 percent of that flexion strength and is measured with the elbow at 90 degrees of flexion. Pronation is usually governed by the force of the pronator teres and the pronator quadratus. Supination is a function of the biceps and the supinator (Table 18-2). Supination strength is normally about 15 percent greater than pronation. Flexion of the wrist is controlled by the flexor pronator group, while extension of the wrist is controlled by the extensor carpi radialis longus and brevis and the extensor digitorum communis. Strength testing becomes important in testing for problems to this area, including "tennis elbow" injuries.

Instability Test

The bony architecture of the elbow does provide a measure of inherent stability; however, both acute and chronic ligament injuries do occur. Elbow subluxations or dislocations may result from vigorous arm tackling or a fall on the outstretched arm. Repetitive valgus stresses during pitching or batting may cause a chronic ligament insufficiency.

Due to the close proximity of the structures on the medial side of the elbow, it is often difficult to determine by palpation alone whether there is injury to the important ligamentous stabilizing structures, such as the medial collateral ligament. Dynamic testing for determining stability of the medial collateral ligament is important in the examination of elbow stability in athletes. To properly assess integrity of the collateral ligament, the elbow should be flexed to about 20 to 30 degrees. This flexion relaxes the anterior capsule and unlocks the olecranon from its bony fossa on the distal humerus. Valgus stress is then applied with the humerus in full external rotation, which brings the medial epicondyle anteriorly. This will enable the examiner to eliminate any rotation of the humerus as a valgus force is applied to the elbow. At the same time, the examiner palpates the medial joint line to assess for any distraction that would indicate an injury to the anterior bundle of the medial collateral ligament, its most functional portion (Fig. 18-8). The degree of valgus as well as presence or absence of an end point should be noted. The severity of the instability may be graded I to III, defined by 5-mm increments of medial opening. When there is suspicion of a lateral collateral ligament injury, a similar test is performed with the arm in full internal rotation, allowing the examiner to apply varus stress and eliminate rotation of the humerus. The examiner

Table 18-2   Muscle Examination and Normal Range of Motion

Motion	Muscle Groups	Innervation	Normal ROM End Point (degrees)
Flexion	Brachioradialis Biceps brachii Brachialis	Musculocutaneous Radial	140
Extension	Triceps	Radial	0
Pronation	Pronator teres Pronator Quadratus	Median	90
Supination	Biceps Supinator	Musculocutaneous Radial	90

ROM, range of motion.

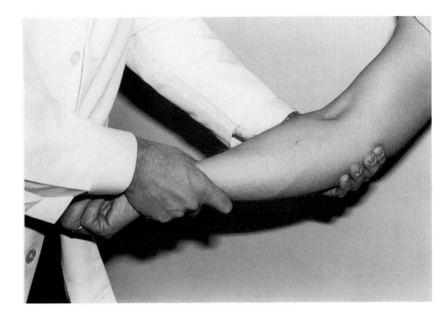

Figure 18-8 When assessing for medial instability, the arm should be positioned with the humerus fully externally rotated. The medial joint line should be palpated while a valgus stress is applied to the forearm.

then palpates along the lateral joint line, assessing for any opening.

Provocative Tests

In the differential diagnosis of medial elbow pain, it is important to eliminate other sources of injury. Injury to the flexor pronator tendon origin or medial epicondylitis (commonly seen in golfers and baseball pitchers) can be elicited by having the athlete flex the wrist and fingers against resistance, producing pain at the flexor pronator tendon or at the medial epicondyle. Pain about the epicondyle is commonly attributed to repetitive indirect injury with irritation and/or partial tendinous detachment; however, violent forces may also cause avulsion of the flexor pronator origin or intramuscular tears (Fig. 18-9). Palpation over the medial epicondyle may help differentiate an avulsion injury from a flexor pronator tendonitis, depending on the location of the tenderness. In addition, the examiner may extend the wrist and fingers passively and also produce pain by stretching the common tendon origin at the medial epicondyle. Intramuscular tears in throwing athletes occur during eccentric muscle contraction and may heal with nodule formation. The location of these nodules varies with the predominant type of pitch thrown. Curveball pitchers tend to injure the finger and wrist flexor muscles, while the pronator teres muscle is more commonly injured when throwing a slider.

Injury to the flexor digitorum sublimis muscle can be determined by holding the wrist in neutral extension and applying passive extension to the fingers or flexion of the fingers against resistance (Fig. 18-10). Forearm pain elicited with these maneuvers would indicate a tear in the flexor digitorum sublimis muscle. We have seen this in several baseball catchers who sustained the injury making snap throws. A large forearm hematoma results, and one must be watchful for an evolving compartment syndrome.

Ulnar nerve compression or neuritis may be another cause of medial elbow pain. The elbow flexion test consists of full elbow flexion for 5 minutes and is con-

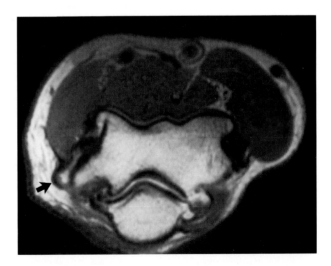

Figure 18-9 MRI of a professional baseball pitcher demonstrating fluid *(arrow)* between the pronator teres and medial epicondyle consistent with tendon avulsion.

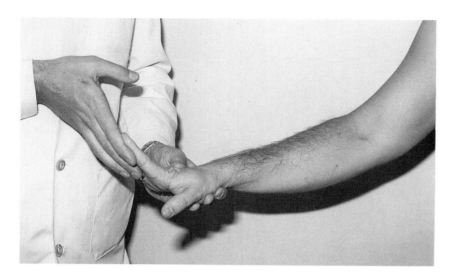

Figure 18-10 Forearm pain upon passive finger extension suggests flexor digitorum sublimis muscle injury.

sidered positive when it elicits symptoms such as pain, paresthesis, or numbness along the distribution of the elbow nerve to the small finger and half of the ring finger. Another finding is recurrent dislocation or subluxation of the ulnar nerve from the cubital tunnel as the elbow is taken from complete extension to full flexion.[4] The nerve is more susceptible to direct trauma or friction neuritis in athletes with nerve hypermobility (see Chs. 3 and 4).

When assessing ulnar nerve compression about the elbow, several etiologies must be considered. Compression may occur proximally by the lateral intermuscular septum. The valgus strain encountered by throwing athletes commonly leads to scarring within the cubital tunnel with secondary nerve compression. Occasionally a discrete constriction may cause a bulbous expansion of the nerve proximal to the tunnel[5] (Fig. 18-11).

Distally, compression may occur as the nerve passes between the muscle bellies of the flexor carpi ulnaris. We have seen this in a pitcher with muscle hypertrophy caused by wrist curls. The location of Tinel's sign is very helpful in rotating the anatomic site of compression.

Tennis elbow is the most common diagnosis of lateral elbow pain. Symptoms may be reproduced by either direct pressure or maneuvers that increase tension at the site of origin of the extensor carpi radialis brevis muscle. If one holds the elbow in full extension and passively flexes the wrist, pain will be elicited at the lateral epicondyle (Fig. 18-12). Another diagnostic test is resistance against active dorsiflexion of the wrist, with the elbow in full extension, which produces pain. One must also remember that radial nerve compression may be the etiology of a recalcitrant tennis elbow,

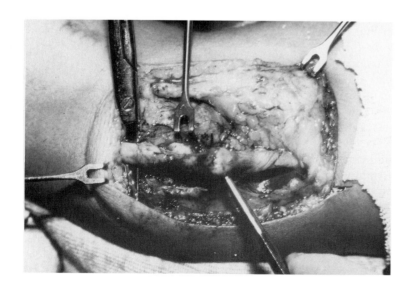

Figure 18-11 Bulbous expansion of ulnar nerve proximal to area of constriction within cubital tunnel.

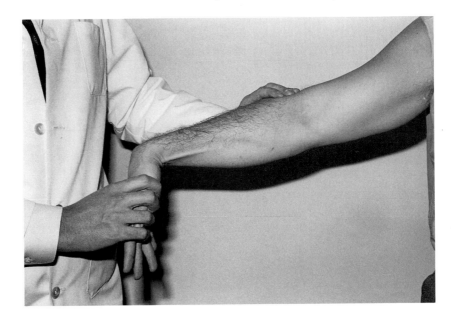

Figure 18-12 Passive wrist flexion, with the elbow in extension, produces pain laterally with tennis elbow.

especially when tenderness is present over the supinator.

There are two tests to rule out radial nerve pathology. When the examiner finds increased pain on resisted active supination of the forearm, this may indicate compression of the radial nerve in the area of the arcade of Frohse. The second test to differentiate radial tunnel syndrome is the middle finger test described by Lister.[6] The patient is instructed to extend the elbow, wrist, and middle finger and then hold the middle finger extended against resistance. In the case of radial nerve entrapment, all pain is referred to the point of the entrance of the radial nerve into the area of the supinator (Fig. 18-13).

Valgus stress in throwing sports can initiate degenerative wear through impingement of the olecranon on the posteromedial aspect of the distal humerus or olecranon fossa.[7] To test for this valgus overload, the partially flexed elbow is brought into a valgus position and then forcefully extended to abut the olecranon against its medial fossa to reproduce symptoms (Fig. 18-14). It is important to rule out any bony tenderness along the proximal portion of the olecranon. Stress fractures have been known to occur in throwers, weight lifters, and gymnasts.[8] In addition, it is also important to perform active triceps extension against resistance to rule out any injury to the triceps tendon.

Injury to the lateral stabilizing complex, specifically the lateral ulnar collateral ligament, may produce posterolateral elbow instability. The pivot shift test is a provocative maneuver used to diagnose this entity.[9] With the humerus stabilized, the fully supinated fore-

Figure 18-13 Radial nerve compression may be diagnosed by pain on resisted long-finger extension.

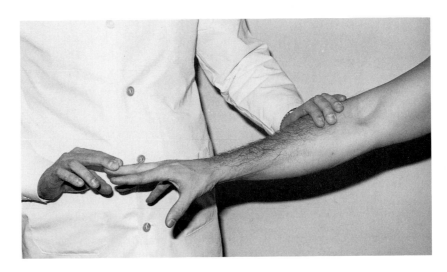

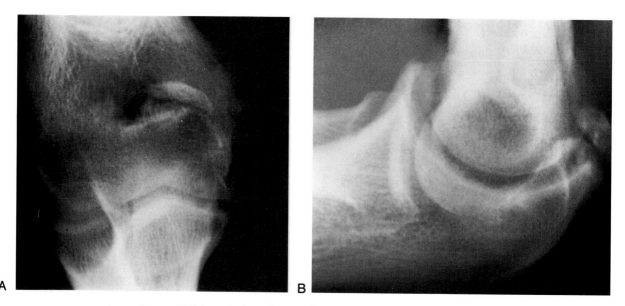

Figure 18-14 **(A)** AP-view and **(B)** lateral-view elbow radiographs demonstrate an olecranon stress fracture in a professional baseball outfielder.

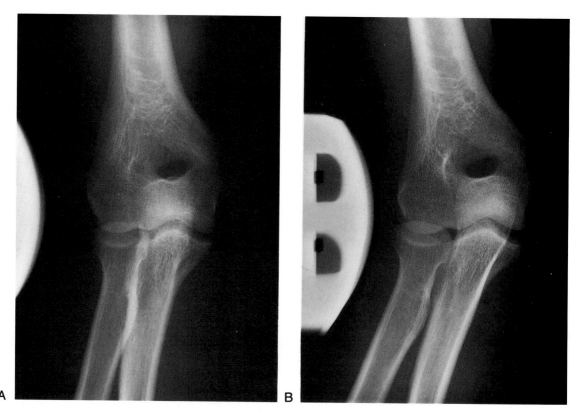

Figure 18-15 Valgus stress radiographs **(A)** control **(B)** medial opening consistent with medial collateral ligament insufficiency. (Courtesy of Dr. Arie M. Rijke, University of Virginia.)

arm is brought from flexion to extension while valgus and axial compressive movements are applied to the elbow. If instability is present, the ulnohumeral joint will rotate about the intact medial collateral ligament, and the radial head will sublux posteriorly. Relocation accompanied by a palpable pop is produced with subsequent elbow flexion and represents a positive test. With disruption of the annular ligament, the biceps pull results in anterior subluxation of the radial head.

Finally, anterior problems such as median nerve entrapment, vascular injury, or biceps tendon pathology must be ruled out. Proximal forearm pain may be increased by resistance to pronation and elbow flexion along with flexion of the wrist, producing a dull proximal forearm pain with this maneuver. Pain in the proximal forearm that is increased by resistance to supination is suggestive of compression of the median nerve by lacertus fibrosis. Resistive active long-finger flexion produced by the flexor digitorum sublimis may produce pain of the proximal forearm when compression of the median nerve is at the flexor digitorum superficialis arch.

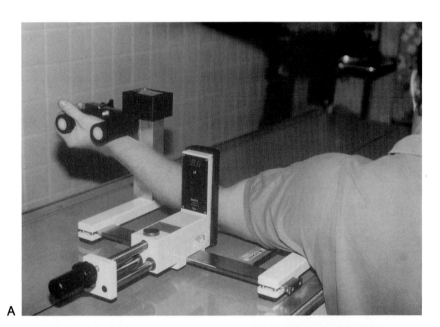

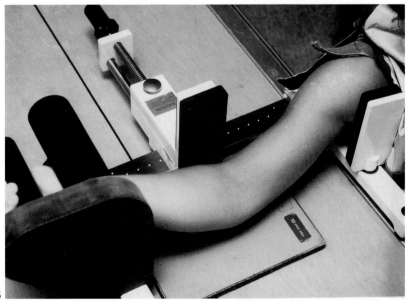

Figure 18-16 (A & B) Telos stress device for elbow radiography. (Courtesy of Dr. Arie M Rijkje, University of Virginia.)

Ancillary Studies

The history and physical examination should form a narrow differential diagnosis for most elbow injuries. Ancillary studies, usually done routinely, should be used for diagnostic confirmation.

Radiographs in the anteroposterior, lateral, and oblique planes comprise the standard elbow views. When there is suspicion of ulnar neuritis, a cubital tunnel view may be obtained in the search for osteophytic impingement. Stress views of the elbow may aid in quantifying instability (Fig. 18-15). A Telos stress device (Fig. 18-16) shields the technician from exposure and applies a reproducible force. Comparison views with the opposite elbow are often helpful.

Arthrography, though mildly invasive, is useful for assessment of articular contours. Physeal fractures,[10] osteochondral fractures, and radiolucent loose bodies may all be seen.

Magnetic resonance imaging (MRI) may provide information on soft tissue injuries not apparent on plain radiographs. Tendon and ligament injuries as well as ulnar neuritis produce characteristic signal changes on MRI. Electromyography and nerve conduction velocity testing is best reserved for complex cases with diagnostic ambiguity (see Ch. 3 and 4). While not necessary in all cases of nerve compression, electromyography and nerve conduction velocity may be beneficial when a double crush syndrome is suspected (see Ch. 1).

An accurate diagnosis of elbow injuries in athletes follows from a careful history and physical examination. Many injuries will be apparent, while others, such as instability, may be quite subtle. If a complete examination becomes routine for the examiner, these subtle abnormalities will be more easily recognized.

REFERENCES

1. Morrey BF, Askew LJ, An KN, Chaso EY: A biomechanical study of normal functional elbow motion. J Bone Joint Surg [Am] 63:872, 1981
2. Kirby RL, Simms FC, Symington: VJ: Flexibility and musculoskeletal symptomatology in female athletes and age-matched controls. Am J Sports Med 9:160, 1981
3. Williams M, Stutzman L: Strength variation through the range of motion. Phys Ther Rev 39:145, 1959
4. Childress HM: Recurrent ulnar nerve dislocation at the elbow. Clin Orthop 108:168, 1975
5. Cabrera JM, McCue FC III: Nonosseous athletic injuries of the elbow, forearm and hand. Clin Sport Med 5:681, 1986
6. Lister G: The radial tunnel syndrome. J Hand Surg 4:52, 1959
7. Wilson RD, Andrews JR, Blackburn TA, McCluskey G: Valgus extension overload in the pitching elbow. Am J Sport Med 11:83, 1983
8. Hulkko A, Orava S, Nikula P: Stress fractures of the olecranon in javelin throwers. Int J Sports Med 7:210, 1986
9. O'Driscoll SW, Bell DF, Morrey BF: Posterolateral rotatory instability of the elbow. J Bone Joint Surg [Am] 73:440, 1991
10. Marzo JM, d'Amato C, Strong M, Gillespie R: Usefulness and accuracy of arthrography in management of lateral humeral condyle fractures in children. J Pediatr Orthop 10:317, 1990

19

Acute and Chronic Performance-Related Injuries of the Elbow

R. Maxwell Alley

Arthur M. Pappas

Successful participation in most athletic activities requires skilled coordination of the upper extremities. The elbow is susceptible to injury by a number of mechanisms depending on the specifics of a given sport. The three clinical stages of injury (acute, recurrent, and chronic) and the related cellular and functional performance changes determine the ultimate impact of the injury. Every athlete presents individual tissue physiology along with individual performance characteristics that influence each of these stages in similar anatomic areas. For example, the cocking/acceleration phase of a baseball pitch imposes multiple forces concurrently and sequentially on the multiple structures of the medial side of the elbow and the performance effect will vary. Acute and repetitive stress to the medial elbow's multiple structures must be specifically evaluated in light of an injury to the structures. If the stress of the medial collateral ligament is increased, and the athlete possesses a lax ligamentous structure, he or she will present with medial ligamentous instability. This ligamentous laxity may cause some changes of ulnar nerve function, resulting in progressive ulnar nerve symptomatology. The repetitive strain on the muscles originating from the medial epicondyle can cause an increase in inflammatory and fibrous tissue,

clinically represented as acute and progressing to chronic medial epicondylitis. The cartilage of the articular surface may respond with the formation of osteophytes or osteochondral disruption.

The degree of injury can range from normal microinjury associated with each performance to a more significant macroinjury caused by an abnormal biomechanic force. A certain degree of microtrauma occurs with every major exertional performance, immediately manifested by swelling, sensitivity, and a recovery interval. Tissue recovery may be influenced by incomplete rehabilitation, the incomplete or incompetent reparative tissues that vary among individuals, and the age and physical demands of the athlete. The spectrum of repetitive and microimpact activity ranges from growth and development changes of the skeletally immature athlete to acute and recurrent inflammatory and fibrous repair in the younger skeletally mature athlete to ultimately the diminished recovery potential and gradual degeneration in the senior athlete. If additional moderate to severe micro- or macroinjury occurs, there may not be a normal healing response in addition to a more significant change in tissue structure and a negative effect on future athletic performance.

A change in performance may predispose the athlete to a specific focal area of discomfort. For example, if a baseball pitcher slips from the mound during a pitch delivery or attempts to throw a maximum output pitch with a slight alteration of his pitching sequence, a significant injury may occur (i.e., macrotrauma). When cyclic strain to a previously injured area is continuous, the subsequent healing and performance potential of the tissues may be altered. The cellular changes may include progressive neuropathy, more chronic inflammatory tissue, limited or excessive flexibility of ligamentous and muscle tissues, or additional articular cartilage and subchondral bone alterations. These tissue changes will influence the athlete's standard of performance as well as the ability to continue each performance for an extended period, characteristics both reflective of the chronic nature of performance-related injuries. The time necessary for tissue healing, rehabilitation, and functional recovery will vary, depending on the relative acute or chronic nature of the injury and the specific tissues involved. Regardless of the severity of the injury, there will be some residual effect on all the involved tissues, resulting in fibrosis and loss of normal excursion and flexibility as well as articular and bony changes. The remainder of this chapter follows a correlative anatomic and functional approach to acute and chronic performance-related injuries of the elbow in athletes. An anatomic regional basis will focus on the anterior, lateral, posterior, and medial quadrants of the elbow as well as related intra-articular factors. The pathologic changes associated with specific acute and chronic performance-related clinical problems will be presented to correlate with known anatomic changes (see Ch. 8).

While discussing each injury individually, it is important to recognize and emphasize the interactive nature of these injuries. Often disruption of one structure will make other structures more prone to injury. This domino effect may be especially difficult to sort out in chronic conditions.

FRACTURES AND DISLOCATIONS

Since many athletic events include contact between competitors, a variety of fractures and dislocations may be seen in the athletic population. Many elbow fractures sustained by football players, jockeys, and sports vehicle drivers are more appropriately considered multiple trauma than sports injuries. The following is a brief discussion of the more commonly encountered elbow fractures and dislocations seen in athletes. For a complete discussion, the reader should refer to the appropriate texts.[1,2]

Fractures

Radial Head Fractures

Radial head fractures are typically seen in collision sports and gymnastics. The usual mechanism is a fall on the outstretched arm or an axial force to the elbow, which combined with angular and rotational forces contribute to an anatomic definition of injury. There is a range of injury severity, and accurate diagnosis and treatment are imperative for the athlete to regain full motion and stability.

The athlete will complain of pain laterally over the elbow, especially with pronation and supination of the forearm and local pressure applied to the radial head area. The interosseous space and distal radioulnar joint should be inspected for tenderness, which when

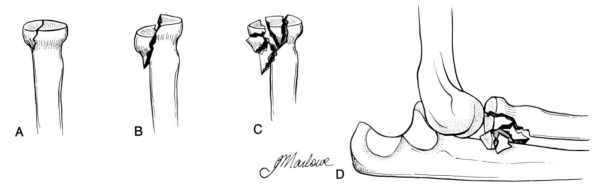

Figure 19-1 Classification of radial head fractures. **(A)** Type I, nondisplaced; **(B)** type II, displaced; **(C)** type III, comminuted; and **(D)** type IV, any with associated elbow dislocation.

present, reveals a more significant disruption of the interosseous linkage. Elbow range of motion on flexion-extension and pronation-supination should be assessed. The presence of a bony block changes the character of the fracture and will impact on recommended treatment. Wrist examination and radiographs should always be obtained when pain is present distally.

Classification of radial head fractures (Fig. 19-1) by Mason[3] and Johnston[4] is as follows:

Type I: nondisplaced fractures

Type II: displaced marginal fractures

Type III: comminuted displaced fractures

Type IV: any with elbow dislocation

Radiographs in the anteroposterior and lateral planes are usually sufficient to delineate the fracture. The presence of displaced fat pads may be the only abnormality seen in type I fractures. Trispiral polytomography or computed tomography may be quite useful when judging displacement and planning internal fixation. Initially, joint aspiration and injection with 2 ml of local anesthesia will relieve much of the acute discomfort. Treatment for type I fractures consists of symptomatic care in a sling, with early motion encouraged and periodic radiographic checks.

Type II fractures should be operatively repaired if a mechanical block to motion is observed. If motion is unrestricted, then early range of motion is encouraged. Elbow instability is much more of a concern when treating type III fractures. In comminuted radial head fractures (type III), no bony resistance to valgus instability exists. The medial collateral ligament is often disrupted during posterior dislocation (type IV).

Early surgical excision of the radial head is recommended, with some method to provide joint stability also recommended. Josefsson and colleagues[5] noted restricted range of motion, instability, and late osteoarthritis in patients treated by radial head excision alone. They recommended medial and lateral ligamentous repair combined with 3 to 4 weeks of immobilization. In patients with accompanying wrist or forearm pain, with suspected injury to the interosseous membrane, percutaneous pinning of the radius to the ulna for 4 to 6 weeks may be indicated to prevent proximal migration of the radius.

Olecranon Fractures

Due to its subcutaneous position, the olecranon is susceptible to fracture by a direct blow, (e.g., a hockey check). Since the fracture is intra-articular, displacement should not be accepted. In truly nondisplaced

fractures, stability should be checked with flexion and extension radiographs. If the fragment remains nondisplaced, nonoperative treatment with a limited motion hinged orthosis may be utilized. More commonly, the fracture is unstable and requires open reduction internal fixation. A tension band construct is recommended for uncomplicated fractures. When comminution is present, a plate provides more secure fixation. Another option exists when severe comminution intervenes between the proximal tip and the remainder of the olecranon. Since the radius of curvature of the trochlear notch is constant, the comminuted region may be excised, and the proximal fragment advanced and fixed. This technique yields a stable, congruous joint. Early motion in a hinged orthosis should be encouraged in postoperative rehabilitation. Protective orthoses for contact sports should be used for several months following radiographic evidence of osseous union.

Dislocations

Elbow dislocations are common athletic injuries, often sustained by a fall on the outstretched extremity, such as during a "take down" in wrestling or during floor exercise in gymnastics. The olecranon serves as a fulcrum, and as the joint hyperextends, the anterior capsule and often the medial collateral ligament fail under tension. The extent of associated soft tissue injury and fractures depends on several factors. Accompanying rotatory and valgus movements during hyperextension commonly result in associated fractures and ligamentous disruptions. The momentum of the athletic activity at the time of injury also plays a role in the spectrum of injury severity. Thus, a headfirst slide into second base may result in a simple posterior elbow dislocation, while a fall during a 90-m nordic ski jump may leave the athlete with a comminuted radial head fracture, coronoid process avulsion, and medial epicondyle avulsion complicating the dislocation. The relative incidence of posterior dislocations complicated by associated fractures of the radial head, coronoid process, or humeral epicondyle is 5 to 10 percent, 10 percent, and 12 percent, respectively.[6] These fractures may dictate the course of initial management and rehabilitation. Initial assessment should include a thorough neurovascular assessment of the extremity. A detailed distal motor and sensory examination should identify nerve injuries. Signs of arterial injury include excessive swelling, diminished distal pulses, sensory alteration, pallor, and, most specifically, pain with passive finger extension. The presence of distal pulses does not preclude the presence of an intimal injury of the brachial artery. When any question exists, an arteriogram should be promptly obtained. As ischemia time increases, irreversible muscle damage may occur, especially within the volar compartments. A spectrum from subtle muscle deficits to the profound disability of a Volkmann's contracture may result.

Case Study I

A 16-year-old high school wrestler suffered a posterior elbow dislocation during a match (Fig. 19-2A). Diminished radial and ulnar pulses were observed both prior to and following successful closed reduction. An arteriogram demonstrated disruption of the brachial artery at the elbow with collateral circulation providing distal perfusion (Fig. 19-2B).

A vein interposition graft was performed and the elbow statically splinted for 2 weeks to protect the arterial repair. Doppler signals in both the ulnar and radial arteries remained normal. Protected range of motion was encouraged at 2 weeks. Resistive exercises were instituted 6 weeks postinjury. The patient ultimately lacked 5 degrees of extension but was able to successfully return to wrestling the following season.

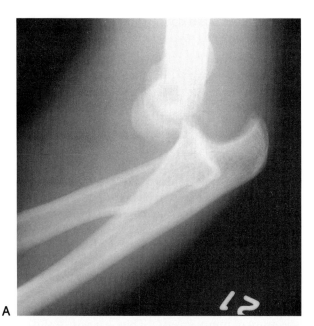

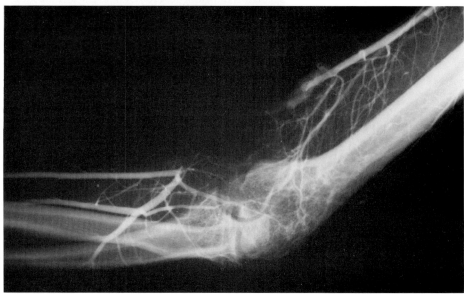

Figure 19-2 (A) Posterior elbow dislocation. (B) Arteriogram demonstrating brachial artery disruption. (Courtesy of David Kahler.)

Plain radiographs should be obtained to assess any associated fractures prior to and after reduction. Classification includes posterior, anterior, and divergent, with the vast majority posterior. A variety of reduction maneuvers have been described, but all require adequate analgesia for a minimally traumatic reduction. We favor placing the patient prone on a stretcher, with the arm positioned dependent over the side. One person holds the forearm fully supinated and applies pressure against the volar aspect. Another person stabilizes the brachium and applies a constant posteriorly directed force. Occasionally, gentle pressure over the palpable olecranon tip is also required. Closed reduction may be prohibited by associated fractures or more rarely, by interposed soft tissues such as the annular or collateral ligaments.[7] If the reduction is difficult, an olecranon wire may also be used for direct traction. The reduction maneuver is reversed for anterior dislocations. Gentle longitudinal tractions and downward pressure on the forearm accompanied by anterior pressure on the brachium usually achieves reduction. The integrity of the extensor and flexor mechanism must be checked following reduction.

Following successful reduction, the neurovascular status and stability of the elbow should be reassessed and radiographs of the fractures should be repeated. Ulnar and medial nerve entrapments have been reported following reduction of elbow dislocations.[8] Passive range of motion of the joint should be performed, and the position at which redislocation occurs (if at all) should be noted. Most elbows are stable following reduction, though disruptions in the brachialis may cause redislocation in extension. Acute valgus instability is common. This is in accord with high reported rates of medial (ulnar) collateral ligament rupture in elbows which have been surgically explored.[9] Fortunately, this ligament injury usually heals, and surgical repair acutely has not yielded superior clinical outcomes.[10]

Postreduction immobilization consists of a posterior splint at 90 degrees of flexion. Circumferential padding should be avoided, as swelling may result in constriction and vascular compromise. In elite athletes whose sport absolutely requires full elbow extension (e.g., gymnasts), immobilization in near-full extension may be beneficial.[6] Frequent radiographic checks are necessary to monitor for early redislocation when this method is chosen. For the simple posterior dislocation that was judged stable at the initial reduction, total immobilization should be discontinued at 3 to 7 days, and protected monitored progressive active flexion and extension of the elbow is then allowed. Patients who demonstrate a tendency to redislocate following reduction are placed in a hinged brace with an extension block. In individuals who demonstrate acute valgus instability, a hinged brace with progressive flexion and extension is used for at least 3 weeks. Chronic instability after posterior elbow dislocation is uncommon; however, some loss of full extension is often observed. Restriction of range of motion may be pronounced when heterotopic ossification is present (Fig. 19-3). For a gymnast or backstroke swimmer, this motion limitation may be quite problematic. Dynamic splinting is encouraged during the first several months if a return of elbow extension is delayed. When heterotopic ossification does occur, it must be allowed to "mature" over 12 to 18 months prior to considering excision. Early excision predisposes to recurrence.

Radial head fractures, associated with elbow dislocations and termed type IV, are treated in a similar manner as when no dislocation exists (see earlier section). Early surgical excision of the radial head is recommended in comminuted radial head fractures; however, some method to provide joint stability is also required. Radial head replacement is another consideration when treating comminuted fractures with accompanying elbow dislocation. (Fig. 19-4). Silicone prostheses have been most widely used; however, there have been reports of implant fracture and synovitis.[11] If utilized, it is generally accepted that the silicone implant should be removed after sufficient soft tissue healing has occurred (6 weeks). Knight and coworkers[12] have reported encouraging results utilizing a

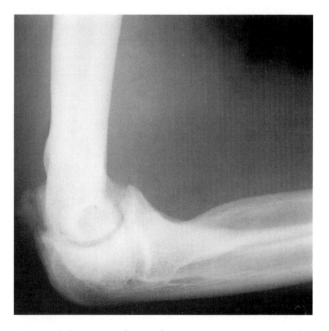

Figure 19-3 Lateral-view radiograph obtained 4 months following posterior elbow dislocation in a 17-year-old gymnast. Heterotopic ossification is present anteriorly, medially, and posteriorly, resulting in a total flexion-extension arc of 30 degrees.

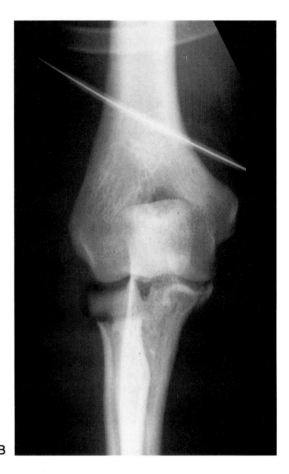

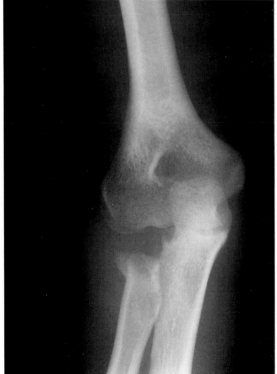

Figure 19-4 (A) A 19-year-old wrestler suffered an elbow dislocation with an accompanying comminuted radial head fracture and coronoid fracture. **(B)** The radial head fracture could not be repaired, and a silastic implant was used to restore stability. **(C)** Six weeks postoperatively, the implant was removed. The joint remained stable, and full motion was regained.

metallic radial head prosthesis following elbow dislocations. Biomechanically, the vitallium implant demonstrated superior resistance to proximal radial migration compared with the silicone implants. The long-term effect upon the capitellar articulation is unknown; therefore, it would seem prudent in the competitive athlete to utilize this as a temporary spacer implant.

In patients with accompanying wrist or forearm pain with suspected injury to the interosseous membrane, percutaneous pinning of the radius to the ulna for 4 to 6 weeks may be indicated to prevent proximal migration of the radius.[8] Aggressive therapy to avoid pronation supination contractures is instituted following pin removal.

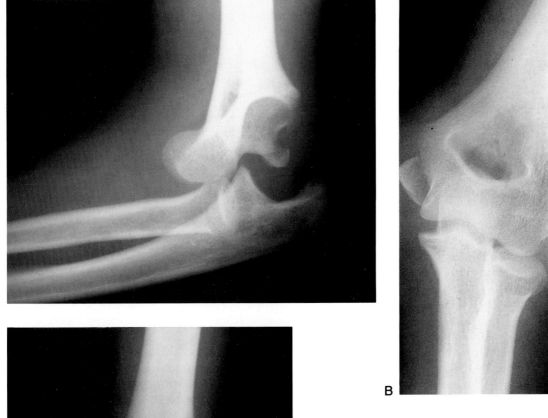

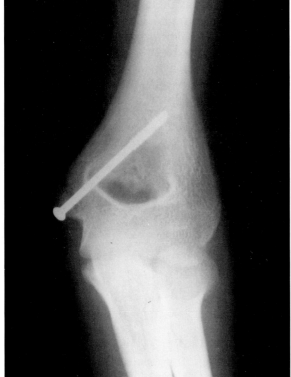

Figure 19-5 (A) A 16-year-old gymnast sustained a posterior elbow dislocation with accompanying fracture of the medial epicondyle while vaulting. **(B)** Postreduction radiographs demonstrated the epicondyle to be displaced and rotated. Valgus elbow instability was also present. **(C)** Open reduction and internal fixation with a single screw restored joint stability. The fractures healed uneventfully, and full motion with return to competition followed. (Courtesy of William E. Hooper, M.D.)

Pure hyperextension injuries resulting in posterior elbow dislocations may be accompanied by an avulsion fracture of the coronoid process of the ulna. Such injuries are commonly seen in gymnasts during vaulting or floor exercise, as the elbow is axially loaded while in full extension or hyperextension. The anterior bundle of the medial collateral ligament, the anterior joint capsule, and the brachialis muscle all have insertions on the coronoid process. Reagan and Morrey[13] have proposed a radiographic classification that has prognostic value as well. Type I fractures are small avulsions from the tip of the process; type II fractures involve less than

50 percent of the process; type III fractures comprise greater than 50 percent. From their retrospective analysis, several trends were noted. Functional outcomes diminished as the grade of the fracture increased. Moreover, recurrent dislocations or subluxations were associated with type III fractures. Early motion within 3 weeks is recommended for type I and type II fractures. Open reduction and internal fixation, followed by early motion, is optimal for type III fractures.[13]

Elbow dislocations may also be complicated by avulsion fractures of the medial epicondyle of the humerus. Though commonly seen in children and adolescents, this fracture is rare in athletes over the age of 20. Four potential complications can occur: (1) incarceration within the joint, (2) ulnar nerve injury, (3) instability, and (4) flexor-pronator weakness. Operative management is required when the fragment is lodged within the joint following reduction of the dislocation. Displacement greater than 1 cm or gross instability are relative indications for surgical treatment. Smooth wires or screws may be used to fix the fragment; if it is too small, it can be excised and the ligament and muscle origins repaired directly to bone (Fig. 19-5). Symptoms of ulnar nerve irritation is another indication for surgical exploration. Rockwood and colleagues[1] state that stiffness rather than instability is more common and advocates nonoperative management. Recommended immobilization consists of a splint holding the elbow and wrist flexed with the forearm pronated for 10 to 14 days, reducing tension in the flexor-pronator groups. Active motion is then encouraged. Hyperextensive taping or a hinged orthoses should be used on return to sport for a minimum of 6 months.

ANTERIOR INJURIES

Distal Biceps Tendon Rupture

Distal biceps tendon disruptions most often occur during heavy resistance weight training with biceps curls. Power lifters who perform biceps curls with heavy weight may develop tenderness and swelling over the tendon consistent with a tendonitis. The patient often feels a "pop," with accompanying pain in the anterior elbow. Clinically, ecchymosis is often present in the antecubital fossa, and the muscle will retract proximally. A palpable defect may be apparent (Fig. 19-7). Degenerative changes are often seen on pathologic inspection of the tendon.[14] Moreover, radiographic changes due to traction on the bicipital tuberosity may also be present, indicating chronic or recurrent stress of the biceps tendon at the insertion of the radial tuberosity (Fig. 19-8).

When the history is suggestive of a distal biceps disruption but a defect is not palpable, a partial tendon rupture or strain of the lacertus fibrosis should be suspected. Activity should be limited during this inflammatory phase, given the risk of subsequent tendon rupture. Acute elbow hyperextension against a contracted biceps, such as may occur during a football tackle or wrestling takedown, may also cause complete or partial disruption of the biceps tendon. Flexion strength is greatly diminished with a complete rupture but may be near-normal with a partial rupture.[15] Nonoperative treatment with immobilization or (Fig. 19-6) operative completion of the disruption and reattachment of the entire tendon are both acceptable options.

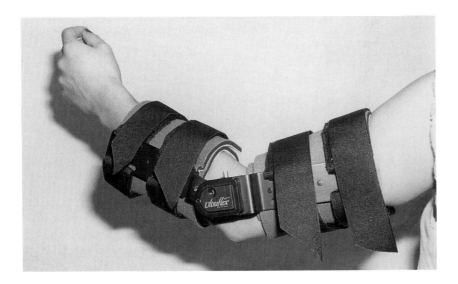

Figure 19-6 Extension block splinting may be used in the treatment of partial bicep ruptures and in rehabilitation of surgically corrected complete tears.

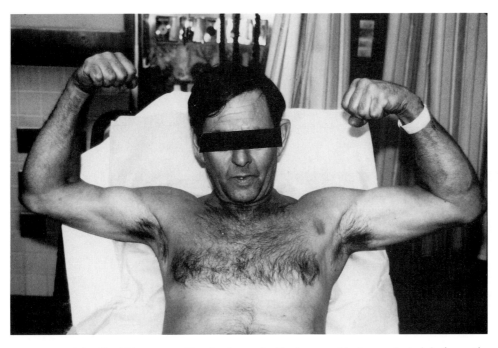

Figure 19-7 Acute right distal biceps tear. Proximal muscle displacement is demonstrated during active elbow flexion.

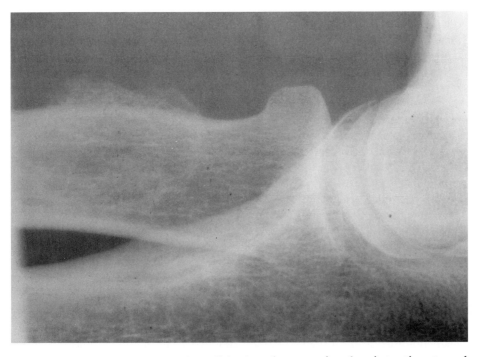

Figure 19-8 Mineralization adjacent to the radial tuberosity suggesting chronic traction stress changes at the biceps tendon insertion.

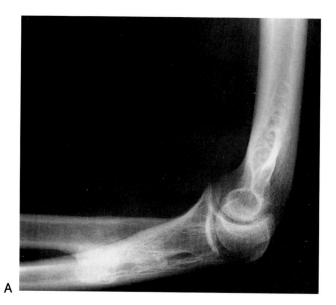
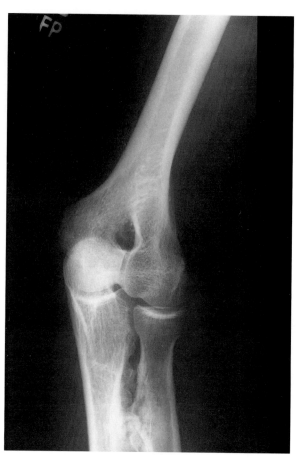

Figure 19-9 **(A)** AP and **(B)** lateral radiographic views demonstrating radioulnar proximal synostosis following repair of a distal biceps rupture using a two-incision technique.

For a complete distal biceps rupture, the procedure of choice is prompt surgical reattachment of the tendon to its insertion on the radial tuberosity. The anterior approach when used alone risks nerve injury. Boyd and Anderson[16] have described a two-incision technique where the second incision is made over the dorsal forearm. This provides excellent exposure of the radial tuberosity, which eases trough formation and tendon reattachment; however, there is a risk of proximal synostosis with this technique (Fig. 19-9). This observed risk of ectopic bone has prompted recent reports of techniques returning to a single anterior incision. Pull-out sutures or suture anchors have been utilized in tendon reattachment.[17,18] Radial and musculocutaneous nerve injury have both been reported, tempering the usefulness of these techniques.

Postoperative rehabilitation includes the use of a static splint at 90 degrees of flexion for 3 weeks, followed by active extension and passive flexion in a hinged orthoses for an additional 3 to 6 weeks. Challenging athletic activities are discouraged until 6 months postoperatively (see Ch. 4).

Traction Spurs

Traction spurs of the coronoid process are commonly seen in throwing athletes. The brachialis has a broad insertion at the base of the coronoid, and anterior band of the medial collateral ligament and eccentrically contracts to control arm deceleration during follow-through. The resultant traction spur may become sufficiently large enough to impinge within the coronoid fossa and thus limit elbow flexion (Fig. 19-10). This impingement may be relieved by arthroscopic burring or open resection of the spur. Fracture of the spur may result in intra-articular loose bodies, which can be removed arthroscopically.

MUSCLE AND TENDON PROBLEMS

Afflictions of the muscles and tendons of the lateral and medial elbow are generally termed "tennis elbow." Symptoms seen in racquet sport athletes (tennis, squash, ping-pong) most commonly are referable to the

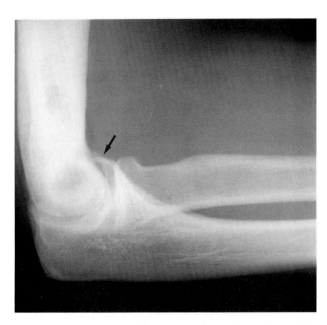

Figure 19-10 Lateral radiographic view of the elbow of a professional baseball pitcher showing a hypertrophic coronoid osteophyte *(arrow)*. Flexion produced anterior elbow pain, which was relieved following excision.

lateral elbow. Repetitive microtrauma to the wrist extensor muscle origin during the backhand groundstroke is the usual etiology. Repetitive elbow extension, maximal pronation, and wrist flexion result in eccentric overload and "lateral epicondylitis" in wheelchair athletes, especially racers and marathon racers. The pathologic findings, which are best described by Goldie[19] and Nirschl and Pettrone[20] report more chronic and degenerative changes rather than primary inflammatory changes. The structure most frequently implicated on the lateral elbow is the extensor carpi radialis brevis with associated but lesser involvement of the extensor carpi radialis longus and extensor carpi ulnaris. At the medial elbow, the anatomic location is more generally localized at the anterior aspect of the epicondyle; the origin of the pronator teres and the flexor carpi radialis (see the section, *Medial Elbow*).

Nirschl[20] has characterized this degeneration and fibroblastic change as angiofibroblastic proliferation. The terminology of tendonosis rather than tendinitis would be more appropriate. The systemic tendency toward other tendonopathies would indicate a predilection for some athletes with characteristic tissue changes. In other instances, it is clear that there is a correlation with intensity and duration of activity in addition to other performance-related factors (e.g., the strength and force required, equipment utilized, and other aspects of biomechanics of performance). Nirschl[20] has recognized three categories of chronic severity (Table 19-1). The pathologic findings correlate with progression from acute to chronic clinical presentations. The treatment alternatives range from traditional nonoperative options for the initial acute stages with associated equipment and performance changes for recurrent, to the ultimate, surgery for chronic problems.

On physical examination, the athlete will localize pain to the area of the lateral epicondyle. Resisted wrist extension and passive wrist flexion will reproduce symptoms. Acutely, the athlete should refrain from aggravating activities and use ice and NSAIDs to control inflammation. When symptoms persist, cortisone injection placed beneath the common extensor origin and deep massage may be helpful. A continuing program of stretching and muscle strengthening should be included.

An analysis of stroke mechanics by a teaching professional should accompany an athlete's return to sport. Alterations in racquet grip, head size, weight, and string tension may help relieve eccentric forces transmitted to the extensor musculature. Moreover, a counterforce brace worn at the proximal forearm limits muscular contraction and thus provides a protective effect (see Ch. 6).

Surgery should be considered for athletes whose symptoms are not improved with rest, rehabilitation, NSAIDs, and technique modifications. Specific indications include duration of symptoms of 1 year, and persistent symptoms despite three cortisone injections.

Table 19-1 Categories of Severity

	Pathology	Symptoms	Treatment
Category I (acute)	Acute inflammation	Minor pain with activity	Rest/rehabilitation
Category II (recurrent)	Partial angiofibroblastic invasion	Intense pain with activity which may resolve with prolonged rest	Rest/rehabilitation ± surgery
Category III (chronic)	Pronounced angiofibroblastic invasion with partial or complete tendon rupture	Constant pain Night pain Athletic activity not possible	Surgical

Approximately 85 percent of athletes can expect a good to excellent return to sport.[20,21]

The standard operative technique utilizes a lateral incision centered over the lateral epicondyle. The extensor digitorum longus is reflected anteriorly, revealing the brevis origin. The granular, degenerated tendon is debrided and the epicondyle decorticated to enhance vascular ingrowth. If any radiocapitellar mechanical symptoms are present, a small arthrotomy is made and the radiocapitellar joint is inspected. Occasionally, a synovial tongue will be present within this joint. This synovium should be resected and its base cauterized. An alternate procedure utilizes percutaneous release of the common extensor origin. This technique has limited morbidity, and a reported 90 percent success rate.[22]

Rupture of the lateral extensor musculature is much less common than medial flexor-pronator injuries. Macrotrauma caused by sudden wrist extension or forced wrist flexion may cause intramuscular tears or acute avulsion from the lateral epicondyle (Fig. 19-11). Nonoperative treatment with the use of splint, rest, and anti-inflammatory medications are indicated, unless a palpable defect is recognized.

Lateral Collateral Ligament Injuries

The lateral collateral ligament structures have not been recognized as major areas of complaint and performance alterations in the athlete. In some instances,

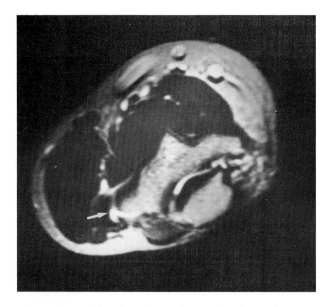

Figure 19-11 T2-weighted MRI image showing an increase in signal intensity at the origin of the common extensor tendon consistent with a partial tear *(arrow).*

these structures are associated with major trauma, while in other cases, the etiology is more likely related to repetitive overload.

We have focused on the medial overload with the cocking to acceleration phase of the baseball pitch. After ball release, much of the force is directed toward the lateral elbow, particularly in the combination of extension and pronation. The collateral complex (which includes the annular ligament) (Fig. 19-12) is frequently the site of the clinically evident problem as discomfort associated with performance forces and ligamentous hyperlaxity and articular hypermobility. It may appear as if there is true subluxation of the radial head with the pronation rotational force. An additional note of caution is warranted with all operative procedures on the lateral elbow, particularly for chronic tennis elbow so the potential for an iatrogenic varus pronation instability is not created. Nestor and associates[23] have described a surgical procedure for lateral rotatory instability of the elbow.

Lateral Intra-articular Injuries

The radial head and capitellum comprise the most complex articulation of the elbow joint. The dynamics of the radial head motion on the capitellum must be considered in light of concurrent motion of the humeroulnar and radioulnar joints. The composite of rotation, compression, axial, and angular forces are concomitantly affecting the radiocapitellar articular surfaces. The changes in the radiocapitellar joint are observed in the skeletally immature athlete as osteochondrosis, Panner's disease, potentially healing or progressing to the fragmentation of an articular surface, resulting in an osteochondritis (osteochondrosis) dissecans with loose body formation[24] (see Ch. 8). If the articular surface is intact, the treatment is directed to a bone graft of the subchondral area to provide biologic support with an attempt to preserve a normal articular configuration. The graft may be performed from the lateral epicondyle approach. Although often associated with Little League athletes, osteochondritis dissecans and acute osteochondral shear fractures are also prevalent in gymnasts.[25]

In the skeletally immature athlete, the initial pathology appears to be from the subchondral osseous area, whereas in the skeletally mature it seems to be more from the subchondral and chondral articular surface. The forces that appear to be most significant are progressive medial varus, compression, rotation, and shearing during the later stages of throwing, causing

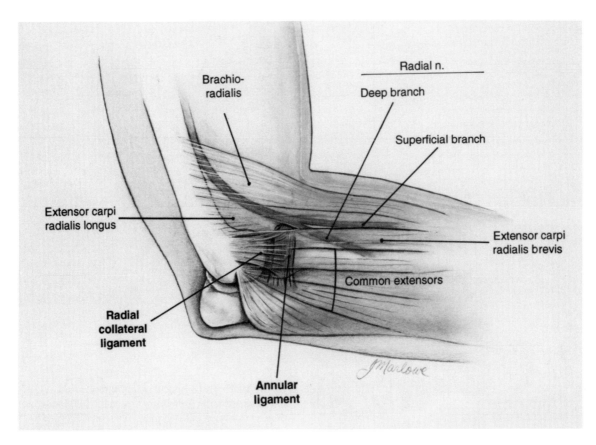

Figure 19-12 Ligaments of lateral elbow.

impact during the final few degrees of elbow extension and pronation. The effect of these forces is directed more toward the inferior and medial aspect of the capitellum and the anteromedial region of the radial head (Fig. 19-13). The clinical effect is articular impact injury, fibrillation of the articular surface, and subchondral osseous changes. The fibrillation may result in cartilaginous fragments within the joint that become osteochondral fragments, or in continuous loss of the articular surface and progressive evidence of degenerative joint disease.

The transition from fibrillated cartilage to osteochondral fragments is unpredictable. The symptoms may include discomfort with performance, associated with joint incongruity or simply the discomfort of a degenerative arthrosis. If there is a free osteocartilaginous fragment, the athlete will complain of intermittent incomplete motion or a true locking. The diagnosis may be evident on plain radiographs (Fig. 19-14). However, if the fragments remain cartilaginous and the symptomatology is suggestive of interarticular fragments, the lack of ossification may not be identified on plain radiographs and therefore other forms of image evaluation will be necessary (e.g., CT or arthrogram) (Fig. 19-15).

The treatment of symptomatic fragments is either an open or arthroscopic technique for removal of the fragment and débridement of the fibrillated area; if the defect is identifiable, it should be débrided and the base drilled to stimulate bleeding and fibrocartilage healing. If the articular surface injury is associated with macrotrauma and a large osteochondral fragment is present, then relocation or replacement of the fragment with appropriate fixation is indicated to assure articular congruity and ultimate function.

ACUTE POSTERIOR INJURIES

Triceps Tendon

Rupture or avulsion of the triceps tendon was noted in 1949 to be "the least common of all tendon injuries."[26] With increasing athletic participation by indi-

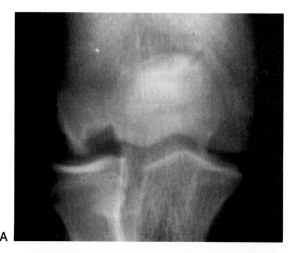

A

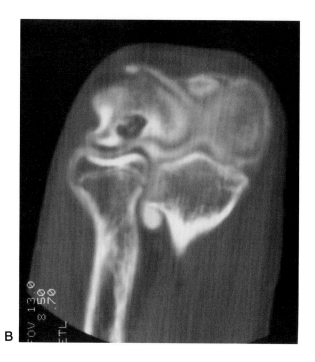

B

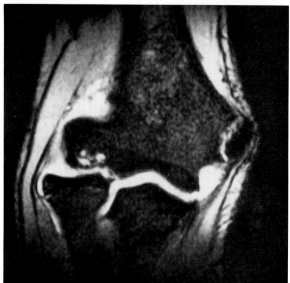

C

Figure 19-13 **(A)** AP-view radiograph demonstrating notch-like deformity of capitellum consistent with osteochondritis dissecans. **(B)** Cystic changes seen on CT scan. **(C)** Joint effusion, thinning of articular cartilage, and subchondral bone changes demonstrated on gradient echo MR image.

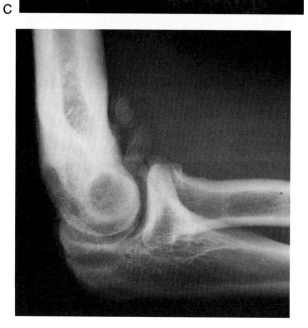

Figure 19-14 Lateral-view radiograph of the elbow demonstrating multiple loose bodies anteriorly within the joint of a veteran baseball infielder.

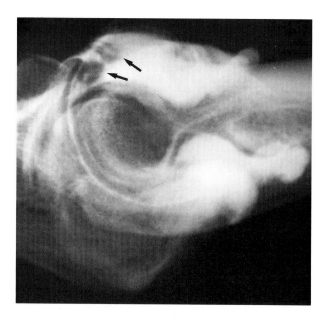

Figure 19-15 Loose bodies *(arrows)* demonstrated anteriorly on arthrogram that were not evident on plain radiograph.

viduals with coexisting medical conditions such as renal osteodystrophy[27] and osteogenesis imperfecta,[28] reports of triceps and olecranon injuries are becoming more common.

Case Study II

A 12-year-old boy with osteogenesis imperfecta presented with pain and swelling after injuring his elbow. He cast a lure while fishing and felt a pop in his elbow. Radiographs demonstrated a displaced olecranon fracture (Fig. 19-16). Open reduction and internal fixation with a tension band construct was performed. The fracture healed uneventfully and the patient recovered full function of the extremity and returned to fishing, his primary sport.

Injury to the triceps mechanism may occur as an intrasubstance tear. The injury occurs with either forced flexion of the elbow with eccentric triceps contraction or a direct blow to the elbow. On physical examination, local discomfort, ecchymosis, swelling, and the inability to completely extend the elbow against resistance is found. Viegas[29] has described a modification of the Thompson test (Achilles tendon), for diagnosis of an acute disruption wherein the triceps is squeezed while the elbow is supported at 90 degrees of flexion. The absence of passive elbow extension demonstrates tendon disruption.

When considering treatment, it should be determined whether the disruption is partial or complete. Patients with partial tears, demonstrated by diminished extensor strength, may be treated with hinged extension block splinting. Complete disruptions are best treated by primary open repair. The tendon avulsion is treated by reattachment with nonabsorbable sutures through drill holes in the olecranon. A tension band wire technique is utilized if a fragment of olecranon has also been avulsed.

The traumatic separation of an unfused ossification center is uncommon; however, it must be treated more aggressively than a traumatic avulsion fracture of the olecranon. Radiographically, the proximal fracture fragment will have a smooth, sclerotic margin. Contralateral elbow radiographs have been normal in all reported cases. Histologically, the "fracture" surface is comprised of hyaline and fibrocartilage, most likely consistent with an unfused physis. Primary bone grafting with open reduction internal fixation is recommended[30] (see Fig. 8-31).

Triceps tendon disruption is also seen following elbow dislocations. If a longitudinal rent is formed in the triceps, the bellies may sublux medially and laterally, greatly diminishing extension power. Reduction and repair of the subluxed muscle was successful in a chronic case seen in a wrestler.

Postoperative rehabilitation should focus on early return of motion. A hinged brace which allows passive extension and active flexion is utilized following wound healing. Minor flexion contractures can occur and may be disabling for some athletes, such as gymnasts.

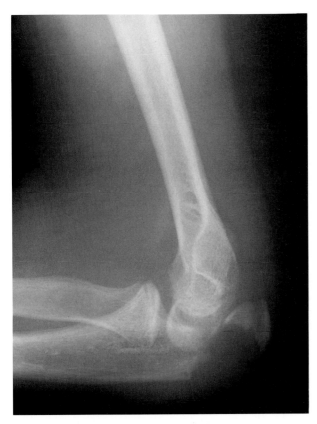

Figure 19-16 Displaced avulsion fracture of the olecranon.

Chronic Posterior Injuries

Performance-related pathology of the posterior compartment of the elbow is most commonly seen in throwers. The medial valgus and lateral compressive forces imparted to the elbow during baseball pitching have been well-described.[31,32] Flexion contractures and cubitus valgus deformities are seen in up to 50 percent of professional baseball pitchers. In pitchers, the spur is symptomatic during late deceleration, as it impacts within the olecranon fossa. A flawed pitching motion or subtle imbalance between flexors and extensors may accentuate this impingement.

Two distinct styles of javelin throwing exist, each with its own characteristic injury pattern. During the "side arm" throw, major valgus forces are applied to the elbow, and medial elbow injury results. The second throwing technique utilizes a more upright delivery. The flexed elbow leads the arm and lies in the same sagittal plane as the shoulder. Forceful elbow extension and shoulder flexion then propel the javelin. The medial collateral ligament is protected with this technique; however, traction and impingement of the olecranon within the fossa during elbow hyperextension result in degenerative spur formation posteriorly on the olecranon.[33] Radiographically, the spur often is separated from the olecranon by a radiolucent line, resembling a nonunion (Fig. 19-17). Repetitive impact on the degenerative spur may cause fragmentation and loose body formation. Treatment consists of arthroscopic or open resection of the spur and removal of loose bodies.

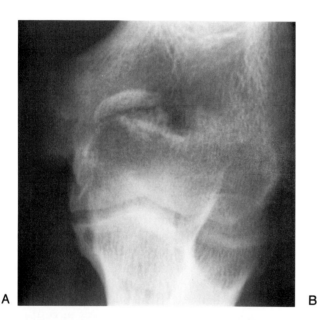
A

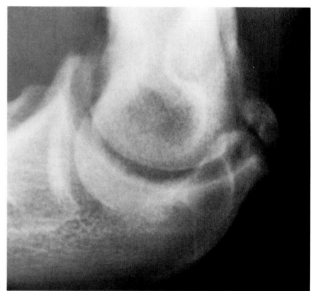
B

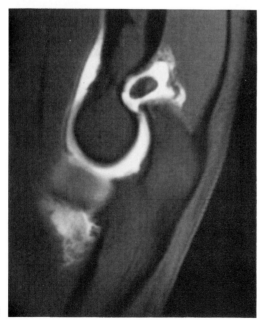
C

Figure 19-17 (A & B) Plain radiographs and (C) sagittal MRI image demonstrating posterior olecranon osteophyte in a 30-year-old outfielder.

Case Study III

A 27-year-old professional baseball pitcher developed chronic posterior elbow pain with subsequent decreased performance over the course of one season. A 15-degree flexion contracture was present. Radiographs (Fig. 19-18) demonstrated posterior olecranon proliferative spurring with associated loose bodies. Open surgical excision of the spur and loose bodies was performed (Fig. 19-19B). Recovery progressed during the off-season and he competed successfully without pain the following year.

A second pattern of spur formation appears along the posteromedial margin of the olecranon. Resulting from traction forces, this posteromedial spur is a common sequelae of the repetitive medial distractive forces imparted during baseball pitching, and discomfort may be secondary impingement of this spur on the olecranon(Fig. 19-19). Indelicato and colleagues[34] and King and colleagues[31] have implicated the acceleration phase of pitching for maximal posteromedial wedging of the olecranon within the fossa. Wilson and Associates[35] introduced the term *extension valgus overload* to describe the syndrome produced by the degenerative changes about the posteromedial olecranon. Symptoms of valgus extension overload include pain posteriorly during forced valgus extension of the elbow.

When performance-related symptoms occur, conservative treatment has not been successful. Open or arthroscopic excision of the posterior osteophyte and its medial extension has been successful.[35] Generous removal of this reactive bone is recommended to prevent further impingement. Recurrence due to osteophyte reformation has been reported.

MEDIAL ELBOW INJURIES

Any sport that requires use of the upper extremity in an overhead or forceful side arm manner presents the potential for medial elbow problems. Of all athletic activities, the baseball pitch is perhaps the most potentially stressful to the medial elbow structures. (The phases of baseball are described in Chs. 9 and 17).

The most stressful part of the pitch as it relates to the elbow is in the final stages of cocking and in the progression to acceleration. The combination of forces that result in posterior medial elbow valgus traction stress during a baseball pitch are most significant at the completion of the cocking phase, when the shoulder is maximally externally rotated, and the beginning of the acceleration phase, when the shoulder is initiating explosive internal rotation. At that moment, the elbow is flexed to approximately 100 degrees, and the forearm is supinated. The composite of anatomic positions and explosive forces of acceleration and the impact of these on the medial elbow account for the traction stress of angular valgus, axial extension, and rotatory supination to pronation. These forces affect all anatomic structures on the posterior and medial side of the elbow and causes recurrent traction stress injury (Fig. 19-20). All the structures as identified on the medial side of the elbow are susceptible to both acute and chronic performance-related injuries. Acute injuries of the elbow may be the first phase that progresses to a recurrent and ultimately career-threatening chronic performance-related injury. The concept of extensible tissue and traction and eccentric forces is critical in the discussion of medial elbow injuries. Ligaments and muscles are subjected to tension and eccentric contraction repeatedly during a pitching performance. This microtrauma initiates an inflammatory response. Healing is promoted by rest and anti-inflammatory medications. Tissue repair and regeneration results in a decline of tissue extensibility, and postinjury tissue is more prone to rein-

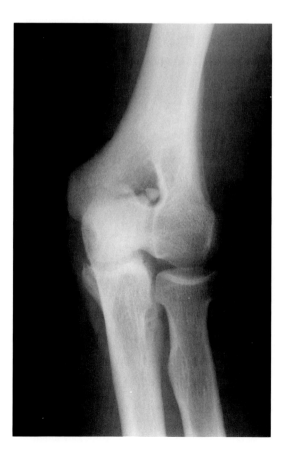

Figure 19-18 Preoperative posterior olecranon spurring with associated loose body in 23-year-old pitcher.

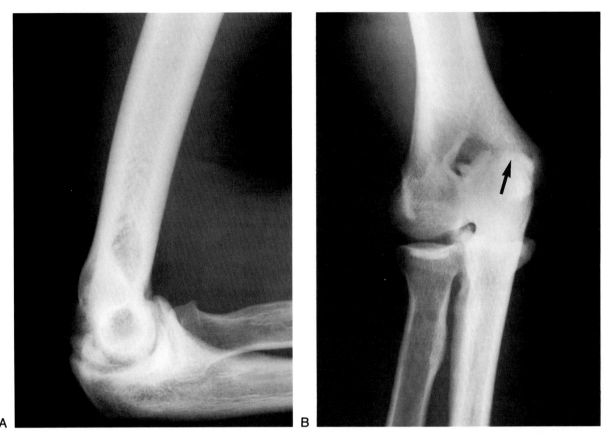

Figure 19-19 (A) AP and (B) lateral radiographic views of elbow demonstrating posteromedial olecranon spurring *(arrow)* and radioulnar arthroses. The pitcher showed signs of valgus extension laxity on physical examination.

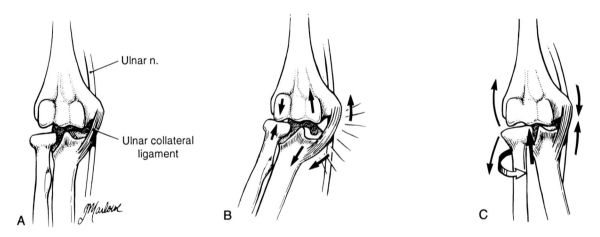

Figure 19-20 (A) Neutral position. (B) Forces on elbow at time of maximal cocking to early acceleration. The valgus force that stresses all medial structures—medial collateral ligament, ulnar nerve, posterior medial insertion of triceps, and pronator flexor muscles originating from medial epicondyle. The varus compression force across radiocapitellar articulation, with elbow flexed and supinated. During this phase the forearm is supinated. (C) After ball release, late acceleration to deceleration, the valgus force is directed to lateral elbow (much less than earlier medial valgus force) and the radial head pronates and impacts on the inferomedial capitellum.

jury, thus creating a cyclical progression to chronicity pattern.

Acute Medial Injuries

The two specific intramuscular injuries that are most frequently associated with the medial epicondyle are those of the pronator teres and the common flexor muscle group. A pronator teres injury is most prevalent in baseball pitchers who throw a majority of forceful rotational pitches (e.g., sliders, screwballs). An eccentric injury results in palpable sensitive nodules within the body of the pronator teres following athletic performance. It is not uncommon for this acute or chronic problem to be primary or secondary in relation to a medial collateral ligamentous injury. Thus the treatment is in part determined by the examination of the medial collateral ligament. If in fact there is no evidence of acute sensitivity of the medial collateral ligament, then a course of rest, ultrasound, massage, NSAIDs, and occasional intermuscular steroidal injection should be instituted. If the pronator teres problem is associated with a medial collateral instability, the treatment regimen discussed for the medial collateral ligament is appropriate.

Intermuscular tears in the proximal area of the flexor muscles are most frequently associated with baseball pitchers throwing curve balls. This usually manifests more as a specific acute injury, although whenever fibrosis occurs in the muscle, the possibility of there being subsequent disruptions are likely. Most veteran pitchers who have sustained a flexor muscle injury will recover and do well throughout the season. However, as they resume their forceful pitching activity the following spring, the damaged area repaired with less extensible tissue will be noted, and these pitchers will experience recurrent symptoms while regaining their muscle extensibility.

Acute discomfort at the flexor pronator origin is most commonly seen in golfers, though it also occurs in athletes engaged in racquet sports and baseball batters. The injury may result from a rapid unexpected deceleration during a golf swing (hitting a rock or wet turf). The manner in which the club is gripped also may predispose to injury at the flexor pronator origin. A "strong" (supinated) right hand will leave the clubface open at impact, resulting in a slice. To counteract this, the player will forcefully pronate the forearm before impact, thereby squaring the clubface and hoping to keep the ball on the mowed grass. Pain is exacerbated by passive wrist extension or wrist flexion against resistance. During the acute stage of medial epicondylitis, treatment focuses on rest, anti-inflammatory mea-

sures, physical rehabilitation, and technical performance modifications.

Chronic Medial Injuries

In most instances, the symptoms of chronic conditions are insidious in onset, usually manifested by incremental medial elbow discomfort at the region of the medial epicondyle. This is associated with a decrease in the rate of activity as well as in the standard of performance. For example, the baseball pitcher may achieve less control with certain pitches and most likely will throw fewer effective pitches in a game (i.e., lasting fewer innings than he had in the past). Or the tennis player may sustain a loss in the motion and location of the serve. The usual finding in these individuals is degeneration of the flexor origin at the medial epicondyle (Fig. 19-21). The area of the injury heals with functionally incompetent reactive fibrous tissues. Generally, individuals who do not respond to conventional therapeutic regimens will improve with an excision of the reactive tissue and return of the flexor origin to a bed of freshened cancellous epicondylar bone.

Immediately beneath the flexor pronator muscle group is the medial collateral ligament and the medial capsule of the elbow. The anterior band of the medial collateral ligament is the stronger component and a significant contributor to the medial stability (Fig. 19-22). The valgus stress in the cocking phase of throwing, or in the swinging of a racquet, bat, or club frequently challenges the medial collateral ligament. The repetitive action of these activities or an unusual force (e.g., a

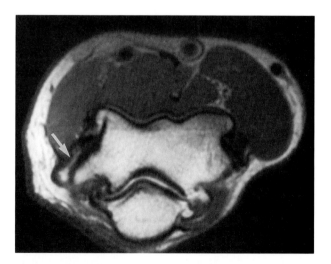

Figure 19-21 Axial MRI reveals inflammation and separation of the flexor-pronator origin at the medial epicondyle, consistent with medial epicondylitis *(arrow).*

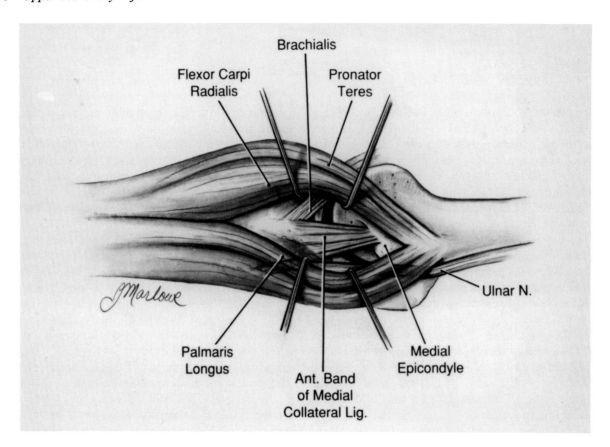

Figure 19-22 The anterior bundle of the medial collateral ligament provides the greatest resistance to the valgus force of overhead pitching activity.

poorly performed activity or one that is abruptly interrupted) may result in injury. The acute injury may initiate the beginning phases of performance-related injury or may represent a significant disruption of the medial collateral ligament.

These stages of progressive chronicity are usually discussed as a continuum that ultimately leads to attenuation and a lax ligament or a frank disruption of a damaged ligament. In general, the pathology for all early ligamentous stress and overuse injuries and tendonopathies are classified in stages of focal edema, inflammation, and minor tissue damage that resolves with rest, treatment, and rehabilitation. If the injury recurs as a result of incomplete rehabilitation, lack of disability time, or too-early return to performance, then future performance will result in additional injury with laxity, fibrosis, and calcification within the ligament (Fig. 19-23). A longer period of rest, rehabilitation, and treatment may possibly permit the athlete to continue at this stage. At this stage, it should be determined if specific intervention for the medial collateral ligament should be undertaken.

Several radiographic modalities are available to diagnose medial collateral ligament incompetence.

Stress radiographs may demonstrate medial joint distraction. Injury to the anterior band of the medial collateral ligament is well-visualized by MRI (Fig. 19-24). Dye extravasation during arthrography is also consistent with a ligament disruption (Fig. 19-25).

In the rare instance of an acute avulsion from the medial epicondyle, the ligament is repaired through drill holes to a cancellous base on the epicondyle. More commonly, the ligament has undergone degeneration, and reconstruction is recommended rather than a repair.

Jobe and colleagues[36] have described a reconstruction utilizing autograft tendon passed through drill holes in the coronoid process and medial epicondyle. This figure-of-eight configuration mimics the native ligament. Palmaris longus tendon from the contralateral side is preferable, though a strip of Achilles tendon, plantaris, or a toe extensor may be substituted. As 40 percent of patients with medial collateral ligament insufficiency have associated ulnar nerve symptoms, an anterior transposition (which also facilitates exposure) is included in the procedure.

The ulnar nerve is also involved in the valgus stress to the medial elbow. Symptoms of ulnar neuropathy may

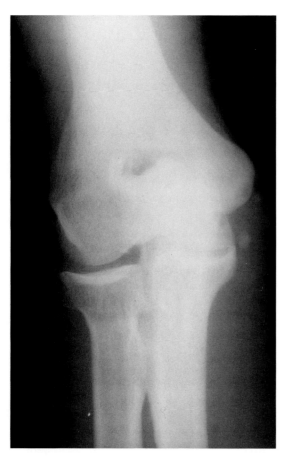

Figure 19-23 Calcification within the medial collateral ligament, suggesting chronic instability.

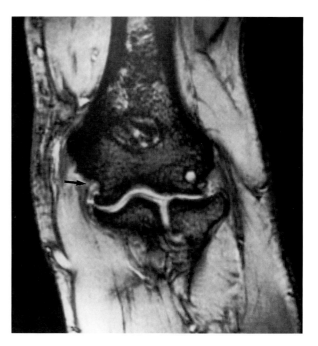

Figure 19-24 Coronal MRI demonstrating edema at the flexor origin consistent with injury. Additionally, disruption of the anterior band of the medial collateral ligament is evident *(arrow)*.

be associated with direct trauma or more likely associated with the repetitive valgus, external rotation supination stress overload mechanism. The cause may be excursion limitation of the ulnar nerve or an anatomic entrapment that results in compression of the ulnar nerve. It is possible that these two mechanisms may act in combination. The clinical complaint is usually one of sensitivity in the area of the ulnar nerve and paresthesias in the sensory distribution of the ulnar side of the ring and the little finger. When no such paresthesias are noted, it may be difficult to make the diagnosis in an athlete who complains of a dull ache medially. Edema about the nerve may be seen on MRI (Fig. 19-26). Elbow discomfort after several innings pitched, other repetitive activity, or with continued performance is a common complaint. The anatomic site of the problem may be located proximal to the medial epicondyle at the region of the intermuscular septum, an aberrant band of the triceps, adjacent to the arcade of Struthers, an aberrant band from a supracondylar process. Compression within the cubital tunnel may be secondary to a hypertrophied ligament or calcific deposits within or adjacent to a chronic injury of the medial collateral ligament. If the overlying compressive force is evident, there is usually a bulbous expansion of the nerve just proximal to the cubital tunnel or arcuate ligaments. There may be a distal source of etiology, usually in the region of the bifurcated area of the flexor carpi ulnaris where motion restriction causes

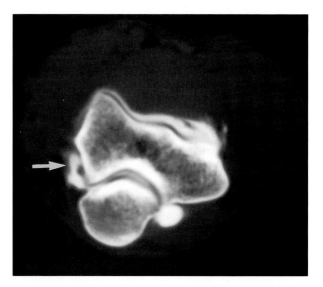

Figure 19-25 Axial CT arthrogram demonstrating dye extravasation along the course of the medial collateral ligament.

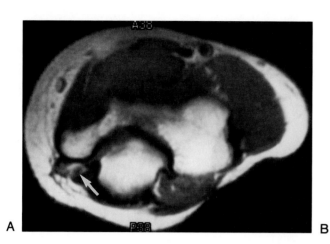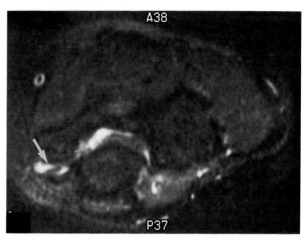

Figure 19-26 (A) Axial fast spin echo, proton density (TR 5,416/TE 30) at the level of the proximal cubital tunnel shows mildly bulbous ulnar nerve with distortion of the overlying cubital tunnel aponeurosis and adjacent subcutaneous fat. **(B)** Axial STIR image at the same level shows perineural inflammation manifested by circumferential increased signal *(arrows)*.

symptoms. Muscle hypertrophy may also constrict the nerve between the heads of the flexor carpi ulnaris (see Ch. 17).

Recurrent subluxation or dislocation from the cubital tunnel may also produce ulnar nerve symptoms. Childress[37] noted that the nerve may sublux and rest on the medial epicondyle (type A) or completely dislocate anteriorly (type B) during elbow flexion. The type A nerve is vulnerable to direct trauma, while the dislocating nerve, type B, may develop a reactive friction neuritis.

There are three stages of ulnar neuropathy. Stage 1 is the acute with local symptomatology and radiculopathy. Stage 2 is the recurrent phase (i.e., symptoms recur with attempts to return to athletic performance following the initial incident). Neurodiagnostic tests usually do not show any evidence of abnormality at either of these stages. Tinel's sign, however, is a helpful indicator for diagnostic location of ulnar neuropathy (see Ch. 3). If there is evidence of recurrent symptomatology with activity, it is recommended (in the majority of cases for high-demand upper extremity athletes) that nerve exploration and transposition be performed. Anterior transposition must allow for thorough decompression from extrinsic etiologies and, moreover, it diminishes tension within the nerve position as it takes the "high road" relative to the medial epicondyle. Stage 3 is a more chronic stage that is associated with persistence of sensory changes and muscle weakness of the ulnar innervated wrist and hand structures. Typically if one waits for these findings, which will be associated with neurodiagnostic changes, it is less likely that there can be a reversal of symptoms as would be expected with an earlier intervention.

When performing anterior ulnar nerve transposition, the nerve may be placed in a subcutaneous or submuscular position. There are advantages to each technique. The subcutaneous transfer involves less dissection and does not violate the flexor-pronator muscle origin. The submuscular positioning of the nerve, however, does provide more protection from direct trauma. Regardless of the technique used, it is imperative to sufficiently mobilize the nerve proximally and distally. A generous incision is made with the arcade of Struthers released at its location proximal to the medial epicondyle. The medial intermuscular septum must be excised, otherwise the transposed nerve will directly overlie it and another source of irritation or entrapment will persist. During the procedure, the sensory branches should be identified and preserved. Distally, the nerve is traced between the heads of the flexor carpi ulnaris muscle to the point where its motor branches are identified. Once the transposition is performed, one should recheck to assure that no proximal or distal compression or kinking exists.

Case Study IV

In an effort to increase the movement on his slider, a 24-year-old professional baseball player began a vigorous off-season program of forearm strengthening utilizing 35-lb wrist curls. A profound hypertrophy of the flexor carpi ulnaris muscle resulted. During the following season, the pitcher complained of medial elbow pain and paresthesias in the ulnar two digits. A Tinel's sign was present over the proximal portion of the flexor carpi ulnaris. Conservative measures were ineffectual.

At surgery, the ulnar nerve was found to be compressed as it passed between the hypertrophied heads of the flexor carpi ulnaris. Following decompression transposition and education regarding weight training, a full return to major league baseball followed.

Just below the ulnar nerve, the capsule between the humerus, the olecranon, can be identified. At times, if there is a forceful valgus maneuver, this area of the capsule will be torn. It is not uncommon to identify a disruption at this level in association with a collateral ligament tear (Fig. 19-25). However, it is also possible to see this as a single problem causing recurrent elbow discomfort and occasionally ulnar nerve symptomatology.

ARTHROSCOPY

The initial report by Burman[38] in 1931 (in the U.S. literature) indicated that the elbow was unsuitable for arthroscopic examination. Since then, the advances in arthroscopic technology and the specific attention to anatomic detail during portal placement have made elbow arthroscopy valuable and advantageous. The arthroscopic observations of interarticular anatomy and function of the multiple ligaments and articular components of the elbow have contributed to our knowledge of athletic performance and injury.[39]

The indications for elbow arthroscopy in the athlete are increasing as the diagnostic and therapeutic advantages are recognized. A prearthroscopic evaluation utilizing plain radiographs, arthrography, computed tomography, scintigraphy, and MRI is helpful regarding the anticipated problems to be observed and treated. The two most common indications for an arthroscopic procedure are the removal of loose bodies and the removal of osteophytes (Fig. 19-27). Other indications include the treatment of osteochondritis dissecans, chondroplasty, focal synovitis, and arthrolysis.[40] Frequently, a loose osteocartilaginous fragment will be attached and localized; on other occasions, if it is not attached, it may move to another portion of the joint, either prior to the intra-articular mobility or due to the fluid currents during the arthroscopic procedure. Although the image studies are particularly helpful, the systematic inspection of the entire joint is imperative whenever a loose body is suspected. The opportunity to manipulate the joint and observe the majority of the intra-articular areas is advantageous in the location and extraction of loose bodies. If the loose body is semi-

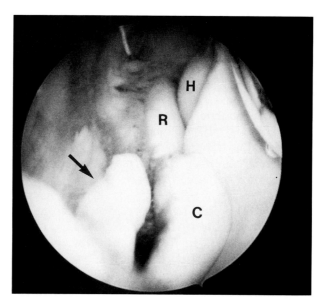

Figure 19-27 Arthroscopic view from the anteromedial portal in the right elbow of a professional baseball catcher. Symptoms included intermittent locking. A loose body *(arrow)* is visualized anterior and distal to the coronoid process. Symptoms resolved following arthroscopic removal of the loose body. R, radial head; H, capitellum; C, coronoid.

or firmly attached to an intra-articular region, then additional partial synovectomy or arthrolysis can be included as part of the procedure. Additional treatment can be undertaken if the loose body is associated with a known area of osteochondrosis or osteochondritis dissecans. For example, if the periphery of the fragment is partially attached to the articular cartilage and the subchondral bone is evident on the underside of the fragment and in the crater, a combined procedure of partial debridement, drilling, and pinning of the fragment may provide long-term preservation of the articular surface. If the fragment is free or if there is not adequate subchondral bone to permit such a procedure, then the fragment can be removed and the sclerotic crater curetted and drilled. This procedure is performed to promote bleeding for the stimulation of reparative fibrocartilage, which will maintain congruity of the articular surface.

In the skeletally mature individual (frequently a baseball pitcher), fraying of the articular cartilage may be noted, in some cases associated with loose body formation and in other cases, a source of traumatic synovitis. A chondroplasty can be performed to remove this frayed articular cartilage. The biology of such a procedure may provide short-term symptomatic relief. However, on a long-term basis it is likely that the progressive articular degeneration will lead to degenerative joint disease.

The arthroscopic removal of intra-articular osteophytes is now recognized as a beneficial procedure. The osteophytes may be secondary to traction, such as medial valgus stress resulting in posteromedial olecranon traction osteophytes. The posterior olecranon osteophytes may be associated with a combination of triceps traction and posterior olecranon humeral impaction. A comprehensive visualization of the involved area is possible as the elbow is directed into various planes. The osteophytes can be readily removed with the use of an osteotome and motorized burr.

The role of elbow arthroscopy should be recognized as a standard procedure that provides significant advantages for treatment as well as rehabilitation of the athlete's elbow. The appropriate prearthroscopic evaluation with necessary image studies will prove helpful in planning the operative procedure. Knowledge of elbow anatomy and topographic portal placements is critical to avoid potential complications.

REHABILITATION

The rehabilitation process after injury or surgery must start with a team of health care professionals who share common knowledge of the anatomic structures involved and the anticipated recovery time to achieve athletic goals. In addition, the details of specific tissue healing, external protection, guided motion, and gradual functional goals must be understood by all members of the health care team. The details of the proposed rehabilitation program must be shared with the athlete regarding the anatomy of the injury or surgery. The goals of each phase of rehabilitation will complement the efforts of the athlete and the team of health professionals. In addition, the educational process will enhance the program of self-administered or assisted therapeutic function. The overall program should be defined and designed to concurrently increase elbow activity while maintaining adequate protection of the injured postoperative area. The phases described in Chapter 2 should be referred to for the goals of elbow rehabilitation.

Highly motivated athletes should be monitored to prevent overzealous rehabilitation, thus achieving a compromised result in too short a period of time. With every rehabilitation program, there should be a review of the continued expectations of the athlete's performance.

While elbow rehabilitation is proceeding, there is also the need to maintain overall conditioning. The protected elbow is usually maintained within a sling. This frequently contributes to the arm positioned in internal rotation and adduction at the shoulder and scapular protraction, accounting for anterior shoulder contractures and posterior shoulder weakening. As soon as possible, a maintenance shoulder program should be incorporated into the elbow rehabilitation program. Maintenance of wrist-hand-finger mobility and strength should also be included in the rehabilitation goals.

Phase I

The objectives of phase I, the acute phase, should include protection of the injured or postoperative site, pain control, minimizing atrophy, and edema management. The use of splints, bivalved casts, and hinged orthoses may be beneficial. If a significant aspect of the surgical procedure was arthrolysis or bone excision, the planned early incorporation of constant passive motion is advised. The characteristics of the injured tissues will determine the rehabilitation process and potential for surgery (i.e., tendon to bone reconstruction, osteophyte excision, and ulnar nerve transposition require significantly different periods of acute phase protection).

Phase II

As soon as the transition to phase II, initial rehabilitation, is possible, the goals must be defined: limiting contracture, increasing motion, initial muscle activity and strengthening. A limited guided active-assisted (progressing to active) range of motion program is appropriate to achieve these goals. If muscle activity is limited, electric stimulation may be helpful. The benefit of frequent periods of therapy and the supplemental use of continuous passive motion (CPM) are important factors to achieve mobility within the earliest and safest period of protected immobilization. The achievement of maximum elbow flexion and extension and forearm pronation and supination are the prime goals of this phase. The frequent periods of therapy should be monitored to assure proper techniques of exercise and progression of motion. For example, substitution of shoulder motion to avoid elbow motion is a common protection mechanism by the athlete. If there is a residual limitation of motion, neurofacilitated exercises should be included and the possible use of dynamic splints.

Phase III

As tissue healing progresses and range of motion improves, the goals of phase III, intermediate rehabilitation, will be directed to maximal active range of all elbow motions with progressive resistive therapy exercise (i.e., isotonic programs). It is during this phase that joint mobilization techniques (which maintain motion and strength), neuroproprioceptive patterns, plyometics, and the initial concepts of limited skill integrative functions, should be introduced. The baseball pitcher would slowly practice the wind-up and delivery motion without ball release while being observed by the health professional. There should be a focus on shoulder-elbow combination patterns.

Phase IV

The progression to phase IV, integrated functions, will include continued comprehensive range of motion, muscle strengthening and endurance, and additional skill exercises. At this point, isokinetic and resistive tube/band therapeutic exercises are of major value. The simulation of skill performance (i.e., progressive demands on the shoulder or elbow) and gradual transition to limited, not competitive, performance would be encouraged and guided by the health care professionals and the athletic coaching staff. The baseball pitcher would progress to long toss, pitching practice, and a simulated game, while the monitored rehabilitation process continued (see Ch. 17). At each step of the progression, the elbow should be examined and the physical findings and motions recorded (e.g., ultimate motion without pain; strength; patterns of function). In addition, it is critical to determine the need for (and then type of) external supports. If continued protection is required, the athlete should participate in the selection of these devices, noting the effect on performance, both mobility and protection. If a football or basketball participant had experienced a dislocation or severely hyperextended elbow, a hinged orthosis or specific hyperextension limiting tape would be indicated.

Phase V

When the athlete is ready to enter phase V, return to sport, there should be a programmed transition from the health care team to the coaching staff. The continued aspects of rehabilitation, motion, strength, and protection must be emphasized and supervised by both the health care and coaching staffs. If anti-inflammatory medication and physical therapeutic modalities are used, they must be monitored and integrated with the return to participation program. The need and use of protective devices must be reviewed with the athlete. The return to competition must be carefully planned with limited playing at maximal performance and a gradual return to unlimited competitive performance,

jointly determined by health professionals and coaching staff as indicated by examination and performance skills. Athletes will often feel restricted and attempt to participate without protection at an increased risk. The required continued rehabilitation and maintenance exercise program will require frequent review between the health care professional and the athlete.

REFERENCES

1. Rockwood CA, Green DP, Bucholz RW: Fractures in Adults. 3rd Ed. JB Lippincott, Philadelphia, 1991
2. Browner BD, Jupiter JB, Levine AM, Trafton PG: Skeletal Trauma: Fractures, Dislocations and Ligamentous Injuries. WB Saunders, Philadelphia, 1992
3. Mason ML: Some observations on fractures of the head of the radius with a review of one hundred cases. Br J Surg 42:123, 1954
4. Johnston GW: A follow-up on one hundred cases of fracture of the head of the radius with a review of the literature. Ulster Med J 31:51, 1962
5. Josefsson PO, Gentz, CF, Johnell O, Wendenberg B: Dislocations of the elbow and intra-articular fractures. Clin Orthop 246:126, 1989
6. Lincheid RL, O'Driscoll SW: Elbow dislocations. p. 441. In Morrey BF (ed): The Elbow and its Disorders. WB Saunders, Philadelphia, 1993
7. Strong ML: Irreducible posterolateral dislocation of the elbow without fracture. Report of two cases. Contemp Orthop 11:69, 1985
8. Pritchard DJ, Linscheid RL, Svein JH: Intra-articular median nerve entrapment with dislocation of the elbow. Clin Orthop 90:100, 1973
9. Tullos HS, Bennett J, Shepard D, Nobel PC, Gable G: Adult elbow dislocations: mechanism of instability. AAOS Instr Course Lect 35:69, 1986
10. Josefsson PO, Gentz CF, Johnell O, Wendeberg B: Surgical versus nonsurgical treatment of ligamentous injuries following dislocation of the elbow joint. J Bone Joint Surg [Am] 69:605, 1987
11. Worsing RA, Engber WD, Lange TA: Reactive synovitis from particulate Silastic. J Bone Joint Surg [Am] 64:581, 1982
12. Knight DJ, Rymaszewski LA, Amis AA, Miller JH: Primary replacement of the fractured radial head with a metal prosthesis. J Bone Joint Surg [Br] 75:572, 1993
13. Regan W, Morrey B: Fractures of the coronoid process of the ulna. J Bone Joint Surg [Am] 71:1348, 1989
14. Davis WM, Yassine Z: An etiologic factor in the tear of the distal biceps brachii. J Bone Joint Surg [Am] 38:1368, 1956
15. Bourne MH, Morrey BF: Partial rupture of the distal biceps tendon. Clin Orthop 291:143, 1981
16. Boyd HB, Anderson MD: A method for reinsertion of the distal biceps brachii tendon. J Bone Joint Surg [Am] 43:1041, 1961

17. Louis DS, Hawkin FM, Eckenrode JF, Smith PA, Wojtys EM: Distal biceps brachii tendon avulsion: a simplified method of operative repair. Am J Sports Med 14:234, 1986

18. Norman WH: Repair of avulsion of insertion of biceps brachii tendon. Clin Orthop 193:189, 1985

19. Goldie I: Epicondylitis lateralis humeri. Acta Chir Scand [Suppl] 339:7, 1964

20. Nirschl RP, Pettrone F: Tennis elbow: the surgical treatment of lateral epicondylitis. J Bone Joint Surg [Am] 61:832, 1979

21. Coonrad RW, Hooper WR: Tennis elbow: its course, natural history, conservative and surgical management. J Bone Joint Surg [Am] 55:1177, 1973

22. Baumgard SH, Schartz DR: Percutaneous release of the epicondylar muscles for humeral epicondylitis. Am J Sports Med 10:233, 1982

23. Nestor B, O'Driscoll SW, Morrey BF: Surgical stabilization for lateral rotatory instability of the elbow. J Bone Joint Surg [Am] 74:1235, 1992

24. Pappas AM: Elbow problems associated with baseball during childhood and adolescence. Clin Orthop 164:30, 1982

25. Priest JD: Elbow Injuries in gymnastics. Clin Sport Med 4:73, 1985

26. Waugh RL, Hathcock TA, Elliot JL: Ruptures of muscles and tendons. Surgery 25:370, 1949

27. Farrar EL III, Lippert FG III: Avulsion of the triceps tendon. Clin Orthop 161:242, 1981

28. Match RM, Corrylos EV: Bilateral avulsion fracture of the triceps tendon insertion from skiing with osteogenesis imperfecta tarda. Am J Sports Med 11:99, 1983

29. Viegas SF: Avulsion of the triceps tendon. Orthop Rev 19:533, 1990

30. Kovach J II, Baker BE, Mosher JF: Fracture separation of the olecranon ossification center in adults. Am J Sports Med 13:105, 1985

31. King JW, Brelsford HJ, Tullos HS: Analysis of the pitching arm of the professional baseball pitcher. Clin Orthop 67:116, 1969

32. Pappas AM, Zawacki RM, Sullivan TJ: Biomechanics of baseball pitching: a preliminary report. Am J Sport Med 13:216, 1985

33. Miller JE: Javelin Throwers Elbow. J Bone Joint Surg [Bh] 42:788, 1960

34. Indelicato PA, Jobe FW, Kerlan RK, Carter VS, Schields CL, Lombardo SJ: Correctable elbow lesions in professional baseball players: a review of 25 cases. Am J Sports Med 7:72, 1979

35. Wilson FD, Andrews JR, Blackburn TA, McCluskey G: Valgus extension overload in the pitching elbow. Am J Sport Med 11:83, 1983

36. Jobe FW, Stark H, Lombardo SF: Reconstruction of the ulnar collateral ligament in athletes. J Bone Joint Surg 68:1158, 1986a

37. Childress HM: Recurrent ulnar nerve dislocation at the elbow. Clin Orthop 108:168, 1975

38. Burman MS: Arthroscopy or the direct visualization of joints. J Bone Joint Surg 13:669, 1931

39. Andrews JR, Soffer JR: Elbow Arthroscopy. CV Mosby, St. Louis, 1994

40. Johnson LL: Elbow Arthroscopy in Arthroscopic Surgery Principles and Practice. p. 1446. Mosby, St. Louis, 1986

20

Wrist Anatomy and Function

William J. Morgan

The wrist is a joint that allows an almost infinite number of motions while providing for the hand's ability to grasp, release, and balance. These functions are necessary for any athlete (e.g., a javelin thrower, a catcher, a racquet player) to successfully compete. The osseous, ligamentous, and musculotendinous structures of the wrist are complex, thus constituting a difficult joint to fully evaluate and treat. An understanding of the anatomy, kinematics, and function of the wrist in its normal state is critical before diagnosis and treatment of a wrist injury in the athlete can occur.

The ability of athletes to position their hands in any spatial orientation is dependent on the combined motion of the distal radioulnar joint, the radiocarpal and midcarpal joints, and the carpometacarpal joints. The forces imposed upon the pitcher's wrist in acceleration, deceleration, and rotation are in marked contrast to the repetitive forced extension stresses imposed upon the wrist of a volleyball player.

The nature of a wrist injury implies a failure (sprain, strain, or fracture) within the intrinsic and extrinsic structures of the joint. It should be recognized that all of these structures work together and rarely sustain isolated injuries. For example, a fracture of the scaphoid that displaces will cause abnormal kinematic changes at the lunate and triquetrum due to the intrinsic influences of the interosseous ligaments. Likewise, a fracture to the distal radius in an athlete may be associated with injuries to the ligamentous structures of the wrist.

OSTEOLOGY

Radius

The distal radius articulates with the proximal carpal row to form the radiocarpal joint and with the distal ulna to form the distal radioulnar joint. The distal radius has an average radial inclination of 22 degrees with a radial length averaging 9 mm and a volar tilt of 11 degrees (Fig. 20-1). The normal carpal height ratio is 0.54 ± 0.03. This is calculated by dividing the height of the carpus by the length of the long-finger metacarpal (Fig. 20-2). This becomes important in the assessment of carpal instabilities (see Ch. 24). The articulation of the radiocarpal joint is comprised of two concave surfaces representing articulations with the carpal scaphoid and lunate—termed the scaphoid and lunate fossae. Along the ulnar border of the radius is a concavity where the distal ulnar head articulates, known as the sigmoid notch (Fig. 20-3).

Carpus

The carpus is composed of eight carpal bones with the majority of surface area comprised of articular cartilage to accommodate the multiple complex articulations. The distal carpal row is made up of the trapezium, trapezoid, capitate, and hamate (Fig. 20-4). The

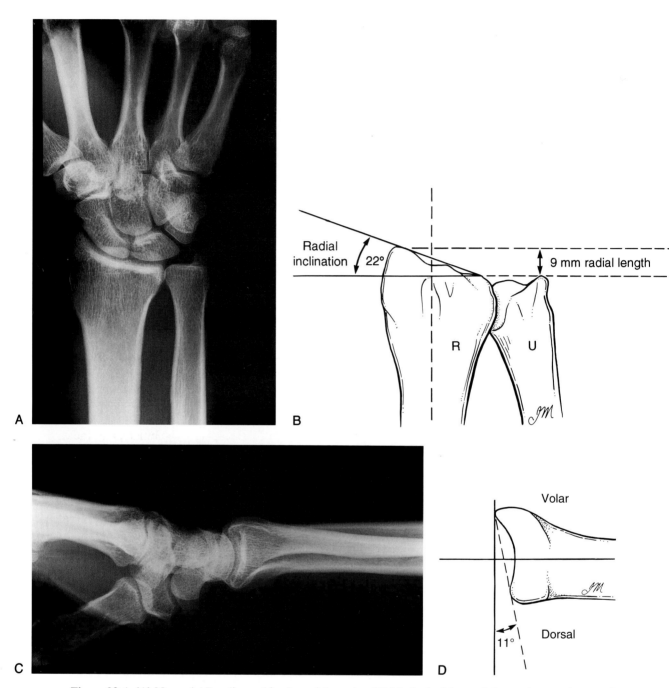

Figure 20-1 **(A)** Normal AP radiographic view of the wrist. **(B)** Method of determining and normal values for radial inclination and length. **(C)** Normal lateral radiographic view of wrist. **(D)** Method of determining and normal value for volar tilt.

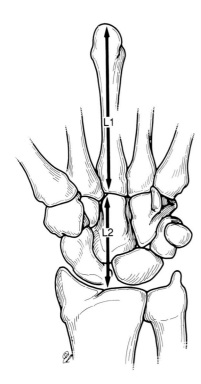

Figure 20-2 Techniques of measurement of carpal height index L_2/L_4. This is performed by measuring long-finger metacarpal (L_1) and carpal height (L_2). Normal ratio: 0.54 ± 0.03

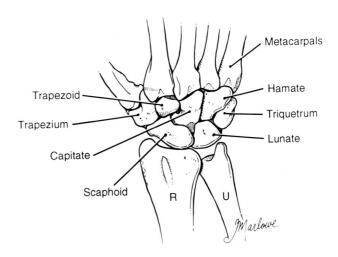

Figure 20-4 Osseous and articular anatomy of carpus.

trapezium forms a "saddle joint" articulation with the base of the thumb allowing for multiplanar motion. The index and long-finger metacarpals form rigid articulations with the trapezoid and capitate, while the ring and small-finger metacarpals form less rigid articulations with the hamate, allowing increased motion in the volar dorsal plane. The proximal carpal row is composed of the scaphoid, the lunate, and the triquetrum (Fig. 20-4). The scaphoid forms a link between the proximal and distal carpal rows (Fig. 20-5). The pisiform is a sesamoid bone within the substance of the flexor carpi ulnaris tendon that articulates with the triquetrum, completing the proximal carpal row. The carpus is stabilized by intrinsic and extrinsic carpal ligaments (see the following section).

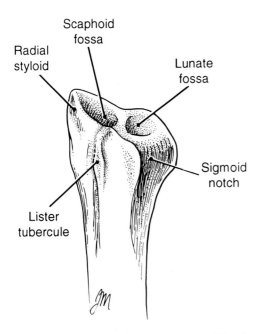

Figure 20-3 Osseous and articular anatomy of distal radius.

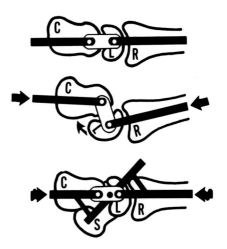

Figure 20-5 Scaphoid functions as a link mechanism between proximal and distal carpal rows preventing collapse.

LIGAMENTOUS ANATOMY

The ligaments of the wrist are complex structures that provide support to multiple articulations, yet allow freedom of motion in a multiplanar direction both actively and passively. Anatomy of the wrist ligaments has been well described by Taleisnik[1] and categorized as intrinsic and extrinsic. The volar extrinsic ligaments are larger than the dorsal extrinsic ligaments and provide the majority of wrist support.

Extrinsic Ligaments

The volar extrinsic ligaments are classified as radiocarpal and ulnocarpal (Fig. 20-6). The majority of the radiocarpal ligaments originate from the radial styloid. The radioscaphocapitate ligament extends from the radial styloid to the capitate, forming a sling across the waist of the scaphoid. The radiolunate ligament extends from the radial styloid to the lunate but often may have extensions to the triquetrum. The radioscapholunate ligament extends from the distal radius to the scapholunate ligament. These structures play a critical role in maintaining carpal stability and preventing ulnar drift. The radioscaphocapitate ligament fails to maintain its integrity at tension forces of 30 lb (151 N), while the radiolunate ligament fails at 21 lb (107 N); both may elongate 30 percent before rupture. (For information on the ulnocarpal ligaments, see Ch. 22.)

Intrinsic Ligaments

The intrinsic ligaments include the interosseous ligaments and the deltoid or V ligament. The interosseous ligaments connect the carpal bones and are named by their articulation. The distal carpal row is connected by the trapeziotrapezoidal, trapezoid capitate, and the capitohamate ligaments. The intrinsic ligaments of the distal carpal row rarely fail clinically and therefore have little clinical applicability. The proximal carpal row is less rigidly connected by the scapholunate and lunotriquetral interosseous ligaments. These ligaments have been shown to fail at tensile forces of 45 lb (232 N) and 75 lb (353 N), respectively. They also may elongate 50 to 100 percent prior to rupture and become incompetent. This concept is important when assessing carpal instability injury patterns. Finally, the proximal and distal carpal rows are connected by the scaphotrapezial and triquetrohamate ligaments forming a ring (Fig. 20-7).[2]

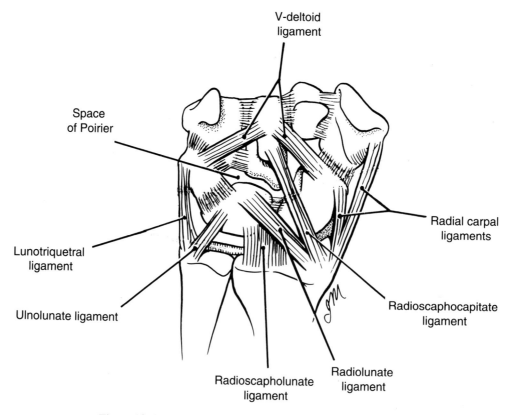

Figure 20-6 Volar extrinsic ligamentous anatomy of the wrist.

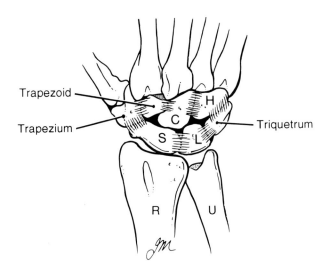

Figure 20-7 Intrinsic ligamentous anatomy of the wrist (see text).

The deltoid or V ligament extends from the capitate distally, where it forms the apex of an inverted V and projects proximally to the scaphoid and the triquetrum. This inverted configuration leaves a relatively weakened area volarly at the capitolunate articulation (space of Poirier) (Fig. 20-6).

DISTAL RADIOULNAR JOINT

The distal articulation of the forearm, consisting of the radius and ulna, composes the distal radioulnar joint. The ulnar head is covered by articular cartilage spanning approximately 240 degrees of its circumference and is articulated with the shallow sigmoid notch of the radius. Rotation of the forearm occurs as the radius rotates around the stable ulna. As the radius rotates into pronation, it crosses the ulnar shaft and is functionally shorter. While in supination, the shafts of the radius and ulna are parallel and thus the radius appears elongated at the distal radioulnar joint (Fig. 20-8) (this is important in understanding the radiographic assessment of the distal radioulnar joint). The shallow sigmoid notch affords a large arc of motion but little skeletal stability to the distal radioulnar joint. Due to the shallow articulation of the sigmoid notch, the wrist rotates up to an arc of 180 degrees (Fig. 20-9). It is also due to this shallow arc that the athlete is at risk of injury if the dorsal or volar ligamentous restraints are disrupted, for example, by falling onto the pronated extended wrist, allowing subluxation of the distal radioulnar joint.

The primary intrinsic stabilizer of the distal radioulnar joint is the triangular fibrocartilage complex, associated with the volar and dorsal marginal ligaments and

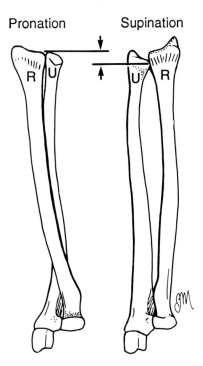

Figure 20-8 Change in wrist ulna variance as the forearm rotates from supination to pronation.

the volar and dorsal distal radioulnar joint capsule. Secondary (or extrinsic) support is rendered by the pronator quadratus, flexor and extensor carpi ulnaris, and the interosseous membrane. The triangular fibrocartilage complex is comprised of the articular disc with associated volar and dorsal marginal ligament (TFC), the ulno-carpal ligaments and the floor of the ECU. The TFC originates at the ulnar border of the lunate fossae of the radius and inserts at the base of the ulnar styloid (fovea) (Fig. 20-10). The triangular fibrocartilage is bordered volarly and dorsally with the volar and dorsal radioulnar marginal ligaments, which also insert into the fovea of the ulna. The ulnolunate and the ulnotriquetral ligaments extend from the volar radioulnar ligament and insert into the lunate and tri-

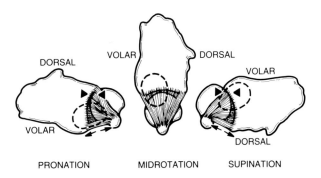

Figure 20-9 Rotation of distal radius about the stable ulna of 180 degrees from supination to pronation.

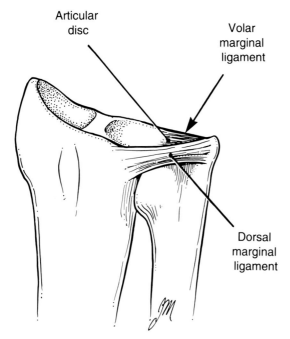

Figure 20-10 Articular disc with volar and dorsal marginal ligaments making up the triangular fibrocartilage.

quetrum. The ulnar collateral ligament merges with the meniscus homologue at the fovea and inserts distally into the triquetrum, hamate, and the base of the fifth metacarpal. Dorsally, the sheath of the extensor carpi ulnaris forms the roof of the triangular fibrocartilage complex (Fig. 20-11).

EXTRA-ARTICULAR ANATOMY

The extra-articular anatomy of the wrist is comprised of multiple musculotendinous units, many of

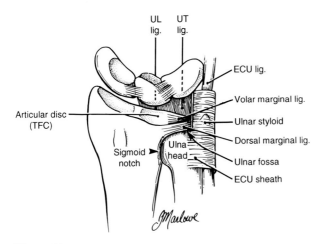

Figure 20-11 Additions of the volar ulnocarpal ligaments and dorsal extensor carpi ulnaris tendon sheath illustrates the three-dimensional nature of the triangular fibrocartilage complex.

which are encased in a fibro-osseous tunnel, providing for optimal mechanical function. These same restraints, however, also offer the potential for overuse, inflammation, or failure. The wrist provides a conduit for the median and ulnar nerves to supply sensation and fine intrinsic function of the hand. As noted for musculotendinous units, however, these same enclosed conduits in an overuse or abnormal state may produce abnormal stressors, manifested by nerve entrapment syndromes. This section introduces the normal anatomy of these structures to provide a better understanding of how injury patterns develop.

To provide for wrist motion (including circumduction), there are several musculotendinous motor units arranged in specific patterns to allow vector forces that translate into pure flexion extension moments or rotational movements. The direct wrist motor musculotendinous units are comprised of the flexor carpi radialis, flexor carpi ulnaris, extensor carpi radialis brevis, extensor carpi radialis longus, and extensor carpi ulnaris. Further motion of the wrist, however, is augmented indirectly by musculotendinous units in the form of the finger flexors and extensors as they cross over this intercalated joint, providing for some increased motion and strength at the wrist joint.

The dorsal surface of the wrist is comprised of an extensor retinaculum, which spans from the radial styloid to the ulnar styloid. Within this extensor retinaculum are six compartments that form separate fibro-osseous tunnels housing the wrist and finger extensors (Fig. 20-12). The first extensor compartment is located along the radial border of the radius just proximal to the radial styloid and contains the abductor pollicis longus and extensor pollicis brevis tendons. This is a common location for tenosynovitis in the athlete (see Ch. 23). More ulnarly is the second extensor compartment containing the extensor carpi radialis longus and extensor carpi radialis brevis. Just ulnar to Lister's tubercle is the third extensor compartment, consisting of the extensor pollicis longus tendon. On the mid-dorsum of the wrist over the ulnar surface of the radius lies the fourth extensor compartment, which contains the extensor digitorum communis tendons and the extensor indicis proprius. More ulnarly, at the level of the distal radioulnar joint, lies the fifth extensor compartment, consisting of the extensor digit minimi. Finally, most ulnarward in the notch at the ulnar styloid is the extensor carpi ulnaris in the sixth extensor compartment (Fig. 20-12).

In the athlete requiring repetitive extensor motions of the wrist (e.g., the batter or racquet player), inflammation of these fibro-osseus tunnels is seen. These anatomic landmarks must be kept in mind when assessing the athlete with dorsal wrist pain (see inflammatory section).

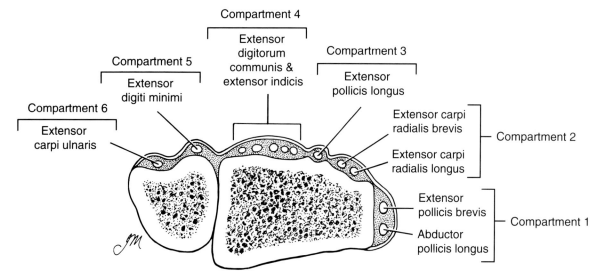

Figure 20-12 Six extensor compartments and their anatomic contents (see text).

Along the volar surface of the wrist and most radial lies the flexor carpi radialis tendon as it traverses just ulnar to the scaphoid tubercle beneath the trapezial ridge and inserts into the base of the second metacarpal. The palmaris longus tendon lies in the midvolar aspect of the wrist as it inserts into the palmar fascia. The palmaris longus may be absent in approximately 15 percent of individuals. Most ulnarly lies the flexor carpi ulnaris tendon as it inserts into the pisiform and extends distally into the hamate and the base of the fifth metacarpal. Lying more deeply are the flexor profundus, flexor sublimis, and flexor pollicis longus tendons as they traverse the carpal tunnel en route to their respective fingers and thumb. The median nerve travels between the muscle bellies of the sublimis and profundus musculotendinous units and emerges into the palm beneath the transverse carpal ligament within the carpal tunnel. This is the location where the median nerve may become injured in the athlete as a result of direct trauma or an entrapment neuropathy within the carpal tunnel. Thus, any one of these structures may be a source of inflammation and should be considered during the assessment of the athlete whose sport requires repetitive wrist flexion, such as in racquet ball.

The ulnar nerve runs parallel with and beneath the flexor carpi ulnaris tendon until it enters Guyon's canal, where it traverses between the pisiform and hamate and divides into the deep motor and sensory branch of the ulnar nerve within the palm (Fig. 20-13). It is at the level of the hamate and pisiform within Guyon's canal that the ulnar nerve may become injured simultaneously with injury of the ulnar carpus, particularly the hook of the hamate and pisiform.

KINEMATICS AND FUNCTION OF THE DISTAL RADIUS

The distal radius is a multiplanar joint with articulations occurring with the carpus and the ulna. Its multiple articulations enable the wrist to move in 80 to 90 degrees of wrist flexion, 70 to 90 degrees of wrist extension, 15 degrees of wrist radial deviation, 30 to 45 degrees of wrist ulnar deviation, 85 to 90 degrees of forearm supination, and 85 to 90 degrees of forearm

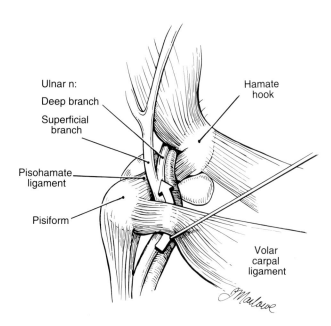

Figure 20-13 Anatomy of Guyon's canal.

pronation. The functional or resting position of the wrist is 20 to 35 degrees of extension and 10 to 15 degrees of ulnar deviation, enabling the fingers to flex with minimal resistance from the extensor antagonists.

KINEMATICS AND FUNCTION OF THE CARPUS

The wrist is capable of motion in essentially any direction due to its multiple shallow articulations and the intercalated segment located within these articulations, the proximal carpal row. The intercalated nature of this segment implies that there are no direct motors inserting into this segment but that the free floating segment is balanced by ligaments and influenced by the motor units that insert more distally. The proximal carpal row is linked to the distal carpal row by the scaphoid, allowing for complex multiplanar motion. The proximal carpal row has no musculotendinous insertions and relies solely upon extrinsic and intrinsic ligaments for support. Although the distal carpal row also has no musculotendinous insertions, it acts less as an intercalated segment by nature of its firm capsuloligamentous attachment to the proximal metacarpals.

The geometry of the carpal bones plays a role in the normal and abnormal kinematics of the wrist. The scaphoid is an S-shaped bone, which forms a link between the proximal and distal rows of the carpus with greater than 80 percent of the surface covered by articular cartilage. The ulnar border of the scaphoid is concave where it articulates with the capitate; its proximal one-third is convex and articulates with the radius.

Distally, there is another convex articulation with the trapezium and trapezoid. Dorsally, there is a spiral groove for capsular attachments (Fig. 20-14) (see Ch. 24). The scaphoid forms the base of the thumb ray, and, if unrestrained by normal extrinsic and intrinsic ligament forces, assumes a more flexed (vertical) position (Fig. 20-15). The lunate has a broader volar surface than dorsal, which encourages a dorsiflexed position in the nonrestrained state (Fig. 20-15). The helicoidal articulation of the triquetrohamate joint causes the triquetrum to rotate volarly and distally on the hamate in ulnar deviation and dorsally and proximally in radial deviation. The trapezoid and capitate and, to a lesser degree, the hamate, form a rigid articulation with the metacarpals, allowing for little motion. The trapezium acts more in the motion of the thumb ray with some influence of scaphoid motion.

As the forearm rotates in pronation, there is a mild volar translation of the radius on the ulna, resulting in increased tension of the triangular fibrocartilage complex volar marginal ligaments and the dorsal capsule of the distal radioulnar joint. Conversely, as the wrist rotates in supination, there is a mild dorsal translation of the distal radius on the distal ulna, resulting in tension of the triangular fibrocartilage complex dorsal marginal ligament and the volar capsule of the distal radioulnar joint (Fig. 20-16). This illustrates the importance of obtaining a detailed history from the athlete following a fall onto the wrist. For example, if a football player falls onto his extended pronated wrist, he is likely to sustain an injury to the dorsal capsule of the distal radioulnar joint as well as the volar marginal ligaments of the triangular fibrocartilage complex, pos-

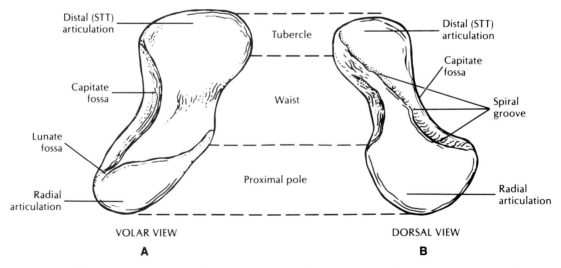

Figure 20-14 Dorsal anatomy of scaphoid demonstrating spinal groove for capsular attachments.

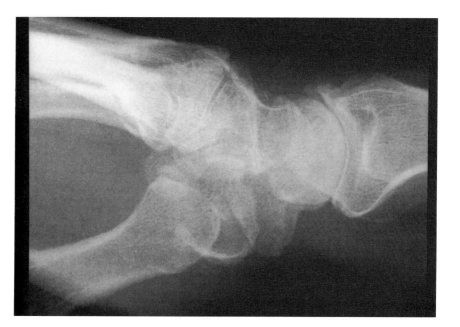

Figure 20-15 Radiograph demonstrating abnormal (nonrestrained) position of the scaphoid and lunate (DISI). Note dorsal subluxation of capitate on hamate (white arrow) and vertical position of scaphoid (black arrows).

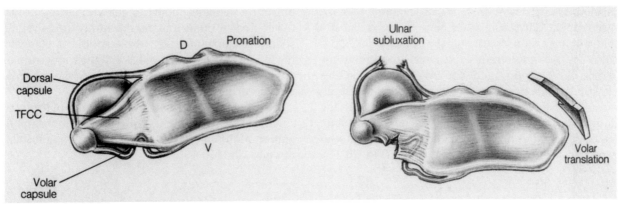

A

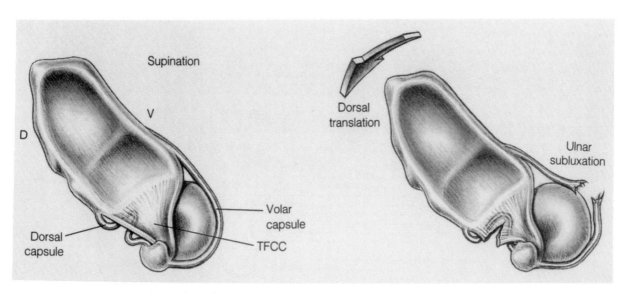

B

Figure 20-16 Changes in tension of the dorsal (D) and volar (V) capsule and marginal ligament of the distal radioulnar joint as the forearm rotates into **(A)** pronation and **(B)** supination (see text). In extremes of rotation, note failure of capsule and marginal ligaments.

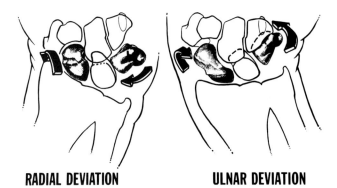

RADIAL DEVIATION   **ULNAR DEVIATION**

Figure 20-17 As the wrist moves into ulnar deviation, the proximal carpal row naturally extends with an elongated appearance of the scaphoid, trapezoidal appearance of the lunate, and overlap of the triquetrum and hamate. In radial deviation, the scaphoid appears foreshortened as it assumes a flexed position, the lunate appears triangular, and the triquetrum moves proximal to the hamate.

sibly resulting in dorsal subluxation or dislocation of the distal radioulnar joint.

Due to the interosseous ligaments providing an internal restraint, the proximal and distal carpal rows tend to move as a unit in both flexion extension and ulnar and radial deviation. In radial deviation, to make room for the narrowing space between the radial styloid and trapezium, the scaphoid assumes a flexed position by the interosseous ligaments, the lunate assumes a volar tilt, and the triquetrum migrates proximal to the hamate. Radiographically, the scaphoid appears foreshortened with a ring sign due to the double density of overlapping cortical bone; the lunate appears triangular in shape and the triquetrum is seen proximal to the hamate and radiograph (Fig. 20-17).

The triquetrum migrates distally and volarly to the hamate in a helicoidal pattern to make room for the shortening between the distal ulna and the fifth metacarpal in ulnar deviation. Due to the interosseus ligamentous restraint, the lunate tilts in a dorsally flexed position and the scaphoid extends with the lunate to fill the void as the trapezium migrates away from the radial styloid. Radiographically, the scaphoid is elongated, the lunate appears trapezoidal, and the triquetrum migrates distal in relation to the hamate where overlapping cortical margins are seen (Fig. 20-17).

Any disruption of this intricate balance of the intrinsic interosseous ligaments will result in abnormal migration of the corpus as manifested by carpal instabilities (see Ch. 23).

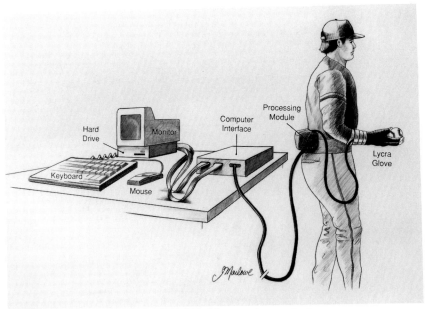

Figure 20-18 Design of pitching motion analysis system.

Table 20-1 Phases of the Pitch

	Cocking	Acceleration	Deceleration	Recovery
Range of motion (degrees)	32.4 (±7.8)	94.2 (±1.8)	43.4 (±3.3)	91.0 (±10.2)
Time (ms)	218.9 (±40.1)	105.2 (±10.8)	863.3 (±40.3)	582.7 (±91.6)
Angular velocity (degrees/second)	148.5 (±25.8)	1084.9 (±121.5)	50.2 (±2.9)	165.3 (±15.2)

KINEMATICS OF THE WRIST DURING PITCHING

The wrist functions in three planes of motion: flexion extension, ulnar and radial deviation, and pronation and supination. It may also function as a composite of all three arcs of motion (i.e., circumduction). During any one of these arcs of motion, various forces are imparted upon the intrinsic and extrinsic structures of the wrist joint, which may lead to intra- or extra-articular injuries in the athlete.

To better understand the kinematic changes seen at the wrist during throwing, the flexion extension arc of the wrist was studied over time in the professional baseball pitcher, utilizing a computerized motion analysis system[3] (Fig. 20-18). In the assessment of kinematics of the wrist during the pitching cycle, four phases have been reproducibly identified. The first phase of the cocking phase demonstrates the motion of the wrist as it moves into maximum extension. In this phase, the wrist is moved into extension by the radial and ulnar wrist extensors with synergistic flexion of the long-finger flexors. The proximal and distal carpal rows rotate into extension. This is then followed by the acceleration phase, which is an explosive transition of the wrist from extension to flexion. This is associated with contraction of the flexor-pronator mass with flexion of the wrist and fingers, and pronation of the forearm. The proximal and distal carpal rows rotate into flexion. At ball release, there is deceleration of the wrist as it progresses into maximum flexion. At this point, cocontraction of the wrist extensors occurs as the contraction of the flexors diminishes, thus slowing the progression of flexion of the wrist. The proximal and distal carpal rows continue to move into flexion, but at a decreasing rate. Finally, this is followed by the recovery phase, during which the wrist slowly assumes a neutral or extended position (Table 20-1 and Fig. 20-19).

Extremes of motion are imposed on the wrist over a short period of time during the throwing cycle. This

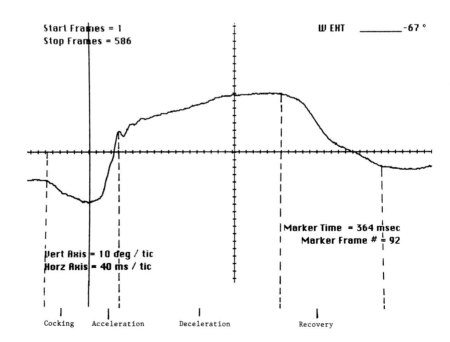

Figure 20-19 Graphic representation of wrist motion during pitching.

requires extremes of flexor acceleration and extensor deceleration in conjunction with intrinsic wrist stabilizers (previously described intrinsic and extrinsic ligamentous supports). Further study of the kinematics of the wrist will be helpful in a better understanding of injury patterns in the throwing athlete.

The wrist is anatomically comprised of multiple articulations balanced by intrinsic and extrinsic ligamentous and musculotendinous restraints. This delicate balance allows for a variety of motions to take place but also lends itself to various pathology, especially in the competitive athlete. The subsequent chapters review the diagnosis, treatment, and rehabilitation of this pathology as applied to individual athletes and their sports.

REFERENCES

1. Taleisnik J: The ligaments of the wrist. J Hand Surgery 1:110, 1976
2. Lichtman DM, Schneider JR, Swafford AR et al: Ulnar midcarpal instability: clinical and laboratory analysis. J Hand Surg 6:515, 1981
3. Pappas AM, Morgan WJ, Schulz LA, Diana R: Wrist kinematics during pitching: a preliminary report. Am J Sports Med, in press

21

History, Physical Examination, and Diagnostic Testing of the Wrist

William J. Morgan

The clinician evaluating a wrist injury in the athlete must consider physical stresses and functional expectations imposed on the wrist from a sport-specific perspective. A gymnast is required to possess extreme flexibility and stability about the wrist in flexion, extension, and circumduction. By contrast, for the swimmer, stability of the wrist joint in a neutral position provides for water displacement during a power stroke. This variability of athletic functional demand, along with the intricate nature of wrist joint dynamics, offers a diagnostic challenge to the sports health care provider.

To provide for the complex motion of the wrist (i.e., flexion, extension, circumduction, supination, and pronation), there must be a balance between multiple shallow articulations and the intrinsic (ligaments) and extrinsic (musculotendinous units) stabilizers. A detailed history should be obtained from the athlete who presents with wrist pain and should include the following: (1) the age and preexisting or associated medical conditions; (2) the time of injury: onset and presentation; (3) the position of the wrist at the time of injury; (4) a list of the activities that aggravate, re-create, or improve the pain; and (5) the sport, the level of competition or skill, time involved in the sport, and previous treatment.

Time spent with the athlete in developing rapport is invaluable to the diagnostic process. This is especially important in adolescent athletes who, from fear of competition or dislike of their sport, may develop symptoms referable to the wrist, particularly if the use of their wrist is primary to their sport. It is critical that this psychological factor be considered before unnecessary invasive testing or surgery is scheduled. It is not uncommon in a sport such as gymnastics, where the training is rigorous and the competition is intense, for a young athlete to present with wrist pain. In this case, while taking the history, it is often noted that the pain is exclusively related to gymnastics and always relieved by a break from the sport, only to be reexacerbated on return to participation. This behavior may be manifested by a display of pain out of proportion to the provocative maneuver (e.g., pulling away with light wrist palpation). Other manifestations noted may include frequent giving way to strength testing or an active range of motion inconsistent with the passive range of motion. These adolescents can often successfully complete other athletic activities without pain. The physical examination is generally quite benign (if not normal) and pursuing further testing, particularly if invasive, should be done with caution.

Historical reports of how the injury affects the athlete's performance are helpful for the subsequent evaluation. For example, the batter whose performance is altered due to a painful "clunk" upon ulnar deviation of his wrist is apt to have a (midcarpal) wrist instability. Conversely, the batter whose performance is altered due to pain at the base of his thumb in extremes of ulna deviation is likely to have an extra-articular inflammatory condition, such as de Quervain's stenosing tenosynovitis or a superficial radial neuroma.

HISTORY

Preexisting or Associated Medical Conditions

Preexisting medical conditions such as ulcerative colitis, psoriasis, and spondyloarthropathies create a predisposition to synovitis within overused joints. In the adolescent athlete, the relationship of intermittent joint effusions and synovitis to the use of certain anti-acne medications has recently been noted (e.g., isotutinoin [Accutaine]).

The use (and overuse) of medications by the athlete in the past and present should be accurately recorded, including narcotic analgesics, nonnarcotic analgesics, nonsteroidal anti-inflammatory medications, steroids (both anabolic and corticosteroids), stimulants, and other prescription medications. This documentation is necessary to control drug interaction as well as to prevent any potential misuse of medications.

Onset of Injury

Understanding the onset of an injury to the wrist is helpful in distinguishing traumatic from inflammatory conditions. The golfer who presents with an insidious onset of wrist pain that slowly worsens over time may be predisposed to an inflammatory condition such as tendinitis or synovitis. By contrast, the golfer who complains of a sudden onset and persistence of ulnar-sided wrist pain following a "fat swing" will in all likelihood have sustained an acute sprain or fracture, such as a fracture of the hook of the hamate (see Ch. 24).

Time of Injury Versus Time of Presentation

In obtaining a history from the athlete, it is important to know the amount of time that has elapsed from the time of injury to presentation. The timing of the injury will have an impact on the presenting symptoms of the athlete as well as the treatment options.

Injuries can be classified as acute (1 to 14 days), subacute (more than 2 weeks, less than 3 months), and chronic (more than 3 months). Defining the time from injury to treatment is imperative in treating both bony and soft tissue injuries. Chronic untreated ligamentous ruptures will retract, fibrillate, and become inoperable with time, while an untreated fracture may go on to nonunion or pseudoarthrosis.[1] For example, bone healing of a distal radius fracture in a football player should be evident by 6 weeks and, if seen acutely, may be treated best by cast immobilization. The same athlete who presents 3 months postinjury may have a delayed union, a nonunion, or a malunion and a poor prognosis for healing with cast immobilization alone. In this case, open reduction internal fixation and/or bone grafting would be warranted.

The athlete with an acute or subacute ligamentous disruption of the wrist may be a candidate for repair of the ligament tear. The athlete with the same injury but of a chronic nature, however, is unlikely to have a successful repair due to ligamentous scarring and retraction. This athletic injury would require a more complex procedure in the form of a reconstruction or arthrodesis, resulting in prolonged rehabilitation and a less optimal result.

Wrist Position

If possible, an accurate history from the athlete on wrist position at the time of injury is important in developing the diagnosis. If the examiner accepts the athlete's history as "I fell onto my wrist," critical diagnostic information will be lost. Important questions regarding the injury must be asked: Was the wrist flexed or extended? Were there forces in radial or ulnar deviation? Was the position of the forearm in pronation or supination? Was the injury the result of a direct blow? A hyperextension injury of the wrist may result in a carpal instability pattern or fractures to the scaphoid or the distal radius, whereas a hyperflexion injury or rotational injury of the wrist may cause damage to the distal radioulnar joint and triangular fibrocartilage complex.

Etiology of the Pain

As mentioned previously, obtaining a history of activities or positions which re-create, aggravate, or improve the pain is helpful in further devising a plan to determine the etiology of the pain. A weight lifter who notes pain only on extreme forced hyperextension of the wrist and who duplicates it for the clinician by the same motion may have a dorsal impingement or occult ganglion of the wrist. Often a diagnosis can be formed by carefully listening to the athlete's history of a reproducible position of pain.

Previous Treatment

Many athletes (particularly veteran athletes) experience recurrent problems about the wrist that are usually inflammatory in nature and due to overuse or deviations from proper technique. It is not uncommon for the senior golfer or tennis player to present on multiple occasions with recurrent ulnar dorsal wrist pain. This area of the wrist is a source of repetitive trauma due to the extension and ulnar deviation of the wrist in both of these sports. This may be manifested as an ulna impaction syndrome with tenosynovitis about the triangular fibrocartilage complex or may be secondary to inflammation about the flexor carpi ulnar's tendon sheath. In the young gymnast, repetitive hyperextension of the wrist results in a dorsal impaction syndrome of the lunate and ulna. This is often successfully treated by a semirigid dorsal extension block splint. Many of these problems can be successfully treated by splint or use of an anti-inflammatory medication. It is therefore imperative that the treating provider inquire about successful and unsuccessful previous treatment. Often, reinstitution of the same or similar treatment program (if previously successful) will bring the presenting complaint to an end.

PHYSICAL EXAMINATION

Observation

Prior to any physical contact by the examiner, the athlete's ability to use the involved extremity should be observed. Ideally, this is best undertaken in the athlete's sports environment, noting gestures of discomfort as well as an inability to perform certain sport-specific activities. If this is not possible, observation should be made as the athlete presents to the office or sports health care facility. Pain or limited motion should be assessed as the athlete enters the room and performs typical activities such as removal of a coat, getting out of a chair, and posturing of the extremities. Ability or willingness to shake hands is a valuable tool in assessing the potential degree of injury and discomfort. This is an opportune time to assess the athlete's range of motion, strength, and potential degree of pain before he or she is aware that the assessment has begun, as it will minimize any "performance" that may otherwise occur during the examination.

Inspection

A visual inspection of the limb should occur prior to any provocative maneuvers that may be painful to the athlete. Both upper extremities should be clearly visualized from shoulder to fingertips and an assessment of atrophy, discoloration, or asymmetry should be made. It must be kept in mind that the athlete's dominant extremity may be somewhat hypertrophied due to conditioning relative to the nondominant extremity, particularly in the throwing athlete.

A careful visual examination should be performed by comparing the symptomatic and the nonsymptomatic wrist; this is best achieved by having the athlete seated in front of the examiner and comparing both hands in supination and pronation. Areas of ecchymosis (suggesting a recent traumatic injury) and erythema (indicating inflammation) should be noted and correlated with the underlying soft tissue and osseous anatomic structures. For example, erythema and swelling noted overlying the dorsal radial aspect of the wrist in a racquet ball player may correlate with the first extensor compartment and suggest de Quervain's tenosynovitis. In the wrists and hands, loss of skin creases will be a subtle indication of swelling and should be compared to the uninvolved limb. Areas of atrophy should be inspected, particularly along the thenar eminence, indicating a median neuropathy, or along the first dorsal interosseous muscle, indicating involvement of the ulnar nerve. Subtle fasciculation may be noted in the thenar or hypothenar eminences, suggestive of muscle denervation. Long-standing neurogenic problems and changes in the sweating patterns of the hand may be noted, and there may be atrophic changes in cases of long-term neuropathies. Less subtle changes such as obvious deformity (particularly when associated with pain) should be assessed radiographically (Fig. 21-1) to rule out an underlying fracture that may be worsened or displaced by any provocative maneuvers or physical examination.

Palpation

Most wrist injuries will present as a somewhat diffuse painful wrist by history, and it is not until the examiner specifically palpates the underlying landmarks that possible diagnoses can be established. There must be an awareness of the underlying osseous, tendinous, and ligamentous structures to correlate the physical findings with the anatomy. Once key topographic landmarks are recognized and palpation is carried out systematically, the examiner will find it a useful tool in the diagnostic process.

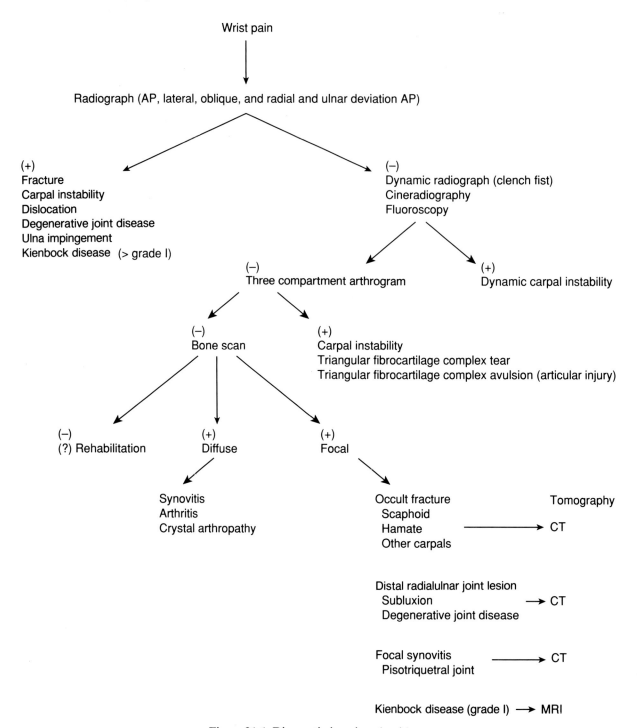

Figure 21-1 Diagnostic imaging algorithm.

Palpation should begin at a landmark easily recognizable by the examiner and performed in a systematic fashion. The athlete should be seated opposite the examiner, with the elbow supported and the wrist in a relaxed position within the examiner's hands. An excellent beginning point is Lister's tubercle, since it is an easily palpated prominence on the dorsal radial aspect of the distal radius and a helpful point for identifying osseus, ligamentous, and tendinous structures. If palpation begins just distal to Lister's tubercle, one can palpate the area of the scapholunate ligament from which further palpation of the osseous structures can be performed. Similarly, in palpating Lister's tubercle, one is able to palpate the third extensor compartment on the ulnar aspect of Lister's tubercle and the second extensor compartment on the radial aspect of Lister's

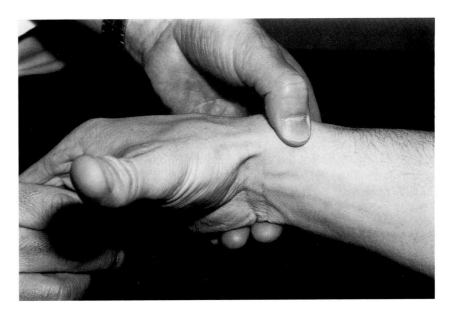

Figure 21-2 Palpation of the first extensor compartment (abductor pollicis longus and extensor pollicis brevis tendons).

tubercle, thus establishing a guide to the six extensor compartments.

As the examination continues, palpation should progress from the least sensitive area to the most sensitive area to prevent the examination ending abruptly because of pain.

Radial Styloid

The radial styloid is easily palpated as the bony prominence just proximal to the base of the thumb. Tenderness to palpation in this area may suggest contusion or fracture of the radial styloid. Palpation 1 cm proximal to the radial styloid (Fig. 21-2) will reveal the first extensor compartment containing the abductor pollicis longus and the extensor pollicis brevis tendons in a fibro-osseous tunnel. Pain to palpation in this area

suggests inflammation or a tendinitis (e.g., de Quervain's tenosynovitis), which may be seen in sports requiring repetitive radial and ulnar deviation such as racquetball.

Second Extensor Compartment

Between the radial styloid and Lister's tubercle is the second extensor compartment, which is a fibro-osseous tunnel, containing the extensor carpi radialis brevis and the extensor carpi radialis longus. Pain to palpation of this area suggests a tendinitis of these two radial wrist extensors. Approximately 3 cm proximal to the second extensor compartment overlies the intersection of the extensors carpi radialis brevis and carpi radialis longus with the abductor pollicis longus and the extensor pollicis brevis musculotendinous junction

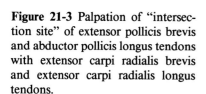

Figure 21-3 Palpation of "intersection site" of extensor pollicis brevis and abductor pollicis longus tendons with extensor carpi radialis brevis and extensor carpi radialis longus tendons.

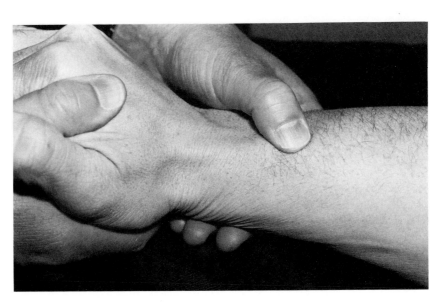

(Fig. 21-3). Pain to palpation in this area suggests an intersection syndrome at the crossroads of these two tendon sheaths (see Ch. 23).

Lister's Tubercle

Palpation just ulnar to Lister's tubercle involves the fibro-osseous tunnel of the extensor pollicis longus tendon. Pain to palpation of this area suggests a tendonitis of the underlying extensor pollicis longus tendon (Fig. 21-4). In the event of a nondisplaced distal radius fracture, exquisite tenderness at this level may represent an impending or existing rupture of the extensor pollicis longus tendon.

Fourth Extensor Compartment

Ulnar to the extensor pollicis longus tendon is a broad and thickened fibro-osseous tunnel consisting of the extensor digitorum communis tendons and the extensor indicis proprius tendon. Pain to palpation of this area represents a tendonitis of the long-finger extensors. With extensor tendonitis, palpation may also elicit crepitation with active motion of the extensor tendons.

Since the fourth extensor compartment is localized along the middorsal of the wrist, care must be taken to exclude other causes of middorsal wrist pain when examining for a common extensor tendonitis. These other causes include an occult ganglion at the radiocarpal joint, injury to the underlying scapholunate ligament, Kienbock disease, or fractures of the underlying

carpus, or dorsal impingement syndrome, as commonly seen in gymnasts.

Distal Radioulnar Joint

The distal radioulnar joint is easily palpated as a sulcus just ulnar to the fourth extensor compartment. While palpating the area, it may be better appreciated during supination and pronation, as the radius can be felt to rotate about the ulna. Pain to palpate over the distal radioulnar joint may suggest a synovitis, instability, or degeneration of the underlying joint. Care must be taken in palpating this area to distinguish the distal radioulnar joint from the triangular fibrocartilage origin at the ulnar aspect of the radius (see the section, *Triangular Fibrocartilage Complex*).

Fifth Extensor Compartment

The fifth extensor compartment overlying the distal radioulnar joint along the radial border of the ulnar contains the fibro-osseous tunnel and holds the extensor digiti minimi tendon. This compartment rarely presents as a clinical problem in the athlete.

Sixth Extensor Compartment

The sixth extensor compartment is palpated in the ulna groove, which is a sulcus just radial to the palpable ulnar styloid and contains the extensor carpi ulnaris tendon (Fig. 21-5). Tenderness to palpation in this area may suggest an extensor carpi ulnaris tendinitis or a

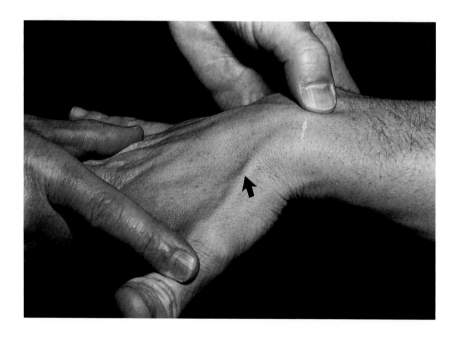

Figure 21-4 Palpation of the third extensor compartment (extensor pollicis longus tendon). Note the tendon as the thumb is extended against resistance *(arrow)*. Examiner's left thumb is just ulnar to Lister's tubercle.

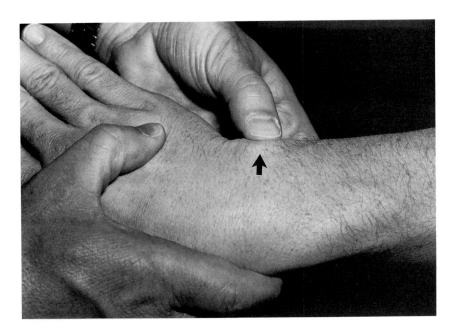

Figure 21-5 Palpation of the sixth extensor compartment (extensor carpi ulnaris tendon).

subluxing extensor carpi ulnaris tendon. Provocative maneuvers to distinguish the subluxation is discussed later in this chapter.

Anatomic Snuffbox

Moving radially, the anatomic snuffbox is defined as a large sulcus just distal to the radial styloid and bordered radially by the abductor pollicis longus and extensor pollicis brevis tendon and ulnarly by the extensor pollicis longus tendon (Fig. 21-6). The anatomic snuffbox also contains the radial artery and the radial

collateral ligament. Pain upon palpation of the anatomic snuffbox generally suggests an injury to the scaphoid, such as a fracture, nonunion, or a scapholunate ligament injury. Provocative maneuvers to distinguish these two entities are presented later in this chapter.

Scapholunate Interosseous Ligament

The scapholunate interosseous ligament is easily palpated just distal to Lister's tubercle at the radiocarpal joint. This is facilitated by flexion of the wrist,

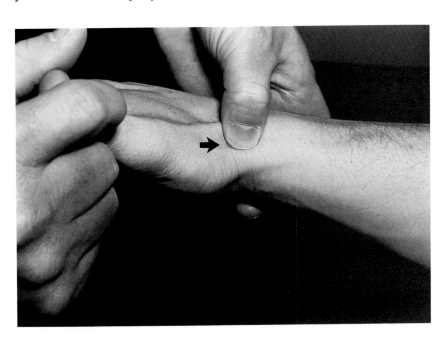

Figure 21-6 Palpation of the anatomic snuffbox.

which will bring the articulation of the scaphoid and the lunate out of the concavity of the distal radius (Fig. 21-7). Pain to palpation in this area suggests an injury to the scapholunate ligament that may be complete or incomplete. Other entities, such as an occult ganglion at the scapholunate ligament or a dorsal impingement syndrome, will also present as tenderness to palpation in the area of the scapholunate ligament (see the section, *Provocative Maneuvers*).

Lunate

The lunate is easily palpated and visualized in hyperflexion of the wrist. It is a bony prominence just ulnar to the scapholunate ligament. Pain to palpation over the lunate may suggest a bone bruise, osteocartilaginous undisplaced compression fracture, a dorsal impingement syndrome, or Kienbock disease.

Lunotriquetral Ligament and Triquetrum

The lunotriquetral ligament will be palpated just ulnar to the lunate. The triquetrum is most easily identified by placing the thumb over the dorsum of the wrist and the index finger over the volar aspect of the wrist at the pisiform. As these two bones articulate, they can be easily palpated together. Upon palpating the lunate with the right hand and the triquetrum with the left hand, ballottment can be used in this area to assess a lunotriquetral instability (see the section, *Provocative Maneuvers*).

Triangular Fibrocartilage Complex

Once the distal radioulnar joint has been identified, the radial origin of the articular disc of the triangular fibrocartilage complex as well as the dorsal distal radioulnar joint ligament can be palpated at the level of the radiocarpal joint, just distal to the distal radioulnar joint (Fig. 21-8). This area is often painful in acute type I tears along the radial border of the triangular fibrocartilage complex articular disc, which may result from a hyperextension injury to the wrist such as a backward fall in basketball. It will also be tender in acute subluxation of the dorsal ligaments of the distal radioulnar joint. It can then be palpated more ulnarward at the base of the ulnar styloid (i.e., the fovea of the ulna) (Fig. 21-9). In partial dorsal capsular tears or partial avulsion to the triangular fibrocartilage complex, this area will be tender to palpation.

Carpometacarpal Joints

The metacarpal-trapezial joint is best palpated by placing the thumb ray in flexion. The sulcus of the thumb metacarpal-trapezial joint can be palpated. In situations of inflammation secondary to sports, this will prove quite painful to palpate (Fig. 21-10). These conditions must, however, be differentiated from an acute capsular sprain or fracture to the base of the metacarpal or trapezium.

The index and long-finger carpometacarpal joints can be palpated at the base of the respective metacarpal. As the examiner's thumb is pressed along the dorsal aspect of the metacarpal, it is brought proximally

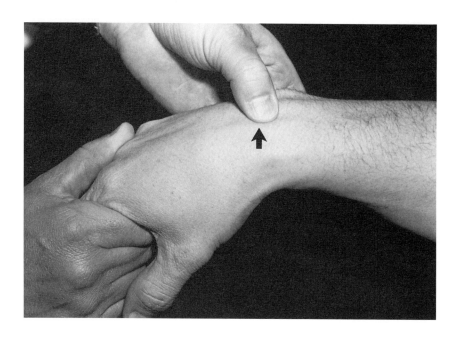

Figure 21-7 Palpation of the scapholunate interosseous ligament. Examiner's thumb is distal to Lister's tubercle palpating scapholunate interosseous ligament while the wrist is in flexion.

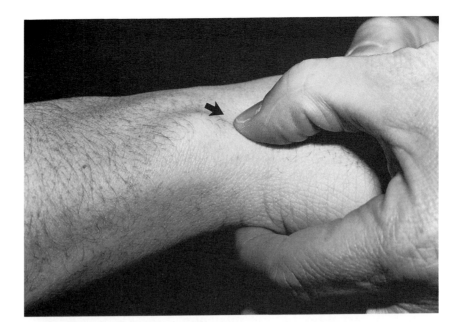

Figure 21-8 Palpation of the radial origin of the triangular fibrocartilage complex.

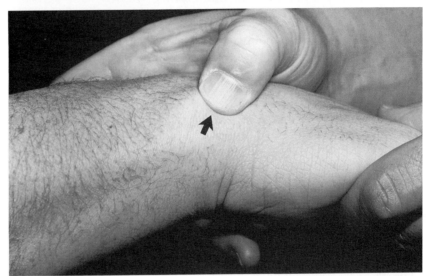

Figure 21-9 Palpation of the insertion of the triangular fibrocartilage complex into the ulnar fovea.

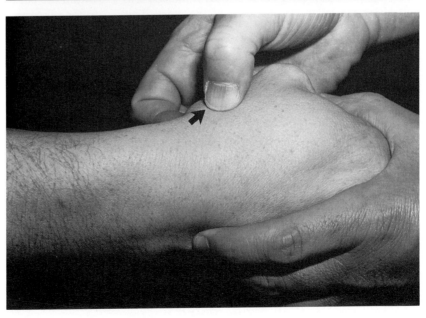

Figure 21-10 Palpation of the thumb metacarpal trapezial joints.

and the metaphyseal flair will end at the carpometacarpal joint. This may be quite prominent in situations of carpal bossing secondary to boxing and hockey. An injury to these joints is often overlooked, yet is common in athletes who frequently apply an axial force to the band metacarpals, such as in boxing or the martial arts. Injury to the carpometacarpal joints of the index (II) and long fingers (III), secondary to a sprain or interarticular fracture, will be present on palpation. Pain may be produced by the *Linscheid test.*[2] The Linscheid test is performed by supporting the metacarpal with the contralateral thumb and pressing the metacarpal head in a volar and dorsal direction (Fig. 21-11). This will elicit pain when injury to the carpometacarpal joint is present.

Carpometacarpal Joint of the Small and Ring Fingers

A significant increase in motion of the ring (IV) and small-finger (V) carpometacarpal joints compared to the long and index fingers is a normal finding. Pain on motion will suggest injury to the carpometacarpal joints (Fig. 21-12). These joints can be palpated via the dorsal metacarpal proximally until its articulation with the hamate is reached. Pain will suggest either a subluxation or sprain to the dorsal ligaments, a fracture, or degenerative arthritis. Injuries to this joint usually are a result of high-energy forces, such as an accident in competitive auto racing.

Volar Scaphoid Tubercle

The scaphoid tubercle is identified and palpated just along the distal course of the flexor carpi radialis tendon along the volar radial aspect of the wrist. This prominence represents the trapezium in its articulation with the scaphoid. Pain to palpation along this prominence may suggest injury to the scaphoid such as fracture or scapho-trapezial synovitis or arthritis. Pain may also be secondary to a scapholunate dissociation when palpating the scaphoid tubercle. Both of these injuries arise out of hyperextension of the wrist with great force as seen in high-contact sports such as football or skiing. Palpation of the scaphoid tubercle or the trapezial ridge just ulnar to the tubercle reveals the insertion of the flexor carpi radialis through the tunnel of the trapezial ridge—a common source of tendonitis in the athlete (Fig. 21-13).

Pisiform

The pisiform is palpated along the ulnar border of the volar aspect of the wrist, just at the distal extent of the distal wrist crease. This can also be located by palpation of the flexor carpal ulnaris tendon insertion into the pisiform. Pain to palpation at this level may represent a contusion or fracture to the pisiform or a flexor carpi ulnaris tendonitis at the level of the pisiform. Pain to palpation of the pisiform, particularly when associated with crepitation, may suggest an underlying arthrosis of the pisotriquetral joint, best noted by palpating the pisotriquetral joint along the ulnar border of the pisiform (Fig. 21-14). This is most frequently seen in cyclists who apply prolonged pressure to the hypothenar eminence.

Hook of the Hamate

The hook of the hamate is a structure situated deep within the palm, approximately 1 cm radial and distal to the pisiform, and it is easily felt on firm palpation.

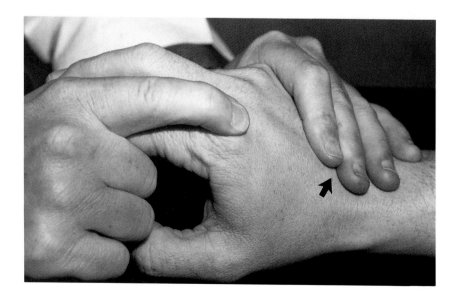

Figure 21-11 Linscheid test for carpometacarpal joint sprain. Pain will be elicited at the base of the metacarpal *(arrow).*

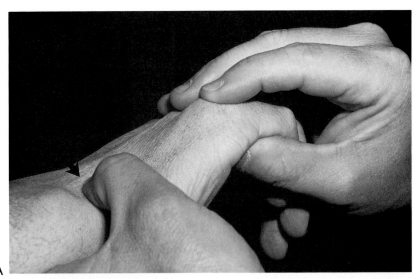

A

Figure 21-12 (A & B) Palpation of the small-finger carpometacarpal joint *(arrow)*, with the metacarpal extended **(A)** and flexed **(B)**.

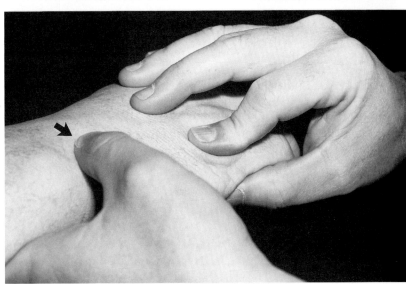

B

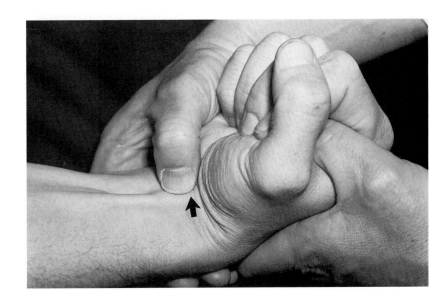

Figure 21-13 Palpation of the flexor carpi radialis tendon at the trapezial ridge *(arrow)*.

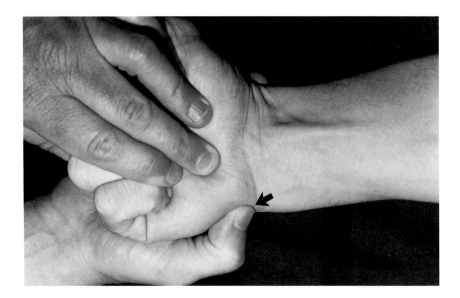

Figure 21-14 Palpation of the piso-triquetral joint *(arrow).*

Pain to palpation usually suggests a fracture or nonunion of the hook of the hamate from a previous injury (Fig. 21-15) (see Ch. 24). It may also represent a contusion to the hook of the hamate when a fracture is not present. The area between the hook of the hamate and the pisiform is Guyon's canal, which contains the ulnar nerve and ulnar artery. A contusion neurapraxia of the ulnar nerve at this level may also be appreciated by pain to palpation.

Range of Motion

The patient's wrist motion should be observed for flexion, extension, ulnar and radial deviation, and supination and pronation. The wrist should be examined for active and passive range of motion and compared to the contralateral uninjured limb. Restriction of motion either secondary to pain or due to mechanical dysfunction should be noted. Loss of range of motion is a sensitive indicator of underlying injury to the wrist. Careful assessment of all planes of motion should be made during the examination.

I find it easiest to assess passive range of motion and to compare it to the normal contralateral wrist in the following manner. The athlete is seated in front of the examiner and is asked to place the palms together and abduct the elbows, thus causing flexion of the wrist, normally 80 to 90 degrees and symmetric. In a similar manner, the dorsal aspect of the hands are placed together and flexion of the wrist is assessed, normally 70 to 90 degrees and symmetric. Supination and prona-

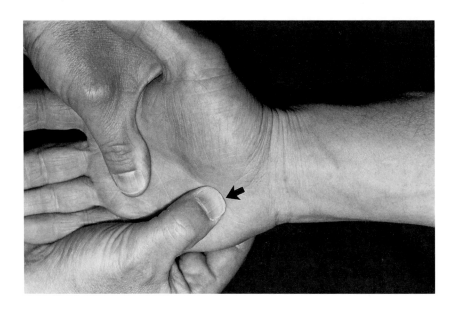

Figure 21-15 Palpation of the hook of the hamate *(arrow).*

tion is best tested when the athlete is in a sitting position and elbows placed at the side. The athlete is asked to show both palms and dorsal aspects of the hand, which should be parallel to the floor, thus demonstrating 80 to 90 degrees of both supination and pronation. Once again, it is important to assess the symmetry of this motion. Finally, radial and ulnar deviation can be assessed by placing the wrist flat on the examiner's table. Ulnar deviation should be symmetric with the contralateral limb and measure approximately 25 degrees. Radial deviation should be assessed in a similar manner and should be symmetric, measuring approximately 15 degrees.

If there is a known motion deficit, documentation should be made if motion is limited secondary to a mechanical obstruction, pain, or both. This can be visually assessed by the athlete's nonverbal behavior.

Motor and Neurovascular Examination

At the end of the physical examination, a complete manual muscle examination of the wrist flexors and extensors should be performed. Differentiation of the ulnar and radial wrist flexors can be accomplished by asking the athlete to flex the wrist in a volar radial or volar ulnar direction. If there is weakness of the radial wrist flexors, simple wrist flexion will result in ulnar deviation of the flexed wrist by overpowering of the intact ulnar flexors. This can also be applied to the wrist's radial and ulnar extensors.

Neurologic examination of the wrist is best performed during the hand examination. It must be kept in mind during the examination that some wrist pain, particularly in the aging athlete, may be a manifestation of a cervical radiculopathy. For example, aging athletes complaining of chronic dorsal radial wrist pain may in fact be manifesting a C6 radiculopathy, and further evaluation should be undertaken once local etiologic factors such as de Quervain's tendonitis or superficial radial neurapraxia have been ruled out. This may be observed in the aging football player who has experienced multiple "burners" in the past and now manifests symptoms of cervical spondylosis.

PROVOCATIVE MANEUVERS

Scaphoid Shift Test (Scapholunate Instability)

The athlete's wrist is placed in ulnar deviation and the examiner's thumb is placed on the scaphoid tubercle. The index finger of the examiner is placed on Lister's tubercle dorsally. A dorsal stress is applied to the scaphoid tubercle, and, while maintaining an axial load on the wrist, the wrist is brought into radial deviation. A positive test reveals a palpable and often audible "clunk" associated with pain (Fig. 21-16). This implies disruption of the scapholunate ligament, which should be investigated by fluoroscopy, arthrography, or other diagnostic procedures as outlined in the section *Wrist Imaging* in Chapter 23.

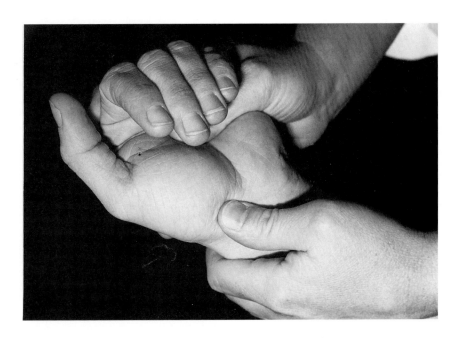

Figure 21-16 Scaphoid shift test.

Lunotriquetral Ballottement Test (Lunotriquetral Instability)

The lunate is palpated just distal and ulnar to Lister's tubercle, the triquetrum is palpated dorsally, and the index finger of the examiner is placed on the pisiform volarly. In this position, the lunate and the triquetrum are grasped between the two hands and compressed. A positive test shows the ability to move the lunate relative to the triquetrum with associated pain. A positive test implies disruption of the lunotriquetral interosseus ligament and thus a lunotriquetral dissociation (Fig. 21-17).

Pisiform Shear Test

The pisiform is grasped along the ulnar volar aspect of the wrist and pressure applied toward the triquetrum with a shear stress. A positive test identifies pain and often palpable crepitation as the pisiform is forced against the triquetrum. This positive test implies synovitis or degeneration of the pisotriquetral joint and there should be further exploration regarding a pisotriquetral arthritis (Fig. 21-18) (see Ch. 23, the section, *Wrist Imaging*).

Distal Radioulnar Joint Grind Test

The radius and ulna are grasped by the hand of the examiner so as to compress the distal radioulnar joints.

While maintaining compression across the distal radioulnar joint, supination and pronation movements are performed. A positive test identifies pain and often crepitation at the distal radioulnar joint during this rotational motion. A positive test also denotes an abnormality about the distal radioulnar joint, usually degenerative changes, or subluxation.

Triangular Fibrocartilage Complex Load Test

The wrist is placed in ulnar deviation, axially loaded, and passively stressed, dorsal and volar. A positive test indicates pain and crepitation along the dorsal ulnar aspect of the wrist. These symptoms imply inflammation in the area of the triangular fibrocartilage complex most likely represented by a tear or the evolution of such a tear by an ulnar impaction syndrome due to an ulna positive wrist (Fig. 21-19).

Extensor Carpi Ulnaris Tendon Subluxation Test

The wrist is placed in supination and extension, and the athlete is asked to actively deviate the wrist, both ulnar and radial. Palpable and often audible subluxation of the extensor carpi ulnaris tendon suggests a disruption of the sixth extensor compartment.

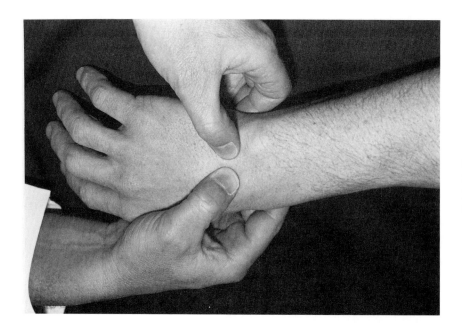

Figure 21-17 Lunotriquetral ballottment test. The examiner's left thumb is palpating the triquetrum, left index finger, the pisiform. The right thumb palpates the lunate and both are sheared in relationship to each other.

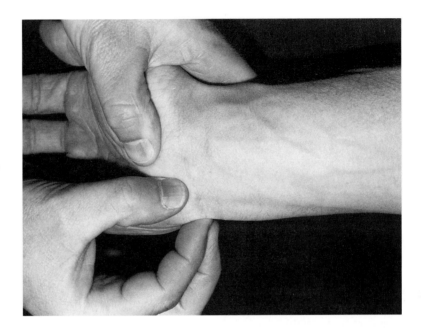

Figure 21-18 Pisiform shear test.

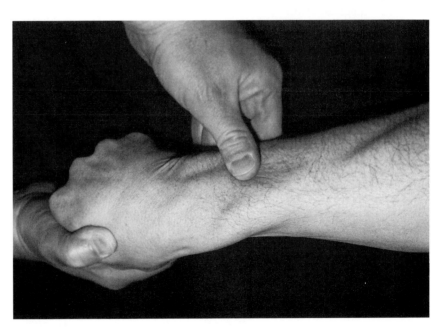

Figure 21-19 Triangular fibrocartilage complex load test.

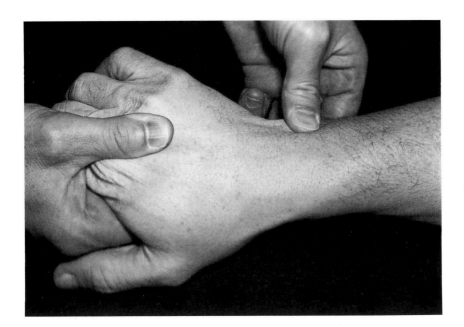

Figure 21-20 Piano key ballottment test of the distal radioulnar joint. The distal ulna is translated volarly and dorsally with respect to the radius.

Piano Key Test

The distal ulna is grasped in relation to the radius and then stressed dorsally and volarly (Fig. 21-20). Abnormal motion relative to the contralateral normal limb suggests an injury to the distal radioulnar joint dorsal and/or volar ligaments. Conversely, upon complete disruption of the distal radioulnar joint ligament, the carpus may supinate on the forearm. Reduction can be performed by placing the examiner's thumb on the pisiform and the fingers on the ulna, and pushing the pisiform dorsally, thus reducing the wrist.

REFERENCES

1. Woo S.L-Y, Bukwalter JA (eds): Injury and repair of the musculoskeletal soft tissues. American Academy of Orthopedic Surgeons Symposium, 1987, Park Ridge, IL
2. Beckenbaugh RD: Accurate evaluation in management of the painful wrist following injury. An approach to carpal instability. Orthop Clin North Am 15:289, 1984

22

Injuries of the Distal Radius and Distal Radioulnar Joint

William J. Morgan
Brian D. Busconi

One of the most common injury sites in the athlete is the distal end of the radius, often associated with injury to the distal radioulnar joint (DRUJ), including the triangular fibrocartilage complex. The distal radius and DRUJ are closely associated structures providing for flexion, extension, radial and ulnar deviation, supination, pronation, and circumduction of the wrist. Given this position between the forearm and the hand, the potential of injury in any athletic activity is high. Distal radius fractures represent approximately 75 percent of all fractures in the forearm[1] and comprise one-sixth of all fractures treated in the emergency room.[2] Fractures of the distal radius present as a broad-spectrum injury. Simple low-impact fractures with minimal displacement or comminution occur in low-contact athletic activities such as racquet sports and track and field. High-impact, intra-articular fractures of both radiocarpal and radioulnar joints occur in high-contact sports such as auto racing, equestrian events, and football. It is common to note a subluxation or instability of the DRUJ associated with fractures of the distal radius. DRUJ injuries can occur as isolated ligamentous injuries or in conjunction with injuries to the forearm or carpus. This may include bony injuries of the ulnar head, sigmoid notch, or ulnar styloid. The triangular fibrocartilage complex comprises the major stabilizers of the DRUJ, and injury may occur to the dorsal or volar marginal ligaments, the volar ulnocarpal complex, or the triangular fibrocartilage articular disc (Fig. 22-1).

Achieving and maintaining an anatomic reduction in fractures of the distal radius is imperative in the athlete, since maintenance of range of motion and strength are critical. Many classification systems categorize methods of treatment of the various fractures of the distal radius, including the AO classification (our preference), Malone's classification, and the Frickman classification.[3-5] This chapter reviews the diagnosis, treatment, and rehabilitation of these injuries in the athlete.

MECHANISM OF INJURY

The most common mechanism of injury to the distal radius and DRUJ results from the instinctive reaction to protect oneself by outstretching the hand during a fall — often seen in running and contact sports such as football, basketball, and lacrosse. As the hand is planted onto the ground, the wrist hyperextends and

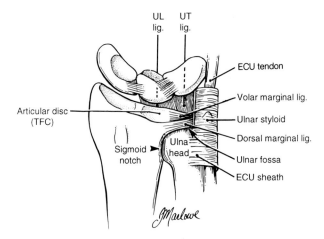

Figure 22-1 The triangular fibrocartilage complex is the major stabilizer of the DRUJ via the dorsal and volar marginal ligaments and ulnocarpal ligaments. UL, ulnolunate; UT, ulnotriquetral; ECU, extensor carpi ulnaris.

with rotation of the forearm on the hand, injuries of the ligamentous complex of the DRUJ occur. With further hyperextension and axial compression, fractures of the distal radius occur. Sometimes, what appears to be a minimally significant fracture of the radial styloid may be part of a fracture and ligament disruption combination (e.g., a perilunate dislocation). It is therefore important to rule out associated ligamentous injuries about the carpus.

PHYSICAL EXAMINATION AND DIAGNOSIS

Fractures of the distal radius usually present with deformity, whereas intra-articular fractures may present without deformity but with pain and limited radiocarpal motion. The health professional should maintain a high degree of suspicion for nondisplaced intra-articular distal radius fractures. Examination of the elbow is critical with a DRUJ injury, since there may be an associated proximal radioulnar joint injury. In an acute injury to the DRUJ, there will be swelling and tenderness with palpation over the volar or dorsal surface of the DRUJ or at the fovea of the ulna styloid. Limited and painful pronation or supination is usually noted. Dorsal subluxation or dislocation may present as a prominence of the distal ulna, particularly in pronation. Volar DRUJ subluxation and dislocation may manifest itself as a dorsal sulcus out of proportion to the uninjured limb.

Most DRUJ injuries will present as subtle subluxations, grade I or II sprains with incomplete tears to the dorsal and volar radioulnar ligaments and/or the ulnocarpal complex.

Instability of the DRUJ is noted by a positive piano key test, and the distal ulna will be freely subluxable volarly or dorsally. The lunotriquetral interosseous ligament is commonly the site of associated injury which should be tested by the lunotriquetral ballottment test.

Chronic injuries of the DRUJ may cause pain with extreme pronation or supination, or may be associated with clicking during rotational activity. A loss of pronation or supination proportional to the direction and degree of the subluxation is usually noted. For example, an athlete with an incompletely treated Galeazzi fracture, with a chronic dorsally dislocated distal ulna, will demonstrate full pronation but little supination. Long-term injury or subluxation may progress to degenerative post-traumatic arthritis of the DRUJ due to incongruous tracking of the joint with rotational activities.

Early and accurate diagnosis of a DRUJ injury in the athlete is critical; initial closed treatment is more likely to be successful. If these injuries become chronic, reconstructive procedures may become necessary with less favorable outcomes.

RADIOGRAPHIC EXAMINATION

The standard posteroanterior (PA) and lateral radiographic views provide most of the radiographic measurements needed to anatomically evaluate the distal end of the radius and DRUJ (see Ch. 20).

Although PA and lateral radiographic views may be sufficient, it is recommended that oblique-view radiographs be obtained to assess subtle displacements such as those in the vicinity of the DRUJ, which can go unnoticed on plain PA and lateral radiographic views. With marked comminution of the distal radius, there is usually significant collapse and overlap of the radius and carpal fragments. Distraction applied across the wrist (usually with the use of finger traps and a counterweight) will separate the fragments by ligamentotaxis, that is, the separation of periarticular fragments by traction through their attached ligaments. Radiographs taken in this position will better demonstrate the degree of fracture comminution and associated carpal injuries. While assessing the distal radius radiographically, care must be taken to assess the carpus for associated fractures or dissociation (see Ch. 23).

If intra-articular pathology warrants further radiographic examination, computed tomography (CT) scanning should be performed at 2- to 3-mm intervals. If a subtle subluxation of the DRUJ is suspected, the imaging technique of choice is a CT scan of the DRUJ in full supination and pronation; subtle dorsal or volar subluxation can be visualized on coronal imaging. CT

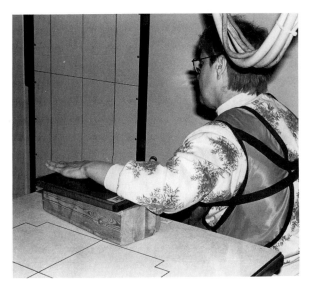

Figure 22-2 Standardized view of wrist with shoulder abducted 90 degrees and elbow in 90 degrees of flexion. This maintains neutral rotation of the forearm.

scanning is also useful to assess the extent of suspected DRUJ arthrosis following injury.

One common late complication of distal radius fractures is radial shortening, with subsequent ulnar impingement and limitation of pronation and supination.[2] Therefore, at initial presentation, ulnar variance should be measured and compared with the contralateral uninjured limb. Ulnar variance is represented by the distance between two perpendicular lines from the longitudinal axis of the radius, one at the head of the ulna and one drawn from the ulnar aspect of the distal radius; on average, this is neutral or 0 mm. When assessing ulnar variance radiographically, standard views must be obtained of the injured wrist and the uninjured wrist for comparison. Standard views are taken in neutral rotation by abducting the shoulder 90 degrees and flexing the elbow 90 degrees (Fig. 22-2). Standardized radiographs consistently place the forearm in neutral rotation and thus provide no change in ulnar variance with different examinations.

ACUTE ISOLATED INSTABILITY

Acute disruptions around the DRUJ may be associated with a fracture or may occur as an isolated instability of the triangular fibrocartilage complex, resulting in volar or dorsal subluxation or dislocation of the distal ulna with respect to the distal radius.

In dorsal subluxation and dislocation, reduction is achieved by supination of the forearm. In volar subluxation or dislocation, reduction is achieved by prona-

tion of the forearm. Once reduction is achieved, the accuracy and stability of the reduction should be assessed clinically. If the DRUJ remains unstable or impossible to reduce during these maneuvers, open reduction and ligamentous repair should be considered. In the majority of isolated injuries to the triangular fibrocartilage complex, closed reduction will be successful, and treatment by immobilization in a long-arm or Muenster cast in either pronation or supination should be complete by 6 weeks.

Case Study I

A 16-year-old gymnast fell from the uneven bars onto her right hand, sustaining a twisting and hyperextension injury of the wrist. She had swelling and pain localized to the DRUJ and the fovea of the distal ulna. A slight prominence dorsally of the distal ulna was easily reducible when the forearm was brought into supination. Plain radiographs were normal but magnetic resonance imaging (MRI) demonstrated dorsal subluxation of the ulna with respect to the radius on pronation that was reduced in supination (Fig. 22-3).

The gymnast was treated in a long-arm cast in supination for 6 weeks. Upon removal, she was protected in a thermoplastic splint and range of motion exercises were initiated to improve pronation. At this point, the DRUJ was quite stable to examination. At 3 months from the time of her injury, she had full range of motion and was allowed to begin gentle workouts to improve her endurance. Full sport activity was not allowed until 6 months from the time of her injury. Upon return to full sport, she was advised to use a hyperextension block splint (see Ch. 2).

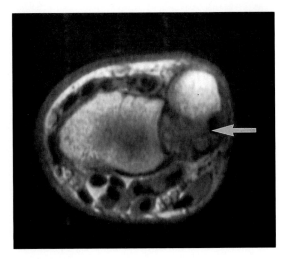

Figure 22-3 MRI of DRUJ in pronation. Note dorsal subluxation of ulna out of the sigmoid notch *(arrow)*.

ACUTE INSTABILITY ASSOCIATED WITH ULNA STYLOID FRACTURE

If an associated ulna styloid fracture is large enough to include the fovea of the ulna styloid, an avulsion of the triangular fibrocartilage complex with the dorsal and volar ulnar ligaments should be suspected (Fig. 22-4). If the DRUJ appears unstable by a positive ballotment test, a radiograph should be obtained to evaluate if an ulna styloid fracture is present. In these cases, acute treatment consists of open anatomic reduction of the large styloid fragment and rigid immobilization either by tension band wire techniques or screw fixation (Fig. 22-5).

If the associated styloid fragment is comminuted or too small for fixation, excision of the fragment may be undertaken with fixation (or reinsertion) of the ligamentous complex into the distal ulna. In this circumstance, there should be immobilization in neutral rotation for approximately 6 weeks.

CHRONIC INSTABILITY

An athlete frequently will present with difficulties about the DRUJ following an injury that occurred several months prior to presentation. Typically the athlete will have been diagnosed with a sprain at the time of

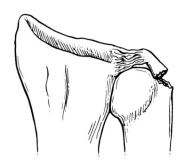

Figure 22-4 Large ulna styloid fracture fragments may have triangular fibrocartilage complex, including dorsal and volar marginal ligaments attached. This will normally be associated with instability of DRUJ.

acute injury and given a wrist splint, with no attention directed to the DRUJ. This late presentation poses both a significant diagnostic and a therapeutic problem.

The athlete generally presents with progressive loss of forearm rotation. With gross instability, radiographs may reveal widening of the DRUJ and dorsal subluxation of the ulna. In more subtle presentation, radiographs may appear normal, but the clinical examination will demonstrate loss of rotation and ballottment of the DRUJ. In these cases, MRI may reveal detachment of the triangular fibrocartilage complex from the ulna fovea. Wrist arthroscopy is also helpful in establishing a diagnosis, since the articular disk of the trian-

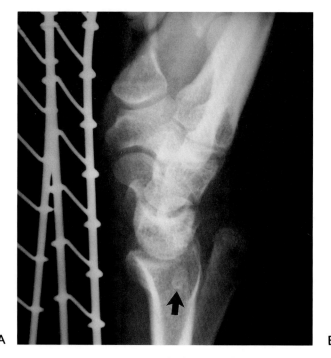
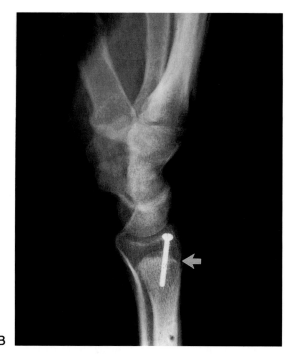

Figure 22-5 (A) Ulna styloid fracture with subluxation of ulna; note large styloid fragment remains adjacent to sigmoid notch *(arrow)*. **(B)** Following ORIF of ulna styloid facture. Note reduction of ductal ulna *(arrow)*.

gular fibrocartilage complex will show significant laxity to palpation, suggesting an avulsion of these ligaments from the fovea.

Treatment of chronic instability of the DRUJ focuses on reestablishing the integrity of the dorsal and volar marginal ligaments with the fovea of the ulnar styloid. Since these injuries are chronic, they are best treated by open debridement of scar from the ulnar fovea and repair of the triangular fibrocartilage complex ligaments into the ulna after reduction of the DRUJ. This procedure can be performed arthroscopically. The DRUJ is pinned percutaneously in a reduced position and in neutral rotation for 6 weeks.

Case Study II

As he was snowboarding, a 19-year-old man fell on a mogul, planted his left hand into semisoft snow, and noted 180 degrees rotation of his forearm and body about the planted hand. He had swelling at the time of his injury and, upon examination, was advised that the radiographs were normal and that he had sustained a "wrist sprain." It was recommended that he wear a volar wrist splint for 2 weeks. His acute pain improved, but during the summer, he experienced several episodes of pain about the DRUJ as well as clicking with rotation.

The examination revealed a prominence of his left ulna, particularly in pronation. He had a positive piano key sign and his carpus appeared supinated on his forearm, reducible with upper pressure on his pisiform. There was crepitation from pronation to supination at the DRUJ with some mild discomfort. In supination, his distal ulna reduced into the sigmoid notch.

Plain radiographs suggested a slight dorsal subluxation of the ulna on a true lateral-view radiograph (Fig. 22-6A). MRI demonstrated avulsion of the triangular fibrocartilage complex, including the volar and dorsal marginal ligaments from the fovea of the ulna (Fig. 22-6B). An area of scarring was also noted at the fovea of the ulna.

Due to the elapsed time since injury, an open repair was performed by advancing the triangular fibrocartilage complex into the fovea of the ulna, using a suture anchor. The DRUJ was pinned percutaneously in neutral rotation with one C-wire and the athlete's upper extremity placed in a long-arm cast for 6 weeks. Following this period of time the pin was removed and he was placed in a protective orthoplast splint. Therapy was initiated with gentle active-assisted supination and pronation exercises. Once full range of motion was reestablished, strengthening was begun and the athlete resumed snow-boarding 3 months postoperatively. It was recommended, however, that he wear a wrist splint while snow-boarding until 6 months from the time of his injury.

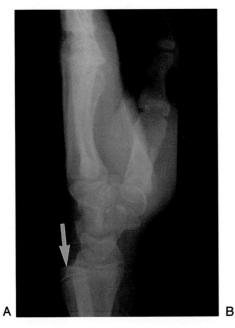 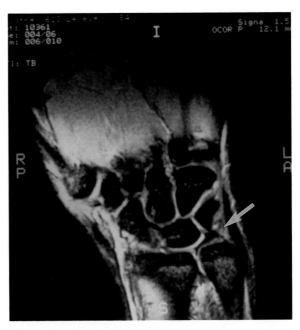

Figure 22-6 **(A)** Lateral-view radiograph demonstrating mild dorsal subluxation of the ulna following injury to the DRUJ *(arrow)*. **(B)** MRI demonstrating avulsion of the triangular fibrocartilage complex from the ulna fovea *(arrow)*.

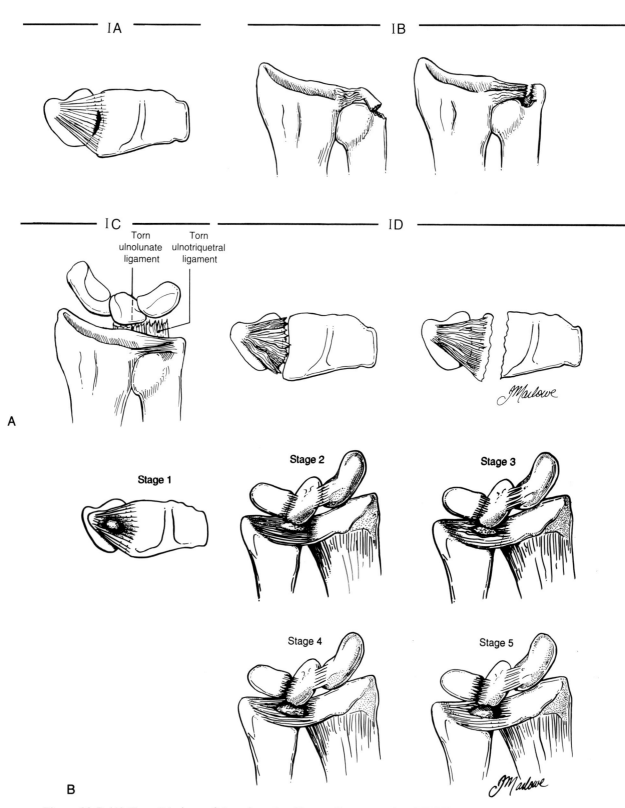

Figure 22-7 (A) Type I lesions of the triangular fibrocartilage complex (TFCC): Ia, central perforation; Ib, avulsion from ulna with or without ulna styloid fracature; Ic, disruption of ulnocarpal ligaments; and Id, avulsion from radius with or without fracture of the sigmoid notch. **(B)** Type II lesions of the TFCC: Stage 1, TFCC tear; stage 2, 1+ lunate and/or ulna chondromalacia; stage 3, TFCC perforation and lunate and/or ulna chondromalacia; stage 4, 3+ lunotriquetral ligament rupture; and stage 5, 4+ ulnocarpal arthritis.

CLASSIFICATION AND TREATMENT OF LESIONS OF THE TRIANGULAR FIBROCARTILAGE COMPLEX

Injuries to the triangular fibrocartilage complex (TFCC) are generally associated with pain to palpation over the radial insertion of the articular disk. There may be a palpable or audible snap with rotation of the DRUJ or ulnar deviation and extension of the wrist combined with axial compression.

Lesions of the triangular fibrocartilage complex have been grouped as Type I or II[6] (Fig. 22-7). Type I lesions are traumatic in origin and are more often associated with the competitive athlete.[7] Type II lesions are degenerative in origin and may be seen in the senior athlete or the athlete with an ulnar positive variance. Most type I and II lesions are amenable to arthroscopic treatment, except type Ic lesions, which may require open repair, and type II lesions, which may require ulna shortening.

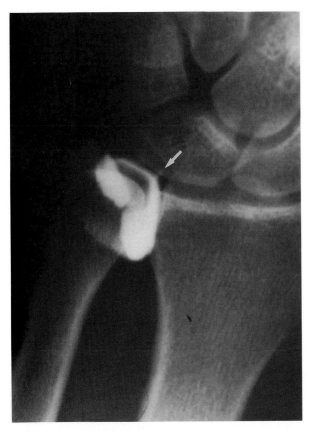

Figure 22-8 Three-compartment arthrogram. Note radiopaque material passing through a tear in the triangular fibrocartilage complex *(arrow).*

Case Study III

A baseball player stealing second base dove head-first into the bag with his arms outstretched. He struck the thenar eminence of his hand onto the bag with hyperextension and pronation of his wrist. Although discomfort was noted, he continued to play. Following the game, an examination did not reveal swelling, but there was discomfort to palpation at the ulnar border of the radius and in extremes of pronation and supination. He was placed in a wrist splint and rested for 1 week with resolution of symptoms. Upon return to baseball, he noted discomfort and clicking occasionally about the distal ulna with rotational activities. Although he could complete the season, his symptoms remained.

After the season, three-compartment arthrography revealed a tear in the triangular fibrocartilage complex adjacent to the radius (Fig. 22-8). At the time of arthroscopy, a flap—type 1A—tear of the triangular fibrocartilage complex was noted and debrided, maintaining the integrity of the dorsal volar marginal ligaments (Fig. 22-9).

Range of motion exercises were started immediately and once range of motion was full (2 weeks), progressive strengthening and training as tolerated was begun. The symptoms of ulnar-sided pain and clicking were both resolved.

DEGENERATIVE CHANGES OF THE TRIANGULAR FIBROCARTILAGE DISC

These injuries are usually associated with an ulnar plus variance (see the section, *Ulnar Impaction Syndrome*). Type IIa and IIb lesions demonstrate fibrillation of the triangular fibrocartilage complex without perforation, suggesting early evidence of impaction. When associated with chrondromalacia of the ulnar aspect of the lunate and the ulna head, significant ulnar impaction is implied, and procedures resulting in ulna shortening should be considered. If left untreated, these partial lesions may progress to lesions which include the perforation of the triangular fibrocartilage articular disc necessitating debridement. Types IId and IIe lesions are usually associated with partial or complete ruptures of the lunotriquetral complex (see Ch. 23).

ULNAR IMPACTION SYNDROME

Persistent ulnar pain is a diagnostic challenge and may be a source of frustration for the treating clinician as well as the athlete. This entity is typically seen in

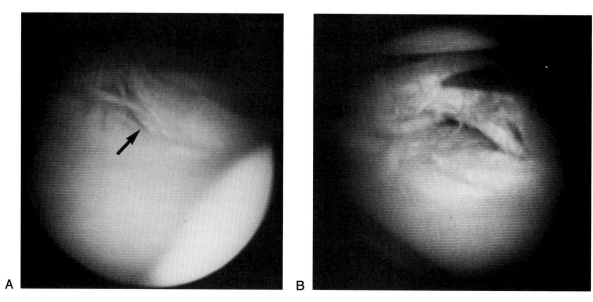

Figure 22-9 (A) Type I a tear of the triangular fibrocartilage complex as seen arthroscopically *(arrow).* **(B)** Triangular fibrocartilage articular disc after débridement. Note stable margins.

athletes who perform repetitive wrist extension and ulnar deviation maneuvers (baseball, golf, racquet sports). The differential diagnosis is a prolonged process, requiring careful clinical and radiographic evaluations. A clinical examination in the acute phase will demonstrate mild swelling over the DRUJ and the lunotriquetral articulation. Pain results from extremes of extension and ulnar deviation. These signs must be differentiated from DRUJ arthrosis through clinical tests described in Chapter 21.

Unlike many of the previously described injuries about the wrist, the ulnar impaction syndrome is generally not an acute injury but rather a chronic, insidious condition. It is typically manifested by swelling and pain about the ulnar dorsal aspect of the wrist, particularly with wrist extension and ulnar deviation. The pathogenesis is impaction of a prominent ulnar head into the triangular fibrocartilage complex and the ulnar carpus, resulting in degenerative midsubstance tears of the triangular fibrocartilage complex, chondromalacia of the ulnar aspect of the lunate and the ulnar head, and, in prolonged cases, may cause attenuation of the lunotriquetral ligament (Fig. 22-10).

The ulnar impaction syndrome can frequently result from a prior injury, such as a malunited distal radius fracture with shortening or dorsal angulation, resulting in an ulnar positive variance. This ulnar positive variance may also be the result of a prior radial head excision with shortening of the radius. Growth arrest of the distal radius with resultant ulnar impaction has been reported in gymnasts.[8]

Radiographic assessment should include standardized radiographs of the wrist, with comparison views of the contralateral or the uninjured limb. Positive or neutral ulnar variance should be noted. Often with long-term cases of ulnar impaction syndrome, flattening of the articular cartilage with cyst formation along the proximal ulnar border of the lunate may be noted (Fig. 22-11). Arthrography may demonstrate a central disc tear of the triangular fibrocartilage complex.

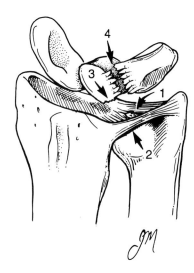

Figure 22-10 Progression of ulna impaction syndrome: 1, perforation of triangular fibrocartilage articular disc; 2, chondromalacia of ulna head; 3, chondromalacia of ulnar border of lunate; and 4, rupture of lunotriquetral ligaments.

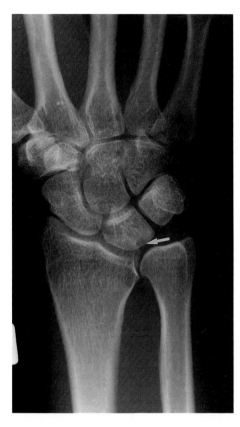

Figure 22-11 AP radiographic view of a patient with chronic ulna impaction syndrome. Note flattening and subchondral cyst on ulna border of lunate *(arrow).*

Diagnostic arthroscopy for chronic ulnar-sided wrist pain can be invaluable. Chondromalacia of the ulnar aspect of the lunate and ulna head may be noted, as the ulnar head can be visualized through a large midsubstance tear (type II) of the articular disc. The integrity of the lunotriquetral ligament can also be visualized and probed.

Initial treatment of ulnar impaction syndrome should be conservative and consist of splint immobilization, nonsteroidal anti-inflammatory drugs (NSAIDs), and rest from the sport. In athletes who do not have significant mechanical impingement secondary to a significant positive ulnar variance, conservative treatment may be successful. In athletes with markedly positive ulnar variance, surgical intervention may be necessary. In these cases, once the athlete's symptoms have resolved, a progressive return to full sport activity is allowed.

In athletes with ulnar impaction syndrome secondary to a malunion of the distal radius, osteotomy and correction of the malunion of the distal radius should be the initial treatment. In athletes with ulnar impaction syndrome secondary to either congenital positive ulnar variance or a previously resected radial head, the treatment is an ulnar shortening procedure. In the young athlete involved in aggressive sports, this should be performed with compression plate fixation (Fig. 22-12).

In cases of ulnar impaction syndrome associated with DJD of the DRUJ, the Suave Kapindje procedure is the procedure of choice, since fusion of the distal ulna will resolve the pain due to DRUJ degenerative joint disease (DJD) while maintaining the structural ulnocarpal support via the triangular fibrocartilage complex. Other procedures such as a Darrach or hemiresection arthroplasty are less predictable in the athlete.

Case Study IV

A 55-year-old golfer had pain and occasional swelling along the dorsal ulnar aspect of her wrist during and after a round of golf, most notably at the end of a full swing. At presentation, she noted that NSAIDs had previously relieved her symptoms, but the pain became persistent enough that she could no longer play golf.

Her examination demonstrated normal range of motion about both wrists with tenderness to palpate over the distal ulna and the ulnar margin of the distal radius. A lunotriquetral ballottment test was negative, but there was pain to axial compression and ulnar deviation of the wrist.

Plain radiographs demonstrated an ulnar positive variant with some mild sclerosis on the ulnar border of the lunate. Arthroscopy demonstrated full-thickness articular wear and tear at the ulnar border of the lunate as well as chondromalacia and articular wear of the ulna head. There was a large midsubstance degenerative tear in the triangular fibrocartilage complex, which was debrided to stable dorsal and volar marginal ligaments, and the prominent ulnar head was recessed, taking care not to involve the DRUJ (Fig. 22-13).

Postoperatively, the golfer was placed in a supportive splint and immediate active-assisted range of motion as tolerated was begun. Three weeks postoperatively, she was allowed to hit balls at the driving range, and her golf game progressed as tolerated. Six weeks postoperatively, she resumed her game without signs of impingement.

INSTABILITY ASSOCIATED WITH DISTAL RADIUS FRACTURES

Associated injuries to the DRUJ are common with distal radius fractures and may include fractures of the sigmoid notch or ulnar head or an impaction syndrome

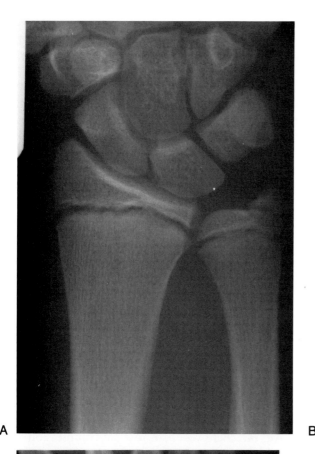

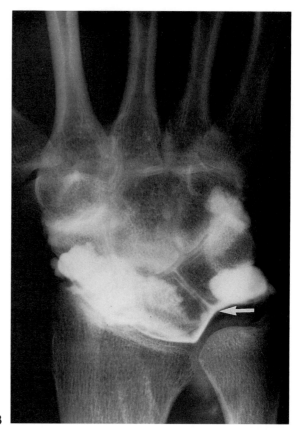

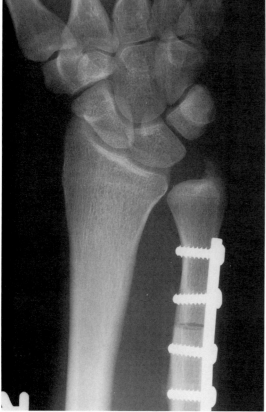

Figure 22-12 **(A)** AP radiographic view of skeletally immature gymnast with clinical findings of Salter I fracture of distal
radius. Also noted is an ulna styloid fracture. **(B)** Two years
later, the gymnast presents with ulna wrist pain. Arthrogram
demonstrates that the patient has suffered a growth arrest of
the radius and is now ulna positive. Note compression of
triangular fibrocartilage disc by the ulna head as well as communication between the radiocarpal and midcarpal joints via
the lunotriquetral interosseous space *(arrow)*. **(C)** Postoperative radiograph after ulna shortening.

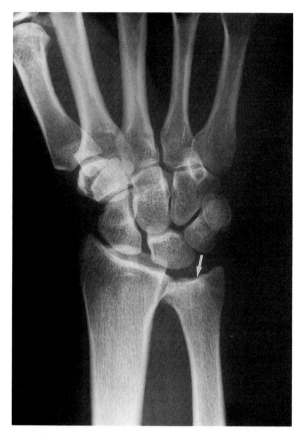

Figure 22-13 Postoperative radiograph following arthroscopic recession of the ulna head. Note flat recession of the ulna head without compromise to the DRUJ *(arrow)*.

GALEAZZI FRACTURES

A Galeazzi fracture is an extremely unstable fracture of the distal one-third of the radius associated with instability of the DRUJ.[9] This instability may manifest itself with frank dislocation or more subtle subluxation about the DRUJ. It is typically encountered in high-contact sports (e.g., skiing, biking, auto racing) with the mechanism of injury involving a high-energy force to the wrist positioned in hyperpronation and hyperextension.

The instability of this fracture dislocation complex results from the forces of the pronator quadratus and the brachioradialis pulling the distal radius fragment proximally and volarly, and avulsion of the triangular fibrocartilage complex from the distal ulna, which may or may not include a fracture of the ulna styloid (Fig. 22-14). With complete disruptions of the triangular fibrocartilage complex from the distal ulna, there often is greater than 5 mm of proximal radius migration and widening of the DRUJ.[10] It is critical to assess the degree of instability to the DRUJ, which is best achieved after open reduction internal fixation and stabilization of the distal radius.

The radius fracture should be anatomically reduced and surgically stabilized, best accomplished by compression plate fixation. Once reduction of the distal radius has been obtained, stability of the DRUJ is assessed clinically and by intraoperative radiographs. If significant instability is present and associated with an ulnar styloid fracture, internal fixation of the ulnar styloid is recommended. If marked instability is present

and ulnar subluxation secondary to distal radius malunion.

Fractures of the ulnar styloid often occur in conjunction with distal radius fractures. Often, the large ulnar styloid fragment will remain attached to the dorsal and volar triangular fibrocartilage complex marginal ligaments, thereby causing instability of the distal ulna. In the low-demand wrist, a fibrous union of the ulnar styloid may offer reasonable stability for daily activity. In the high-performance athlete, however, demands of the wrist usually supersede the stability of a fibrous union.

A displaced fracture (>2 mm) of the ulnar styloid with associated instability of the DRUJ implies an avulsion of the dorsal and volar marginal ligaments with the large ulnar styloid fragment. To ensure wrist stability, these fractures should be treated by open reduction and internal fixation either with lag screw fixation or tension band wiring techniques.

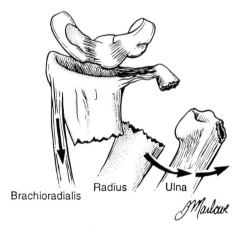

Figure 22-14 Galeazzi fracture and dislocation demonstrating soft tissue deforming forces. Note instability of DRUJ due to disruption of triangular fibrocartilage complex *(arrow)*.

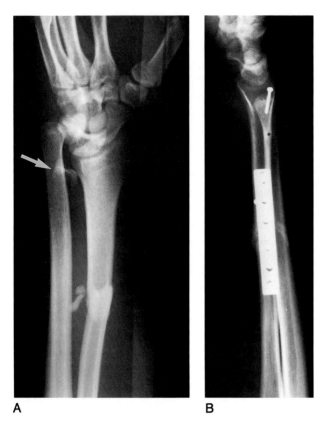

Figure 22-15 (A) AP radiographic view of a downhill skier after a severe fall. Note radius fracture, proximal migration of the radius, and widening of DRUJ. Note ulna styloid fracture (attached to triangular fibrocartilage complex at sigmoid notch) *(arrow).* **(B)** Postoperative lateral radiograph of Galeazzi fracture in skier. Note open reduction internal fixation of radius with stabilization of the DRUJ by fixation of ulna styloid (with associated volar and dorsal marginal ligaments).

The health professional should maintain a high degree of suspicion when examining an athlete with a radial head fracture, and should carefully examine the DRUJ under these circumstances, checking for swelling and pain with palpation and motion. Radiographic assessment of a suspected Essex Lopresti fracture should consist of PA and lateral radiographic views of the elbow as well as standardized PA radiographic views of both wrists.

Treatment consists of repair of the radial head and DRUJ ligamentous complex. The radial head should be internally fixed to maintain the length of the radius. Excision of the comminuted fragments is contraindicated, since there will be marked migration of the radius proximally and continued instability of the DRUJ. In cases where it is impossible to reconstruct the radial head and an excision is the only alternative, temporary placement of a radial head prosthesis is recommended to maintain the length of the radius while the DRUJ ligamentous disruption is healing. In a significantly unstable DRUJ, the joint should be opened and the triangular fibrocartilage complex repaired. This should be performed in conjunction with pinning of the DRUJ in a neutral position to maintain a normal ulnar variance, as described for Galeazzi fractures.

Postoperative immobilization should be in a long-arm cast in neutral rotation for 2 weeks. If stable fixation of the proximal radius has been obtained, or if prosthetic replacement has been necessary, it is then converted to a Muenster cast to allow a gentle arc of flexion extension of the elbow while prohibiting rotation of the forearm for another 4 weeks. At that time, the DRUJ pin is removed, and gentle rotational exercises are initiated.

without an ulna styloid fracture, open repair of the avulsed triangular fibrocartilage complex should be performed in conjunction with stabilization of the DRUJ using a .062 C-wire. Six weeks of immobilization in a long-arm cast in neutral position is necessary to allow proper ligamentous healing of the triangular fibrocartilage complex (Fig. 22-15).

ESSEX-LOPRESTI FRACTURE DISLOCATIONS

The Essex-Lopresti fracture includes a radial head fracture and instability of the DRUJ, implying a partial or complete injury to the interosseous membrane, with injury to both the proximal and distal radioulnar joints. This is an uncommon injury, created by a large amount of axial rotatory force, which results in an extremely unstable fracture-dislocation complex (Fig. 22-16).

MANAGEMENT OF DISTAL RADIUS FRACTURES

Fractures of the distal radius can involve a wide spectrum of injuries from nondisplaced extra-articular fractures to complex displaced intra-articular fractures. In the evaluation of distal radius fractures in the athlete, a distinction should be made between stable and unstable fractures. There are certain factors suggestive of unstable injuries: excessive comminution and severity of fracture displacement, angulation of the radial articular surface greater than 20 degrees, articular fragment separation greater than 2 mm, and, finally, comminution of both volar and dorsal metaphyseal cortices.

It is only through restoration of normal radial alignment, length, and preservation of articular congruity that successful recovery can be achieved. If there is

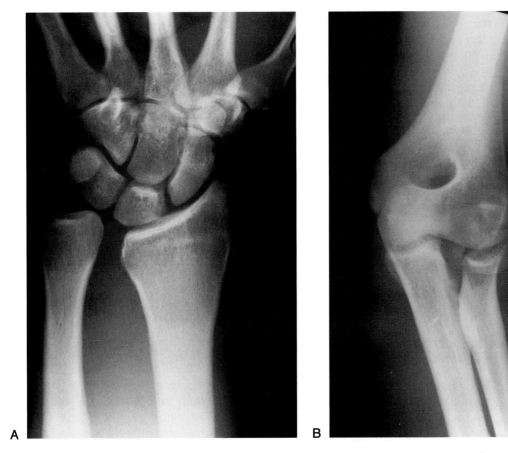

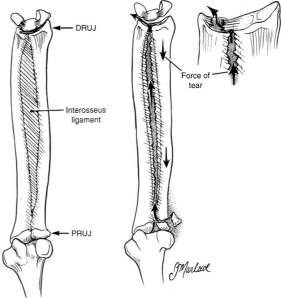

Figure 22-16 **(A)** AP radiographic view of the wrist of 24-year-old motorcycle racer following a collision. Note shortening of radius and widening of DRUJ. **(B)** AP radiographic view of the elbow in the same athlete, demonstrating comminuted fracture of the radial head. **(C)** Illustration of intrinsic instability in Essex-Lopresti fracture with disruption of proximal and distal radioulnar joints and interosseous membrane.

greater than 10 degrees of dorsal angulation or 5 mm of radial shortening after closed reduction and manipulation, either remanipulation or supplemental fixation will be necessary. In the following section, treatment and rehabilitation of distal radius fractures will be categorized into extra-articular (simple) and intra-articular (complex) fractures of the distal radius.

EXTRA-ARTICULAR FRACTURES OF THE DISTAL RADIUS

Extra-articular fractures of the distal radius are the most commonly seen fractures, generally occurring in the skeletally immature athlete involved in low-impact athletic events. Clinical presentation is typically pain and swelling about the distal radius, which may be associated with a dorsal and often radial deformity at the wrist (silver fork deformity). Generally, there is retention of a periosteal hinge dorsally, which will aid in guiding the reduction (Fig. 22-17).

Once reduction has been accomplished, the majority of extra-articular fractures can be supported in an external cast or splint. In fractures involving marked comminution of the dorsal cortex, care must be taken to perform a three-point fixation mold on the cast to maintain the reduction. With unstable fractures, fixation may be augmented by placing the forearm in pronation with the elbow flexed in a long-arm cast. If extreme instability is noted, percutaneous wire fixation should be considered (at times, in conjunction with

external fixation). It is rarely necessary to stabilize these fractures with plate fixation.

Protection of extra-articular radius fractures by cast immobilization is generally necessary for a period of 4 to 6 weeks. In many cases, particularly in running sports, the athlete may be allowed to continue competing while protected in the cast, or may be allowed to continue with total body conditioning. Once healing of the fracture has been obtained by note of callus formation on radiographs and clinical stability on examination, the athlete's extremity is placed into a protective removable splint and active-assisted range of motion is begun.

Case Study V

A 32-year-old rugby player was tackled and extended his left wrist to protect his fall. He noticed immediate onset of pain and deformity as his body weight came down on his hyperextended wrist. A clinical deformity at the wrist was noted with full sensation and motion of the fingers present. A radiograph demonstrated a dorsally displaced extra-articular distal radius fracture (Fig. 22-18A). A hematoma block was placed and the fracture was reduced (Fig. 22-18B).

Cast immobilization was maintained for 4 weeks, whereupon there was early radiographic evidence of healing. Clinically, the fracture fragments were not mobile, and the athlete did not experience pain to palpation of the fragments. He was placed in a removable volar orthoplast splint and began range of motion and progressive strengthening exercises as tolerated. Three months postinjury, the athlete had full return of strength and range of motion and was allowed to return to rugby with a protective splint.

NONCOMMINUTED INTRA-ARTICULAR FRACTURES OF THE DISTAL RADIUS

Noncomminuted intra-articular fractures of the distal radius are categorized by fractures composed of two large fragments extending into the joint. These fractures are the result of shear forces from either a dorsal or volar direction of the respective lips of the radius, with intra-articular fracture and displacement, as may occur from wrist hyperextension during a fall while skiing. Reduction of these fractures is usually accomplished by reversal of the deformity, but maintenance of reduction is extremely difficult by closed means.

In dorsal Barton's fractures, once reduction has been obtained, percutaneous pinning may be helpful in

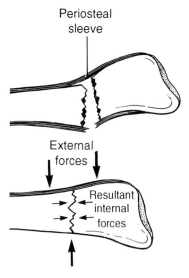

Figure 22-17 Dorsally displaced fracture of the distal radius. Note how the retained dorsal periosteum can be utilized as a "hinge" to aid in reduction.

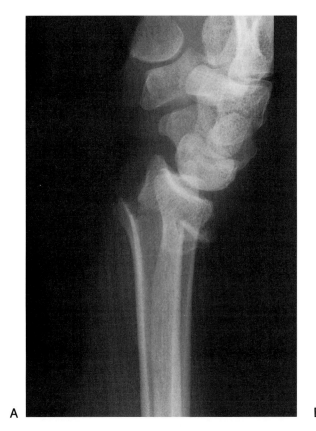
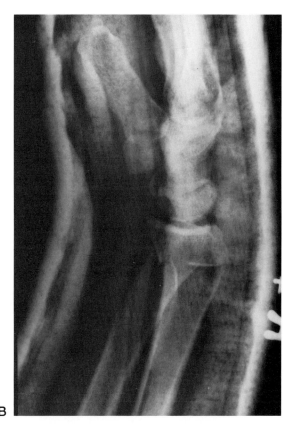

A   B

Figure 22-18 **(A)** Dorsally displaced distal radius fracture. **(B)** Reduction with three-point fixation in AP splints.

maintaining the reduction of the fracture. In stable dorsal Barton's fractures, reduction may be maintained by a well-molded cast. With decreasing stability, augmentation by percutaneous pinning, external fixation, or internal fixation via dorsal plating may be necessary.

In volar Barton's fractures, maintenance of reduction by a cast alone is not possible, and percutaneous pinning is generally prohibited by the presence of flexor tendons and the median nerve (Fig. 22-19). Successful treatment is usually accomplished by open reduction and rigid internal fixation, using a volar buttress plate (Fig. 22-20). Internal fixation allows for active-assisted range of motion only, and the athlete should be reminded to refrain from aggressive activities. Protection of these fractures is recommended for 4 to 6 weeks with range of motion, strengthening, and rehabilitation protocols as discussed in the section *Rehabilitation* below.

Other noncomminuted intra-articular fractures at the distal radius include a fracture of a large portion of the radial styloid, usually the result of avulsion and rotational forces by way of the extrinsic radial carpal ligaments. This can occur in football when the hand is planted on the turf and the body is rotated with an axial load. These fractures are potentially unstable due to the deforming force of the brachioradialis insertion at the radial styloid (Fig. 22-21). If these fractures are minimally displaced, percutaneous pinning through the radial styloid and augmentation by cast immobilization should be the treatment of choice.

COMPLEX INTRA-ARTICULAR FRACTURES OF THE DISTAL RADIUS

Athletic injuries to the distal end of the radius associated with a high-energy axial impact result in the carpus (primarily the lunate) being driven into the

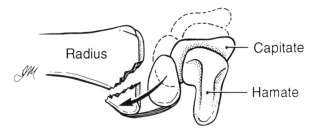

Figure 22-19 Mechanism of displacement of volar Barton's fracture.

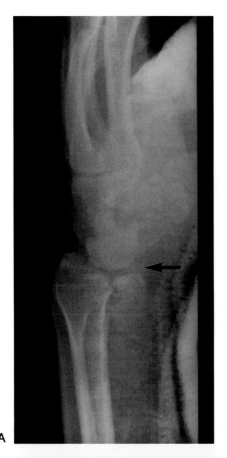

A

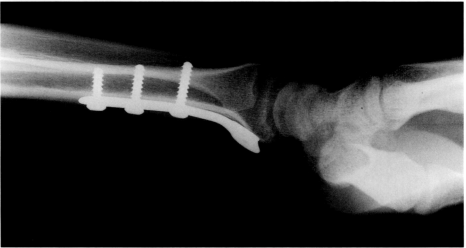

B

Figure 22-20 (A) Displaced volar Barton's fracture; note volar subluxation of carpus with volar fragment *(arrow)*. **(B)** Radiograph after open reduction and internal fixation.

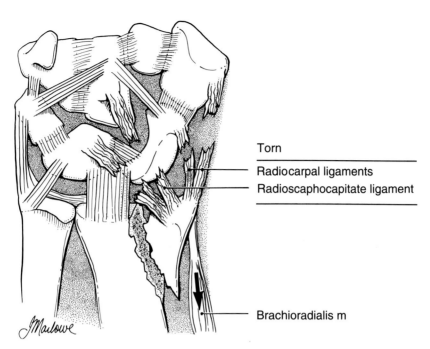

Torn
Radiocarpal ligaments
Radioscaphocapitate ligament

Brachioradialis m

Figure 22-21 Soft tissue-deforming forces such as the brachioradialis promote instability of the large radial styloid fractures.

radius articular fossa, subsequently causing comminution of the articular surface. These fractures have an inherent tendency for shortening and articular collapse secondary to the comminution of the dorsal cortex and subchondral bone.

If articular fractures have minimal displacement (<2 mm) and meet the previously described accepted indices, long-arm thumb spica cast immobilization is maintained for 4 weeks, at which time the limb may be placed into a short-arm cast for the remaining 2 to 4 weeks. Decisions on changing from a long-arm to a short-arm cast and total time of immobilization should be based on clinical and radiographic findings of stability.

As these fractures are markedly unstable, early and close observation after reduction is necessary, since shortening and loss of reduction may occur. If a 2- to 3-week period is allowed to pass without radiographic reassessment of the fracture and settling has occurred, time for remanipulation will have been lost and the athlete will have a suboptimal result.

Due to the precarious stability of these fractures, external fixation alone is inadequate and limited internal fixation is recommended. Displaced intra-articular fractures may be reduced by distraction and ligamentotaxis of fracture fragments, and maintained by external fixation. If articular reduction is incomplete, then further invasive manipulation must be performed. Arthroscopy may be helpful since it allows visualization

for an anatomic reduction. Impacted fragments may be disimpacted through a small extra-articular incision and subchondrally elevated during arthroscopic-assisted reduction. If a bony deficit is evident, it can be bone-grafted with regional (distal radius) or iliac crest autogenous bone graft, or cancellous allograft. Fracture fragment stability may be further gained by fluoroscopic-assisted percutaneous pinning (Fig. 22-22).

Fractures whose complex intra-articular patterns and subsequent displacement, rotation, or impaction are not amenable to limited operative exposure or arthroscopic-assisted reduction or external fixation must be treated by open reduction and internal fixation (Fig. 22-23). Restoration of normal articular anatomy is critical and should be achieved in an arthroscopic-assisted or an open reduction and internal fixation. It is especially critical to identify a median or ulnar neuropathy which may indicate an impending or established compartment syndrome and warrant immediate decompression.

REHABILITATION

After the critical treatment and period of immobilization, the athlete should follow a tissue-specific rehabilitation program consisting of the five phases of rehabilitation (acute, initial, progressive, integrated

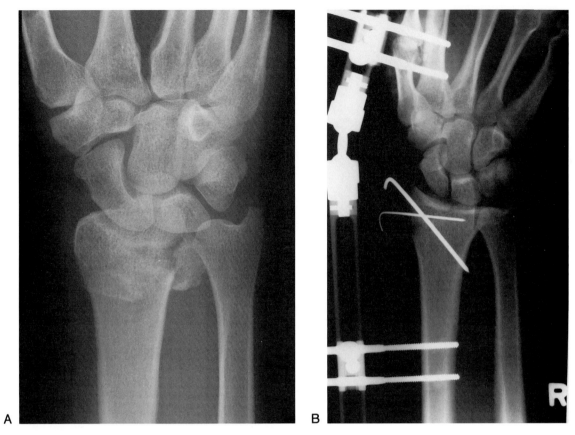

Figure 22-22 (A) A 20-year-old collegiate basketball player fell onto one hand and sustained an intra-articular displaced distal radius fracture. **(B)** After arthroscopic-assisted reduction and percutaneous pinning with placement of external fixator.

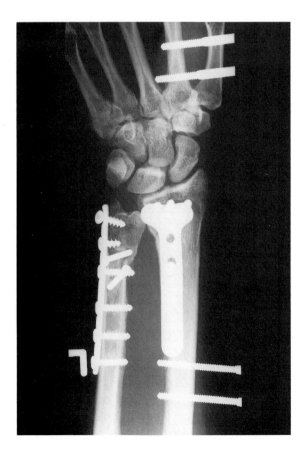

Figure 22-23 Severely comminuted fractures of the distal radius and ulna after open reduction and internal fixation augmented by cancellous bone graft.

functions, and return to sport). The characteristics of the rehabilitation depend on the healing process of the injury (i.e., bone, ligament, triangular fibrocartilage complex, and articular surface) and upper extremity demands of the athlete. Certain injuries will require longer protection in phase I (reduction of swelling and pain relief) and phase II (progressive pain-free range of motion). When the athlete is ready to return to sport (phase V), the use of protective equipment will vary, depending on the injury and the sport.

Injury-Specific Rehabilitation

Extra-articular Fractures

Extra-articular fractures of the radius are held in a cast for 4 to 6 weeks until healed. The athlete's wrist is then supported in a thermoplastic splint while phases II through V of rehabilitation are accomplished (generally 4 to 6 weeks further). Full return to upper extremity intensive sport without protection is not allowed prior to 3 months from the time of injury. If the sport allows, the athlete may participate in a playing cast while rehabilitation proceeds.

Simple Intra-articular Fractures

Fractures with Rigid Internal Fixation

Simple intra-articular fracture with rigid internal fixation (e.g., volar, Barton's) may be protected by a thermoplastic splint with early active-assisted range of motion encouraged. Upper extremity strengthening and sport activities are not allowed until there is clinical and radiographic evidence of healing (4 to 6 weeks). At this time, protection in a thermoplastic splint is continued, but rehabilitative phase III is begun. Full upper extremity sport activity is not allowed before 3 months have elapsed, unless the sport can be played with a playing cast.

Fractures without Rigid Internal Fixation

Simple intra-articular fractures without surgical internal fixation (e.g., percutaneous pins) are treated and rehabilitated as for extra-articular fractures (discussed above).

Comminuted Intra-articular Fractures

Most comminuted intra-articular fractures are extremely unstable and require a combination of internal and external fixation to maintain the length and integrity of the articular surface. These fractures are immobilized for 6 to 12 weeks, depending upon the degree of comminution. The efficacy of articulating external fixation has not been clearly defined but may have a role in the future for early mobilization of intra-articular fractures while maintaining distraction.

After removal of the external fixator or cast, thermoplastic splint protection is continued and active-assisted range of motion is begun. The athlete will invariably have difficulty regaining motion, and full range of motion is unlikely to be obtained. Three months after fracture, if stability is ensured clinically and radiographically, dynamic splinting may be initiated as well as a strengthening program. Light sport-specific training is initiated at this time, but full return to the upper extremity sport of the high-demand athlete is discouraged until 6 months from the time of injury.

Triangular Fibrocartilage Complex Injuries

Articular Disc

The athlete treated for a triangular fibrocartilage tear of the articular disc (type Ia or type II degenerative tears) is rehabilitated symptomatically. After arthroscopic debridement, the athlete's wrist is held in a splint for 1 week until suture removal. Following this, the athlete progresses through phases II through V as tolerated.

Triangular Fibrocartilage Complex Peripheral Tears or Avulsion

These injuries are soft tissue and ligamentous by nature and require prolonged immobilization and protection. Following repair of the tear or avulsion (either arthroscopically or open), the athlete's arm is placed into a long-arm cast for 6 to 8 weeks. Following this, the arm is protected in a long-arm thermoplastic splint as active-assisted range of motion is begun. Dynamic splinting and strengthening may be initiated 3 months after injury, and light sport-specific upper extremity activities begun (throwing a tennis ball, light racquet volley against a wall). It is not recommended that the high-contact athlete return to sport with a playing cast at this time. Full return to sport is not allowed until a minimum of 6 months from repair, and not until the athlete has demonstrated adequate return of strength, motion, and flexibility.

Galeazzi and Essex-Lopresti Fracture-Dislocation

The Galeazzi and Essex-Lopresti fracture-dislocations represent serious bony and ligamentous injuries with prolonged rehabilitation and unpredictable out-

comes. After fracture fixation, the treatment and rehabilitation for the remaining soft tissue injuries are as
described in the subsection *Triangular Fibrocartilage
Complex Peripheral Tears or Avulsions*. The exception
is the Galeazzi fracture-dislocation that is repaired by
rigid internal fixation of both the radius and large ulna
styloid fragment, which contains attachments of the
triangular fibrocartilage complex. In this case, early
protected range of motion may be initiated with a thermoplastic splint protector. This will hasten rehabilitation phase II, and phases III through V are begun when
healing is noted (6 to 8 weeks). Return to sport in this
case may be 12 weeks from repair.

On the other end of this spectrum, the Essex-Lopresti
fracture-dislocation will require prolonged rehabilitation (up to 12 months), and the prognosis for return to
high-demand upper extremity sport is poor.

REFERENCES

1. Owen RA, Melton JJ Jr, Johnson A et al: Incidence of
   Colles fracture in North American community. Am J
   Public Health 72:605, 1982

2. Jupiter JB: Current concepts review fractures of the distal end of the radius. J Bone J Surg [Am] 73:461, 1991
3. Muller ME, Nazarian S, Kich P: Classification AI des
   Fractures: Les Os Longs. Springer-Verlag, Berlin 1987
4. Melone CP Jr: Articular fractures of the distal radius.
   Orthop Clin North Am 15:217, 1984
5. Frykman G: Fracture of the distal radius including sequelae, shoulder hand finger syndrome, disturbance in
   the distal radioulnar joint and impairment of nerve function: a clinical and experimental study. Acta Orthop
   Scand [Suppl] 108:1, 1967
6. Palmer AK, Werner FW: The triangular fibrocartilage
   complex of the wrist: anatomy and function. J Hand
   Surg 6:153, 1981
7. Heiple KB, Freehafer AA, Van't Hof A: Isolated traumatic dislocation of the distal end of the ulna or distal
   radioulnar joint. J Bone Joint Surg [Am] 44:1387, 1962
8. Roy S, Came D, Singer IC: Stress changes of the distal
   radial epiphysis in young gymnasts. Am J Sports Med
   13:301, 1985
9. Mikic DJ: Galeazzi fracture dislocation. J Bone Joint
   Surg [Am] 57:1071, 1975
10. Moore EM: Three cases illustrating subluxation of the
    ulna in connection with Colles fracture. Med Rec
    17:305, 1880

23

Ligamentous Injuries of the Wrist

William J. Morgan

Ligamentous injuries about the wrist joint, resulting in carpal instabilities and dislocations, are frequently encountered in the athletic population. Despite continued research in this area, the diagnosis and therapeutic management of carpal instabilities continue to pose a significant dilemma for the treating physician. This chapter is intended for the health care provider treating athletic wrist injuries and offers current recommendations on treatment. A comprehensive understanding of carpal instabilities will decrease the therapeutic challenges of these disorders.

Knowledge of carpal anatomy and kinematics, including the intrinsic and extrinsic ligaments, is critical in the accurate diagnosis and treatment of carpal instabilities. The preferred treatment for acute ligamentous disruptions is restoration of normal anatomy, stabilization to allow ligamentous healing, and appropriate rehabilitation. Ligamentous instabilities that are allowed to become chronic leave few options for optimistic treatment. Late ligament reconstruction or intercarpal fusions are associated with limited success, particularly in the high-performance athlete. A realistic approach to treatment and expected outcomes must be maintained by the physician and conveyed to the athlete. The outcome of these injuries, although relative to the severity, chronicity, and treatment of the wrist instability, in many cases may be career-threatening to the athlete.

CLASSIFICATION

Many classification systems on carpal instabilities have evolved, including classifications based on anatomic location of the injury or radiographic findings (static versus dynamic instabilities). More recently, classification schemes have evolved that more clearly outline the subtle variations seen in location and severity of carpal instabilities.[1] These have been further modified by Green.[2]

MECHANISM OF INJURY

Most athletes who sustain an injury to their wrist do so by falling onto an outstretched arm either in front of themselves (e.g., breaking a fall while being tackled in football) or behind themselves (e.g., falling backward onto a basketball court or ice-skating rink), resulting in extreme wrist hyperextension.

Depending on the severity of the hyperextension, subtle "sprains" of the interosseous ligaments to more extreme perilunate fracture dislocations may result. Mayfield[3] has attempted to describe the progression of severity of injury by using stages to detail the progression of injury about the lunate. These continuing ligamentous injuries about the lunate have been termed *progressive perilunar instabilities*, the four stages of which are outlined in Table 23-1.

Table 23-1 Progressive Perilunar Instability

Stage 1
Injury to the scapholunate interosseous ligaments and the volar radioscaphocapitate extrinsic ligament, resulting in a scapholunate dissociation

Stage 2
Progressive injury and subluxation of the capitate on the dorsal pole of the lunate through the space of Poirier

Stage 3
Includes stages 1 and 2 as well as injury to the lunotriquetral interosseous ligaments and the extrinsic volar carpal ligaments; at this stage, there may be a complete dorsal dislocation about the lunate presenting as a perilunate dislocation

Stage 4
A composite of stages 1, 2, and 3 with rupture of the dorsal radiolunate ligaments resulting in volar dislocation of the lunate

Perilunate instabilities involving only the interosseous and extrinsic ligaments will result in a "lesser arc" perilunate injury. Perilunate ligamentous injuries may also involve fractures of the radial styloid, scaphoid, proximal pole of the capitate and triquetrum, and the ulna styloid, resulting in "greater arc" injuries (Fig. 23-1) (see later sections of this chapter).

Progressive perilunate instabilities resulting in perilunate or lunate dislocations require extreme forces of hyperextension and are usually seen in injuries resulting from a fall from a great height or a motor vehicle

accident. Most athletic injuries will be the result of a less forceful injury and will usually present as early stages (i.e., stage 1 or stage 2 perilunate instabilities). The presentation of stage 1 or 2 perilunate injuries may be very subtle, often presenting with normal radiographs. Therefore, a high index of suspicion must be maintained when the athlete presents with wrist pain or swelling following a hyperextension injury about the wrist. Subtle radiographic changes, such as a fracture of the radial styloid, should alert the health care provider to assess for further intercarpal injury, such as scapholunate dissociation. The severe perilunate instability will be obvious in the clinical and radiographic evaluation; however, the more subtle carpal instability will be the more common presentation in the athletic population and, if left undiagnosed and untreated, may progress to a chronic instability with a much less favorable outcome.

Along with an improved understanding of the pathophysiology of carpal instabilities, there has also been progress in the diagnostic modalities available to assess these injuries. It must be recognized, however, that these technological modalities represent only an adjunct to diagnosis and treatment and should not be a substitution for a careful history and physical examination. For complete information on history, diagnosis, and physical examination, see Chapter 21.

CLINICAL DIAGNOSIS

The athlete who presents with a potential instability about the wrist following an acute injury often may also have swelling and diffuse discomfort. Palpation and provocative maneuvers should be performed to more precisely locate the potential site of ligamentous disruption. An acute wrist injury must be carefully evaluated to avoid the nonspecific diagnosis of "wrist sprain," which may imply a less serious injury than actually exists. Even with the presence of normal radiographs, a high index of suspicion for ligamentous injuries in the athlete must be maintained until further diagnostic tests prove otherwise.

Radiographic Evaluation

Standard radiographs in the evaluation of wrist pain should include posteroanterior and true lateral views. On the PA view, the carpal alignment should be noted, and there should be particular attention directed to Gilula's lines[4] (Fig. 23-2), which should follow smoothly contoured arcs of both the proximal carpal and midcarpal rows. Abnormal spaces or diastases be-

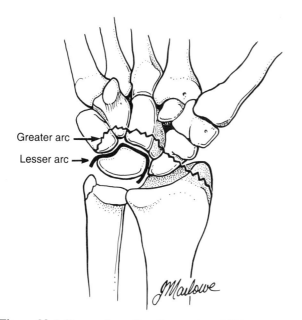

Greater arc
Lesser arc

Figure 23-1 Progression of perilunate instabilities may be purely ligamentous *(lesser arc)* or may evolve via fractures of the radius, scaphoid, capitate, triquetrum, and ulna styloid consecutively *(greater arc)*.

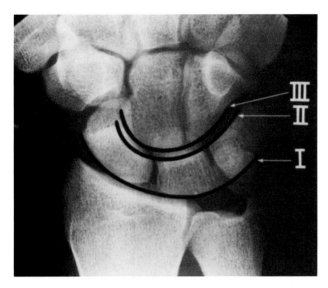

Figure 23-2 Gilula's lines should follow as smooth arcs contouring the proximal and distal carpal rows. Any break in the congruity strongly suggests a ligamentous instability at the site of incongruity.

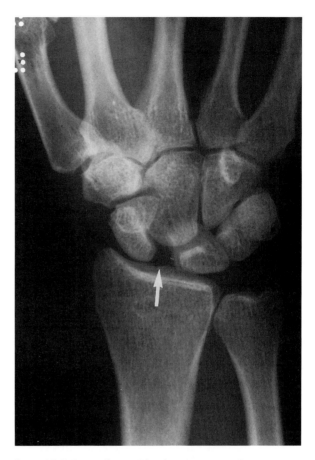

Figure 23-3 PA radiographic view demonstrating an abnormal diastasis (> 3 mm) *(arrow)* between the scaphoid and lunate indicating a scapholunate dissociation.

tween the carpal bones should be noted, particularly at the level of the scapholunate joint. Diastases in this area are generally defined by a separation of greater than 2 to 3 mm (Fig. 23-3). In some athletes (particularly adolescents), a small degree of normal ligamentous laxity may manifest itself by a diastasis of 2 to 3 mm between the scaphoid and the lunate. In these cases, contralateral comparison views should be obtained to assess for asymmetry. In cases where carpal instability is suspected, but standard AP and lateral radiographic views are normal, oblique and PA views in radial and ulna deviation may reveal an instability pattern.

PA views of the wrist in ulnar and radial deviation are extremely valuable in assessing the kinematics of the wrist without the use of fluoroscopy. In radial deviation, the height of the scaphoid decreases, and a ring sign appears at the distal pole of the scaphoid (see Fig. 20-1). This occurs as the scaphoid assumes a volar flexed position, allowing the thumb ray to approach the radial styloid. In ulnar deviation, the scaphoid is noted to increase in height as it assumes a more extended or neutral position as the thumb ray travels away from the radial styloid. In radial and ulnar deviation, any abnormal diastases along the proximal carpal row or at the triquetrohamate junction should also be noted.

A true lateral view is critical for the assessment of carpal instability patterns. In the normal lateral view, the radius, lunate, and capitate are noted to be colinear. More accurate assessment can be made of this by measurement of the radiolunate and capitolunate angles. The normal radiolunate angle is 0 to 30 degrees, the

normal capitolunate is 0 to 15 degrees. The position of the long axis of the lunate relative to the long axis of the scaphoid (i.e., the scapholunate angle) is also noted on the true lateral radiographic view. Although there is some discrepancy as to the measurement technique, in addition to interpretation variability, it is generally agreed that a normal scapholunate angle is 30 to 60 degrees (Fig. 23-4A). A scapholunate angle of greater than 60 degrees represents a rotatory subluxation of the scaphoid and strongly suggests a scapholunate dissociation. This has further been categorized by Linscheid and colleagues[5] into dorsal intercalated segment instability (DISI) and volar intercalated segment instability (VISI) patterns.[3] In a DISI pattern, the lunate is noted to be dorsiflexed and the capitate is noted to be subluxed dorsally on the lunate (Fig. 23-4B).

A DISI conformation on the lateral-view radiograph suggests an injury to the scapholunate ligament and may also be seen in a displaced scaphoid fracture. A VISI pattern is noted with the lunate tilting in a volar-flexed position with some mild volar subluxation of the

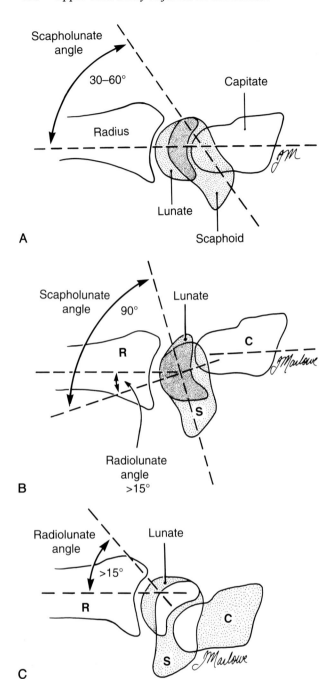

Figure 23-4 (A) Diagrammatic representation of the technique of the measuring the scapholunate angle. **(B)** Diagram of DISI (dorsal intercolated segmental instability). Note abnormal radiolunate, capitolunate, and scapholunate angles. **(C)** Diagram of VISI (volar intercolated segmental instability). Note abnormal radiolunate and capitolunate angles. The scapholunate angle will usually be normal.

capitate (Fig. 23-4C). A VISI pattern may be seen in injuries to the lunotriquetral ligaments or midcarpal injuries (triquetrohamate).

Further assessment of potential wrist instability can be made by the carpal height index. This is a ratio of the height of the carpus as measured from the distal radius to the base of the third finger metacarpal divided by the length of the long-finger metacarpal (see Fig. 20-2). This is normally a ratio of 0.54 ± 0.03.[6] Ratios less than this normal value indicate carpal collapse. In subtle and early injuries resulting in carpal instabilities, the carpal height index will be normal and other methods must be used to determine an early carpal injury.

Fluoroscopy and Cineradiography

Fluoroscopy and cineradiography are useful adjuncts in the evaluation of wrist instability patterns. With the use of fluoroscopy, the dynamic motion of the proximal and distal carpal rows can be monitored. Recording the fluoroscopic image is helpful (cineradiography): repeated evaluation can be made, and the speed of the image can be reduced, thereby allowing observation of subtle abnormalities. The carpus can be loaded by a clenched fist, further exacerbating any instabilities. Radial and ulnar deviation can be observed for abnormal "jumps" that may occur in the carpus, often associated with an audible or palpable "clunk" and pain. Correlations can then be made of the abnormal carpal segment to further identify the source of instability.

Arthrography

Wrist arthrography is indicated in cases that present with normal plain radiographs but where a dynamic instability is suspected. We utilize the three-compartment method as described by Palmer and coworkers.[7] (Fig. 23-5), which minimizes the incidence of false negatives that result from a valvular-type tear of the interosseous ligament. Positive results are indicated by leakage of dye from a radiocarpal injection into the midcarpal joint through the scapholunate or lunotriquetral interval, and/or leakage of dye from the midcarpal joint injection into the radiocarpal joint through the scapholunate or lunotriquetral interval. In this technique, the radiocarpal joint is injected, the joint stressed, and an evaluation is made. One hour is allowed for dye resorption, and separate injections are then made into the midcarpal and distal radioulnar joints, allowing for further observations. This technique offers the advantage of visualizing interosseous ligamentous tears or triangular fibrocartilage tears, which may be valvelike and therefore not always visualized on a unicompartmental injection. This technique also offers the advantage of better assessment of the articular surfaces of the midcarpal and distal

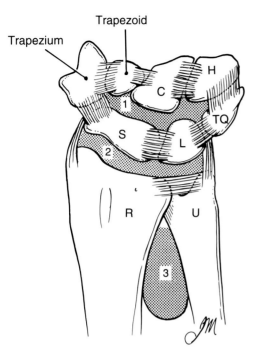

Figure 23-5 Diagram of three separate wrist compartments. The midcarpal compartment is separated from the radiocarpal compartment by the proximal carpal row and its associated intact interosseous ligaments. The distal radioulnar compartment is separated from the radiocarpal by the intact triangular fibrocartilage complex. Any alteration of the integrity of these structures will be shown by passage of dye from one compartment to another.

radioulnar joint, and the identification of avulsion injuries of the triangular fibrocartilage complex that would not be observed on radiocarpal injection alone.

Tomography and Computed Tomography

Tomography and computed tomography (CT) have limited utilization in purely ligamentous injuries to the carpus. It is, however, useful in distinguishing otherwise occult scaphoid fractures or ligamentous avulsion fractures that may be associated with carpal instability patterns. CT is indicated in the diagnosis of distal radial ulnar joint instability, degeneration, or dislocations by providing transverse sections of the sigmoid notch.

Bone Scintigraphy

A technitium bone scan is a highly sensitive modality, though not very specific. It offers some diagnostic information on occult injuries that are not readily apparent on the aforementioned studies. It may also prove helpful in localizing an area of injury that may be investigated further by more invasive studies such as

arthroscopy. For example, an athlete may present with vague dorsal wrist pain and normal radiographs. A bone scan may demonstrate increased uptake in the lunate, indicating further evaluation of a potential bone contusion or impaction fracture.

Magnetic Resonance Imaging

With the development of surface coils for the wrist, there has been a marked improvement in the ability of magnetic resonance imaging (MRI) to visualize normal and abnormal anatomy about the wrist. Injuries to the carpal interosseous ligaments may be noted on MRI, which may not be apparent on routine radiographs or arthrography. Injury to the capsular structures, extrinsic ligaments, and triangular fibrocartilage complex may also be demonstrated by MRI. Other subtle articular injuries and joint effusions may be evaluated by this method. The value of MRI in assessing bone viability has been shown in the early diagnosis of Kienbock disease. The use of MRI should be reserved only to answer those questions that cannot be satisfactorily answered by more conventional and less costly modalities.

Arthroscopy

Wrist arthroscopy has evolved into a valuable diagnostic and therapeutic modality for ligamentous injuries about the wrist. It is preferable to wrist arthrotomy, particularly in the athlete, as "downtime," morbidity, and rehabilitation are markedly lessened. Wrist arthroscopy is helpful in diagnosing partial tears of the interosseous ligaments, as well as in assessing the integrity of the volar extrinsic ligaments. Incomplete or partially healed tears of the intrinsic ligaments or the triangular fibrocartilage may go unnoticed by arthrography, but are usually visualized by arthroscopy. During arthroscopy, the extrinsic and intrinsic ligaments can be probed to further assess not only their integrity but the potential laxity of these structures.

Arthroscopic-assisted reduction and percutaneous pinning of acute carpal instabilities and distal radius fractures is beneficial, since there can be direct observation of the congruity of reduction, with minimal disruption of associated soft tissues.

SCAPHOLUNATE DISSOCIATION

Scapholunate dissociation is the most common of the carpal instabilities and is seen in essentially any running sport. The mechanism of injury is a fall onto the thenar eminence of the extended hand, with resultant wrist hyperextension, ulna deviation, and intercarpal supination.[3]

The athlete should be observed for middorsal swelling of the wrist. There will be pain on palpatation of the scapholunate interval dorsally and the scaphoid shift test may be positive (see Ch. 21). Since the clinical presentation may be mild and the symptoms minimized by the athlete, a high index of suspicion by the health professional should be maintained. Outcomes of treatment in the athlete, particularly range of motion and strength, are significantly more favorable when treatment is initiated acutely, and generally poor when the treatment is instituted in a chronic scapholunate dissociation.

AP and lateral radiographic views are imperative in the evaluation of the athlete with suspected scapholunate dissociation. Any evidence of a scapholunate diastases of greater than 2 to 3 mm should be noted. Presence of a "cortical ring sign" of the distal pole of the scaphoid should also be noted, since this occurs as the scaphoid assumes a volar-flexed position, suggesting damage to the scapholunate interosseous ligament (Fig. 23-6). It must be noted, however, that many scapholunate dissociations, particularly those presenting acutely, will present as dynamic instabilities. These will not become apparent on plain radiographs. Under these circumstances, AP and lateral radiographic views should be obtained in a stress or "clenched fist" position. In the clenched fist position, the axial loading of the capitate at the scapholunate junction is markedly increased, thereby causing a diastasis at the scapholunate interval and a rotatory subluxation of the scaphoid if the scapholunate ligament is not intact.

Treatment options for scapholunate dissociation are varied and related to the time from injury until institution of treatment. These represent a serious injury in the high-demand upper extremity athlete, and time should be spent with the athlete and family discussing treatment options, expected outcome, and potential for return to his or her sport competitively.

Partial Tears

Partial tears of the scapholunate interosseous ligament (grades I and II) present with middorsal wrist pain but generally have normal radiographs and arthrogram. MRI may be positive for edematous changes in the ligament. Arthroscopy is extremely valuable in this situation, as a definitive diagnosis can be made. At the same time, the partially torn ligament, which may cause a mechanical block, can be excised with a small-

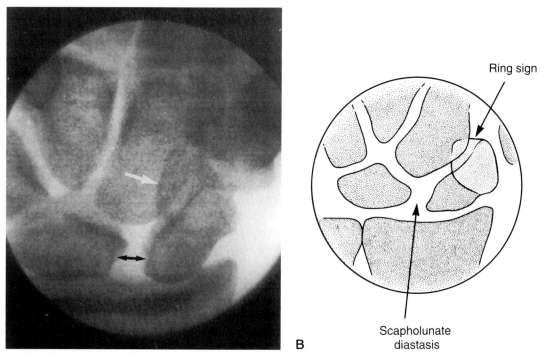

Figure 23-6 **(A)** AP fluoroscopic image of scapholunate dissociation. Note cortical ring sign of scaphoid although the wrist is not in radial deviation *(white arrow)* and diastasis of scapholunate interval *(black arrow)*. **(B)** Diagram of scapholunate diastasis and cortical ring sign.

joint shaver. Associated hypertrophic synovium may be removed as well. The wrist position that provides the least tension of the ligament can be determined, arthroscopically, and the wrist can be immobilized in this position for 4 to 6 weeks. If the sport allows, the athlete may continue to participate in a playing cast during this period. Range of motion and strengthening exercises should begin after cast removal, but the wrist should be protected while participating in sports until 3 months after the injury. An excellent outcome can be expected with partial tears.

Acute Complete Scapholunate Tears

Complete tears of the scapholunate interosseous ligament (grade III) are best treated by early recognition and repair of the ligament. Arthroscopy is an excellent means of achieving and evaluating reduction. Some authors advocate arthroscopic reduction and percutaneous pinning of acute scapholunate dissociation and report good results.[8] Treatment of complete tears of the scapholunate ligament should not be undertaken by cast immobilization alone, since it is impossible to maintain a proper alignment of the scaphoid and lunate without pinning.

In most upper extremity-intense athletes, however, it is preferable to perform open reduction and repair of the torn ligament with pinning of the carpus in an anatomic position.[9] Open repair may be performed as long as there is reparable ligament substance and ability to easily reduce the scaphoid[10,11] (usually within 6 months of injury). This repair is augmented by a dorsal capsulodesis similar to that described by Blatt.[12]

After ligament repair and pinning, the wrist is immobilized in a cast for 8 to 10 weeks. Following cast removal, protection in a thermoplastic splint is imperative as the athlete rehabilitates with range of motion only during the first 2 weeks. Once maximum comfortable motion has been obtained, strengthening procedures should begin, but not until at least 3 months after surgery. Participation in sports without the use of a cast or splint should not be allowed for a minimum of 6 months postsurgery.

Case Study I

A collegiate gymnast missed her dismount from the parallel bars, and fell onto her outstretched right hand. Following this injury, she noted full range of motion with some mild middorsal swelling and continued discomfort. The initial diagnosis was a "wrist sprain," and she was placed into an Ace wrap. With an attempt to return to sport within the following

days, she had continued pain about the wrist and a sensation of "catching" in her wrist on range of motion, particularly hyperextension.

On examination 1 week postinjury, there was little swelling about the wrist but tenderness to palpation over the mid-dorsum of the wrist at the level of the scapholunate interosseous ligament. A scaphoid shift test was positive, with subluxation of the carpus both palpable and audible associated with pain. Plain AP and lateral radiographic views were normal, but fluoroscopic stress views revealed a diastasis at the scapholunate interval with the suggestion of a rotatory subluxation of the scaphoid. A three-compartment arthrogram showed leakage of dye through the scapholunate interval (Fig. 23-7).

Open reduction and repair of the interosseous ligament with dorsal capsulodesis was performed, followed by 8 weeks of cast immobilization. At 8 weeks the pins were removed and the patient was placed in a thermoplastic thumb spica splint. She started an active-assisted range of motion program, and strengthening was initiated at 12 weeks. At that time, a sport-specific rehabilitation program was instituted, and she was allowed to return to gymnastics 6 months postoperatively. It was noted that she continued to have occasional discomfort about the dorsum of the wrist, particularly with hyperextension maneuvers of the wrist. A hyperextension block

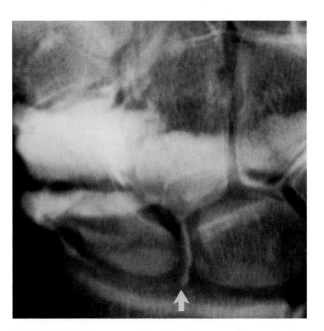

Figure 23-7 Three compartment arthrogram demonstrating flow of contrast from midcarpal to radiocarpal joint through the scapholunate interval indicating a rupture of the SL interosseous ligament *(arrow).*

splint was helpful in minimizing these symptoms (see Ch. 2).

CHRONIC SCAPHOLUNATE INSTABILITIES

Once the scapholunate injury has become chronic (>6 months), treatment options are limited and unpredictable in outcome, particularly in the competitive athlete. Many attempts have been made in the past for interosseous ligament reconstruction by free tendon grafts with variable outcomes.[13,14] Most have resulted in stretching of the ligamentous reconstruction and recurrence of the initial dissociation. Blatt[12] has described a dorsal scaphoid capsulodesis with good early results. This procedure is particularly indicated in the skeletally immature athlete with a chronic scapholunate dissociation. Care must be taken to ensure that there is no evidence of preoperative degeneration at the scaphoid fossa before proceeding with the dorsal scaphoid capsulodesis.

In the competitive athlete with extensive upper extremity demands, more predictable outcomes can be obtained with the use of limited intercarpal arthrodeses. To stabilize the volar-flexed scaphoid in a chronic scapholunate dissociation, the scaphotrapezium trapezoid arthrodesis has been utilized. In this arthrodesis, the scaphoid is brought into a more extended position and pinned to the capitate prior to arthrodesis at the scaphotrapezium trapezoid joint. Care must be taken not to overextend the scaphoid, which will result in increased morbidity and further loss of wrist motion.

Scaphocapitate or scaphocapitolunate fusion is used more often to obtain the same result of further scaphoid extension and carpal stability. This arthrodesis is more predictable and is technically easier. Care must be taken when decorticating between scaphoid and capitate to maintain volar cortex and cartilage, so that normal anatomic distances between the carpus are not altered (Fig. 23-8). Reduction is maintained by internal fixation, preferably power staples or interosseous screws. The patient is then placed in a thumb spica short-arm cast until a radiographic fusion is apparent (generally 6 weeks). This is then substituted with an orthoplast splint and a hand therapy program for range of motion, followed by strengthening and a sport-specific upper extremity rehabilitation program, combined with the athlete's general training program. Full return to sport without a playing cast is not allowed for 6 months.

SCAPHOLUNATE ADVANCED COLLAPSED WRIST

It has been previously noted that the natural history of untreated scapholunate dissociations may result in a scapholunate advanced collapsed (SLAC) wrist.[15] Due to abnormal radioscaphoid and intercarpal motion, there is noted degeneration of the radioscaphoid joint followed by degeneration of the capitolunate juncture; as the carpus degenerates, the radiolunate joint is spared. At this point, however, joint motion is painful and markedly limited. Treatment options are described in Chapter 24.

INSTABILITIES

Ulnar Wrist Instabilities

Pain isolated to the ulnar aspect of the carpus has been referred to as the "low back pain of the wrist" because the diagnosis is often elusive. These injuries often manifest as ulnar-sided pain and an abnormal clicking or shucking of the wrist in ulnar and radial deviation. Differential diagnosis includes midcarpal instabilities, lunotriquetral instabilities, triangular fibrocartilage complex tears and/or avulsions, ulnar impaction syndrome, distal radioulnar joint subluxation, or combinations of the above. Care must be taken when performing a physical examination to localize areas of pain and to subsequently perform the appropriate diagnostic maneuvers to differentiate the aforementioned injury potentials.

Lunotriquetral Instabilities

Instability of the lunotriquetral joint results from rupture of the lunotriquetral interosseous ligament, causing pain overlying the lunotriquetral articulation and snapping when the wrist is moved in ulnar and radial deviation. This injury is usually seen in high-impact sports such as rugby, football, and hockey, and is the result of a significant force to the hypothenar eminence, associated with wrist hyperextension.

In the diagnosis of lunotriquetral instability, pain is noted on palpation over the lunotriquetral joint. There is also a positive lunotriquetral ballottment test as described by Reagan et al.[16] On plain radiographs, a VISI configuration on the lateral-view radiograph may be noted.

A three-compartment arthrogram is helpful in further delineating a lunotriquetral interosseous tear with

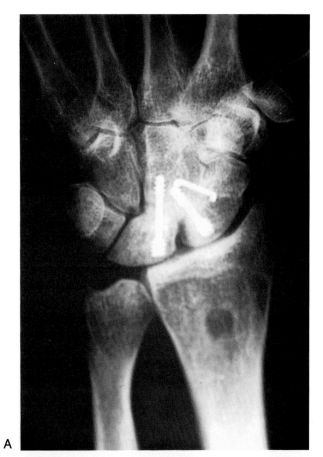

Figure 23-8 (A) AP and (B) lateral limited intercarpal fusion (scaphocapitolunate) for scapholunate dissociation.

A

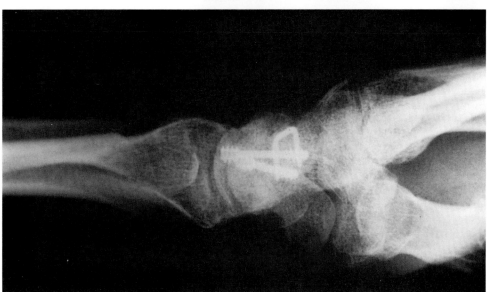

B

leakage of dye into the midcarpal joint on radiocarpal injection or into the radiocarpal joint on midcarpal injection.[7] MRI may play a role in the diagnosis of a rupture of the interosseous ligament, but the sensitivity and cost effectiveness are yet to be determined. Arthroscopy has become increasingly helpful in the diagnosis of ulna-sided wrist injuries. Through arthroscopy, the lunotriquetral interosseous ligament can be assessed directly and observations for other sources of ulna-sided wrist pain, such as ulna impaction syndrome, can be made (see Ch. 22).

If noted acutely, treatment is cast immobilization for 6 weeks, providing there is anatomic reduction. If a static instability is present, then reduction should be obtained and held by percutaneous pinning. Chronic instabilities of the lunotriquetral interval are not amenable to ligamentous reconstruction, particularly in the competitive athlete. Lunotriquetral arthrodesis is the treatment of choice. Postoperative cast immobilization is provided by a short-arm cast for 6 weeks, followed by a thermoplastic splint and hand therapy for 6 weeks. Sport-specific rehabilitation should then begin in conjunction with the usual rehabilitation program. Return to vigorous sport activities should not be recommended for 6 months from the time of surgery, and after confirmation (by tomography) of a solid fusion.

Midcarpal Instabilities

Although somewhat rare, midcarpal instability has been observed in the competitive athlete.[17] Most often, it is seen in the athlete who is required to perform frequent ulnar and radial deviation, particularly while supplying an axial load to the wrist, for example, follow-through in baseball batting and various racquet sports with backhand motion and ulnar deviation. Midcarpal instability is considered to be the result of a rupture of the triquetrohamate ligament, and the capitotriquetral arm of the arcuate extrinsic ligament, causing a loss of the normal smooth helicoidal motion as the triquetrum descends relative to the hamate in ulnar deviation. This produces a sudden snapping of the proximal carpal row into dorsiflexion as the wrist is brought from radial to ulnar deviation. Care must be taken to distinguish midcarpal hypermobility from midcarpal instability. In the young female athlete with joint hyperlaxity, an asymptomatic "clunk" may occur with radial and ulnar deviation but may not be associated with pain. When assessing midcarpal symptoms, the contralateral limb of the athlete should be examined for similar joint hyperlaxity. When this is seen in the young female gymnast, for example, overtreatment should be prevented and symptomatic treatment only

should be provided with intermittent splint use and nonsteroidal anti-inflammatory medications.

Plain radiographs are generally normal, although on the true lateral view there may be a note of a mild VISI deformity. Cineradiography is the most useful modality in the diagnosis of midcarpal instabilities. The athlete is asked to make a clenched fist, (thus loading the wrist in an axial direction), then bring the wrist from radial to ulnar deviation. With midcarpal instability, a "clunk" and pain overlying the ulnar aspect of the carpus are noted. Often a radiopaque marker can be used by the athlete to point toward the area of pain, which is generally in the triquetrohamate joint area. On cineradiography, a sudden snapping of the proximal carpal row into dorsiflexion is noted when proceeding into ulnar deviation. There is a sudden but congruous movement of the entire proximal carpal row into dorsiflexion. There may also be an abnormal widening at the triquetrohamate junction on ulnar and radial deviation. Arthrography may further help in confirming this diagnosis if there is leakage of dye at the triquetrohamate junction following a midcarpal injection.

Treatment of chronic midcarpal instability should be symptomatic and sport-specific. Midcarpal instabilities associated with infrequent snapping, but with pain related to localized synovitis, may be treated by a local corticosteroid injection and rest. Splints have been devised that may help hold the midcarpal joint reduced in sports not requiring frequent radial and ulnar deviation or grasping maneuvers. Earlier reports of ligament reconstruction have demonstrated less than optimal results.[18] Triquetrohamate arthrodesis has been the treatment of choice. Postoperative cast immobilization is through a short-arm cast for 6 weeks, followed by an orthoplast splint and hand therapy for 6 weeks. Sport-specific rehabilitation should then begin in conjunction with the athlete's usual rehabilitation program. Return to vigorous sport activities should not be recommended prior to 6 months from the time of the surgery.

Case Study II

A 22-year-old minor league baseball player noted a painful and audible "clunk" in his left wrist on attempts to swing a bat. He recalled no precipitating event but did sustain multiple "wrist sprains" in the past. This current problem was severely affecting his ability to hit.

On examination, he had no swelling about the wrist, had full range of motion, flexion, extension, rotation, and ulnar and radial deviation. He had no neurovascular deficits but was noted to have a mildly decreased grip strength. On clenched fists and with radial and ulnar deviation motions, there was a sudden jump in the wrist associated with an audible clunk and pain. Plain radiographs were normal. Fluoroscopy was obtained with clenched fist and radial and ulnar deviation, and the proximal carpal row was noted to suddenly jump from volar flexion to extension, nonsynchronized with the distal carpal row, indicating a midcarpal instability.

Attempts to prevent a recurrence were unsuccessful since the athlete was unable to wear the splints during batting. After explaining to the athlete that there would be a loss of some degree of motion in all planes, stabilization of the proximal and distal carpal rows was recommended via triquetrohamate fusion. A triquetrohamate arthrodesis was performed, and the athlete was placed in a short-arm cast until early evidence of fusion was noted at 8 weeks (Fig. 23-9). He was then placed in a removable orthoplast volar splint and began a graduated range of motion program. Strengthening was allowed at 3 months and full return to athletic activity was allowed after the

athlete plateaued with range of motion and strengthening. The athlete was able to return to baseball 6 months postoperatively at the minor league level, with some difficulties in batting due to limited ulna deviation.

PERILUNATE-LUNATE DISLOCATIONS

Injuries resulting in perilunate dislocation or lunate dislocation are likely to be seen only in high-contact sports such as football, skiing, and auto racing. Progressive instabilities about the wrist appear to follow the sequence described by Mayfield.[3] It is rare that perilunate or lunate dislocations present as either pure greater or lesser arch injuries and instead usually include components of both (Fig. 23-10). Regardless of the presenting radiographs of the injured athlete, perilunate instabilities are extremely unstable, and all potential injury sites of a perilunate dislocation must be checked.

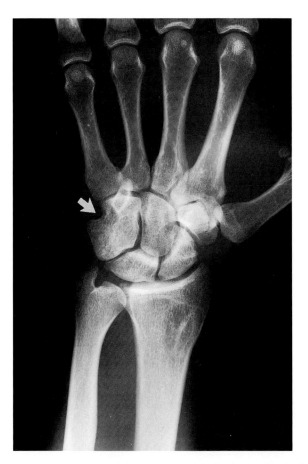

Figure 23-9 Triquetrohamate arthrodesis in a baseball player with symptomatic midcarpal instability *(arrow)*. Note here that persistent pisotriquetral symptoms necessitated pisiform excision.

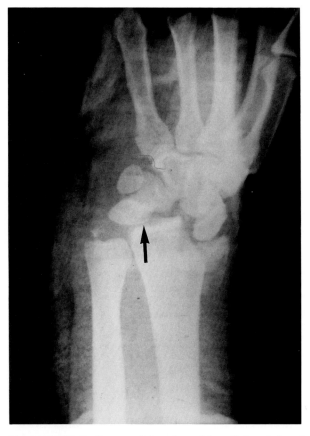

Figure 23-10 Perilunate dislocation with radial and dorsal translocation. Note lunate remains seated on the lunate fossa *(arrow)*.

Most athletes who present with perilunate injuries have marked swelling and clinical deformity. As in all wrist injuries, a complete neurovascular examination of the hand should be undertaken, as many perilunate dislocations present with an acute compartment syndrome of the carpal tunnel that may require release.

Routine radiographs usually demonstrate an overlap of the proximal and distal carpal rows with loss of the normal collinearity of the radius lunate and capitate on the lateral radiographic view (Fig. 23-11). Often there will be associated fractures of the radial styloid, scaphoid, or capitate that may be difficult to visualize on the presenting routine radiographs. I have found distraction radiographs to be invaluable in assessing the degree of injury and instability.

Perilunate dislocations are extremely unstable, and cast immobilization alone is not recommended. If a successful closed reduction of a perilunate dislocation is possible, some authors advocate percutaneous pinning in an anatomic position. Since these results are somewhat unpredictable, it is recommended in the competitive athlete that an open repair of the ruptured interosseous ligaments be performed, and treatment should be the same as that administered for acute scapholunate dissociations. As noted above, gentle traction is helpful in diagnosing the extent of intercarpal injury in the athlete presenting with a perilunate dislocation, and is essential in performing the reduction maneuvers. This is best performed with full muscle relaxation and gentle traction over a 10-minute period. In perilunate dislocations, gentle force on the dorsally dislocated capitate with hyperextension may aid in reduction at the capitate-lunate interval. It is very difficult to reduce a volar lunate dislocation by closed manipulation, therefore open reduction with ligament repair is recommended.

In volar lunate dislocations, most athletes present with a median neuropathy. The lunate dislocation should be volarly approached with decompression of the carpal tunnel and open reduction of the lunate. The lunate emerges from a transverse rent in the volar radiocarpal ligaments, and these should be repaired at the time of reduction. Further augmentation by percutaneous pinning should be performed.

Following ligamentous repair and percutaneous pinning, the wrist should be placed into a thumb spica splint to allow for predictable swelling. This should then be replaced by a short-arm thumb spica cast when the swelling has subsided. Pins are removed at 8 weeks and the patient is placed into a removable thumb spica orthoplast splint and should begin gentle range of motion exercises. Strengthening exercises (including gripping exercises) should begin around 12 weeks from the time of reduction. At that time, a gentle strengthening program and sport-specific rehabilitation should begin. The athlete's full return to sport should not take place until at least 6 months after reduction.

Since perilunate instabilities are susceptible to late carpal collapse, these must be followed for some time after the removal of pins. If the development of carpal collapse occurs after pin removal, then some form of intercarpal or total wrist arthrodesis as described in the previous sections should be recommended.

Perilunate or lunate dislocation may be associated

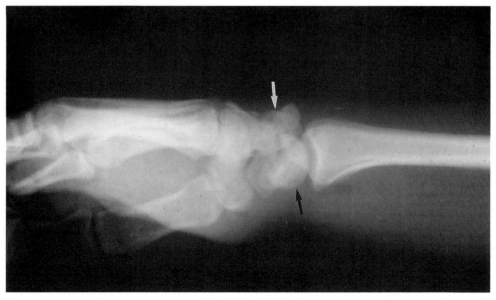

Figure 23-11 Lateral radiograph of perilunate dislocation. Note maintenance of the radiolunate axis *(black arrow),* but dorsal subluxation of the capitate (and remaining carpus) *(white arrow).*

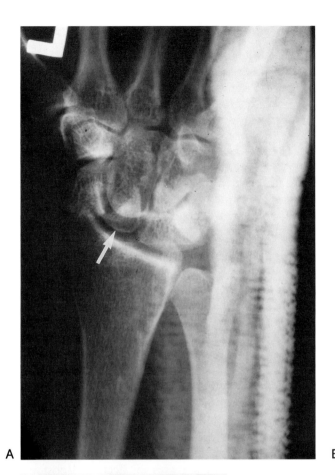

A

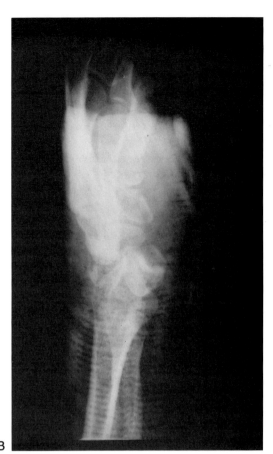

B

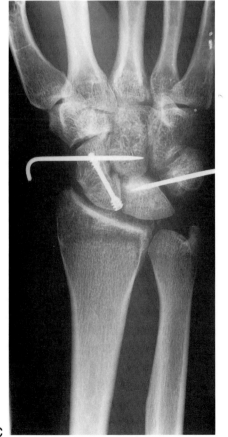

C

Figure 23-12 **(A)** AP and **(B)** lateral radiographic views of transcaphoid perilunate fracture dislocation. Note that proximal pole of the scaphoid remains with the lunate due to maintenance of the integrity of the scapholunate interosseous ligament *(arrow).* **(C)** Treatment is best performed by fixation of the fractured scaphoid and repair and pinning of interosseous ligament ruptures.

with fractures of the radial styloid, fractures to the scaphoid, the capitate, or triquetrum. The transscaphoid perilunate dislocation is most commonly seen (Fig. 23-12).

When assessing the perilunate dislocation during distraction views, these fractures should be diagnosed and an anatomic reduction performed. In the athlete, I would recommend open reduction of a transscaphoid fracture dislocation and internal fixation, preferably with an interosseous scaphoid screw. If there has been no injury to the scapholunate interosseous ligament, this fixation will improve stability to the proximal and distal carpal rows.

With a scaphoid fracture, an associated fracture of the capitate known as the *scaphocapitate syndrome* may occur (see Ch. 24).

Postoperative rehabilitation should be similar to that described for perilunate and lunate dislocations with careful follow-up radiographs to assess the healing of the associated fractures. Observation should continue, since there is the potential for avascular necrosis of the proximal pole of the scaphoid as well as the proximal pole of the capitate if these structures are involved. If the scaphoid progresses to avascular necrosis and/or nonunion, further treatment may be necessary (see Ch. 24).

Dysfunction of the median nerve associated with trauma (e.g., a distal radius fracture) should be considered a compartment syndrome of the carpal tunnel, and open decompression should be used in conjunction with treatment of the distal radius fracture (see Case Study III).

TREATMENT OF CARPAL TUNNEL SYNDROME

Most cases of carpal tunnel syndrome associated with athletic activities, such as grasping a racquet or ball, present as idiopathic and insidiously progress over time. The athlete reports weakness, sensory loss, and an awkward feeling in his or her grip. These symptoms are frequently associated with the classic symptoms of carpal tunnel syndrome, including nocturnal dysesthesias and pain and numbness while at rest.

The treatment of carpal tunnel syndrome should begin conservatively and will depend on the etiology. Initial treatment should consist of a volar splint with the wrist in neutral position and the fingers free for use. The splint should be worn at night and during aggressive activities. A splint should be used in association with nonsteroidal anti-inflammatory medications.

An injection of a corticosteroid into the carpal tunnel is a treatment option, but may only offer transient relief of symptoms. An aqueous corticosteroid solution is preferred to minimize potential complications of intraneural injection. Corticosteroid injection is prescribed in conjunction with the use of a splint as noted above. If the result is favorable, injection may be repeated at 6-month intervals.

In cases where conservative treatment has failed, surgical carpal tunnel decompression is the treatment option. Techniques of both open and endoscopic carpal tunnel decompression can be used. Open decompression is performed through a longitudinal incision just ulnar to the thenar crease. Palmar fascia and the transverse carpal ligament are divided in their entirety with exploration of the carpal canal. Median neurolysis is rarely indicated, and in most cases of idiopathic carpal tunnel syndrome, it is contraindicated.

To minimize palmar tenderness, endoscopic techniques for decompression of the carpal tunnel have been developed. Endoscopic decompression is performed through a transverse incision at the distal wrist crease. The transverse carpal ligament can be visualized from within the carpal tunnel and once the distal extent is identified, can be resected within the carpal tunnel, maintaining the integrity of the palmar fascia. This treatment provides for decreased postoperative pain and an earlier return to athletic activities. Postoperatively, the athlete is placed in a soft sterile dressing for 2 days and is encouraged to perform light range of motion and day-to-day activities as pain tolerance permits. Return to full athletic activity is allowed as the athlete's symptoms warrant, but generally sports requiring extensive use of the hands (e.g., racquet sports, gymnastics, or throwing sports) are difficult to perform for a minimum of 6 weeks postoperatively.

Case Study III

On prolonged riding, a 36-year-old competitive cyclist noted tenderness and numbness about the radial three digits in the midpalm of her hand. She frequently awoke at night with numbness and pain in the radial three digits of both of her hands, with the right worse than her left.

Her examination demonstrated a positive Phalens test on the right at 10 seconds and on the left at 30 seconds, and a positive Tinel's sign at the distal wrist crease bilaterally. Nerve conduction and electromyographic studies demonstrated a prolonged latency across the carpal tunnel bilaterally with no electromyographic changes in the thenar musculature.

Idiopathic carpal tunnel syndrome was diagnosed. The athlete was advised to use bilateral wrist splints on a full-time basis for 1 week, and bilateral corticosteroid injections were administered. One week following injection, her symptoms resolved, and she resumed her usual training program. Three months following injection, the athlete's symptoms of carpal tunnel syndrome returned.

An endoscopic decompression of both median nerves was performed under local anesthesia with sedation. She was placed into a soft dressing and an Ace wrap following her surgery and was given bilateral wrist splints to wear at night as her symptoms warranted. One week postoperatively her sutures were removed, and she was given instructions on activities for range of motion and progressive strengthening of the hands. Her nocturnal dysesthesias resolved, with no pain or numbness in her radial three digits, although deep palpation elicited some tenderness in the midpalm.

Two weeks postoperatively, she attempted to return to cycling and noted some tenderness in the midpalm of both her hands. Cycling gloves with a relief Neopryne pad in the palm were prescribed. Six weeks postoperatively, her tenderness and symptoms were resolved, and she returned to competitive cycling.

INFLAMMATORY CONDITIONS OF THE WRIST

Inflammatory conditions of the upper extremity are commonly seen in sports where the upper extremity is frequently and repetitiously moved (e.g., throwing sports, racquet sports, batting, and golf). These conditions become even more apparent in athletes who are just beginning their season when their tissue conditioning and endurance status has not been fully achieved. Inflammatory problems are also frequently seen in racquet sport athletes who change their grip style (see Case Study IV). The fibro-osseous tunnels of the wrist are lined with synovial sheaths, and repetition, overexertion, or direct trauma may cause swelling within the sheaths, resulting in tenosynovitis or tendinitis.

De Quervain stenosing tenosynovitis results from overuse and repetitious ulnar and radial deviation of the wrist, causing swelling and inflammation of the tenosynovium in the first extensor compartment housing the abductor pollicis longus and extensor pollicis brevis tendons (Fig. 23-13). Frequently there are several septated compartments within the first extensor compartment housing several slips of the abductor pollicis longus and one or two slips of the extensor pollicis brevis.

Diagnosis is confirmed by a positive Finkelstein's test (see Ch. 21) and swelling and pain over the first extensor compartment. Other conditions that may present as de Quervain stenosing tenosynovitis should be ruled out such as arthritis of the thumb metacarpal trapezial joint, scaphoid nonunion or fracture, or intersection syndrome (see below).

The treatment of de Quervain stenosing tenosynovitis in the athlete is rest from the inciting activity. This condition is also frequently seen in the wheelchair athlete and alterations in the method of mobility should be made. The extensor pollicis brevis and abductor pollicis longus tendon are best rested by placing the thumb in a thumb spica splint. The interphalangeal joint of the thumb may be left free, since this extends by way of the extensor pollicis longus and the intrinsic tendons of the thumb. In conjunction with the splint, a nonsteroidal anti-inflammatory medication should be prescribed. This conservative treatment should be attempted for at least 2 weeks.

If the athlete is in midseason and requires an early return to sport or if conservative treatment fails, an injection of a corticosteroid preparation into the first extensor compartment should be given. The injection may frequently lead to a quick resolution of the symptomatology and an earlier rehabilitation. However, in

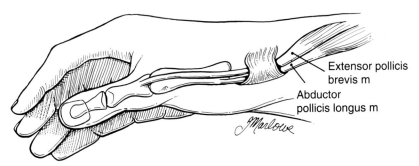

Figure 23-13 Pathoanatomy of de Quervain stenosing tenosynovitis where the APL and EPB cross the wrist extensor tendons. Stenosis of the first extensor compartment results in inflammation and pain with swelling resulting in further stenosis.

many cases of de Quervain stenosing tenosynovitis, septated compartments may require a second injection. In certain cases, the athlete may not be helped by the injection at all.

In athletes with unsuccessful injection and conservative treatment or with recurrent symptomatology, surgical decompression of the first extensor compartment should be considered. Again, great care must be taken by the surgeon to investigate for several septated compartments in that all compartments are released. In the athlete, it may be best to perform a Z lengthening reconstruction of the fibro-osseous tunnel to prevent any subluxation of the abductor pollicis longus or extensor pollicis brevis during subsequent athletic activities. Postsurgically, the patient is placed in a thumb spica splint for 2 weeks until sutures are removed. At this point, gentle range of motion exercises are performed for the following 2 weeks, and then strengthening as tolerated may be initiated. Full return to sport is generally not allowed for 4 to 6 weeks postsurgery.

Case Study IV

A 31-year-old tennis player decided to play squash during the winter months. Two weeks after starting to play, he noted pain and swelling along the dorsal radial aspect of his wrist, most frequently with ulnar and radial deviation mechanics during his shots. These symptoms accelerated to the degree that he had to stop playing and noted pain with day-to-day activity.

His examination revealed warmth and swelling over the first extensor compartment at the dorsal radial aspect of the wrist. He had crepitation in this area when he actively extended and flexed his thumb, and had a positive Finkelstein's test (see Ch. 21). Radiographs were negative and showed no evidence of radial scaphoid arthritis or scaphoid pathology. De Quervain stenosing tenosynovitis was diagnosed and the athlete was placed in a thumb spica splint and began NSAIDs. He was advised not to participate in racquet sports until reevaluation in 1 month.

After 1 month, the athlete stated that his symptoms had resolved. His examination demonstrated no evidence of swelling over the first extensor compartment. His Finkelstein's test was negative, and he had no discomfort out of his splint for over a week.

He was advised to continue with his anti-inflammatory medication and was given exercises for gentle stretching of the radial wrist and thumb extensor tendons. A strengthening program was instituted, and he was allowed to begin short volleying workouts with a tennis racquet. After 1 week, the athlete reported no wrist tenderness. He was then instructed to slowly increase the time of his workouts on an incremental basis over the next month. At that time, he returned to full sport activities with no recurrence of pain.

INTERSECTION SYNDROME

Intersection syndrome is seen in the same sports as listed in the section on de Quervain stenosing tenosynovitis. This condition can also be caused by repetitive flexion extension and ulnar and radial deviation of the wrist. In addition, it can result from a tenosynovitis of the second extensor compartment or more proximally at the level where the extensor pollicis brevis and abductor pollicis longus musculotendinous junction crosses over the extensor carpi radialis brevis and longus. Presentation is usually swelling and pain. Approximately 4 cm proximal to the wrist joint, there may be crepitation in the area where the abductor pollicis longus and extensor pollicis brevis cross over the ECRB and ECRL.

Treatment is similar to de Quervain stenosing tenosynovitis, with conservative treatment consisting of the use of a splint and anti-inflammatory medication. If these measures fail, the next step is injection into the inflamed area, and finally surgical decompression (although this is necessary less often than with de Quervain stenosing tenosynovitis).

Flexor Carpi Radialis Tendinitis

Flexor carpi radialis tenosynovitis is commonly seen in any athlete who is required to perform repetitious and forceful flexion maneuvers of the wrist. The flexor carpi radialis tendon traverses through its sheath approximately 3 cm proximal to the wrist crease but then travels through a tunnel bordered by the trapezial ridge radially, and transverses carpal ligaments volarly to a thick septum along its ulnar border. This is the area where most pain and inflammation occur in the athlete presenting with flexor carpi radialis tendinitis.

Conservative treatment is appropriate in the athlete who is in the off-season. However, the response to splint use and nonsteroidal anti-inflammatory medications alone is somewhat unpredictable and the trial period is prolonged. Therefore in the athlete who is involved in the midseason of his or her sport, a corticosteroid injection into the tendon sheath at the level at the trapezial ridge may be the recommended treatment. In most cases, this will result in a satisfactory response such that the athlete can complete his or her season.

In certain cases, surgical decompression of the flexor carpi radialis sheath may be necessary, followed by immobilization 2 weeks postoperatively, and a gentle range of motion and strengthening program as tolerated. Return to full sport activity is not recommended prior to 6 weeks.

Case Study V

A 28-year-old body-builder wanted to increase the mass of his forearms so they would be consistent with the remainder of his physique. He began a rigorous training program that included frequent repetitious high resistance wrist curls. By the end of the third day of training, he started to notice pain along the volar radial aspect of his wrist, particularly on the morning following his rigorous workout. There was some swelling, and he noted some discomfort along the volar radial aspect with hyperextension of his wrist on attempted push-off. His pain made it difficult to continue with training.

On examination, he had tenderness to palpate over the scaphoid tubercle and trapezial ridge and tenderness to resisted wrist flexion and radial deviation. There was some mild swelling along the volar radial aspect of his wrist. Radiographs did not demonstrate any evidence of articular pathology.

The athlete was diagnosed with a flexor carpi radialis tendinitis. Conservative treatment consisting of rest, the use of a splint, and anti-inflammatory medications were recommended. Since the athlete insisted that he continue training for an upcoming meet, a local anesthetic and corticosteroid were injected into the flexor carpal radialis sheath, with an immediate relief of symptoms. The athlete rested his wrist for 1 week and resumed his training program with a graduated program of light repetitions of wrist curls over a 2-week period. At this point, full weight training was resumed.

EXTENSOR POLLICUS LONGUS AND EXTENSOR CARPI ULNARIS TENDINITIS

Extensor pollicis longus tendinitis is rare. In the athlete presenting with a seemingly benign nondisplaced distal radius fracture but significant middorsal pain, decompression of the extensor pollicis longus tendon should be considered due to the occurrence of extensor pollicis longus tendon rupture in this situation.

Extensor carpi ulnaris tendinitis may be frequently seen in the athlete performing repetitive wrist extension and ulnar deviation, such as in rowing. Treatment is as described for other types of tenosynovitis. Care must be taken in evaluating the athlete with ulnar dorsal wrist pain to differentiate subluxation or dislocation of the extensor carpi ulnaris sheath. Although rare, inflammation of the tendon sheath can occur in essentially any area of the wrist where a tendon traverses a fibro-osseous tunnel, including the extensor digitorum communis, the extensor digiti minimi, and the flexor carpi ulnaris. Treatment depends on the severity at presentation and the stage of competition for that particular athlete and is the same as discussed in the previous sections.

CARPOMETACARPAL BOSS

The carpometacarpal boss is an osteoarthritic spur occurring at the index and/or long carpometacarpal joints. It is clinically manifested as a firm, tender, nonmobile mass. The athlete presenting with a carpometacarpal boss is usually in the third and fourth decades of life and is involved in a sport requiring grasp, usually golf.

The boss is best visualized radiographically with the hand in 40 degrees of supination such that the mass is tangential to the radiographic beam. CT scan or tomography also provides excellent visualization (Fig. 23-14).

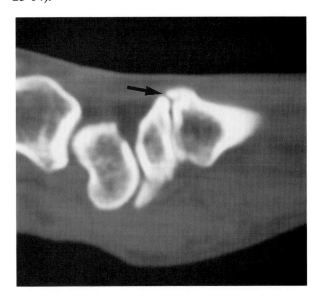

Figure 23-14 A 45-year-old golfer noted pain at the base of his right index metacarpal after 3 or 4 holes of golf. This was associated with swelling. CT scan demonstrated osteophytes bridging the index carpometacarpal joint without fusion *(arrow).* At the time of surgery, the golfer was noted to have an associated ganglion which was excised with the carpal boss. The golfer returned to light putting in 3 weeks and full golf in 6 weeks.

Use of NSAIDs may be helpful in controlling discomfort for day-to-day activities, but is usually ineffective in continuing athletics. Excision is the treatment of choice in the symptomatic athlete with the osteophyte excised to normal joint. Often there is an associated ganglion, which is also excised. Postoperatively, a protective cast is used for 2 weeks, then the athlete is placed in a thermoplastic splint and progressive range of motion and strengthening exercises are begun. Full return to sport is usually accomplished 6 weeks postoperatively.

REFERENCES

1. Amadio PC: Carpal kinematics and instability: a clinical and anatomic primer. Clin Anat 4:1, 1991
2. Green DP: The effect of avascular necrosis on the bone grafting for scaphoid nonunion. J Hand Surg 18A: 597, 1985
3. Mayfield JK: Mechanism of carpal injuries. Clin Orthop 149:45, 1980
4. Belling Hansen HW, Gilula LA, Young LV, Weeks PM: Posttraumatic palmar carpal subluxation: report of two cases. J Bone Joint Surg [Am] 65:998, 1983
5. Lindscheid RL, Dobyns JH, Beckenbaugh RD et al: Instability patterns of the wrist. J Hand Surg 8:682, 1983
6. Yourn Y, McMurthy RY, Flatt AE, Gillespie TE: Kinematics of the wrist. I. An experimental study of radial-ulnar deviation and flexion-extension. J Bone Joint Surg [Am] 60:423, 1978
7. Palmer AK, Levinsohn FM, Kuzma GR: Artrhrography of the wrist. J Hand Surg 8:15, 1983
8. Whipple TL: Arthroscopic Surgery: The Wrist. JB Lippincott, Philadelphia, 1992
9. Lavernia CJ, Cohen M, Taleisnik J: Scapholunate dissociations by ligamentous repair and capsulodesis. J Hand Surg 17A:354, 1992
10. Conyers DJ: Scapholunate interosseous reconstruction and imbrication of palmer ligaments. J Hand Surg 15: 690, 1990
11. Lavernia CJ, Cohen M, Taleisnik J: Treatment of scapholunate dissociation by ligamentous repair and capsulodesis. J Hand Surg 17A:354, 1992
12. Blatt G: Capsulodesis in reconstructive hand surgery: dorsal capsulodesis for the unstable scaphoid and volar capsulodesis following excision of the distal ulnar. Hand Clin 3:81, 1987
13. Palmer AK, Arbyns JH, Lonscherd RL: Management of posttraumatic instability of the wrist secondary to ligament rupture. J Hand Surg 3:507, 1978
14. Almquist FE, Bach AW, Sack JT et al: Four bone ligament reconstructions for treatment of chronic complete scapholunate separation. J Hand Surg 16A:322, 1991
15. Watson HK, Ryu J: Evaluation of arthritis of the wrist. Clin Orthop 202:57, 1986
16. Reagan DS, Linscheid RL, Dobyns JH: Lunotriquetral sprains. J Hand Surg 9A, 502, 1984
17. Lichtman DM, Schneider JR, Swafford AR, Marck GR: Ulnar midcarpal instability clinical and laboratory analysis. J Hand Surg 6:515, 1981
18. Lichtman DM, Schneider JR, Scafford AR, Mark GR: Ulnar midcarpal instability: clinical and laboratory analysis. J Hand Surg 6:515, 1981

24

Carpal Fractures of the Wrist

William J. Morgan
Terry F. Reardon

Many wrist injuries are combinations of fractures with subluxations and dislocations associated with ligamentous injuries. These ligamentous injuries are often difficult to diagnose and treat in such a manner that gives the athlete a completely pain-free, full functional result (see Ch. 23). Isolated fractures of the carpus may be seen in the athlete and also may be difficult to diagnose, although treatment results are usually more successful.

Certain fractures of the carpus are common to specific sports. For example, a fracture of the hook of the hamate is more commonly associated with racquet, batting, or club sports, while scaphoid fractures are often seen in football, soccer, and basketball players. The high occurrence of scaphoid fractures in these players is due to the frequent number of falls onto the outstretched hand. This hyperextension mechanism results in shear stresses imparted to the scaphoid that then lead to fractures.

Fractures of the carpus secondary to a direct blow occur in sports where the hand and wrist are susceptible to crush injuries. For example, a football player's hand may be caught between two helmets during a tackle, resulting in a capitate or hamate body fracture. An ice hockey player who receives a slash to the ulnar border of the gloved hand may sustain a triquetral or hamate fracture.

The differential diagnosis (which includes isolated carpal fractures and associated ligamentous injuries) is determined by the history and physical examination and can be further enhanced by static and specialized radiographic views, including carpal tunnel or clenched fist views, dynamic fluoroscopy, trispiral tomography, computed tomography, magnetic resonance imaging, bone scans, or arthrography (see Ch. 21).

Treatment should be individualized for each athlete with special attention directed to the competition level, requirements and rules of the sport, stability of the injury, support, and stabilization or fixation methods.

The length of treatment is important to the athlete, since this determines both the timing of rehabilitation and time away from competition. Stable anatomic and congruent articular reduction followed by early range of motion in the athlete offers the most favorable results. Rehabilitation programs may start once a sufficient degree of stability is achieved either from a fixation device or biologic healing. For example, athletes with carpal fractures that require open reduction with rigid internal fixation may be allowed early motion and appropriate conditioning in preparation for a return to sports. The functional results of treatment for wrist injuries in the athlete is dependent upon range of motion, (sport-specific) strength, minimal residual pain, and the maintenance of coordinated function.

SCAPHOID FRACTURES

Fractures of the scaphoid constitute 78 percent of all carpal fractures and are second only to distal radius fractures as the most common wrist fracture. Unfortunately, fractures of this small bone can result in prolonged periods of immobilization and increased morbidity; up to 6 months or even longer may be lost from the sport.

Classification System

As with most fractures, a classification system is useful in developing a treatment plan as well as determining the prognosis of the particular fracture. Herbert[1] has devised a fracture classification based on stability of the fracture complex as well as prognosis of healing. Fractures to the scaphoid can further be classified by the location of the fracture along the body of the scaphoid, which may be helpful in determining prognosis. The vascular supply to the scaphoid is thought to be critical for healing and arises dorsally and distally via soft tissue attachments along the spiral groove and dorsal ridge[2,3] (Fig. 24-1). This correlates with a less favorable rate of healing with more proximal fractures of the scaphoid.

Mechanism of Injury

Fractures of the scaphoid occur as a result of a fall onto the outstretched hand with wrist hyperextension (Fig. 24-2A). Midwaist fractures of the scaphoid occur as the radioscaphocapitate ligament acts as a fulcrum volarly, while dorsal forces are imposed on the proximal pole of the scaphoid by the distal radius, resulting in shear forces (Fig. 24-2B). Fractures of the scaphoid tubercle as well as small proximal pole fractures are more likely the result of avulsion forces (Fig. 24-3). Despite the mechanism of injury, associated ligamentous anatomy should be kept in mind when assessing a scaphoid fracture, since the radiographic appearance of a scaphoid fracture may represent a more significant wrist instability for example, a transscaphoid perilunate dislocation that has reduced (see Ch. 23). A delayed union or nonunion may result from a delay in diagnosis or the athlete not seeking treatment, or it may be associated with unrecognized carpal instability.

Diagnosis

In most cases, the athlete will recall a hyperextension injury during an athletic activity. There will be swelling about the dorsoradial aspect of the wrist as well as some loss of wrist motion. Examination of the wrist will demonstrate focal or point tenderness to palpation over the scaphoid tubercle and the anatomic snuffbox.

The health professional should be wary when an athlete presents with pain in the anatomic snuffbox or scaphoid tubercle but with normal-appearing radiographs. It is easy to diagnose this as a "wrist sprain" and treat with only an elastic bandage. Any athlete who presents with clinical suspicion of a scaphoid fracture

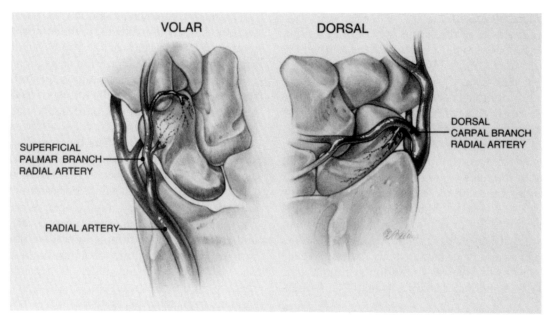

Figure 24-1 Most of the vascular supply of the scaphoid arises distally and dorsally, affecting the healing of the proximal scaphoid fracture.

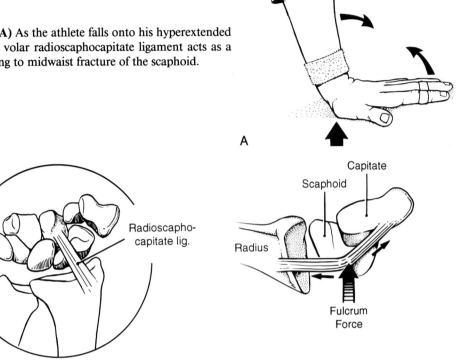

Figure 24-2 (A) As the athlete falls onto his hyperextended wrist, **(B)** the volar radioscaphocapitate ligament acts as a fulcrum leading to midwaist fracture of the scaphoid.

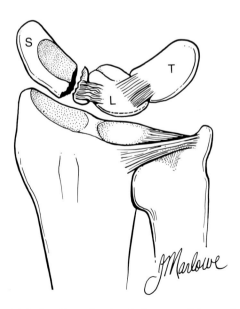

Figure 24-3 Small proximal pole fracture of the scaphoid as a result of avulsion by the scapholunate interosseous ligament.

should be placed in a thumb spica cast and reevaluated in 2 weeks. If at that time tenderness persists, a repeat radiograph should be obtained. Some resorption of the fracture site usually has occurred at this point and will become apparent. In cases where pain persists and ra-diographs appear normal, a bone scan should be obtained.

Although many views have been described for the radiographic diagnosis of scaphoid fractures, the vast majority of fractures can be recognized by four views: anteroposterior (AP), oblique, lateral, and ulnar deviation AP. In the ulnar deviation AP view, the scaphoid assumes an extended position, thus minimizing bony overlap (Fig. 24-4). The lateral view may demonstrate a carpal instability pattern with displaced fractures of the scaphoid. A radioisotope bone scan is extremely sensitive in demonstrating an acute fracture of the scaphoid. In the highly competitive or professional athlete whose routine radiographs are nondiagnostic and whose time is of the essence, a bone scan should be obtained in 48 to 72 hours to establish the diagnosis.[4] With a positive bone scan, trispiral tomography or computed tomography (CT) should then be performed to determine the location and position of the fracture. Although magnetic resonance imaging (MRI) may be useful in the assessment of scaphoid nonunion, it has less value in the evaluation of acute scaphoid fractures.

Case Study I

A 14-year-old basketball player hyperextended her right wrist while falling during a game. She noted some tenderness about the dorsoradial aspect of her

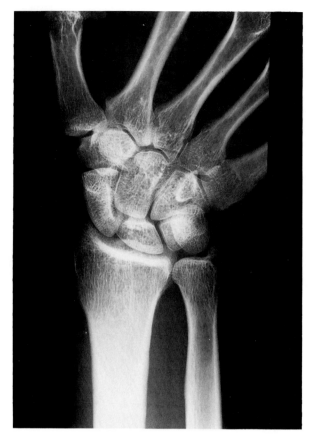

Figure 24-4 AP-view radiograph in ulnar deviation demonstrating extended position of scaphoid.

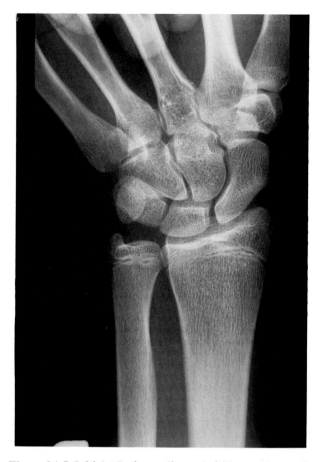

Figure 24-5 Initial AP-view radiograph failing to show evidence of a scaphoid fracture.

wrist but continued to play basketball. One week later, due to persistent pain, she was seen for evaluation. The initial examination demonstrated minimal swelling but pain to palpation over the scaphoid tubercle or the anatomic snuffbox. Range of motion was minimally altered due to the pain. Initial radiographs did not demonstrate any evidence of fracture or instability (Fig. 24-5). Due to the physical findings, however, the athlete was placed in a short-arm thumb spica cast. Two weeks later, follow-up radiographs clearly demonstrated a midwaist nondisplaced scaphoid fracture (Fig. 24-6).

Since this was a nondisplaced stable midwaist fracture, the athlete continued in a thumb spica cast for 6 more weeks. Radiographs at that time demonstrated a healed fracture (Fig. 24-7). The athlete was then placed in a thumb spica orthoplastic splint and instructed on gentle range of motion exercises three times a day. Two weeks later, she essentially had full motion and began a progressive resistance exercise program and was allowed to shoot baskets. Fifteen weeks later, with normal-appearing radiographs, she returned to full athletic activities.

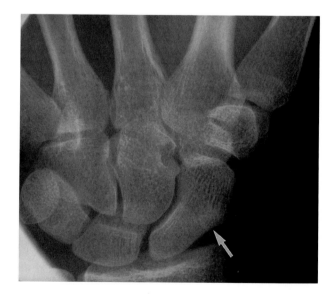

Figure 24-6 AP-view radiograph demonstrating a stable, nondisplaced midwaist scaphoid fracture *(arrows)*.

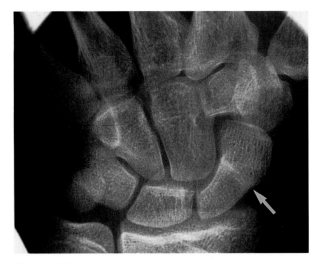

Figure 24-7 AP-view radiograph demonstrating healed scaphoid fracture as indicated by sclerotic line *(arrow)*.

Fractures to the distal third of the scaphoid have a favorable prognosis and tend to have a rapid union and a low incidence of nonunion, most likely due to an abundant blood supply as well as a stable fracture configuration (Fig. 24-8). Fractures of the middle third of the scaphoid, which are most commonly seen, however, hold a less favorable prognosis, since there is a less predictable blood supply, and a more unstable fracture configuration (Fig. 24-9). Fractures of the proximal one-third of the scaphoid have a reportedly poor prognosis with a high rate of nonunion and avascular necrosis due to interruption of the blood supply from distally based vessels and an extremely unstable fracture configuration (Fig. 24-10).

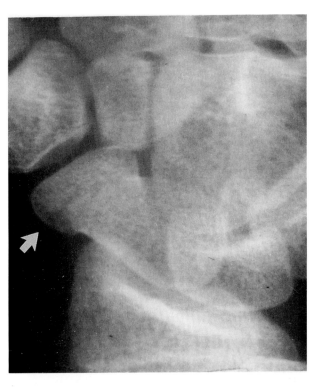

Figure 24-8 Fracture nonunion of the distal one-third of the scaphoid *(arrow)*.

Stable Fractures of the Middle Third of the Scaphoid

There are differing opinions as to what constitutes a stable versus an unstable fracture of the scaphoid.[5] Most authors, however, would agree that nondisplaced and nonangulated acute fractures of the scaphoid are considered stable. Fractures demonstrating displacement equal to 1 mm or more, or associated with angulation or abnormal carpal alignment are considered unstable (Fig. 24-11). These fractures may frequently be associated with other carpal injuries (e.g., perilunate instability) and should be assessed (see Ch. 23).

Acute stable fractures of the scaphoid waist are treated by immobilization in a short-arm thumb spica cast in slight radial deviation and palmar flexion to relax the sling effect of the radioscaphocapitate ligament. Expected healing rates are 90 to 100 percent within 8 to 12 weeks.

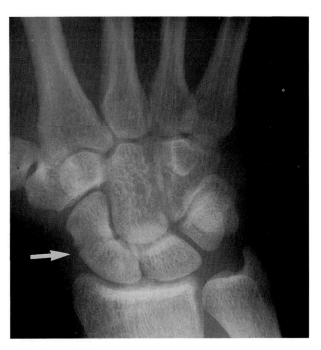

Figure 24-9 Fracture of the middle one-third of the scaphoid *(arrow)*.

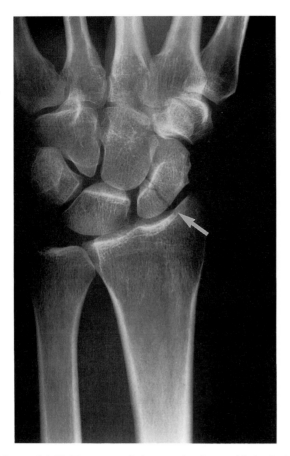

Figure 24-10 Fracture of the proximal one-third of the scaphoid *(arrow).*

The use of internal fixation in the treatment of stable scaphoid fractures can be used, since there is the potential for early range of motion to hasten rehabilitation and early return to sport. Athletes involved in contact sports will still need a playing cast for a minimum of 3 months. These treatment options and their potential risk/benefit ratio should be carefully discussed with the athlete and their families.

Fractures of the scaphoid tubercle represent a stable fracture complex. These fractures are treated in a short-arm thumb spica cast for 4 weeks and then protected in a removable splint while motion and strengthening exercises are begun.

Unstable Acute Fractures of the Scaphoid

Unstable acute fractures of the scaphoid (i.e., fractures displaced > 1 mm or malangulated) have a higher incidence of nonunion or malunion with carpal insta-

bility, and are best treated by open reduction internal fixation (ORIF) (Fig. 24-12). ORIF should be performed as soon as the displacement or malalignment is recognized to prevent the increased possibility of resorption at the fracture site, progressive carpal instability, or malunion.

If comminution is present, augmentation with bone graft is advised. Despite internal fixation, these fractures must be protected from further stresses, including heavy grasping, and splint supplementation is recommended. Active-assisted range of motion is allowed if rigid fixation is obtained with intermittent protection in a thermoplastic thumb spica splint. As previously noted, if the athlete is continuing to participate in his or her sport, then protection in a playing cast is advised. As noted above, protection is continued until clinical fracture healing is confirmed by CT scans or tomography prior to allowing a return to contact sports or power weight training with that upper extremity (approximately 4 to 6 months).

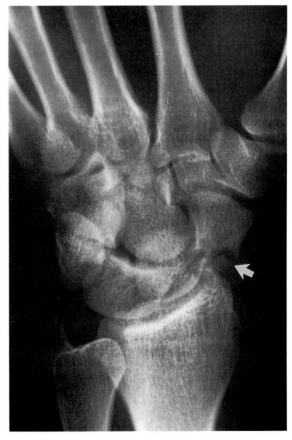

Figure 24-11 Displaced, unstable fracture of the scaphoid *(arrow).*

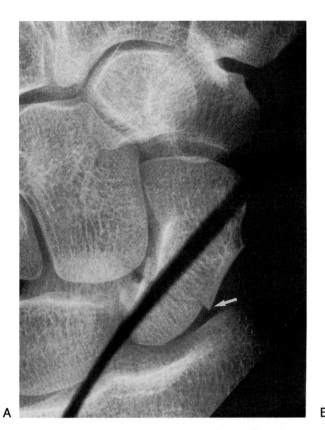

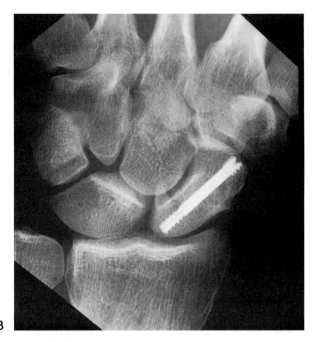

A

B

Figure 24-12 **(A)** Displaced scaphoid fracture *(arrow);* **(B)** S/P ORIF with bone graft.

Scaphoid Nonunions

Scaphoid fracture nonunions are difficult to treat. The natural history of (untreated) scaphoid fractures that go on to nonunion and are left untreated is radiocarpal degeneration.[5] Aggressive primary treatment, therefore, is advised. Since it is unlikely that healing will take place in an established nonunion by simple cast immobilization alone, treatment should consist of ORIF with bone graft.

In treating this nonunion, the fibrous union must be debrided back to bleeding cancellous bone. This will invariably leave a wedge-shaped deficit that must be reconstituted by a wedge-shaped corticocancellous bone graft obtained from the iliac crest. Despite rigid internal fixation following bone grafting of a scaphoid nonunion, the fracture stability should be augmented by a short-arm thumb spica cast until healing of both the proximal and distal margins of the bone graft is demonstrated by tomography (usually 3 to 6 months). Fixation of small proximal pole fractures may be accomplished by retrograde interosseous screw placement by a dorsal approach (Fig. 24-13).

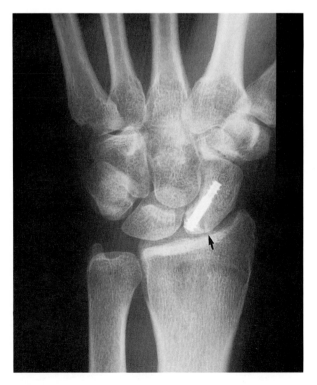

Figure 24-13 Proximal pole nonunion *(arrow)* treated by retrograde (dorsal) Herbert-Whipple screw.

Case Study II

A 22-year-old collegiate football quarterback noted decreasing range of motion of his nondominant left wrist as well as pain along the dorsal radial aspect of the wrist. These symptoms had become worse during the season.

His examination demonstrated decreased flexion extension with pain and mild swelling along the dorsal radial aspect of the wrist. During the previous football season he had fallen onto his left wrist and sustained a hyperextension injury. He noted pain at that time, but radiographs were interpreted as negative, and he was placed in a removable splint and treated for a wrist sprain. Current radiographs 13 months postinjury obtained demonstrated a nonunion of a fracture of the proximal third of the scaphoid (Fig. 24-14).

A scaphoid nonunion was diagnosed and internal fixation with bone grafting was performed through a volar approach utilizing a corticocancellous iliac crest graft and Herbert screw fixation.

The athlete was placed into a short-arm thumb spica cast for 12 weeks. A plain radiograph demonstrated evidence of early union (Fig. 24-15). He was then placed in a removable thermoplastic splint and began an active-assisted range of motion program.

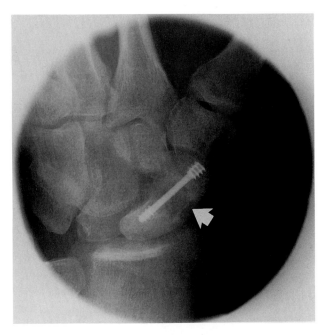

Figure 24-15 AP-view radiograph suggesting early healing of corticocancellous graft following open reduction internal fixation *(arrow)*.

At 16 weeks postoperatively, a sagittal CT scan was taken of the scaphoid, which revealed evidence of union (Fig. 24-16). At this point, the athlete then began a sport-specific strengthening program and returned to his sport the following season.

Avascular Necrosis of the Scaphoid

Established nonunions of the scaphoid can be due to avascular necrosis of the proximal pole, indicating an extremely poor prognosis for healing despite surgical intervention.[2] Unfortunately, it has been difficult to determine the vascularity of the proximal pole preoperatively and therefore difficult to make recommendations on fixation and bone grafting. MRI may prove beneficial in predicting surgical outcome with established nonunions (Fig. 24-17).

Scaphoid Lunate Advanced Collapse (SLAC) Wrist

The natural history of untreated scaphoid nonunions parallels untreated scapholunate carpal instability patterns in the wrist resulting in degenerative arthritis manifested by scaphoid lunate advanced collapse (SLAC wrist). At early presentation, there is noted mild radioscaphoid DJD with narrowing and spurring of the radial styloid (Fig. 24-18). On late presentation, there is marked degeneration and collapse with sparing of the radiolunate joint (Fig. 24-19). In the

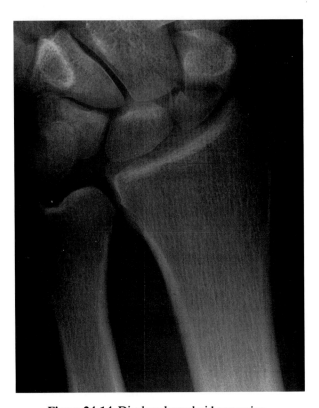

Figure 24-14 Displaced scaphoid nonunion.

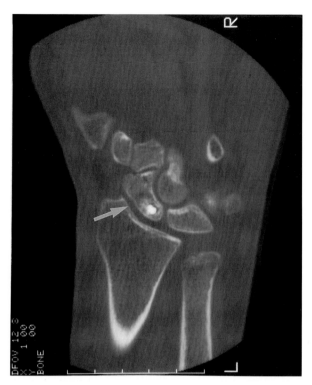

Figure 24-16 Healed scaphoid nonunion following open reduction internal fixation with corticocancellous graft as shown by CT scan *(arrow)*.

then excision of the scaphoid with a four-corner intercarpal fusion should be performed. The athlete will experience 50 to 70 percent loss of normal wrist motion due to the excision of the degenerated radioscaphoid joint and fusion of the degenerated capitolunate joint. Although this procedure may provide pain relief noted with light activity, high-demand upper extremity athletic activity is unlikely due to diminished motion and persistent pain with extremes of motion. Silicone implant arthroplasty of the scaphoid is contraindicated due to the high degree of associated silicone synovitis.

In the early stages of SLAC wrist with degeneration of the radioscaphoid joint but no degeneration of the capitolunate joint, proximal row carpectomy may offer a secondary treatment option in the athlete. In this instance, the articular surface of the proximal pole of the capitate articulates with the lunate fossa after excision of the proximal row. This may afford the athlete better range of motion than with a four-corner fusion.

The final salvage procedure in the SLAC wrist, particularly for the athlete who requires power grip but insignificant flexion extension motion, is a total wrist arthrodesis. In the athlete not requiring wrist motion (e.g., soccer player, broad jumper, track), this provides excellent pain relief.

low-demand or senior athlete, treatment may begin with nonsteroidal anti-inflammatory medications and intermittent use of a splint for comfort.

If conservative treatment is ineffective, manifested by continued pain resulting in limitation of activities,

LUNATE FRACTURES

The lunate is in a relatively well-protected position in the lunate fossa between the scaphoid, capitate, and triquetrum. The lunate is stabilized by several intrinsic

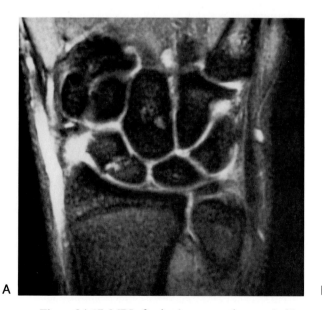

A

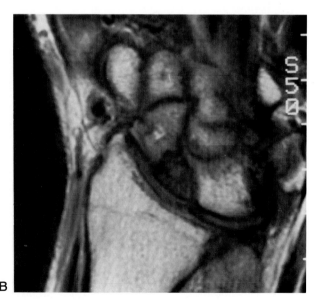

B

Figure 24-17 MRI of wrist demonstrating scaphoid nonunion. **(A)** Normal marrow signal of proximal and distal scaphoid poles. **(B)** Abnormal marrow signal of proximal scaphoid pole, suggesting vascular compromise.

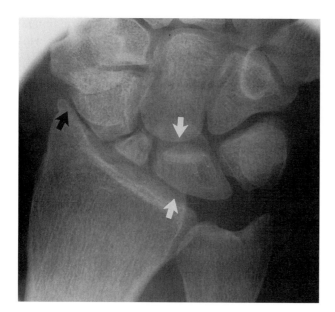

Figure 24-18 Early SLAC wrist. Scaphoid nonunion with small proximal pole fragment. Note narrowing of the radioscaphoid joint *(black arrow),* but the radiolunate and lunocapitate joints are spared *(white arrows).*

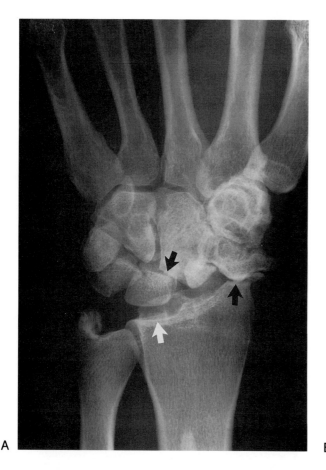

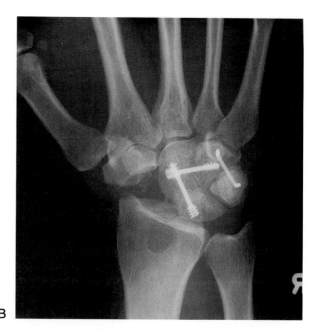

Figure 24-19 **(A)** Advanced SLAC wrist due to a chronic untreated scaphoid nonunion. Note marked degeneration of the radioscaphoid and capitolunate joints *(black arrow),* but sparing of the radiolunate joint *(white arrow).* **(B)** Four-corner fusion for SLAC wrist. Since the radiolunate joint is spared in the SLAC wrist, fusion of the remaining carpus with excision of the scaphoid will decrease discomfort while maintaining partial motion.

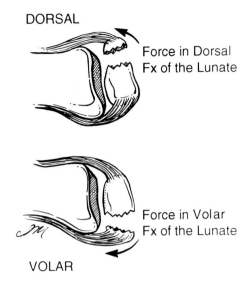

DORSAL

Force in Dorsal
Fx of the Lunate

Force in Volar
Fx of the Lunate

VOLAR

Figure 24-20 Avulsion fractures of the lunate due to pull of the (**A**) dorsal or (**B**) volar ligamentous insertions.

and extrinsic wrist ligaments which include the scapholunate, lunotriquetral, ulnolunate, radioscapholunate and radiolunotriquetral ligaments. These anatomic findings reflect the two common types of lunate fractures: compression and avulsion fractures. A major axial compressive force between the capitate and the distal radius is required to fracture the body of the lunate. This mechanism typically results in a fracture which is transverse in the coronal plane.

Avulsion fractures may be the result of ligamentous or capsular traction type injuries secondary to extremes of motion. These fractures may be classified as either dorsal or volar horn avulsion fractures (Fig. 24-20). Avulsion fractures are best seen on oblique radiographs of the carpus. The treatment of isolated avulsion fractures that are nondisplaced is immobilization for 4 to 6 weeks; ORIF may be necessary if the fracture is displaced.

The treatment of acute isolated lunate body fractures without displacement and not associated with Kienbock disease is immobilization in a short-arm cast for 6 weeks. The risk of avascular necrosis of the lunate following fractures involving the body has not been discussed in the literature, but experimental work on the vascularity of the lunate suggests that even an undisplaced horizontal fracture may be predisposed to avascular necrosis.[6] The majority of lunate fractures, however, heal without resultant avascular necrosis.

KIENBOCK DISEASE

Kienbock disease or avascular necrosis of the carpal lunate is most commonly seen in active young adult men.[7] The clinical presentation of Kienbock disease in the athletic population is quite variable. Most typically, the presenting clinical picture involves nonspecific wrist pain localized to the lunate and decreased range of motion, which is secondary to the synovitis and inflammatory changes incited by the avascular necrosis. Strength of the hand, as indicated by a weakness of grip, is often compromised.

The diagnosis of Kienbock disease may be confirmed with plain radiographs demonstrating avascular changes in the lunate. The radiographic appearance may present as increased density or sclerosis with or without collapse of the lunate. In the earliest stages of Kienbock disease, prior to changes on plain radiographs, the diagnosis may be made with MRI or with bone scintigraphy. Although there is no consensus as to a specific or predisposing event related to the onset of Kienbock disease, many theories about its cause have been published.[8]

Recommendations for the surgical management of Kienbock disease are based on the stage of the disease at the time of presentation (Table 24-1). There is an increased incidence of Kienbock disease in a wrist that has an ulna minus variant (Fig. 24-21). Therefore, the health professional should be suspicious when confronted by the athlete with dorsal wrist pain and ulna minus variant on radiograph.

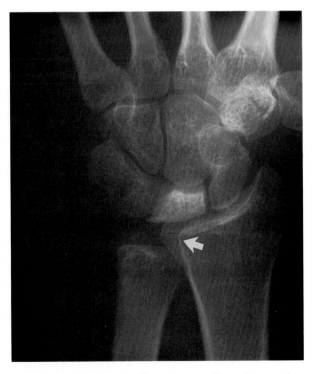

Figure 24-21 Kienbock disease: note ulna minus variant *(arrow)*, and radiographic sclerosis of the lunate.

Table 24-1   Kienbock's Disease

	Stage I	Stage II	Stage III	Stage IV
Symptoms	Wrist pain; mild loss of motion with no evidence of collapse of lunate or carpal instability.	Radiographic sclerosis of the lunate with minimal collapse and no carpal instability	Fracture and/or collapse of the lunate with associated carpal instability	Collapse of the lunate with carpal instability and the development of degenerative changes in the joint
Treatment	Possible cast immobilization in the athlete; with ulna minus variance: joint leveling procedure accomplished by radial shortening or ulna lengthening	Same as stage I	Mild collapse of lunate and mild associated carpal instability patterns: joint leveling procedure; scaphocapitate or STT fusion with or without excision of lunate for more advanced collapse; proximal row carpectomy may be considered if there is no associated degeneration of the proximal pole of the capitate or lunate fossa	Stage III or total wrist arthrodesis

OSTEOCHONDRAL IMPACTION ("BRUISE") OF THE LUNATE

Athletes who sustain a hyperextension injury of the wrist may present with dorsal wrist pain, particularly with attempted hyperextension of the wrist (e.g., when attempting to perform a push-up). The clinical examination is somewhat unremarkable except for pain to palpate over the lunate. Plain radiographs are normal. MRI may demonstrate localized marrow signal changes signifying injury (Fig. 24-22).

These athletes usually respond with 6 weeks of cast immobilization followed by 6 weeks of structured range of motion and strengthening with progression

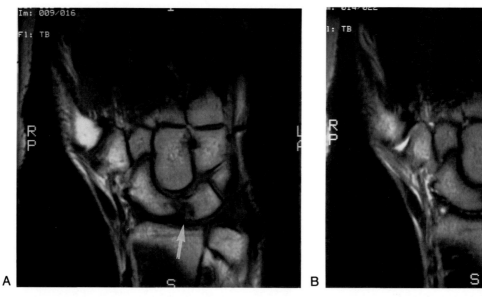

Figure 24-22 MRI of a 26-year-old baseball player with middorsal wrist pain after a hyperextension injury when he ran into the catcher at home plate. **(A)** T1-weighted image demonstrates suppression of normal marrow signal at radial border of the lunate *(arrow)*. **(B)** T2-weighted image demonstrates edema of the radial border of the lunate suggesting an acute injury *(arrow)*.

into their sport. Care must be taken to differentiate this problem from established Kienbock disease, occult dorsal ganglion, or dorsal impingement syndrome.

HAMATE FRACTURES

There are two main types of fractures of the hamate bone: fractures limited to the hook of the hamate and fractures involving the body. A fracture of the hook of the hamate represents approximately 2 percent of all carpal fractures, with a higher incidence in certain sports. These fractures typically occur in sports that require a strong grip on a racquet, bat, or club. The fracture occurs in the hand that grips the butt or base of the club and may be related to a sudden change in direction or a force that is oppositely applied. A golfer who accidently grounds the club while hitting a shot (i.e., a "fat" swing) or a batter with a sudden check swing is at an increased risk for a hamate hook fracture (Fig. 24-23). A fracture through the base of the hamate hook may also result from a fall onto the palm, outstretched and hyperextended.

A history of a racquet sport injury resulting in vague deep-seated hand pain or weakness (which may include paresthesias in the ulnar nerve distribution) is consistent with a hamate hook fracture. The finding, when present, is due to compression of the motor branch of the ulnar nerve passing ulnar to the base of the hamate along with the sensory branch in Guyon's canal.

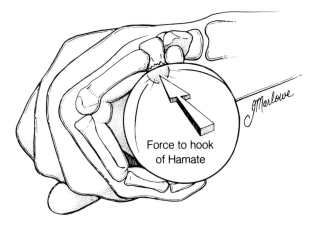

Figure 24-23 Fracture of the hamate hook due to a check swing with the butt of the bat causing compression of the hamate hook.

The physical examination will usually demonstrate hypothenar tenderness in the region of the hook of the hamate, pain with resisted ring- and small-finger flexion, weakness in grip strength measurements, and ulnar nerve paresthesias localized distal to Guyon's canal. A hamate hook fracture is usually not recognized on plain radiologic evaluation and may require carpal tunnel views, fluoroscopy, polytomography, bone scan, or computed tomography for diagnosis (Fig. 24-24).

Cast immobilization for a hamate hook fracture is not recommended in the athlete because it is associated with a high rate of nonunion due to altered blood sup-

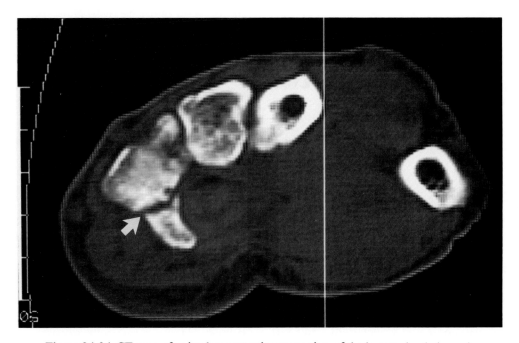

Figure 24-24 CT scan of wrist demonstrating nonunion of the hamate hook *(arrow).*

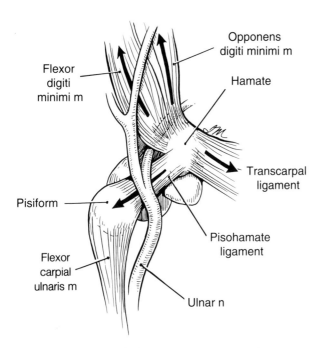

Figure 24-25 Extrinsic forces on hamate hook include the transcarpal ligament, flexor digiti minimi, opponens digiti minimi, and flexor carpial ulnarus. These opposing forces may lead to nonunion.

ply and extrinsic forces imposed upon the hook of the hamate (Fig. 24-25). Open reduction internal fixation of the hook of the hamate has been described with limited success and is not recommended in the competitive athlete. Excision of the hook of the hamate is considered the treatment of choice with a persistent symptomatic nonunion. Following excision, immobilization is necessary only as symptoms warrant. Return to athletic activities with few upper extremity demands may be possible as early as 2 weeks postoperatively. Sports requiring a normal grip strength and a nontender palm (e.g., tennis player, pole vaulter, or baseball player) generally require up to 6 months before there is full return of strength and loss of tenderness at the incision site in the palm.

Case Study III

A 17-year-old left-handed female tennis player presented with a 9-month history of vague ulnar-sided left hand pain. She noted the onset during a tennis game when she fell onto her left palm. She stated that this pain in the palm of her left hand, which grips the base of the racquet, prevented her from swinging racquet normally. She admitted to a weakness of grip compared to her right hand but

denied paresthesias in the median or ulnar nerve distribution. Although a radiograph had been previously interpreted as normal, her hand pain persisted whenever she gripped a tennis racquet during a match.

The physical examination demonstrated pain on palpation in the hypothenar area in line with the base of the ring finger 3 cm distal to the volar wrist crease. Minimal pain was elicited with resisted flexion of the distal interphalangeal joint of the small finger. Plain radiographs included AP and lateral views, which were interpreted as normal; however, a carpal tunnel view showed an ununited fracture at the base of the hamate hook· (Fig. 24-26).

She underwent excision of the ununited hamate hook. The postoperative protocol involved the early use of a splint for comfort followed by hand therapy for range of motion and strengthening exercises with a gradual return to activities by 4 weeks. She was able to return to full athletic activities at 12 weeks.

A fracture through the body of the hamate is described primarily as a coronal fracture of the dorsal aspect of the hamate.[9,10] A variety of mechanisms has been attributed to the fracture of the body of the hamate, which includes direct trauma such as a blow to the ulna aspect of the hand blocking a kick in Tae Kwon Do, extremes of radial deviation or palmar flexion, and compression between the triquetrum with ulnar deviation. When this fracture is related to axial compression of the metacarpal on the hamate caused by striking a solid object such as a wall, jaw, or base of skull with a closed fist, it may be associated with a carpometacarpal fracture dislocation. More commonly, an avulsion fracture of the hamate bone is seen with this type of mechanism.[11]

Treatment of nondisplaced fractures to the body of the hamate consists of immobilization in an ulnar gutter splint for 4 weeks, followed by the intermittent use of a protective splint for 4 more weeks with early rehabilitation (including range of motion and then strengthening by 6 weeks). Return to full athletic activity is possible at 12 weeks postinjury. Treatment of displaced fractures to the body of the hamate with or without associated dislocation of the carpometacarpal joint is open reduction internal fixation. With large fracture fragments, this may be accomplished with interfragmentary lag screws, which provide enough fixation for limited splint use. If the fragments are small, K-wire fixation should be utilized, augmented by a cast as noted above.

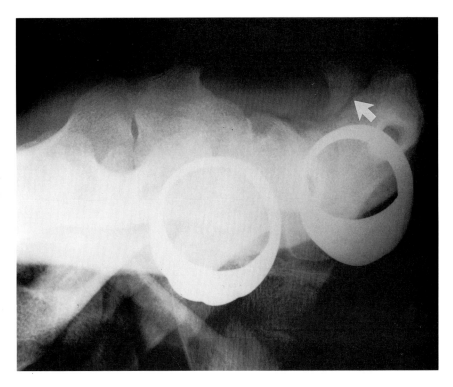

Figure 24-26 Carpal tunnel view demonstrating a fracture of the hamate hook *(arrow)*.

TRIQUETRUM FRACTURES

The triquetrum is the third most commonly fractured carpal bone, although it is rarely displaced. The triquetrum is surrounded by very strong ligamentous structures on its dorsal, volar, and ulnar sides. The broad attachments of these ligaments explain the spectrum of fractures. Fractures of the triquetrum consist primarily of two types—avulsion or impaction injuries and fractures involving the body of the triquetrum.

The most common type of fracture of the triquetrum is noted by a dorsal "chip" on radiograph and may be caused by hyperflexion injuries resulting in dorsal avulsion fractures at the insertion of the dorsal radiocarpal ligament.[12,13] More likely, however, the dorsal chip fracture is produced by impingement of the ulnar styloid or hamate against the triquetrum in a position of extreme extension and ulnar deviation resulting from a fall onto the outstretched hand,[14,15] as seen when a base runner dives head first into second base with resultant hypertension of the wrist on the bag. Failure may also occur within the substance of the ligaments, allowing the force to be further transmitted to the body of the triquetrum. This may be seen during a perilunate dislocation, resulting in a fracture through the body of the triquetrum (i.e., transtriquetral perilunate dislocation). The dorsal compression/avulsion fractures are diagnosed by localized tenderness on physical exami-

nation and are easily seen on the lateral or pronated oblique radiograph. Treatment with immobilization in a short-arm cast in neutral position for a period of 4 to 6 weeks offers an excellent prognosis.

PISIFORM FRACTURES

The pisiform is located within the substance of the flexor carpi ulnaris tendon which inserts into the hamate and metacarpals via the pisometacarpal and pisohamate ligaments. This superficial position of the pisiform subjects it to injuries caused by direct force compressing it against the triquetrum. For example, a pisiform fracture may be seen in a cyclist compressing his clenched hands on the handlebars or in a batter's check swing. Typically, these injuries are minimally displaced due to the enveloping flexor carpi ulnaris tendon (Fig. 24-27). A supinated oblique radiograph should be used in the evaluation of the articular surface following a pisiform fracture.

Cast immobilization of pisiform fractures may be undertaken for 4 weeks, followed by range of motion and strengthening as tolerated. Return to sport is allowed when symptoms resolve. If symptoms persist due to nonunion, malunion, or resulting degenerative arthritis, the treatment of choice is excision of the pisiform. Acute excision of the pisiform should also be

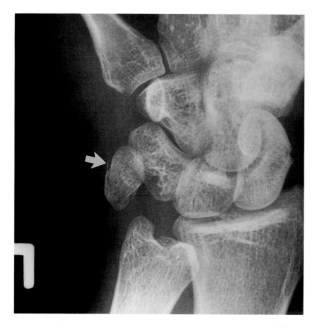

Figure 24-27 Fracture of pisiform body *(arrow).*

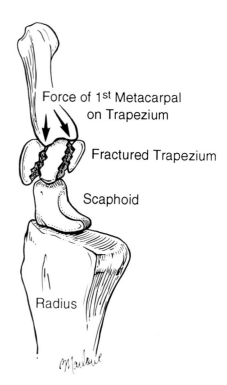

Figure 24-28 Axial load on thumb metacarpals resulting in fracture of the body the trapezium.

considered in the competitive or elite athlete with a displaced pisiform fracture, as the athlete may develop future symptomatology secondary to degeneration of the pisotriquetral joint. Following excision, immediate range of motion is encouraged and return to sport is determined as the athlete's symptoms allow (see the section *Hamate Fractures*).

TRAPEZIUM FRACTURES

Fractures of the trapezium are rare, comprising approximately 4 to 5 percent of all carpal fractures.[16] Generally, trapezium fractures are seen in combination with other injuries such as Bennet's or second metacarpal fractures. Trapezium fractures may involve the body of the prominent palmar ridge, with fractures of the trapezial body seen more often.

The mechanism of a trapezial body fracture is axial force transmitted by the base of the thumb metacarpal to the surface of the trapezium, resulting in either a vertical, longitudinal, or comminuted fracture pattern[17] (Fig. 24-28). The diagnosis of trapezial fractures may require special radiographic assessment such as carpal tunnel view or a bone scan to confirm clinical suspicions. Often, tomography or CT scans aid in the complete evaluation of the trapezial body fracture.

Nondisplaced and avulsion fractures of the trapezium can be treated with thumb spica cast immobiliza-

tion for 4 to 6 weeks followed by a removable thumb spica splint. Range of motion is then encouraged and strengthening begun at 6 weeks postinjury. The intermittent use of a splint may be discontinued at 6 to 8 weeks and full return to sports can occur at 12 weeks. Trapezial ridge fractures that remain symptomatic after a period of immobilization may require excision.

TRAPEZOID FRACTURES

The trapezoid is relatively well protected from fracture due to its keystone-type shape and ligamentous attachments within the carpus. The mechanism of injury is usually a direct axial force transmitted by the index metacarpal to the trapezoid, although this force rarely results in an isolated fracture of the trapezoid (Fig. 24-29). Fractures of the trapezoid are more commonly seen with a dislocation of the index carpometacarpal joint rather than as a isolated injury.

Nondisplaced trapezoid fractures are treated by immobilization in a radial gutter splint for 4 weeks followed by intermittent use of a splint, range of motion and strengthening as tolerated. Return to athletics is sport-specific but usually accomplished within 12

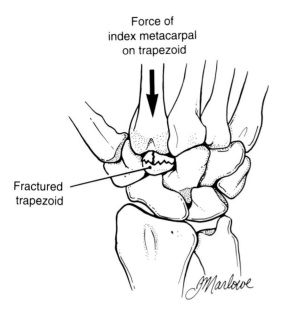

Figure 24-29 Axial load on the index metacarpal resulting in fracture of the trapezoid.

weeks. Displaced fractures of the trapezoid require ORIF, with trapezoid excision not advised.

Case Study VI

A 32-year-old wheelchair marathon racer made a turn at the bottom of a downhill run and tipped his chair, causing entrapment of his right wrist between the wheel and the ground. He noted discomfort at the base of the index finger and was unable to complete the race. There was swelling about the radial dorsal aspect of his hand as he presented for treatment. A physical examination demonstrated tenderness to palpation at the base of the index finger with swelling and ecchymosis at this area. He had full range of motion of his digits with pain in full flexion. There was no malrotation or malangulation of the digits. A radiograph demonstrated a nondisplaced fracture of the trapezoid with no subluxation of the index carpal metacarpal joint (Fig. 24-30).

The athlete was placed into a radial gutter splint to immobilize the index carpal metacarpal joint. At 4 weeks, the cast was removed, and the athlete began a range of motion program followed by strengthening. There was no evidence of tenderness about the carpal metacarpal joint and early radiographic evidence of healing. Eight weeks following the injury, the athlete started to train in his wheelchair, and by 12 weeks had returned to full racing without difficulties.

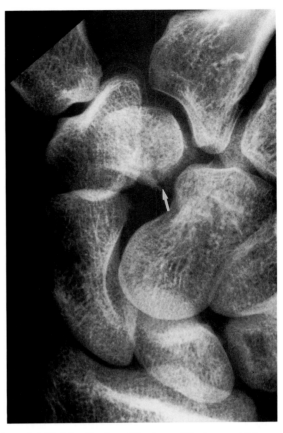

Figure 24-30 Nondisplaced fracture of the trapezoid *(arrow)*.

CAPITATE FRACTURES

Capitate fractures occur in approximately 1 to 2 percent of carpal fractures. The capitate may be fractured in the body or at the level of the capitate neck. The mechanism of injury for capitate fractures is usually high energy, with the wrist in forced extension such as can occur in auto racing. Capitate fractures are more typically seen with other injuries such as perilunar dislocations or the scaphocapitate syndrome. The scaphocapitate syndrome represents a variant of perilunate dislocations (i.e. a transscaphoid transcapitate perilunate dislocation), which may include disruption at the lunotriquetra interval (see Ch. 23).

Due to the displacement of these fractures and the high incidence of avascular necrosis, closed treatment of isolated capitate fractures and the scaphoid capitate syndrome is not recommended. Instead, open reduction internal fixation should be performed, usually with the use of intraosseous screws (Fig. 24-31). If rigid fixation is obtained and there is no associated ligamentous injury, guarded range of motion and intermittent

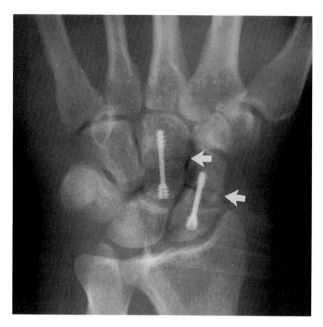

Figure 24-31 Status postdorsal approach to open reduction internal fixation of scaphocapitate syndrome. Note scaphoid and capitate fractures *(arrows)*.

use of a splint is encouraged to minimize wrist stiffness. If rigid internal fixation is not obtained or if there is an associated ligamentous injury, cast immobilization is required for 6 weeks, followed by intermittent use of a splint and a range of motion and strengthening program. Return to full sports activity should not be resumed prior to 6 months from the time of injury.

Due to the lack of soft tissue attachments to the proximal pole of the capitate, a high incidence of avascular necrosis with this type of fracture exists. Avascular necrosis of the proximal pole of the capitate associated with collapse and/or degeneration may be treated by excision of the proximal pole and a fascial arthroplasty.

REHABILITATION

As with other wrist injuries, athletes with carpal fractures should follow the five phases of rehabilitation (acute, initial, progressive, integrated functions, and return to sport) with a focus on the specific sport.

Fractures to the carpus are almost always intra-articular and as such, anatomic positioning and maintenance is a necessity. In the acute phase, cast protection is required until fracture healing (4 to 6 weeks). If rigid internal fixation has been obtained, gentle active range of motion is allowed with intermittent protection in a thermoplastic splint.

In fractures where vascular compromise is common (scaphoid nonunions, mid- and proximal pole scaphoid fractures, proximal capitate fractures, and lunate fractures), extra precautions should be followed, including prolonged immobilization (3 to 6 months), consideration of internal fixation, and confirmation of healing by tomography before progressing to strengthening (phase III).

Following fracture healing, range of motion (phase III) is initiated until a pain-free plateau of motion has been obtained (2–4 weeks). This is followed by strengthening (3 weeks) which progresses into sport-specific light activity (phase IV). Phases III through V (return to sport) should represent a continuum and progress as the athlete demonstrates strength and flexibility goals. However, with "routine" (i.e., minimally significant) carpal fractures, return to full sport should not be earlier than 3 months, and with proximal pole scaphoid fractures and scaphoid nonunions, should not be earlier than 6 months.

When the preferred treatment in the athlete with fractures or nonunions may be excision (hamate hook or pisiform), the hand is protected until wound healing (2 to 3 weeks), and the remaining four phases of rehabilitation are followed as tolerated (usually 6 to 8 weeks).

REFERENCES

1. Herbert TJ: The Fractured Scaphoid. Quality Medical Publishing, St. Louis, 1990
2. Green D: The effect of avascular necrosis on Russe bone grafting for scaphoid nonunion. J Hand Surg 10A:597, 1985
3. Gelberman RH, Menon J: The vascularity of the scaphoid bone. J Hand Surg 5:508, 1980
4. Gavel A, Engel J, Osher Z et al: Bone scanning in the assessment of fractures of the scaphoid. J Hand Surg 4:405, 1979
5. Mack GR, Bosse MJ, Gelberman RH et al: The natural history of scaphoid nonunion. J Bone Joint Surg [Am] 66:504, 1984
6. Gelberman RH, Bauman TD, Merron J, Akeson WH: The vascularity of the lunate bone and Kienbock's disease. J Hand Surgery 5:272, 1980
7. Szabo RM, Greenspan A: Diagnosis and clinical findings of Kienbock's disease. Hand Clin 9:399, 1993
8. Trumble T, Glisson RR, Seaber AV, Urbaninsk JR: A biochemical comparison of methods for treating Kienbock disease. J Hand Surg 11A:88, 1988
9. Loth TS, McMillan MD: Coronal dorsal hamate fractures. J Hand Surg 13A:616, 1988
10. Roth JH, deLorenzi C: Displaced intra-articular coronal fracture of the hamate treated with a Herbert screw. J Hand Surg 13A:619, 1988

11. Cain JE, Shepler TR, Wilson MR: Hamatometacarpal fracture-dislocation: classification and treatment. J Hand Surg 12A:762, 1987

12. Bonnin JG, Greening WP: Fractures of the triquetrum. Br J Surg 31:278, 1944

13. Conwell HE: Injuries of the wrist. Ciba Clin Symp 22:23, 1970

14. Garcia-Elias M: Dorsal fractures of the triquetrum: avulsion or compression fractures? J Hand Surg 12A:266, 1987

15. Levy M, Fischel RE, Stern GM, Goldberg I: Chip fractures of the os triquetrum. J Bone Joint Surg [Br] 61:355, 1979

16. Zemel NP: Carpal Fractures: In Stickland JW, Rettig AC (eds): Hand Injuries in Athletes. WB Saunders, Philadelphia, 1992

17. Botte MJ, Gelberman RH: Fractures of the carpus, excluding the scaphoid. Hand 3:149, 1987

25

Sport-Related Injuries of the Hand

Thomas F. Breen

The hand is the most frequently injured part of the athlete's upper extremity. It has been estimated that roughly one-quarter of athletic injuries are related to the hand and wrist. Most athletic activities require some combination of fine dexterous movement of the wrist and digits with various degrees of strength. The hand is often the least protected of the upper extremity and thus is vulnerable to injury. These injuries represent a complex interaction between the bony pathology and associated soft tissue trauma. Treatment of hand injuries in the athlete generally follows the same guidelines as those in non-sports-related cases. Yet, because of the athlete's high motivation, along with the need for a dexterous functional outcome, specific performance requirements should be considered when choosing the initial treatment modality as well as the most effective rehabilitation program.

An increase in the number of individuals participating in athletic activities has resulted in an increase in the number of injuries. Certain trends have developed over the years with respect to specific injuries being associated with specific sports. Tendon injuries, such as the mallet finger and boutonnière deformity, are associated with sports involving a ball (e.g., football, basketball, or baseball). Closed flexor tendon injuries are often associated with a violent avulsion of the flexor tendon when the hand gets caught in various parts of the uniform (especially a jersey) and is typically seen in football. The most common hand injury associated with skiing is derangement of the metacarpophalangeal joint of the thumb, with the ski pole often implicated. Proximal interphalangeal (PIP) joint derangement with collateral ligament and volar plate

disruption are often seen in sports such as football and basketball where there are often violent collisions between the hand and the ball or another player. Fractures of the hand can be seen in virtually any sport where there is a risk of either a high-energy blunt trauma or a twisting or torquing-type injury to the digits and hand.

Similarly, neurovascular injuries in the athlete (most of the chronic compressive type) are becoming more recognized as sports participation increases. The most popular participation sport in the United States, bowling, is associated with "bowler's thumb" or ulnar digital nerve perineural fibrosis. Nerve compressive problems, especially of the ulnar nerve, are often associated with long-term bicycle riding due to compression against the handlebars (see Ch. 4).

Athletic activities are popular with the skeletally immature population as well. Often this population will present with injuries specific to the immature skeleton, many of which are fractures involving the growth plate (see Ch. 8). This chapter also covers special conditions that may occur during athletic activities, such as human bites and compartment syndromes.

TENDON INJURIES

Mallet Finger

Injury to the extensor mechanism of the digit is often secondary to an axial load to the fingertip. This results in a forceful passive flexion of the digit when it is being actively extended, and, as previously mentioned, is

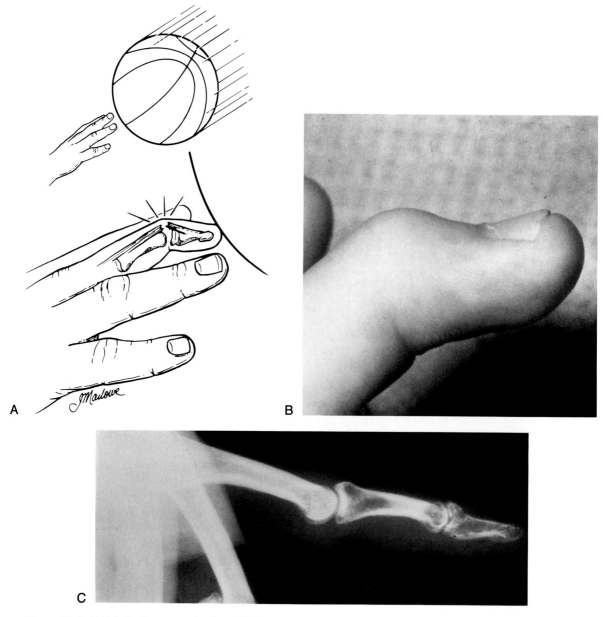

Figure 25-1 **(A)** Mallet finger mechanism of injury with axial load from ball striking digit. **(B)** Flexion posture of distal interphalangeal joint of mallet finger. **(C)** Bony mallet tendon avulsion. *(Figure continues.)*

seen in sports involving a ball (Fig. 25-1). Depending upon the force of the injury and the posture of the finger at the time of impact, either a mallet or boutonnière deformity will follow.

The mallet finger is an avulsion injury of the terminal extensor tendon of the distal interphalangeal (DIP) joint. Clinically, this results in a droop or extension lag at the distal interphalangeal joint of the involved digit. The abnormal posture of the digit will be obvious to the examiner; there will be little (if any) active extension of the joint, although there is generally full passive exten-

sion with accompanying tenderness over the dorsum of the distal interphalangeal joint. When examining a patient with a mallet finger, it is imperative to obtain a radiograph in two planes to rule out a bony avulsion and joint subluxation, or an epiphyseal fracture in the skeletally immature.

The majority of these injuries can be treated nonoperatively (Fig. 25-2). The most common type of mallet finger injury is the type I or midsubstance rupture of the terminal extensor tendon. Type II or bony avulsion injuries are less common but present clinically in the

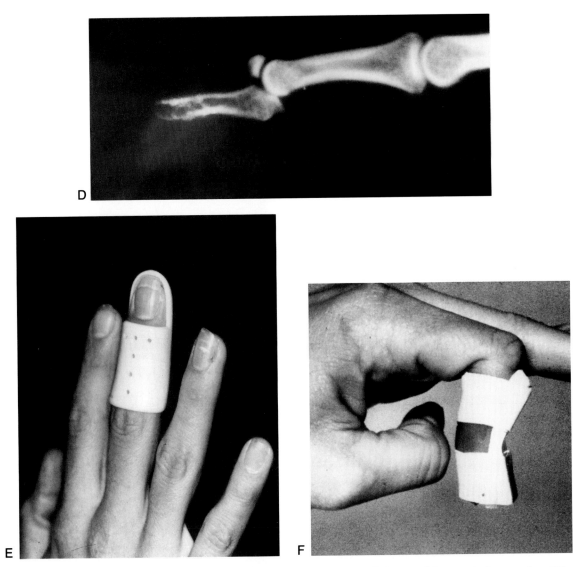

Figure 25-1 *(Continued)* **(D)** Unstable bony mallet with subluxation of joint requiring surgical correction. **(E)** Stack splint for mallet finger. **(F)** Optional aluminum foam splint for mallet finger. Notice that proximal interphalangeal joint is left free while in splint.

same manner, and therefore radiographic examination is necessary. It is critical to assess any degree of distal interphalangeal joint subluxation seen on the lateral-view radiograph. Subluxation of the joint, usually in the palmar direction, is a relative indication for surgical intervention and reflects a more significant injury to both the capsule and collateral ligamentous complex. Often the avulsion will involve a substantial portion of the articular surface of the distal phalanx, resulting in a loss of normal intrinsic joint stability. If detected both clinically and radiographically, the unstable joint and displaced fracture may need to be stabilized with open reduction and internal fixation of the fracture fragment.

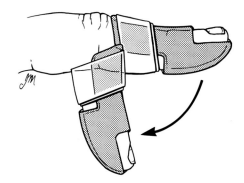

Figure 25-2 Stable splint showing support of distal interphalangeal joint while maintaining mobility of proximal interphalangeal joint.

Most mallet fingers, however, are type I or stable type II bony avulsion types. The majority of these injuries are amenable to close conservative treatment consisting of maintaining the distal interphalangeal joint in extension for 6 weeks while bony union occurs or a midsubstance tendon disruption heals. It is critical that the patient understand the absolute need for continuous splinting of the distal interphalangeal joint in extension. If the patient needs to remove the splint for any reason (e.g., hygiene purposes), he or she should be instructed on a safe method to don and doff the splint to maintain distal interphalangeal extension.

There are a variety of splints that can be used either on the dorsal or palmar aspect (see Ch. 6). When splinting the mallet finger, it is important to keep the proximal interphalangeal joint free to help maintain a supple finger. Any extension lag of the distal interphalangeal joint after 6 weeks of splinting should be resplinted for an additional 6 weeks. Graded active and passive range of motion exercises are initiated at 8 weeks, with exten-

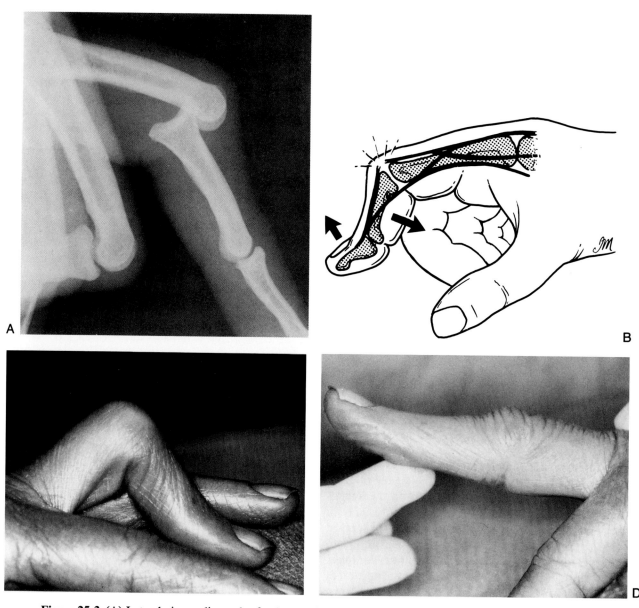

Figure 25-3 **(A)** Lateral-view radiograph of volar proximal interphalangeal joint dislocation with central slip disruption. **(B)** Schematic view of rupture of central slip and boutonnière deformity with volar subluxation of lateral bands. **(C)** Flexion posture of proximal interphalangeal joint in boutonnière deformity with extension deformity at the distal interphalangeal joint. **(D)** Passive correction of deformity. Passive motion is maintained but active extension is lost in boutonnière deformity.

sion splinting continued at night for an additional 4 to 6 weeks. An athlete may return to competition with a dorsal splint if it is necessary for the particular position. If there is still an extension lag after 12 weeks of splinting, the patient should be reevaluated for possible surgical intervention.

Boutonnière Deformity

The boutonnière deformity of the digit is second only to the mallet finger in incidence of sport-related digit extensor tendon disruptions. Whereas the mallet finger is a disruption of the terminal extensor tendon over the distal interphalangeal joint, the boutonnière deformity results from a disruption of the central slip of the extensor mechanism at the base of the middle phalanx as well as a disruption of the triangular ligament (Fig. 25-3). The deformity is proximal interphalangeal joint flexion combined with a hyperextension deformity of the distal interphalangeal joint. The triangular ligament, which is the dorsal stabilizer of the lateral bands, is ruptured, resulting in palmar subluxation of the lateral bands, which converts these structures from extensors to flexors of the proximal interphalangeal joint. This disruption results in the loss of the extensor power of the proximal interphalangeal joint and a relative increase in the extensor power at the distal interphalangeal joint, creating a secondary hyperextension deformity. Clinically, in addition to the posture of the digit, there is tenderness at the central slip insertion dorsally and an inability to actively extend the proximal interphalangeal joint, with a loss of active flexion at the distal interphalangeal joint.

Often, an acute injury to the central slip will not demonstrate any abnormal posture immediately. Over time, a relative imbalance occurs between the extension flexion of the proximal interphalangeal joint, resulting in a boutonnière deformity. Acutely, these patients will be tender at the insertion of the central slip and should be splinted in extension. Also, with a volar dislocation of the proximal interphalangeal joint, a subsequent boutonnière deformity should be looked for carefully. All of these injuries require close follow-up to determine whether there is any developing boutonnière deformity.

Most boutonnière deformities associated with sports are closed injuries. If the central slip has been lacerated, there is a relative indication for primary surgical repair. In the vast majority of sport-related boutonnière deformities, however, the injury is a closed disruption, and treatment should consist of splinting the proximal interphalangeal joint in extension while leaving the metacarpophalangeal joint and distal interphalangeal

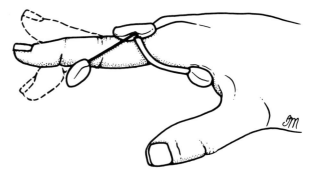

Figure 25-4 Boutonnière splint maintaining passive extension of the proximal interphalangeal joint while keeping the distal interphalangeal joint free.

joint unsplinted (Fig. 25-4). The splint should be worn for 6 weeks. As with the mallet finger, splinting for the boutonnière deformity should be continuous. It is important to leave the distal interphalangeal joint free from any immobilization. While the splint is on the digit, the patient is encouraged to actively flex the distal interphalangeal joint (10 repetitions every waking hour, 8 hours daily) which tends to relocate the traumatically palmarly subluxed lateral bands back to their normal anatomic alignment, dorsal to the axis of rotation of the proximal interphalangeal joint. After 6 weeks, full active range of motion is begun. Night extension splinting is continued for an additional 4 to 6 weeks, and dynamic splinting is used during the day. A progressive resistive exercise program is introduced as a range of motion improves, with resistive exercises to strengthen both the flexor and extensor mechanisms (see Ch. 2). When the athlete returns to competition, taping to an adjacent digit will provide some protection to the previously injured digit.

The extensor apparatus can be traumatized at the level of the metacarpophalangeal joint. The sagittal bands that aid in extension of the metacarpophalangeal joint also centrally stabilize the extensor tendon over the dorsum of this joint. Injury to this sagittal band will cause a subluxation of the extensor tendon to either side between the adjacent metacarpal heads. This is often incurred via an axial load against the metacarpal head with the metacarpophalangeal joint flexed; most typically seen in boxing, this injury is commonly known as *boxer's finger*. The subluxation of the extensor tendon on either side of the metacarpophalangeal joint, due to disruption of the sagittal band, will result in the inability to fully and actively extend the joint; there will also be a tendency for deviation of the finger to the side of the tendon subluxation. On examination, the extensor tendon, which tends to lie in its normal anatomic location in extension, will sublux to the pathologic side upon joint flexion. This tendon subluxation and snapping will be visible when examining the hand. It is best treated with surgical repair of the sagittal band. Protection of the repair with a splint for 4 to 6 weeks is necessary after surgery. After 8 to 10 weeks, there can be gradual return to full activities, with protection used for collision sports.

Flexor Tendon Injuries

Flexor tendon injuries in the athlete can either be lacerated open wounds or closed wounds (resulting in a rupture of the tendon). Ruptured or lacerated flexor tendons are treated like those that are non-sports-related, and treatment depends on the location of the flexor tendon pathology. There should be prompt referral to a physician who is experienced in hand surgery, for primary repair should be performed within 3 to 4 days. The specific examination for the integrity of the flexor digitorum superficialis, flexor digitorum profundus, and flexor pollicis longus are illustrated in Figure 25-5. The presenting resting posture or cascade of the hand digits will often indicate which tendon structures have been lacerated. The normal cascade of the digits can be seen in Figure 25-6. Lacerations of the flexor digitorum profundus or flexor digitorum superficialis tendons will alter this cascade and should always be compared to the assumed normal contralateral hand. It is important to examine each individual tendon in the hand, since a single intact flexor tendon in a digit can still present a flexion posture to the hand and may mask the laceration of the other tendon. A laceration of the flexor digitorum superficialis tendon with an intact flexor digitorum profundus tendon may present with a relatively normal posture of the hand. This is because the long flexor to the tip of the finger is intact and there may be some secondary flexion at the proximal interphalangeal joint of this tendon. It is therefore imperative that each individual tendon be examined. With flexor tendon lacerations, injuries to the digital neurovascular bundle are commonly encountered. In addition to assessing the overall viability of the digit, two-point discrimination on both the radial and ulnar side should be assessed to detect disruption of the digital nerves.

A closed tendon rupture of the digit is more typically associated with athletic injuries to the hand. The rupture of the flexor digitorum profundus (the *rugger jersey* injury) is perhaps the most common. This occurs when the actively flexed digit is caught in the jersey or piece of equipment of another player, and there is a forceful passive extension of the actively flexed digit, resulting in either a midsubstance rupture of the flexor

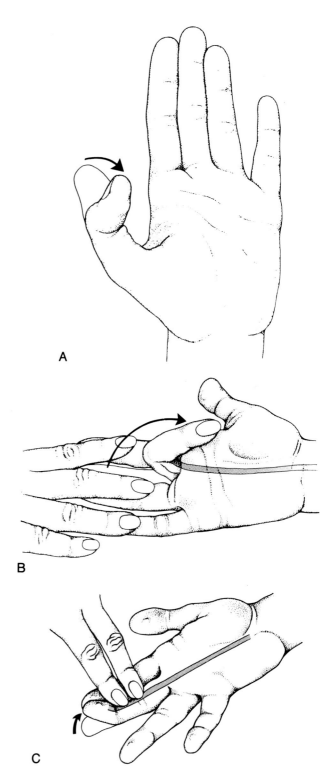

Figure 25-5 (A) Function of flexor pollicis longus. **(B)** Examination for function of the flexor digitorum superficialis of middle finger. **(C)** Examination for flexor digitorum profundus of middle finger.

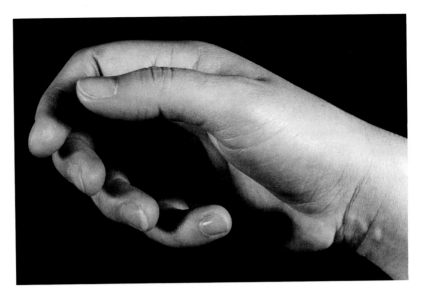

Figure 25-6 Normal cascade of the digits in a normal hand. Notice the gradual increase in flexion of the digits from the index to little finger.

digitorum profundus tendon near the insertion, or a bony avulsion of the tendon of the distal phalanx tendon (Fig. 25-7).

The patient will present with an inability to actively flex the distal interphalangeal joint and will have considerable discomfort over the area of the flexor disitorum profundus insertion. Depending upon the degree of retraction of the flexor tendon, the tenderness over the stump may range from the level of the distal digital flex increase to the palm. With a midsubstance

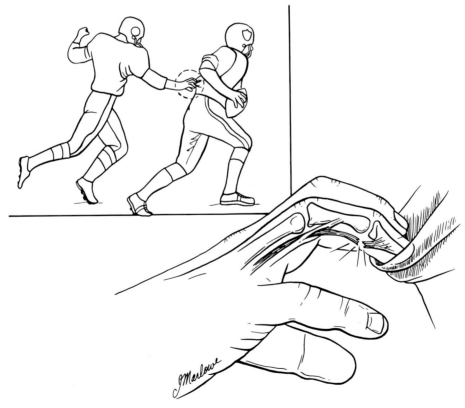

Figure 25-7 Flexor digitorum profundus avulsion injury (jersey finger). Mechanism of injury as the finger gets caught in the jersey and the actively flexed distal interphalangeal joint is suddenly and forcibly passively extended, rupturing the tendon.

rupture of the tendon, retraction of the proximal stump into the palm can occur. Retraction is minimized by intact vinculae and the lumbrical musculature. If the injury is a bony avulsion, there is a fracture fragment attached to the distal portion of the flexor digitorum profundus tendon, which often inhibits proximal retraction. It is therefore critical that both AP and lateral radiographic views are taken of the digit to assess any bony involvement.

Unlike the mallet finger and boutonnière deformity on the extensor side of the digit, flexor tendon disruptions are treated by primary surgical repair. As mentioned previously, these injuries should be treated within 3 to 4 days. The acute treatment consists of a primary repair of the midsubstance tendon disruption or reattachment of the bony avulsion. The treatment of the chronic, neglected flexor disitorum profundus tendon avulsion is an entirely different matter. Because of an intact flexor digitorum superficialis tendon in the digit, there is usually normal proximal interphalangeal motion with absent active distal interphalangeal joint flexion. Surgical treatment at this time should not be undertaken lightly. Depending on the time from original injury, treatment ranges from primary repair to flexor tendon grafting to two-stage reconstruction using Silastic rods and pulley reconstruction. All of these delayed surgical procedures offer less predictable results than acute primary repair, including both achieved active flexion of the distal interphalangeal joint and the unaltered flexor disitorum superficialis tendon function at the proximal interphalangeal joint. Due to these concerns, these injuries should be treated on an acute basis, since the results are superior with primary repair.

The rehabilitation program should be initiated within 24 hours after the tendon has been repaired. A dorsal extension block splint is fabricated with the wrist in 20 to 30 degrees of flexion, metacarpophalangeal joints flexed to 70 degrees, and the interphalangeal joints in extension. This position reduces the tension on the flexor tendon repair. Guarded range of motion exercises are initiated at this time and should be initially supervised by a hand therapist. These are the only exercises allowed until 6 weeks after tendon repair, with resistive exercises not introduced until 8 weeks after repair (see Ch. 2).

INJURIES TO THE LIGAMENT AND JOINT STABILIZERS

Injuries to the soft tissue stabilizers of the joints in the hand range from low grade I stretches of ligaments and capsule requiring only symptomatic treatment to complete disruption of ligaments and capsule requiring surgical repair. These injuries are usually the result of either axial and torsional stresses to the digit from a ball to high-energy blunt trauma secondary to falls or collisions. Early recognition is important before significant swelling has occurred, possibly preventing an accurate examination; it will also enable the provider to initiate more predictable treatment. A radiographic examination should be performed to rule out any bony involvement, especially in intra-articular fractures (Fig. 25-8). The most important area to address is the stability of the joint. If the joint is stable with provocative examination, then the treatment in almost all cases can be nonoperative with splinting. However, if the joint is unstable either in a lateral or dorsal/volar plane, then surgical intervention should also be considered. It should be remembered that this is a spectrum and, while grossly unstable joints should be surgically treated, the mildly unstable joint often can be treated nonoperatively.

Ligamentous Injuries to the Proximal Interphalangeal Joint

Stable (Incomplete)

The proximal interphalangeal joint is one of the most commonly injured joints in the hand. These injuries are incurred secondary to an axial load, resulting in stretching of the collateral ligament or transient dorsal subluxation of the middle phalanx. Forces that laterally angulate or hyperextend the joint may also injure the capsule, as in the classic jammed finger typically seen in athletes. These lesser injuries to the proximal interphalangeal joint do not usually begin with a frank dislocation of the joint.

The collateral ligament should be examined to assess any degree of instability (Fig. 25-9). Because the proximal interphalangeal joint is essentially a hinged joint with some inherent bony instability, there should be no more than 10 degrees of laxity in either a radial or ulnar direction with provocative lateral stress. If there is tenderness above the joint without gross joint instability or a fracture, this injury can usually be treated with buddy taping to an adjacent finger for 3 to 4 weeks. Range of motion is allowed within the confines of the buddy taping. If there is gross instability and/or an avulsion fracture of the collateral ligaments as seen on the AP and lateral radiographic views, then surgical intervention may be considered (Fig. 25-10). Patients with low-grade sprains (treated nonoperatively) often can immediately return to athletic participation with modifications in equipment splinting or protective taping (see Ch. 6).

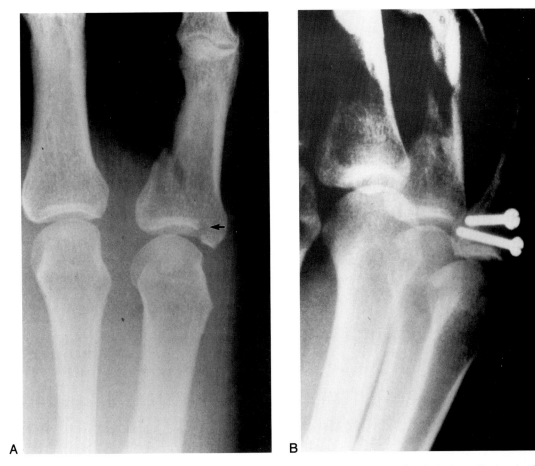

Figure 25-8 (A) AP-view radiograph of an intra-articular fracture of the proximal phalanx. Notice the fracture entering the metacarpophalangeal joint and the step-off and malreduction. **(B)** The same fracture as depicted in Fig. A after open reduction internal fixation. Note the reduction of the fracture and the congruency of the articular surface.

Unstable (Complete)

Unstable or complete injuries to the proximal interphalangeal joint involve a higher degree of force applied to the joint, which almost always results in a transient subluxation or frank dislocation. These injuries can be isolated to the collateral ligaments and volar plate, or they can be associated with fracture dislocations of the base of the middle phalanx. The soft tissue anatomy around the proximal interphalangeal joint is critical for both lateral and dorsal-palmar stability (Fig. 25-9). The proper collateral, accessory collateral, and volar plate constructs provide joint stability in these two planes. Dislocation of the proximal interphalangeal joint, which is most often dorsal, requires careful clinical and radiographic examination.

Often, the dorsally subluxed or dislocated proximal interphalangeal joint will be manipulated by either the coach, trainer, or athlete in an attempt to reduce the

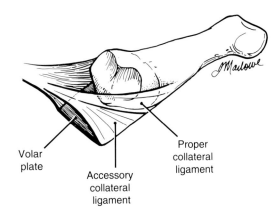

Figure 25-9 Volar plate and associated proper and accessory collateral ligament of the proximal interphalangeal joint.

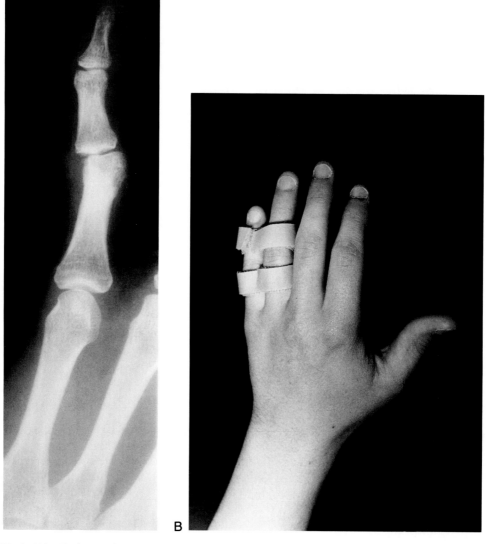

Figure 25-10 **(A)** AP-view radiograph of the little finger showing subluxation of the proximal interphalangeal joint after injury to the collateral ligaments resulting in an unstable joint. **(B)** Same patient with buddy straps to allow protected motion of the proximal interphalangeal joint of the little finger.

joint. This is usually accomplished by longitudinal traction attempting to "snap" the finger back in place. Although common, "on the field" reduction is not routinely recommended because it risks further injury, fracture, or displacement of a previously undisplaced fracture. If the injured joint is not grossly deformed and has minimal swelling, buddy taping to the adjacent finger will provide protection. If there is considerable swelling and/or deformity of the digit, radiographs and a careful clinical examination off the field should be completed so a definitive treatment plan can begin. Low-emission portable x-ray machines are frequently available both in the locker room as well as on the

sidelines in many professional and college programs, facilitating optimal early initial evaluation. After any joint manipulation, especially a relocation, radiographs should be obtained to assess not only the extent and displacement of any fractures but also the congruency of the joint. If the joint is not congruent, it may be a sign of instability. Radiographic evaluation should be combined with the clinical examination to assess overall joint stability.

With dislocation of the proximal interphalangeal joint, at least two structures of the collateral ligament/volar plate complex must be disrupted—usually the volar plate and one of the collateral ligaments (Fig.

25-11). The specific collateral ligament will be determined by the direction of the force. The volar plate disruption can either be midsubstance or an avulsion from the volar base of the middle phalanx. Most often, if there is no bony avulsion associated with this injury, reduction will result in a joint that is congruent and stable enough to warrant conservative therapy. Conservative therapy consists of edema management techniques and active and passive range of motion exercises. The athlete should be protected with buddy taping when returning to practice and competition. If the pathology involves intra-articular avulsion fractures of the middle phalanx, the bony buttress that maintains the congruency of the proximal phalanx head may be lost. Often there will be a (dorsal) drift of the middle phalanx necessitating surgical stabilization (Fig. 25-12).

Proximal interphalangeal joint dislocations, which are essentially volar plate disruptions with collateral ligament trauma without fractures, can usually be treated nonoperatively with dorsal extension block splinting. Because the injured structures are on the lateral and palmar sides of the joint, digital extension results in increased stress to the injured structures. A flexion posture of the finger, therefore, will relieve tension of the involved structures and facilitate healing. The extension block splint allows active flexion in an unrestricted fashion and limits the range of active extension (Fig. 25-13). This treatment should allow (early) protective motion while maintaining a well-reduced joint. A range of motion program within the confines of the splint should be initiated as soon as possible following the injury (ideally within 24 hours). This will minimize joint stiffness and assist with edema reduction. Due to the initial dorsal joint subluxation, the reduced joint is more stable in flexion. The initial position of the proximal interphalangeal joint should

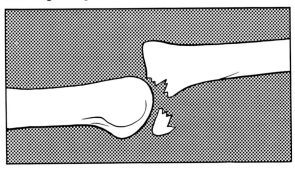

Radiologic image

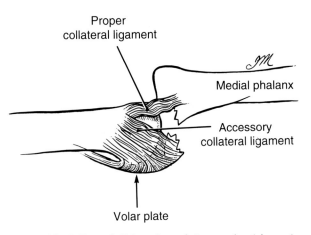

Proper collateral ligament

Medial phalanx

Accessory collateral ligament

Volar plate

Figure 25-12 Dorsal dislocation of the proximal interphalangeal joint with a bony avulsion of the volar plate. **(Top)** The volar plate actually is intact but is pulled away from its bony insertion with a fragment of bone. **(Bottom)** A typical lateral-view radiograph of the digit with the associated fracture.

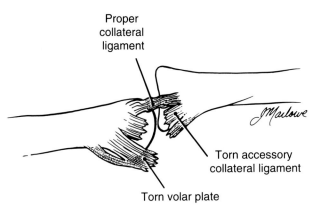

Proper collateral ligament

Torn accessory collateral ligament

Torn volar plate

Figure 25-11 Dorsal dislocation of the proximal interphalangeal joint with tear of the volar plate and accessory collateral ligament.

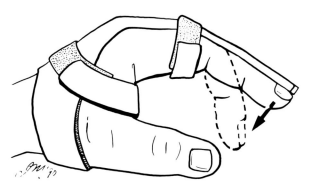

Figure 25-13 Dorsal extension block splint of the proximal interphalangeal joint for treatment of volar plate disruptions, allowing full unrestricted active flexion but restricting active extension of the joint.

be the maximum extension that still maintains a congruent proximal interphalangeal joint, and should be documented with lateral-view radiographs while in the splint. Once the dorsal extension block is in place, active flexion of the proximal interphalangeal joint, and extension of the joint within the confines of the extension block is encouraged.

Follow-up is critical with these injuries. Serial radiographs are obtained on a weekly basis, and the splint is altered, usually to allow 10 degrees more extension each week. After any splint change, radiographs should be obtained to ensure that the joint is still congruent. If the congruency is lost with more extension, the digit should be maintained in the previous degree of extension block. Once the proximal interphalangeal joint has been brought out to full extension, over the course of 4 to 5 weeks, the splint can be discontinued, range of motion is maximized, and gentle strengthening exercises begun. At this point, the joint should be protected with buddy strapping during sports participation (e.g., a volleyball match) for another 6 weeks.

It should be remembered that fracture-dislocations of the proximal interphalangeal joint are essentially avulsion injuries to the distal insertion of the volar plate. These fractures are discussed in the subsection *Phalangeal Fractures.*

Distal Interphalangeal Joint Dislocation

Distal interphalangeal joint dislocations are uncommon in athletes. Injuries to this joint are more typically manifested by the mallet deformity or flexor digitorum profundus tendon avulsions. Frank dislocations of the distal interphalangeal joint are generally associated with open wounds and often with high-energy impact loading. These dislocations are almost invariably dorsal and can be treated with closed reduction and stability assessment as with proximal interphalangeal joint dislocations. It is important to assess any trauma to the nail matrix. If there is subungual hematoma, then the nail plate should be removed to determine any matrix laceration and disruption that will require primary repair. Radiographs are critical prior to reduction to detect not only any fracture but the degree of displacement, which will often give an indication of associated soft tissue injury (i.e., matrix lacerations secondary to displaced fracture fragments). If the dislocation is reduced and the joint is clinically stable, then simple splinting in a stack style splint (see Ch. 6) for 4 to 6 weeks will result in a stable, functional joint. Instability or incongruency of this joint after reduction should signal the potential for intra-articular interposition of

the volar plate or collateral ligament complex and treatment should be surgery.

Metacarpophalangeal Joint Dislocation

Metacarpophalangeal joint dislocations are the result of an axial load and extension force to the digit, and are almost always dorsal (i.e., the phalanx is dorsal to the metacarpal). The articular surface of the proximal phalanx is displaced dorsally and proximally. A rent in the capsule allows dorsal migration of the proximal phalanx and a tear to the volar plate of the metacarpophalangeal joint allows palmar migration of the metacarpal head (Fig. 25-14). The dorsal thumb metacarpophalangeal joint dislocation is more easily reduced by closed manipulation than the metacarpophalangeal joint digit dislocations. Gentle longitudinal traction is used and pressure should be applied to the dorsum of the digit at the base of the proximal phalanx. As the base of the proximal phalanx is brought just distal to the articular surface of the metacarpal, the digit will begin to relocate as the digit is flexed. Prereduction radiographs should always be obtained.

After reduction, it is important to assess lateral joint stability because of possible associated collateral ligament injury. The majority of these injuries can be treated nonoperatively with splinting and immobilizing the digit with the metacarpophalangeal joint flexed to 50 degrees, not only to prevent hyperextension of the digit but to prevent shortening and contracture of the collateral ligaments, which may result in joint stiffness (Fig. 25-15). Immobilization should be with either a

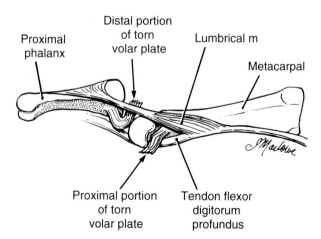

Figure 25-14 Dorsal dislocation of the metacarpophalangeal joint with a tear of the volar plate, showing it interposed between the base of the proximal phalanx and the head of the metacarpal, preventing reduction.

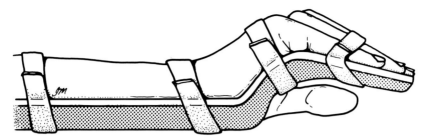

Figure 25-15 Forearm-based resting splint extending to the tips of the fingers.

forearm base thumb spica cast or splint for 4 weeks and supportive taping during athletic activities (e.g., boxing, hockey, skiing, lacrosse) for another 4 weeks. If the dislocation cannot be reduced, it is most likely secondary to volar plate (and/or collateral ligament) interposition and should be explored surgically and reduced (Fig. 25-14). Treatment after surgery should be the same as described above.

The mechanism of injury and the reduction techniques for dorsal metacarpophalangeal joint dislocations of the index, middle, ring, and little fingers are the same as for the thumb. Often, however, these dislocations in the digits will be impossible to reduce due to volar plate intra-articular interposition, and therefore should be surgically reduced. After open reduction, the joint should be maintained in approximately 50 degrees of flexion and immobilized for approximately 4 weeks, with mobilization of the digit to follow (see Ch. 2). After motion has been obtained, the digit should be buddy-strapped to the adjacent digit for protection during athletic activity for an additional 4 weeks.

Carpometacarpal Dislocations

Dislocations or subluxations of the carpometacarpal joints of the hand are relatively uncommon in athletes. They are usually indicative of high-energy injuries and are often associated with an extensive soft tissue swelling in the hand. There is little motion in the carpometacarpal joints of the digits relative to other joints in the hand. Joint stability is maintained by ligamentous supporting structures. Subluxation or frank dislocation of these joints should be assessed with AP- and lateral-view radiographs. Often these injuries can be reduced with closed manipulation but will be unstable, making percutaneous pinning necessary. If the dislocation cannot be reduced or there is residual subluxation, then open reduction internal fixation will be required.

Carpometacarpal joint dislocations of the thumb are a different sort of injury. The carpometacarpal joint of the thumb is an inherently unstable joint. The bony architecture of this joint lends itself to many planes of motion, including flexion extension, abduction, adduction, and circumduction, and a variable degree of rotation. This saddle joint relies on a constellation of soft tissue stabilizers, including dense capsular and ligamentous structures (Fig. 25-16). Disruption of these soft tissue stabilizers can lead to subluxation and/or dislocation. The thumb carpometacarpal joint is more prone to injury because the thumb lies in a different plane from the digits and is not relatively protected by any adjacent digits. Because the thumb is so dependent on capsular ligamentous stabilizers for optimal function, disruption of these structures with a dislocation can lead to symptomatic chronic instability that may significantly compromise activities of daily living as well as athletic activities. This is in contrast to dislocations of the carpometacarpal joints of the digits, which are relatively stable when reduced and have a much more predictable prognosis.

Radiographs are essential to this injury because of the frequent association of intra-articular fractures of the thumb metacarpal, specifically, Rolando's or Bennett's fracture (Fig. 25-17).

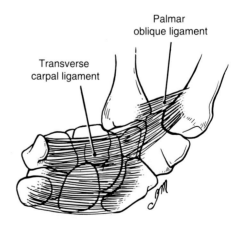

Figure 25-16 The transverse carpal ligament blending in with the palmar oblique ligament to the base of the thumb metacarpal, which provides the primary stabilizing structure of the thumb metacarpal joint.

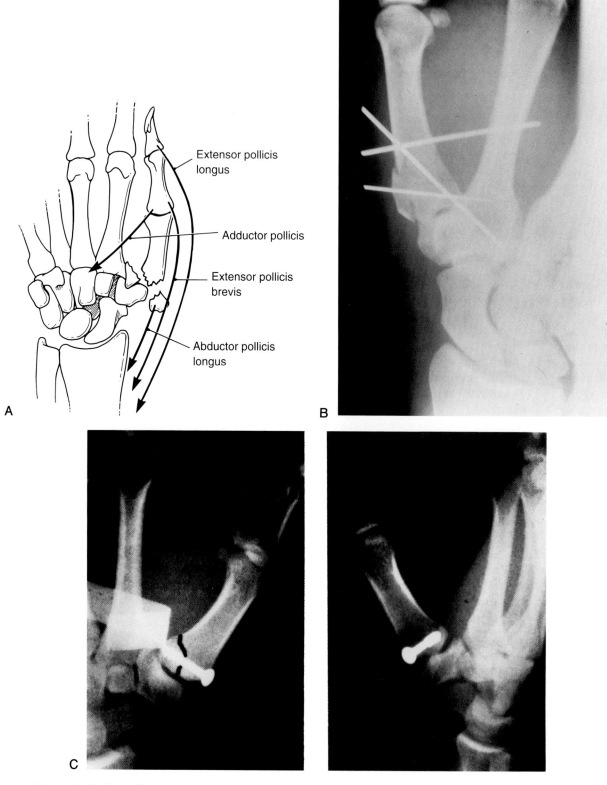

Figure 25-17 **(A)** Deforming forces of Bennett's fracture. **(B)** AP radiographic view of open reduction internal fixation of a comminuted Bennett's fracture. **(C)** Alternative technique of fixation with a screw.

Case Study I

Bennett's Fracture

R.C. is a 20-year-old college baseball player who fell on an outstretched hand while diving for a fly ball in the outfield. He sustained a hyperabduction and axial load injury to his dominant thumb. Radiographs showed a noncomminuted fracture of the thumb metacarpal with a classic Bennett's fracture type of intra-articular extension (Fig. 25-17). Virtually all Bennett's fractures require a reduction and fixation of some sort. Options include percutaneous Kirshner wire fixation or open reduction and internal fixation utilizing screws or pins. Due to the minimal comminution, an open reduction internal fixation was performed with a cancellous screw providing rigid fixation, enabling the player to remain out of a cast and begin early rehabilitation therapy for range of motion. This facilitated his return to playing baseball in 5 weeks. Fixation of the fracture, as shown in Figure 25-17, facilitated early hand therapy, preventing stiffness and disuse atrophy.

If these fractures are detected, surgical fixation and stabilization based on the same criteria used for non-sports-related fractures of this type should be considered. If there are no fractures associated with a carpometacarpal dislocation at the base of the thumb and closed reduction results in a congruent joint, treatment should consist of immobilization in a short-arm thumb spica cast for 4 to 6 weeks. Careful consideration should be given, however, to stabilizing this joint with percutaneously placed pins, assuring a congruent joint and no subluxation within the cast. This is an unstable injury, and subluxation within a cast is an indication for surgical stabilization.

Gamekeeper's Thumb: Metacarpophalangeal Joint Instability

The most common ligamentous injury to the hand is trauma to the ulnar collateral ligamentous complex of the metacarpophalangeal joint, known as gamekeeper's thumb (Fig. 25-18). This injury occurs most often when a skier falls onto an outstretched hand with an abducted thumb. The ski pole has often been implicated as the mechanism that predisposes the thumb to injury. The ski pole maintains the thumb in an abducted position, making it more vulnerable to radial stresses at the metacarpophalangeal joint when the athlete falls (Fig. 25-19). Sprains to the ulna collateral ligamentous complex of the metacarpophalangeal joint also occur in contact sports and in sports where there is a collision between two players. This is typically seen in baseball during a collision between a runner and a fielder. The fielder experiences the injury when he goes to make a tag and suffers a hyperextension abduction injury to his gloved thumb when it impacts a sliding base runner (e.g., the catcher during a collision at homeplate). These injuries result in ulnar laxity of the metacarpophalangeal joint and often dorsal subluxation secondary to palmar plate involvement. Ulnar collateral ligament integrity is essential for a strong pinch. If chronically lax, the patient will complain of

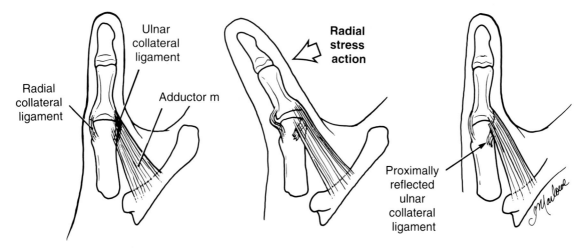

Figure 25-18 Trauma to the ulnar collateral ligament of the metacarpophalangeal joint of the thumb, resulting in a Stenar lesion with a proximally reflected ulnar collateral ligament, with the abductor tendon interposed between it and its insertion.

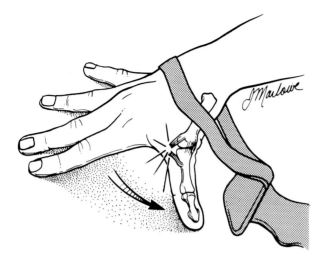

Figure 25-19 The mechanism of injury in skier's thumb resulting in a tear of the ulnar collateral ligament of the metacarpophalangeal joint. The thumb sustains an axial and radial deviating force to this joint in a fall.

weakness in activities that require a strong pinch. In the acute setting, the athlete will have swelling, ecchymosis, and tenderness along the metacarpophalangeal joint on the dorsal ulnar side. Around 95 percent of ligamentous injuries to the metacarpophalangeal joint of the thumb are to the ulnar collateral ligament. Radial collateral ligament injuries are relatively uncommon. If an injury to the ulnar collateral ligament is suspected, radiographic examination is mandatory (Figs. 25-20 and 21). If the ligamentous injury is through its midsubstance, the radiographs will show only soft tissue swelling and possible joint subluxation. Frequently, however, there is bony avulsion of the ulnar collateral ligament insertion at the base of the proximal phalanx.

If the bony fragment is displaced more than 1 mm or involves greater than 10 percent of the articular surface, then primary surgical repair is indicated. If the fragment is anatomically aligned or displaced less than a millimeter, it can be treated conservatively with a short arm thumb spica cast for 6 weeks. If, however, the radiograph shows no bony involvement, the degree of laxity should be assessed with stress radiographs of the thumb metacarpophalangeal joint. A digital block anesthesia with 1 percent plain lidocaine can be used if necessary. Laxity of the ulnar collateral ligament complex greater than 35 degrees on the AP-view radiograph or greater than 15 degrees relative to the contralateral thumb are relative indications for surgical repair (Fig. 25-22). Stress examination of the collateral ligament complex should be performed with the joint in full extension and full flexion. This gives selective exami-

nation to the proper and accessory collateral ligamentous complex. Laxity in extension is indicative of accessory collateral ligament laxity, whereas laxity in flexion suggests trauma to the proper collateral ligament. Stress radiographs are not indicated when there is bony avulsion.

Acute injuries to the ulnar collateral ligament complex, whether treated operatively or nonoperatively, should be immobilized in a short-arm thumb spica cast for about 4 to 6 weeks. Laxity detected 6 weeks after the injury may not be amenable to operative primary repair or may be less predictable when treated nonoperatively compared to the acute situation. Therefore, often with chronic laxity, reconstruction of the ligamentous complex, requiring tendon grafts to reconstruct the ligament, may be necessary. Postoperatively, these patients should be immobilized for approximately 6 weeks in a short-arm thumb spica cast for adequate graft healing. After removal of the cast, whether in an acute or chronic situation, there will be variable amounts of stiffness in the thumb, and this will often

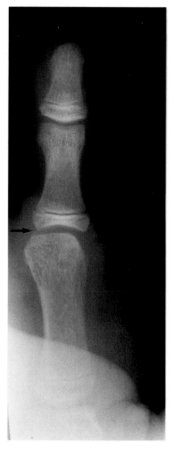

Figure 25-20 Radial subluxation of the metacarpophalangeal joint secondary to a tear of the ulnar collateral ligament complex without bony avulsion.

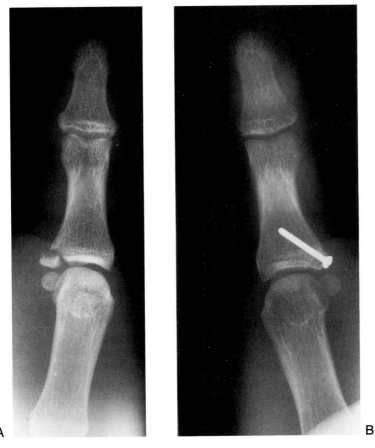

A   B

Figure 25-21 **(A)** Bony avulsion of the ulnar collateral ligament complex with a rotated intra-articular fracture fragment. **(B)** The same patient in **A** after open reduction internal fixation. Note the correction of the alignment of the fracture fragment and reconstitution of the joint.

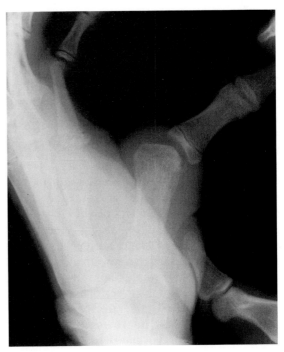

Figure 25-22 AP stress radiographic view of the metacarpo-phalangeal joint of the thumb showing gross subluxation of the joint with stressing of the ulnar collateral ligament complex by the examiner. There is virtual dislocation of the joint.

require post-treatment hand therapy to maximize both return of motion and functional recovery. Once the cast is removed, a protective hand-based short opponens muscle splint is fabricated. The splint is removed for a range of motion program as well as strengthening for grip and pinch. The athlete will need splinting or taping for a safe return to practice or competition (see Ch. 6).

Case Study II

Gamekeeper's (Skier's) Thumb

N.A. is a 31-year-old skier who fell with the ski pole in his right hand. He sustained injury to his thumb, as shown in Figure 25-20. The patient had discomfort about the metacarpophalangeal joint and was very ecchymotic. Stress view radiographs were obtained after installation of local anesthesia (Fig. 25-20). At surgery, a complete tear of the ulna collateral ligament complex was identified and repaired. Postoperatively, the patient was placed in a thumb spica cast for 4 weeks. Hand therapy was started after the cast was removed and a hand-based thumb spica splint was fabricated, allowing the patient to participate in skiing and other sporting activities.

There have been many injuries in skiers. Although the strap on the ski pole may be the culprit, it is believed by most that it is simply having the ski pole grip in the hand which maintains the thumb in an abducted position, making it more susceptible to abduction and hyperextension injuries to the metacarpophalangeal joint of the thumb.

FRACTURES OF THE HAND

When treating fractures of the hand, it is important to consider not only the associated soft tissue trauma but also what effect the chosen treatment will have on the soft tissues. As always, the inherent risks of surgery and the anesthetic technique should be considered relative to the benefits of the proposed surgery. The goal of fracture treatment in the hand is restoration of the normal anatomy and obtaining the most functional outcome. The patient's desire and need to return to athletic competition may, in certain circumstances, influence the choice of treatment for these fractures. For example, closed nonoperative treatment of metacarpal fractures, which would require a minimum of 4 weeks of immobilization prior to the institution of therapy, may result in considerable loss of playing time and stiff digits, resulting in prolonged extensive hand therapy. Immediate rigid internal fixation, however,

would allow immediate range of motion therapy and may return the athlete to an active status sooner. These decisions should be made on an individual basis and are based on good fracture treatment care as well as the individual athlete's expectations (Fig. 25-23).

Case Study III

Phalangeal Fracture

P.M. is a 31-year-old professional bicycle racer who fell during a race, sustaining a comminuted fracture of the proximal phalanx of the right ring finger (Fig. 25-23). This injury occurred at the start of the season and 10 days before the start of a major international race. The patient underwent immediate open reduction internal fixation with supplemental bone graft (Fig. 25-23). Although this fracture would have healed if placed into a cast, rotational alignment was ensured and early fixation gave this fracture immediate stability allowing early return to cycling, which is this patient's livelihood. A thermoplastic splint was worn by the patient while riding. Two days postsurgery (Fig. 25-23), the patient completed his entire season, not missing any races because of his hand. During that time, he received extensive therapy for his range of motion. Six months after the initial surgery, the patient had the hardware removed and a tenolysis was performed to increase active and passive range of motion.

Metacarpal Fractures

Metacarpal fractures are a common injury to the athlete's hand. They are usually the result of a direct blow or a crush to the dorsum of the hand by having it stepped on by another participant or as a result of being hit by a ball. These fractures may also result from a twisting or torsional type of injury to the hand secondary to a fall, and can be in a transverse, oblique, or spiral configuration. Fractures of the metacarpal neck, especially in the ring and little fingers, are often seen secondary to an axial load to the flexed metacarpophalangeal joint, such as punching with a closed fist (Fig. 25-24).

Angular displacement of metacarpal-diaphyseal fractures is almost invariably apex dorsal secondary to the deforming force of the interosseous muscles (Fig. 25-25). Oblique and spiral fractures tend to shorten and override more than transverse fractures. It is critical in the treatment of these injuries to recognize that some degree of rotation and malalignment are often present because the distal fracture fragment tends to shift and rotate relative to the proximal, more immobile frag-

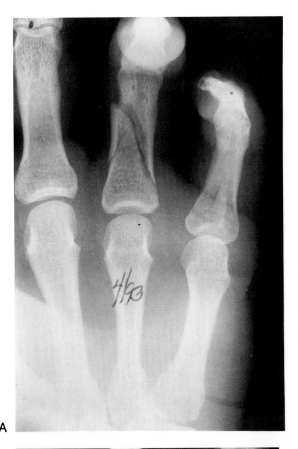

A

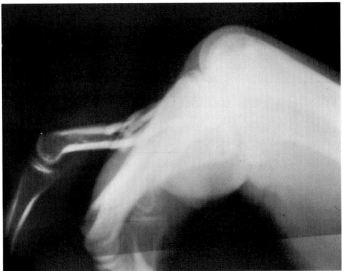

B

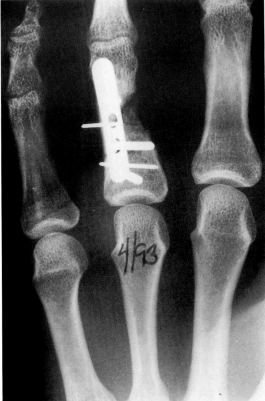

C

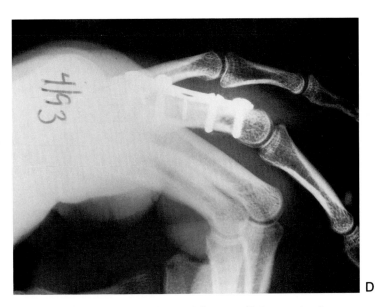

D

Figure 25-23 (A) AP-view radiograph of a comminuted displaced and malrotated fracture of the proximal phalanx of the ring finger. **(B)** Lateral-view radiograph showing the comminution and apex volar alignment. **(C)** AP-view radiograph following open reduction internal fixation with a plate, screws, and Kirchner wires. **(D)** Lateral-view radiograph showing the correction of the malalignment as illustrated in **B**.

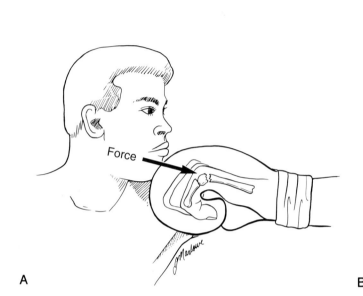
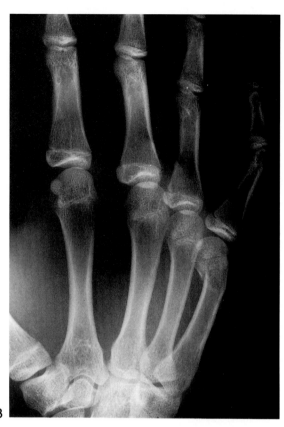

Figure 25-24 (A) The mechanism of injury in a boxer's fracture, resulting in a fracture of the metacarpal neck of the fifth metacarpal. **(B)** AP-view radiograph showing the fracture of the metacarpal neck of the fifth metacarpal.

ment. In addition to angulation, rotational deformities must be correct when assessing the adequacy of a closed reduction maneuver. Shortening and rotation are often secondary to an intrinsic or interosseous muscle pull.

Many of these fractures can be treated nonopera-

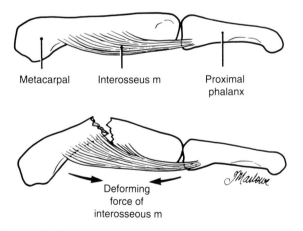

Figure 25-25 Deforming forces of the interosseous muscle on a metacarpal fracture, resulting in an apex dorsal angulation.

tively. Nondisplaced fractures or anatomically aligned fractures with no rotational malalignment can be treated with cast immobilization (Fig. 25-26). The cast should be worn for approximately 4 weeks, followed by a removable rigid splint in the same hand position with gentle active and active-assisted range of motion therapy for the wrist and digits. If treated nonoperatively, the patient should be reexamined within 7 days after initial splinting or cast application to detect any changes in alignment on radiograph and any clinical evidence of rotation malalignment. If the fracture does displace with more than 1 mm of shortening or any rotational malalignment, then open reduction internal fixation should be considered. Transverse fractures that are angulated and displaced should be reduced. Dorsal angulation of 10 degrees of the index and middle metacarpals can be tolerated and 20 degrees of angulation tolerated in the ring and little metacarpals. Initial excessive dorsal angulation which is accepted can result in a cosmetic deformity and palmar hand pain secondary to a prominently displaced metacarpal head — causing discomfort for the patient when gripping objects tightly (Fig. 25-27).

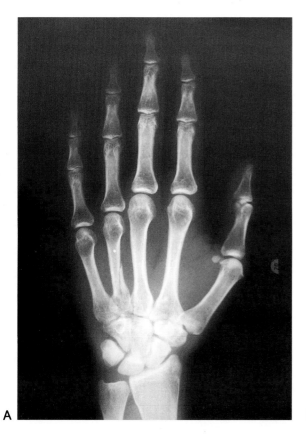 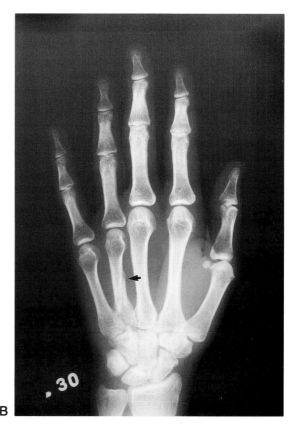

Figure 25-26 **(A)** AP-view radiograph of a stable oblique fracture of the ring metacarpal. **(B)** AP-view radiograph 6 weeks later showing maintenance of reduction and callus formation *(arrow)*. This was treated with a cast and resulted in an excellent clinical result.

Case Study IV

Metacarpal Fracture

J. H. is an 18-year-old high school football player who is 6 ft 4 in., 240 lb. He had received a full football scholarship to start college after his high-school graduation. In the summer that preceded his college entrance, while participating in a high-school All-Star Game, the patient sustained a transverse metacarpal fracture, as depicted in Figure 25-27. The patient had a clinically malrotated digit. There was also considerable concern about the ability of the patient to start his college career. An open reduction internal fixation of this metacarpal fracture was performed to correct and control his malrotation as well as to facilitate an early rehabilitation. Because of the rigid fixation, using plates and screws, the patient was able to return to football practice in 2 weeks and to full contact with a protective splint in 5 weeks. The patient was able to complete his freshman year in college football.

Rotational malalignment is an absolute indication for reduction, and frequently, open reduction internal fixation. Rotational abnormalities will be more easily demonstrated if the digits are in as much flexion as possible during the examination. Examination with the digits in extension often gives a false sense of security because the rotator malalignment will not be as readily detectable (particularly with spiral and oblique fractures). If these abnormalities are treated nonoperatively, they require especially close follow-up to detect alignment changes. If instability is detected and the reduction is inadequate, surgery is then indicated (Fig. 25-27).

Metacarpal fractures associated with significant soft tissue injury to the skin, subcutaneous tissue, and flexor or extensor tendons should be treated more aggressively with open reduction internal fixation to facilitate better treatment and rehabilitation of soft tissue injuries. The rehabilitation program designed to follow open reduction internal fixation of metacarpal fractures should be started immediately. Early mobilization will help to minimize the joint stiffness and tendon

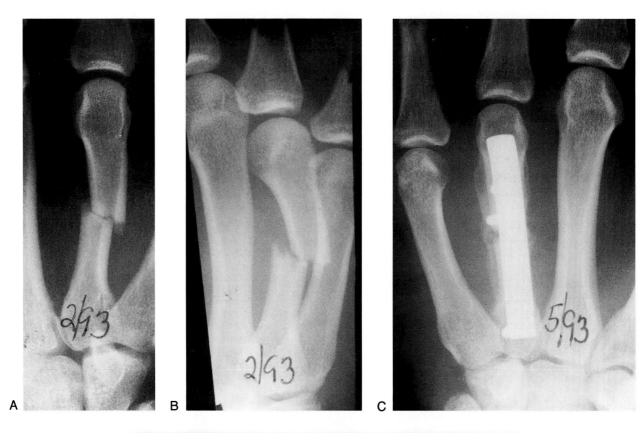

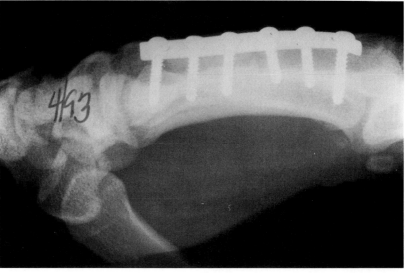

Figure 25-27 **(A)** AP-view radiograph of transverse minimally displaced and slightly malrotated fracture of the midshaft of the ring metacarpal. **(B)** Lateral-view radiograph showing the apex dorsal angulation of the fracture. This is secondary to the deforming forces as outlined in Figure 25-25. **(C)** AP-view radiograph following open reduction internal fixation with plates and screws. Patient has restoration of alignment and has gone on to heal. **(D)** Lateral-view radiograph showing the correction of the apex dorsal angulation with the internal fixation.

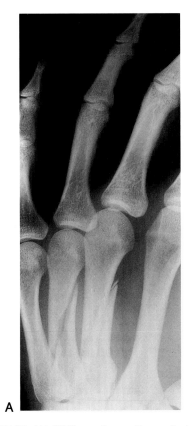 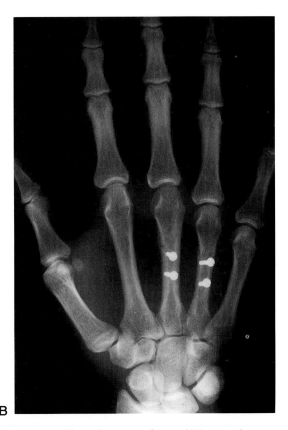

Figure 25-28 **(A)** Oblique-view radiograph showing long oblique fractures of the middle and ring metacarpals with displacement and malrotation. **(B)** AP-view radiograph showing open reduction internal fixation with screws, resulting in an anatomic alignment with rigid fixation, allowing early motion.

adhesions that commonly occur as a result of metacarpal fractures (Fig. 25-28).

Case Study V

Multiple Metacarpal Fractures

M.F. is a 27-year-old competitive ski racer who fell at high speed, sustaining multiple metacarpal fractures depicted in Figure 25-28. Radiographs showed long oblique fractures of the middle and ring metacarpals with some evidence of malrotation; this was also evident clinically with overlapping fingers. Because these fractures were felt to be unstable, there was a long-term concern about malrotation and overall hand function and a short-term concern about returning to competitive ski racing. A decision was made to fix the metacarpal fractures with interfragmentary screws (Fig. 25-28), which prevented the need for a postoperative cast. The patient had a protective splint fabricated to wear over his glove and was able to start skiing within 4 days following the

surgery. The patient had full range of motion within 7 days following the surgery.

Fixation of multiple metacarpal fractures stabilizes an unstable situation when multiple fractures are involved. This facilitates an earlier return to athletic activities and ensures proper alignment and diminishes problems with stiffness and decreased range of motion.

The initial rehabilitation consists of protective splinting (volar wrist splint with metacarpophalangeal block, but interphalangeals free), and gentle range of motion. Edema management is also initiated immediately postoperatively (see Ch. 2).

Metacarpal Neck Fractures

Fractures of the metacarpal neck generally result from impact loading of the metacarpal with the metacarpophalangeal joints flexed (e.g., a closed fist when punching) (Fig. 25-24). The metacarpophalangeal

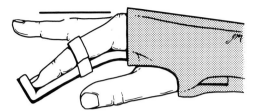

Figure 25-29 Short-arm cast with aluminum foam outrigger splint incorporated into the cast *(arrow),* mobilizing the metacarpophalangeal joint.

joint is displaced palmarly with the apex of angulation directed dorsally, and the fracture is usually impacted. The ring and little fingers are most commonly affected. Due to the overall mobility of the ring and little finger metacarpals, these fractures do well when treated non-operatively, can tolerate less than an anatomic alignment (maximum 20 to 30 degrees of angulation), and are best treated with an ulnar forearm cast and outrigger splint (Fig. 25-29). Similar fractures in the index and middle fingers do not do as well functionally with a less than anatomic alignment and should be carefully considered for open reduction internal fixation (maximum 10 degrees of angulation) (Fig. 25-30). Nondisplaced metacarpal neck fractures of the index and middle fingers and those with angulation less than 10 degrees can be treated with a simple forearm base splint or cast to the tip of the involved finger. Angulation greater than 10 degrees is an indication for reduction and possible open reduction internal fixation as seen on the lateral radiographic view. Angulation as much as 30 degrees can be tolerated in the little finger (the so-called boxer's fracture).

Since an excellent functional result can be obtained with a less than anatomic alignment, open reduction internal fixation is less often used in the treatment of thumb metacarpal extra-articular fractures. Reduction should be performed under hematoma infiltration or local anesthesia followed by a forearm base thumb spica cast for 4 to 6 weeks.

Intra-articular fractures at the base of the thumb require special consideration and are discussed in the

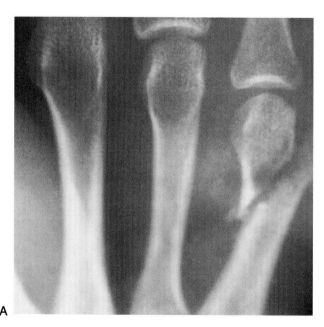

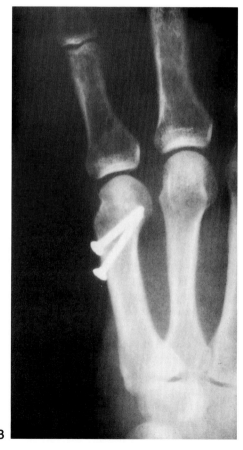

A   B

Figure 25-30 (A) AP-view radiograph of displaced fracture of the fifth metacarpal neck. **(B)** AP-view radiograph following open reduction internal fixation with screws.

Phalangeal Fractures

Fractures of the proximal and middle phalanges are relatively common injuries to the athlete in contact sports (e.g., football) and in those sports that require catching a ball (e.g., basketball, baseball). Occasionally, fractures occur when the athlete falls, such as in cycling, motor cross-racing, skiing, or gymnastics. Basic fracture treatment for these hand injuries is the same as those not associated with athletic activity. The goal of fracture treatment is to restore the normal anatomy and attain the most functional outcome. The patient's desire and need to return to competition may in certain circumstances influence the choice of treatment for these fractures. Intra-articular extension or rotational malalignment are relative indications for surgical intervention. This will facilitate not only fracture healing but a more predictable functional outcome (Fig. 25-23).

Phalangeal fractures are usually secondary to hyperextension or hyperabduction forces and often will involve the proximal interphalangeal or metacarpophalangeal joints. When these fractures are intra-articular,

section *Carpometacarpal dislocations.* As with all intra-articular fractures, fractures involving this area require anatomic alignment, restoration of a congruent joint, and careful rehabilitation.

one should be aware of the possibility of a fracture-dislocation at the time of injury and possible associated joint laxity.

Fractures of the proximal and middle phalanges will typically exhibit a characteristic deformity based on the deforming forces of the intrinsic and extrinsic musculature (Fig. 25-31). These deforming forces must be kept in mind when attempting to reduce these fractures (Fig. 25-32).

Middle Phalanx Fractures

Fractures of the middle phalanx can be treated using the same guidelines as those outlined for fractures of the metacarpal shaft. Often there is significant swelling and contusion of the soft tissue about the phalanx; thus, postfracture scarring of the intrinsic and extrinsic extensor apparatus is common, necessitating hand therapy after the fracture has stabilized in order to regain functional motion (see Ch. 2). It is also imperative that the fracture be realigned in the most anatomic configuration possible to prevent excessive motion limitation and malangulation of the digit. Any clinical malrotation of the digit is unacceptable. The digit should be examined in as much flexion as possible to elicit any malrotation, which implies an unstable fracture. If any malrotation is accepted initially, the digit will only increase its clinical malrotation and will not self-correct.

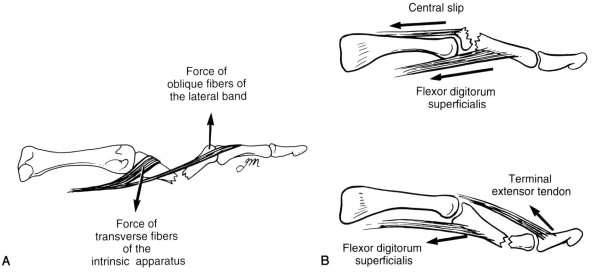

Figure 25-31 (A) Deforming forces of proximal phalanx fracture. The forces of the intrinsic apparatus cross the fracture site, causing an apex volar angulation seen on the lateral view. **(B)** Deforming forces of a middle phalanx fracture. **(Top)** The pull of the flexor digitorum superficialis tendon from the volar side and the central slip from the dorsal side cause an apex dorsal angulation of the middle phalanx fracture near its base. **(Bottom)** The fracture at the distal portion of the middle phalanx is apex volar via the pull of the flexor digitorum superficialis volarly and the terminal extensor tendon dorsally.

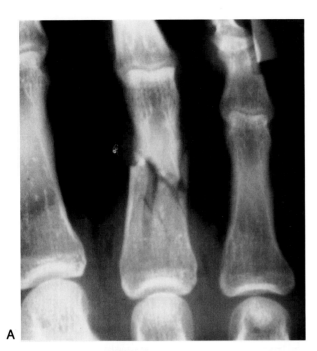

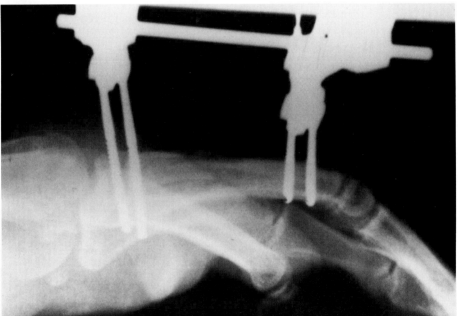

Figure 25-32 **(A)** AP-view radiograph of comminuted fracture of the proximal phalanx of the middle finger. **(B)** Lateral-view radiograph showing alignment after closed reduction and external fixation.

Nonintra-articular fractures without malrotation can be treated nonoperatively if the fracture malalignment is less than 2 mm. If the fracture, however, is intra-articular, anything less than an anatomic alignment is unacceptable. Any step-off of the articular surface will predispose the patient to developing a stiff, painful digit with a propensity for post-traumatic arthritis. The treatment goal for these fractures should be anatomic alignment of the particular surface and facilitation of early mobilization. Thus, any diastasis or step-off of the articular surface should be reduced (open or closed) and internally fixed (Fig. 25-33).

Case Study VI

Intra-articular Fracture Middle Phalanx

E.B. is a 21-year-old college basketball player who sustained an intra-articular fracture at the base of the middle phalanx; the finger sustained an axial load-type injury when struck by the ball (Fig. 25-33).

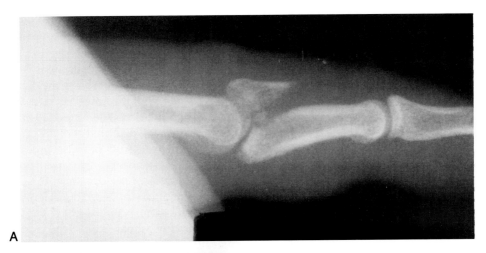

A

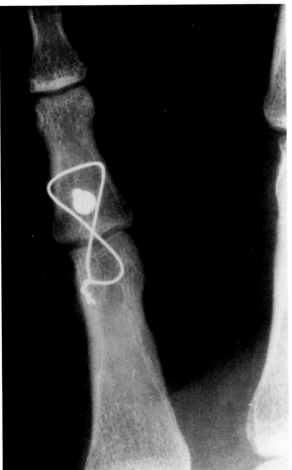

B

Figure 25-33 (A) Lateral-view radiograph of a displaced intra-articular fracture of the base of the middle phalanx with joint incongruency. **(B)** AP-view radiograph following open reduction internal fixation with a screw and tension band wiring.

This fracture, which involves the proximal interphalangeal joint, was very unstable. There was a definite step-off and incongruency of the joint requiring open reduction internal fixation, facilitating not only fracture healing and proper alignment but stabilizes the joint and minimizes the chances for post-

traumatic degenerative arthritis. The patient underwent immediate fixation of the fracture. With rigid fixation, therapy was started immediately consisting of supervised hand therapy three times a week plus a home program. Using a protective hand-based splint for the finger, the patient was able to begin shooting basketballs within the week. Because therapy was started immediately, functional range of motion was obtained quickly with minimal swelling. After 4 weeks, the patient continued to play with simple buddy taping.

This fracture is an unstable one, not successfully treated with nonoperative treatment. Fixation, such as described above, not only facilitates long-term functional recovery but in the short-term also facilitates early return to athletic activities.

Often, long oblique fractures of the middle phalanx will be unstable and will have a tendency to shorten and malrotate, requiring either open or closed reduction and percutaneous or internal fixation. This may be necessary to ensure proper alignment and facilitate early rehabilitation to minimize post-traumatic stiffness and an early return to athletic activities.

One fracture of the middle phalanx that should be highlighted is the commonly seen fracture of the palmar base (Fig. 25-12). This is an intra-articular fracture that results from either a hyperextension injury to the proximal interphalangeal joint and/or a dorsal dislocation/subluxation of the joint, and is typically seen in sports that require catching a ball (e.g., baseball, basketball). This injury of the distal insertion of the palmar plate acts as a palmar stabilizer of the proximal interphalangeal joint, preventing hyperextension. The fracture fragment is best seen on the lateral-view radiograph and is connected to the volar plate, thus making it an avulsion injury. If the fracture fragment involves less than 40 percent of the articular surface, the injury can often be treated nonoperatively. Due to the initial deforming forces in the dorsal dislocation, the reduced joint is more stable in flexion. Treatment should consist of early protected motion while maintaining a congruent joint, accomplished with a dorsal extension block splint (Fig. 25-13).

Unrestricted flexion, permitted with the dorsal extension block splint, will allow the proximal interphalangeal joint to flex, reapproximating the avulsed palmar plate. The initial position of the digit should be in the maximum amount of extension that still maintains a congruent proximal interphalangeal joint and should be documented with lateral-view radiographs. Subsequent management is outlined in detail in the subsection on unstable proximal interphalangeal joint injuries under *Ligamentous Injuries to the Proximal Interphalangeal Joint.*

These fracture dislocations may be associated with a soft tissue laceration on the volar surface of the digit, making it an open or compound fracture. These injuries should be treated with vigorous lavage, loose wound closure, and selected antibiotic treatment.

Proximal Phalanx Fractures

Fractures of the proximal phalanx can occur in a variety of geometric configurations (e.g., transverse, oblique, or spiral), predisposing the digit to angulation or shortening, with the potential for a clinically malrotated digit. If this malalignment is accepted, it may result in a rotated digit that is unacceptable to the athlete, not only in sports but also in activities of daily living. Pitchers who have had finger fractures note permanent changes in performance. It is imperative that the examination occur with the digit in as much flexion as possible, as the extended finger may mask malrotation. The functional hand has little tolerance for malrotated digits, and thus serves as an indication for surgical reduction and fixation.

If no malrotation is detected, a decision can then be made concerning surgical versus nonoperative treatment of the fracture based on the status of the soft tissues, any intra-articular extension of the fracture, or excessive angulation. The maximum amount of acceptable malalignment and fracture offset is the same as for the middle phalanx (see above) with the same indications for open reduction internal fixation (Fig. 25-34).

Fractures of the proximal phalanx tend to angulate because of the pull of the intrinsic tendons (Fig. 25-30). Similar fracture treatment guidelines are recommended for the proximal phalanx as for fractures of the metacarpal shaft. Because of the intimate association of the dorsal extensor apparatus over the dorsum of the proximal phalanx, proper treatment of these fractures is essential to minimize extensor adhesions and the stiff digit. Early mobilization and modality use will facilitate tendon gliding and maximize motion (see Ch. 2).

If the fracture is treated nonoperatively with reduction and cast immobilization, close follow-up must be maintained to recognize any loss of reduction or malrotation (Fig. 25-35). If the fracture proves to be unstable, it should be fixed surgically. Rigid stabilization with precise rotational control of the digit permits early mobilization and an earlier return to athletics.

Case Study VII

Malrotation Proximal Phalanx Osteotomy

B.B. is a 19-year-old martial artist who sustained a long oblique fracture of the proximal phalanx during competition. This fracture was treated nonoperatively with a closed reduction and a splint. The patient's fracture went on to heal, but a malrotated digit (Fig. 25-35) interfered with the patient's normal grip

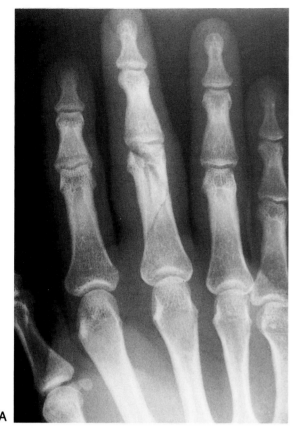
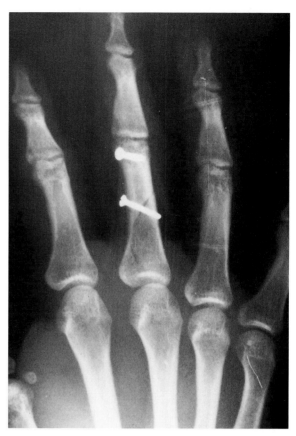

A   B

Figure 25-34 **(A)** AP-view radiograph of the comminuted intra-articular fracture of the proximal phalanx of the middle finger with extension into the proximal interphalangeal joint. **(B)** AP-view radiograph following open reduction and internal fixation, resulting in anatomic reduction and reconstitution of the proximal interphalangeal joint.

and also had an adverse effect on his performance. An osteotomy was subsequently performed to correct the malrotated digit. A derotation osteotomy can be performed either at the site of the fracture (here, in this case, the proximal phalanx) or proximally in the metacarpal. Osteotomy in the metacarpal has certain technical advantages with more predictable healing. A derotation osteotomy performed in the metacarpal and fixed rigidly with plate and screws, enabled the patient to start immediate therapy to maintain range of motion. A protective splint was worn for 1 month during practice. After 1 week, no splint was worn during activities of daily living, which facilitated therapy and return to function.

This case illustrates a problem that arises when a fracture is incurred in the phalanx, which is not recognized as unstable. Careful monitoring of phalangeal fractures is critical for early malrotated detection, as the finger has very little capacity to accommodate for malrotation. Malrotation is quite debilitating and is easier to correct prior to fracture

healing. When the fracture does heal, however, options are available such as those discussed here.

If the fracture is virtually (< 1 mm) anatomically aligned, continued nonoperative therapy is indicated. The immobilization should be with a forearm-based splint or cast with the affected digit immobilized to the tip of the involved finger, the metacarpophalangeal joint in 70 degrees of flexion with the interphalangeal joints extended to 0 degree. The cast should be maintained for approximately 4 weeks with supervised hand therapy instituted at that time. When hand therapy is initiated, protection will be provided by a thermoplastic hand-based resting splint (see Ch. 6), and a range of motion program will be initiated (see Ch. 2). Often an additional 4 weeks will be required for recuperation until the athlete can resume participation in the sport. Internal fixation of these fractures may allow mobilization often during the first postoperative week. This may minimize stiffness associated with prolonged immobilization and can result in an earlier return to activities.

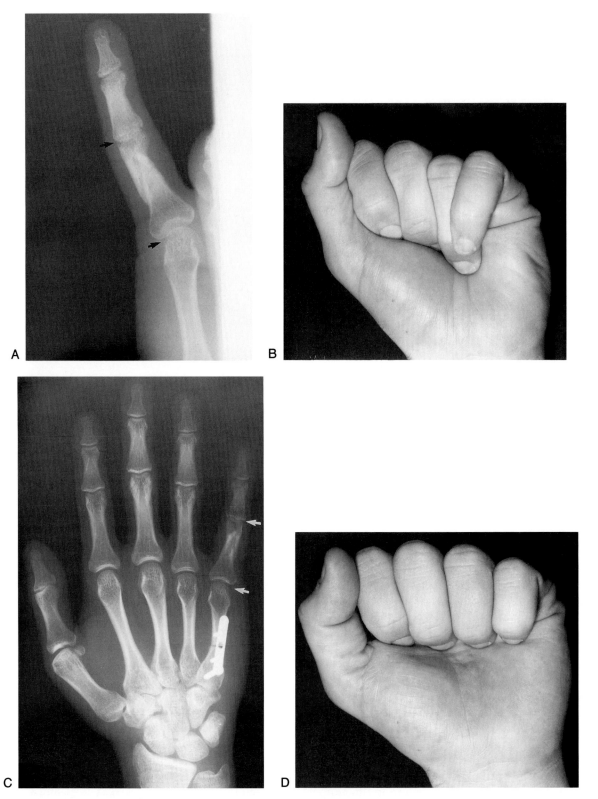

Figure 25-35 (A) AP-view radiograph of a malunited proximal phalanx fracture. There is a rotational deformity of this fracture. **(B)** Malrotation of the fracture exhibited in Fig. A with overlap of the little and ring fingers. **(C)** AP-view radiograph of rotational osteotomy of the metacarpal for correction of the malrotated proximal phalanx fracture. Following the rotation of the metacarpal to correct the clinical malalignment of the digit, one can see a more normal-appearing proximal phalanx, specifically the proximal interphalangeal and metacarpophalangeal joints. This is in contrast to the contours of the joint as seen in Fig. A, before osteotomy. **(D)** Postoperative clinical picture following healing of the osteotomy and correction of the malrotation.

DIGITAL TIP INJURIES

Although common in the general population, digital tip injuries are relatively uncommon in the athlete. These injuries are associated with a crushing type of mechanism secondary to the finger being stepped on (especially with spiked shoes or crushed between two helmets) or violent impact from a ball. As with all injuries to the digits, radiographic examination is necessary to evaluate the presence and extent of any fractures to the distal phalanx. (Fig. 25-36). A close clinical examination is also required to assess the function of the flexor and extensor tendons to the distal interphalangeal joint. Careful examination should be given to any

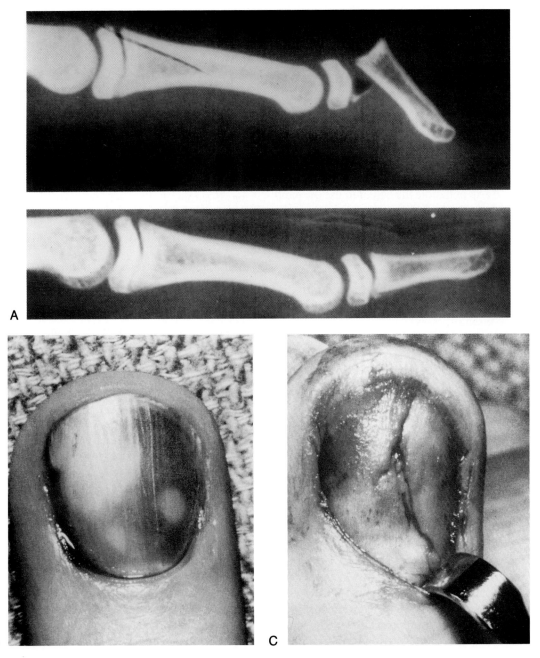

Figure 25-36 **(A)** Lateral-view radiograph of an injury to the tip of the index finger, following an axial load and crush injury. There is a marked dorsal displacement of the distal fragment into the nail matrix. The lower radiograph was done after reduction. **(B)** A subungual hematoma in the patient in Fig. A. This is highly suggestive of a matrix injury secondary to the displaced fracture and blunt trauma. **(C)** After removal of the nail, there is a stellate laceration of the matrix, requiring primary repair for normal nail growth.

subungual hematoma with digital tip crush injuries. Although discomfort secondary to a painful subungual hematoma can be relieved by perforating the nail plate, these injuries may require more extensive treatment. A subungual hematoma that compromises over 50 percent of the nail plate should be examined for a possible matrix laceration. The nail plate can be removed under digital block anesthesia to examine the matrix. Any lacerations should be repaired with fine, 6 or 7–0 absorbable sutures, since this enhances the chances of normal subsequent nail growth. Distal digital tip injuries can result in a loss of varying degrees of soft tissue. Loss of the pulp of 1 cm square or less may be treatable with dressing changes. Any soft tissue loss greater than 1 cm should be considered for possible soft tissue coverage, such as skin grafting or local or regional flap coverage.

Following an injury resulting in soft tissue loss at the fingertip, a common finding is hypersensitivity at the digit tip. Functionally, this may interfere with the athlete's ability to grip or handle the ball or to use the hand for related sports activity. This hypersensitivity can be treated with a structured desensitization program such as the three-phase program developed by the Downey Hand Center, Downey, California. This type of program is designed to bombard the sensitive area with noxious stimuli in order to raise the threshold for discomfort. Patient compliance is a key component of this rehabilitation program.

NEUROVASCULAR INJURIES IN THE ATHLETE

Neurovascular injuries in the athlete's hand occur most frequently secondary to repetitive compression and local blunt trauma. More traditional acute injuries to digital neurovascular structures can occur secondary to lacerations, more commonly seen in the general population (see Chs. 3 to 5).

Neurovascular injuries that are relevant to athletic activities will usually present after repetitive localized blunt trauma. For example, bowlers may complain of discomfort along the distribution of the ulna digital nerve of the thumb with subsequent distal paresthesias and alterations in sensation. This is known as bowler's thumb and is characterized by a perineural fibrosis of the ulna digital nerve secondary to chronic compression and irritation as the thumb rests in the hole of the ball (Fig. 25-37). This is initially treated with rest and a variable amount of time away from bowling until the patient is asymptomatic. Often a padded glove can be worn over the thumb with a more shallow thumb hole in the bowling ball. If this proves to be unsuccessful, then surgery may be indicated to neurolyse the ulnar

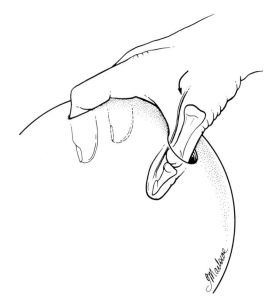

Figure 25-37 Compression of the ulnar digital nerve of the thumb from impingement against the thumb hole in bowling. If chronically irritated, this may result in a bowler's thumb.

digital nerve with resection of the neuroma incontinuity. The overall nerve is intact, but there is scarring between the fascicular bundles. The scar is dissected out under the operating microscope, leaving the overall nerve intact. The goal is maintenance of the nerve integrity to preserve sensation of the involved digit. This may not only restore sensation and reduce discomfort but allows for a return to bowling with diminished symptoms. Postoperatively, it is wise to have the patient use a small pad over the base of the thumb to cushion the thumb hole-thumb interface.

Case Study VIII

Bowler's Thumb

J.G. is a 33-year-old competitive bowler who bowls approximately four times a week. The patient noted discomfort in her thumb, limited to the portion that rested on the edge of the bowling ball thumbhole (Fig. 25-37). She also noted diminution of sensation in the distribution of the ulnar digital nerve of the thumb, with paresthesias in the same distribution when the tender spot on her thumb was palpated or bumped. In addition, she noticed a pea-sized tender mass in her thumb. On examination, she did have Tinel's sign along the ulnar digital nerve between the proximal and distal flexion creases of the thumb, representing a classic bowler's thumb, or a neuroma in continuity of the ulnar digital nerve.

The patient was brought to the operating room for an exploration of the area with the neuroma depicted in Figure 25-38. A microsurgical excision of the neuroma was performed with maintenance of the normal fascicles of the digital nerve. The patient retained her two-point discrimination in the distribution of the ulnar digital nerve. A padded splint was made to protect this area when she returned to bowling 2 weeks later. Often, patients will complain of discomfort in the thumb with no paresthesias and no palpable neuroma. A pad can be worn or the thumbhole can be slightly enlarged to decrease pressure in this area. If, however, the paresthesias persist and/or a neuroma is suspected with Tinel's sign or is palpable, then surgery is indicated.

Repetitive blunt trauma to the neurovascular bundles of the digits, especially the index finger, is seen in baseball players, (particularly catchers) due to repeated contusions from catching the baseball. The modern catcher's mitt is one with a minimal amount of padding to enable the catcher to catch one-handed to protect the throwing hand. This predisposes the catcher to repetitive trauma to the index finger's neurovascular bundles. This condition is also seen in handball players and in athletes who participate in the martial arts.

Athletes will complain of pain and cold intolerance in the digit. The trauma to the neurovascular bundle is at the level of the metacarpal head. Attempts at modifying the equipment by augmenting the padding will occasionally give some symptomatic relief. There has been some attempt to treat this condition with calcium channel blockers, as in the treatment of Raynaud's disease. If symptoms do not lessen, then the provocative activity should be discontinued to prevent a chronic problem. Digital artery sympathectomy, shown to have a beneficial effect in Raynaud's disease, has a theoretical indication in the athlete with this problem. Although the literature supports digital sympathectomy in Raynaud's disease, there has been no conclusive series on this treatment technique for repetitive blunt trauma to the neurovascular bundle in the athlete (see Chs. 3 to 5).

CARPAL TUNNEL SYNDROME

Carpal tunnel syndrome (compression of the median nerve at the wrist) is the most common peripheral nerve compression syndrome in the United States. Although not commonly seen in the athletic population, it may occur when athletes experience chronic repetitive, strenuous motion to their wrists, possibly causing tenosynovitis of the flexor tendons within the carpal tunnel. This may also lead to chronic ischemic changes in the median nerve, resulting in the symptoms of carpal tunnel syndrome. Patients will typically complain of discomfort in the hand and wrist with some discomfort and paresthesias in the median nerve distribution distally. Treatment should include rest, wrist splinting (with the wrist in a neutral position), and a trial of anti-inflammatory medication. If symptoms persist, then an injection of corticosteroid into the carpal tunnel may be considered and should be followed by wrist splinting for 48 hours and a gradual resumption of activities as symptoms permit. If this proves ineffective and symptoms do not diminish, then consideration should be given to decompression of the carpal tunnel by division of the transverse carpal ligament (see Chs. 3 and 4).

TRANSIENT ULNAR NERVE COMPRESSION

Transient ulnar nerve compression in the hand is becoming more of a recognized problem as the number of cyclists increase. Due to the relative extension of the wrist when resting on the handlebars, pressure is applied to the ulnar nerve at the level of Guyon's canal (Fig. 25-39). Over a long ride, cyclists should be encouraged to alter their hand positions to minimize

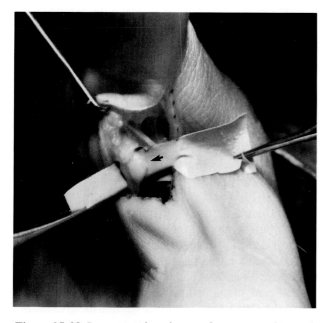

Figure 25-38 Intraoperative picture of a neuroma in continuity. Resection of this neuroma resulted in resolution of the patient's discomfort and maintenance of her distal thumb sensibility.

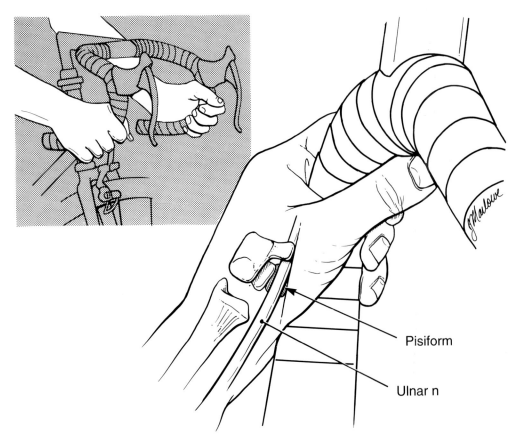

Figure 25-39 The mechanism of injury of chronic compression to the ulnar nerve of a cyclist. The ulnar nerve is impinged between the hook of the hamate, pisiform, and handlebars.

chronic compression. Numbness and paresthesias in the ulnar two digits usually go away within a few minutes or hours following cessation of riding. Occasionally, however, the numbness, which is secondary to transient ischemia to the ulnar nerve, can last for 2 weeks. The prognosis is good and treatment should be conservative. If the paresthesias have been persistent during this period, the patient should not cycle until the ulnar nerve has recovered. Despite the use of padded gloves, these symptoms may still occur. The cyclist should be reassured that, in the majority of cases, the symptoms will resolve with conservative care. If carpal tunnel or ulnar nerve compression symptoms continue for a month or longer, then neurometric studies (electromyogram-nerve conduction velocities) may be helpful to document the location and severity of the compression. It should be noted that some physicians do not wait for a month and order these studies immediately.

BLUNT TRAUMA TO THE ULNAR ARTERY

Repetitive blunt trauma to the hand, especially to the ulnar palm, may result in thrombosis or pseudoaneurysm formation of the ulnar artery. This condition can be the result of simple external repetitive contusion to the ulnar artery or direct injury from a fracture of the hook of the hamate. The athlete will often have pain and tenderness under the hypothenar eminence and may exhibit some cold intolerance. Physical examination usually will elicit pain and tenderness between the hook of the hamate and the pisiform bones and should always include the Allen test to determine the completeness of the superficial and deep palmar arches. The Allen test is performed by having the patient repeatedly clench and unclench his fist as the examiner digitally occludes the radial and ulnar arteries. After this has been done a number of times by the patient and the arteries are occluded, the hand will be pale. The pressure over the ulnar artery is then removed while maintaining occlusion of the radial artery. At this point, the capillary fill of the little finger and the thumb are assessed. If the little finger and the thumb have good capillary fill while the ulnar artery is free and the radial artery is occluded, then one can assume that the ulnar artery, which makes up the superficial palmar arch, will supply not only the little finger but the entire hand, including the thumb. The same technique is repeated a second time, except the radial artery and not the ulnar artery is released, and the same capillary fills in the thumb and the little finger. When the radial artery is decompressed while maintaining occlusion of the ulnar artery, there is expected capillary fill into the thumb, but, if there is continuing capillary fill across the hand into the little finger, then the radial artery is patent, and there is a complete arch allowing flow to proceed across the entire hand from the thumb to the little finger.

If pathology to the ulnar artery in the hand is suspected, Doppler studies and digital plethysmography should be performed (see Ch. 5). Consideration can be given to arteriography of the hand to further delineate the pathologic anatomy. If thrombosis or pseudoaneurysm formation of the ulnar artery is diagnosed, surgery is usually indicated. Operative care consists of either resection of the involved portion of the ulnar artery and ligation if the vascularity of the hand is not compromised or reconstruction with an interpositional vein graft.

Case Study IX

Ulnar Artery Pseudoaneurysm

R.K. is a 36-year-old competitive handball player, who plays five times a week and is actively competing in regional and national tournaments. Pain developed in the palm of the patient's hand, with occasional paresthesias in the ulnar nerve distribution as well as some feeling of weakness in his pinch and grip. The examination at the time of presentation showed a focused, tender area just ulnar to the hook of the hamate in his palm. He also had a mildly positive Tinel's sign. The intrinsic muscles in his hand were slightly weakened. It was thought that this may represent some possible pathology to the ulnar nerve. Because of the nature of his sport, with repetitive blunt trauma to this area, in addition to his symptoms involving both the motor and sensory portions of the ulnar nerve, it was believed that a possible pseudoaneurysm formation of the ulnar ar-

tery could be the primary problem. Angiography was obtained, which showed a classic pseudoaneurysm (Fig. 25-40). The patient had a negative Allen test, suggesting that he had a complete arch in his hand and had an adequate vascular supply to the entire hand from both the ulnar and radial arteries. At exploration, a large pseudoaneurysm was detected (Fig. 25-40) and excised. The ulnar artery in this region often is tortuous and an adequate length was obtained to allow a primary end-to-end anastomosis without the need for a vein graft.

SPECIAL CONSIDERATIONS IN THE JUVENILE AND ADOLESCENT ATHLETE

The skeletally immature athlete is susceptible to many of the injuries outlined in this chapter. However, due to the open physis, fewer pure ligamentous injuries are seen, and there is an increased incidence of fractures, especially involving the physis. It is critical that radiographs be obtained in the skeletally immature athlete. Classic ligamentous and tendon avulsion injuries in the adult, which are often unremarkable on radiographic examination, will show various types of fractures involving the physis in the skeletally immature (see Ch. 8) (Fig. 25-41).

SPECIAL CONDITIONS

Human Bite

In sports that involve contact, there will invariably be instances of human bites to the hand. These bites are usually secondary to an altercation during the contest or an accidental impaction of the hand against an opponent's tooth. These injuries, although initially unimpressive in terms of wound size (Fig. 25-42), can be devastating if inadequately treated, and can result in significant and serious infection, leading to loss of hand function and prolonged time away from participation. Any human bite wounds to the hand should be treated promptly. The hand should be evaluated in the clinic or emergency room immediately for wound assessment and proper treatment. If there is any delay in getting to the treatment center, the hand should be washed with a mild soap and water solution and rinsed thoroughly with running water. A dressing can then be placed over the wound and the patient can be transported to the health care facility for definitive treatment. The most common location is over the dorsum of the hand near

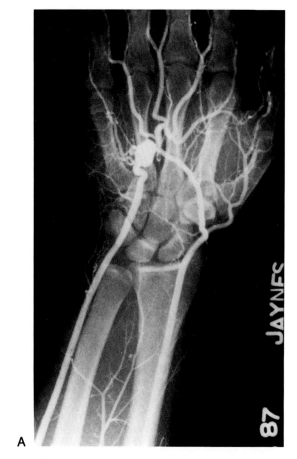 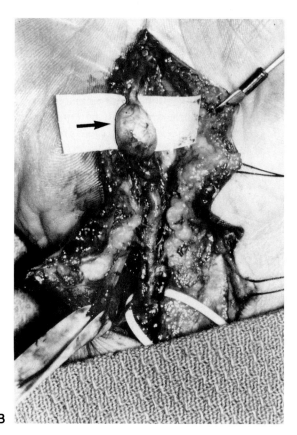

Figure 25-40 **(A)** AP-view radiograph of an angiogram showing a pseudoaneurysm formation of the ulnar artery in Guyon's canal. **(B)** Intraoperative photograph of the pseudoaneurysm of the ulnar artery as depicted in Fig. A. This was resected with complete resolution of the patient's symptoms.

the metacarpophalangeal joint. There may be associated extensor tendon trauma, which must be treated with primary repair, despite the open nature of the wound.

The most important determination is whether the wound is intra- or extra-articular relative to the metacarpophalangeal joint. An intra-articular inoculation of human oral flora can result in a severe septic arthritis, which needs to be treated aggressively with surgical incision, drainage, and antibiotics to minimize articular joint damage. The threshold for surgical debridement and lavage should be quite low. The wound will often have to be extended for adequate exposure and lavage.

Radiographs should be obtained to rule out foreign bodies, associated fractures, and air within the joint (an indication of intra-articular extension). Prior to extensive lavage, the patient should be updated (if necessary) with tetanus toxoid. *Staphylococcus* and anaerobic bacteria, especially *Eikenella corrodens,* are the usual

pathologic organisms; thus, the patient should be prophylactically treated with a cephalosporin and penicillin for 7 to 10 days.

If inspection of the wound shows evidence of intra-articular extension or damage to the extensor apparatus, the patient should undergo surgery for definite repair, debridement, and lavage. For a small puncture or laceration not involving the joint and with no associated structural damage, vigorous lavage within the emergency department and outpatient treatment with antibiotics is appropriate. Close follow-up is necessary in all of these patients to ensure that any infection is under control, and patients should be splinted in a position of rest (a thermoplastic splint with the hand positioned as follows: wrist, 30-degree extension; metacarpophalangeal joints, 70-degree flexion; and interphalangeal joints, neutral) until there is no evidence of infection. After the infection has been controlled, hand therapy should be started to regain motion and function. In addition, active and active-assisted range of

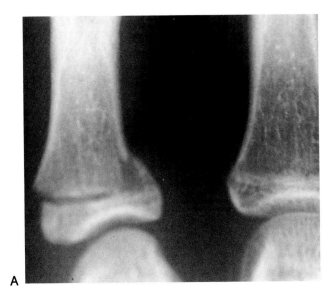

A

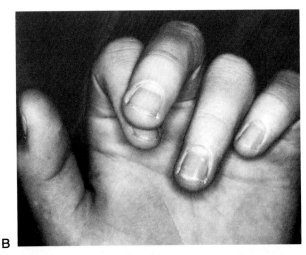

B

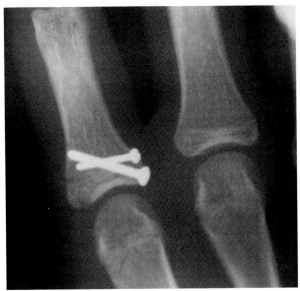

C

Figure 25-41 (A) AP-view radiograph of a displaced Salter-Harris group III fracture of the base of the proximal phalanx of the index finger. (B) Clinical photograph of the patient in Fig. A with a malrotation of the index finger manifested by the crisscrossing of the index and middle fingers. (C) AP-view radiograph following open reduction internal fixation to correct malrotation, resulting in correction of the clinical malrotation.

Figure 25-42 Clinical photograph of a typical wound over the long finger metacarpophalangeal joint secondary to a human bite sustained in an altercation. Frequently, this injury requires surgical incision and drainage, followed by a course of intravenous antibiotics.

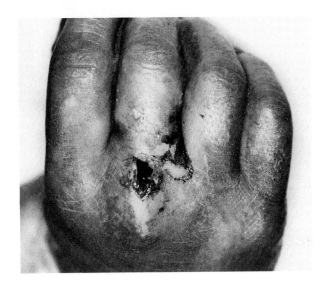

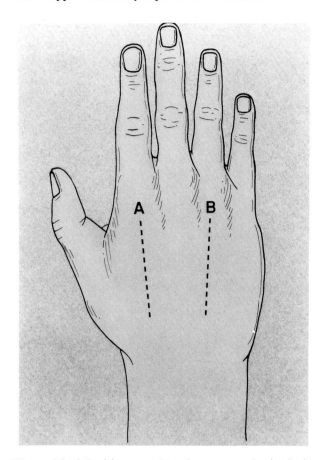

Figure 25-43 Incisions used to decompress the intrinsic compartments of the hand. This is done through two incisions labeled *A* and *B*.

motion exercises should be encouraged to facilitate tendon gliding. Any human bite wound treated in the outpatient setting, which then progresses to suppuration or abscess formation, should be brought to the operating room for definitive incision, drainage, and debridement.

Compartment Syndromes

Compartment syndromes do occur in the hand. As in the lower extremity, exercise-associated dynamic compartment syndromes can develop after chronic, repetitive, and strenuous use. A compartment syndrome should be considered if the athlete is complaining of chronic pain in any of the intrinsic hand compartments, without identifiable structural damage associated with chronic repetitive use. Diagnosis of these dynamic compartment syndromes can be made with indwelling wick-type catheters, which can measure intracompartmental pressures during exercise. If an increase in pressure is documented, then decompression of the compartment is indicated.

More commonly, however, compartment syndromes in the hand occur after trauma. Fractures associated with soft tissue injuries can lead to hemorrhage and edema within a compartment, resulting in a compartment syndrome. Compartment pressures can be measured as in the lower extremity. If a compartment syndrome is suspected clinically, the compartments

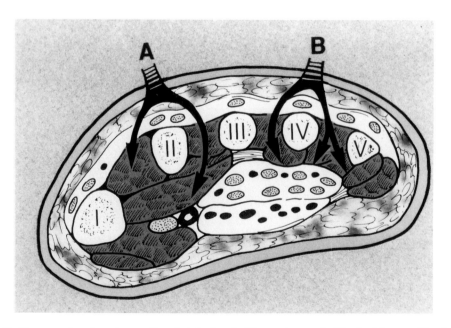

Figure 25-44 Cross-sectional anatomy of hand at the level of the metacarpals. The incisions outlined are labeled *A* and *B*. Through these two incisions, the compartments between all five metacarpals are approached and decompressed.

should be surgically decompressed immediately. Compartments of the hand are illustrated in Figures 25-43 and 25-44.

SUGGESTED READINGS

Mallet Finger

Stark H et al: Operative treatment of intraarticular fractures of the dorsal aspect of the distal phalanx of digits. J Bone Joint Surg [Am] 69:892, 1987

Stern P, Kastrup J: Complications and prognosis of treatment of mallet finger. J Hand Surg 13A: 329, 1988

Wehbe M, Schneider L: Mallet fractures. J Bone Joint Surg [Am] 66:658, 1984

Boutonniere Deformity

Elso R: Rupture of the central slip of the extensor hood of the finger: a test for early diagnosis. J Bone Joint Surg [Br] 68:229, 1986

McCue F et al: Athletic injuries of the proximal interphalangeal joint requiring surgical treatment. J Bone Joint Surg [Am] 52:937, 1970

Souter W: The Boutonniere deformity: a review of 101 patients with division of the central slip of the extensor expansion of the fingers. J Bone Joint Surg [Br] 49:710, 1967

Flexor Digitorum Profundus Avulsion

Bynum D, Gilbert J: Avulsion of the flexor digitorum profundus: Anatomic and biomechanical considerations. J Hand Surg 13A:222, 1988

Chang W et al: Avulsion injury of the long flexor tendons. Plastic Reconst Surg 50:260, 1972

Leddy J, Packer J: Avulsion of the profundus tendon insertion in athletes. J Hand Surg 2:66, 1977

Manske PR, Lesker PA: Avulsion of the ring finger digitorum profundus tendon: an experimental study. Hand 10:52, 1978

Proximal Interphalangeal Joint

Baugher W, McCue F: Anterior fracture-dislocation of the proximal interphalangeal joint: a case report. J Bone Joint Surg 61A:779, 1979

McCue FC, Andrews JR, Hakala M et al: The coaches finger. J Sports Med 2:270, 1974

McCue FC, Baugher WH, Bourland W et al: Hand injuries in athletes. Surg Rounds 1:8, 1978

McCue FC, Baugher WH, Kulund DN et al: Hand and wrist injuries in the athlete. Am J Sports Med 7:275, 1978

McElfresh E et al: Management of fracture-dislocation of the proximal interphalangeal joints by extension block splinting. J Bone Joint Surg [Am] 54A:1705, 1972

Peimer C et al: Palmar dislocation of the proximal interphalangeal joint. J Hand Surg 9A:39, 1984

Rodriguez AL: Injuries to the collateral ligaments of the proximal interphalangeal joints. Hand 5:55, 1973

Distal Interphalangeal Joint

Palmer A, Linscheid R: Irreducible dorsal dislocation of the proximal interphalangeal joint of the finger. J Hand Surg 3:95, 1978

Metacarpophalangeal Joint Dislocation

Becton J et al: A simplified technique for treating complex dislocation of the index metacarpophalangeal joint. J Bone Joint Surg 57A:699, 1975

Cunningham D, Schwartz G: Dorsal dislocation of the index metacarpophalangeal joint. Plastic Reconst Surg 56:654, 1975

Green D, Terry G: Complex dislocation of the metacarpophalangeal joint: correlative pathological anatomy. J Bone Joint Surg [Am] 55:1480, 1973

May J et al: Closed complex dorsal dislocation of the middle finger metacarpophalangeal joint: anatomic considerations and treatment. Plastic Reconst Surg 82:690, 1988

Carpometacarpal Joint Dislocation

Bora F, Didizian NH: The treatment of injuries to the carpometacarpal joint of the little finger. J Bone Joint Surg [Am] 56:1459, 1974

Carroll R, Carlson E: Diagnosis and treatment of injury to the second and third carpometacarpal joints. J Hand Surg 14A:102, 1989

Henderson J, Arafa M: Carpometacarpal dislocation. An easily missed diagnosis. J Bone Joint Surg [Br] 69:212, 1987

Gamekeeper's Thumb

Bowers W, Hurst L: Gamekeeper's thumb. Evaluation by arthrography and stress roentgenography. J Bone Joint Surg [Am] 59:419, 1977

Camp R et al: Chronic posttraumatic radial instability of the thumb metacarpophalangeal joint. J Hand Surg 5:221, 1980

Coonrad R, Goldner J: A study of the pathological findings and treatment in soft-tissue injury of the thumb metacarpophalangeal joint: with a clinical study of the normal range of motion in 1000 thumbs and a study of postmortem findings of ligamentous structures in relation to function. J Bone Joint Surg [Am] 51:1291, 1969

Louis D et al: Rupture and displacement of the ulnar collateral ligament of the metacarpophalangeal joint of the thumb. J Bone Joint Surg [Am] 68:1320, 1986

McCue MW, Andrews JR et al: Ulnar collateral ligament injuries of the thumb in athletes. J Sports Med 2:70, 1974

Stener B: Displacement of the ruptured ulnar collateral ligament of the metacarpal phalangeal joint of the thumb: a clinical and anatomic study. J Bone Joint Surg [Br] 44:869, 1962

Metacarpal Fractures

Burkhalter W: Closed treatment of hand fractures. J Hand Surg 14A:390, 1989

Gross M, Gelberman R: Metacarpal rotational osteotomy. J Hand Surg 10A:105, 1985

Hall R: Treatment of metacarpal and phalangeal fractures in noncompliant patients. Clin Orthop 214:31, 1987

Hastings H: Unstable metacarpal and phalangeal fracture treatment with screws and plates. Clin Orthop 214:37, 1987

Hunter J, Cowen N: Fifth metacarpal fractures in a compensation clinic population: a report of one hundred thirty-three cases. J Bone Joint Surg [Am]52:1159, 1970

Viegas S et al: Functional bracing of fractures of the second through fifth metacarpals. J Hand Surg 12A:139, 1985

Middle Phalanx Fractures

Hastings H: Unstable metacarpal and phalangeal fracture treatment with screws and plates. Clin Orthop 214:37, 1987

Huffaker H et al: Factors influencing final range of motion in the fingers after fractures of the hand. Plastic Reconst Surg 63:82, 1979

Proximal Phalanx Fractures

Belsky MP, Eaton RG, Labe LB: Closed reduction and internal fixation of proximal phalangeal fractures. J Hand Surg 9A:725, 1984

Bilos Z, Eskestrand T: External fixator use in comminuted gunshot fractures of the proximal phalanx. J Hand Surg 4:357, 1979

Burkhalter W: Closed treatment of hand fractures. J Hand Surg 14A:390, 1989

Green DP, Anderson JR: Closed reduction and percutaneous pin fixation of fractured phalanges. J Bone Joint Surg [Am] 55:1643, 1973

Hastings H: Unstable metacarpal and phalangeal fracture treatment with screws and plates. Clin Orthop 214:37, 1987

Mansoor I: Fractures of the proximal phalanx of fingers: a method of reduction. J Bone Joint Surg [Am] 51:1196, 1969

McCue F et al: Athletic injuries of the proximal interphalangeal joint requiring surgical treatment. J Bone Joint Surg [Am] 52:937, 1970

Reyes F, Latta L: Conservative management of difficult phalangeal fractures. Clin Orthop 214:23, 1987

Weckesser E: Rotational osteotomy of the metacarpal for overlapping fingers. J Bone Joint Surg [Am] 47:751, 1965

Widgerow A et al: An analysis of proximal phalangeal fractures. J Hand Surg 12A:134, 1987

Digital Tip Injuries

Beasley R: Fingernail injuries. J Hand Surg 8:784, 1983

Engber W, Clancy W: Traumatic avulsion of the fingernail associated with injury to the phalangeal epyphyseal plate. J Bone Joint Surg 60:713, 1978

Kleinert H et al: The deformed fingernail, a frequent result of failure to repair nail bed injuries. J Trauma 7:176, 1967

Seymour N: Juxta-epiphyseal fracture of the terminal phalanx of the finger. J Bone Joint Surg [Br] 48:347, 1966

Zook E et al: Anatomy and physiology of the perionychium: a review of the literature and anatomic study. J Hand Surg 5:528, 1980

Bowler's Thumb

Dobyns J et al: Bowler's thumb: diagnosis and treatment: a review of seventeen cases. J Bone Joint Surg [Am] 54:7515, 1972

Carpal Tunnel Syndrome

Gelberman R et al: The carpal tunnel syndrome. A study of carpal canal pressures. J Bone Joint Surg [Am] 63:380, 1981

Gellman H et al: Carpal tunnel syndrome. An evaluation of the provocative diagnostic tests. J Bone Joint Surg [Am] 68:735, 1986

Modaver J: Tinel's sign. Its characteristics and significance. J Bone Joint Surg [Am] 60:412, 1978

Pfeffer G et al: The history of carpal tunnel. J Hand Surg 13B:28, 1988

Phalen G: The carpal tunnel syndrome: seventeen years' experience in diagnosis and treatment of 654 hands. J Bone Joint Surg [Am] 48:211, 1966

Seiler J et al: Intraoperative assessment of median nerve blood flow during carpal tunnel release with laser Doppler flowmetry. J Hand Surg 14A:986, 1989

Ulnar Nerve Compression

Kleinert H, Hayes J: The ulnar tunnel syndrome. Plastic Reconst Surg 47:21, 1971

Shea J, McClain E: Ulnar nerve compression syndromes at and below the wrist. J Bone Joint Surg [Am] 51:1095, 1969

Uriburu I et al: Compression syndrome of the deep motor branch of the ulnar nerve (pisohamate hiatus syndrome). J Bone Joint Surg [Am] 58:145, 1976

Ulnar Artery Compression

Conn J et al: Hypothenar hammer syndrome: posttraumatic digital ischemia. Surgery 68:1122, 1970

Green D: True and false traumatic aneurysms in the hand: report of two cases and review of the literature. J Bone Joint Surg [Am] 55:120, 1973

Kalisman M et al: Ulnar nerve compression secondary to ulnar artery false aneurysm at the Guyon's canal. J Hand Surg 7:137, 1982

Kleinert H et al: Aneurysms of the hand. Arch Surg 106:554, 1973

May J et al: Cyanotic painful index and long fingers associated with an asymptomatic ulnar artery aneurysm: case report. J Hand Surg 7:622, 1982

Compartment Syndrome

Imbriglia J, Boland D: An exercise-induced compartment syndrome of the dorsal forearm: a case report. J Hand Surg 9A:142, 1984

Phillips J et al: Exercise-induced chronic compartment syndrome of the first dorsal interosseous muscle of the hand: a case report. J Hand Surg 11A:124, 1986

Sarokhan A, Eaton R: Volkmann's ischemia. J Hand Surg 8:806, 1983

Spinner M et al: Impending ischemic contracture of the hand: early diagnosis and management. Plastic Reconst Surg 50:341, 1972

Juvenile Athlete

Andrish JT: Upper extremity injuries in the skeletally immature athlete. p. 675. In Nicholas JA, Hershman EB (eds): The Upper Extremity in Sports Medicine. CV Mosby, St. Louis, 1990

Burton RI, Eaton RG: Common hand injuries in the athlete. Orthop Clin North Am 4:809, 1973

Emans JB: Upper extremity injuries in sports. p. 46. Micheliaj N (ed): Pediatric and adolescence sports medicine. Little Brown, Boston, 1984

Garrick JG, Requa RK: Injuries in high school sports. Pediatrics 61:465, 1978

Hastings H, Simmons BP: Hand fractures in children. Clin Orthop 188:120, 1984

Figure and
Table Acknowledgments

Table 2-1 from Robbins SL: Inflammation and repair. In Cotran RS, Kumar V, Robbins SL (eds): Pathologic Basis of Disease. 4th Ed. WB Saunders, Philadelphia, 1989, with permission.

Figure 2-1 from, and Table 2-2 adapted from Pappas AM: Rehabilitation. p. 196. In Dyment PG (ed): Sports Medicine: Health Care for Young Athletes. 2nd Ed. American Academy of Pediatrics, Elk Grove Village, IL, 1991, with permission.

Table 2-3 from Flynn JE, Graham JH: The role of tendon in healing with primary repair of tendon transplants. p. 211. In Jupiter JB (ed): Flynn's Hand Surgery. Williams & Wilkins, Baltimore, 1991, with permission.

Table 2-4 adapted from Dyment PG: Rehabilitation. p. 196. In Dyment PG (ed): Sports Medicine: Health Care for Young Athletes. 2nd Ed. American Academy of Pediatrics, Elk Grove Village, IL, 1991, with permission.

Figure 2-5 adapted from Dyment PG: Rehabilitation. p. 196. In Dyment PG (ed): Sports Medicine: Health Care for Young Athletes. 2nd Ed. American Academy of Pediatrics, Elk Grove Village, IL, 1991, with permission.

Figure 2-9 from Lehman JF, deLateur BJ: Therapeutic heat. pp. 611–612. In Lehmann JF (ed): Therapeutic Heat and Cold. 4th Ed. Williams & Wilkins, Baltimore, 1990, with permission.

Figure 3-1 modified from Asbury AK, Johnson PC (eds): In Pathology of Peripheral Nerve: Basic Pathologic Mecha-nisms, Ch. 3. p. 50. WB Saunders, Philadelphia, 1978, with permission.

Figure 5-3 from Rohrer MJ, Cardullo PA, Pappas AM et al: Axillary artery compression of thrombosis in throwing athletes. J Vasc Surg 11:761, 1990, with permission.

Figure 6-2A courtesy of Boston Brace International, Inc.

Figure 6-2B courtesy of Medco Supply Company.

Figure 7-3 courtesy of Sports and Spokes.

Figures 8-6, 8-23, 8-24, 8-29, 8-30, 8-31, and 8-32 from, and Table 8-1 adapted from, Pappas AM: Elbow problems associated with baseball during childhood and adolescence. Clin Orthop 164:30, 1982, with permission.

Figure 8-2 adapted from Pappas AM: Elbow problems associated with baseball during childhood and adolescence. Clin Orthop 164:30, 1982, with permission.

Portions of chapter 9 text adapted from Pappas AM: Biomechanics of baseball pitching. Am J Sports Med 13:216, 1985, and from Pappas AM: Injuries of the shoulder complex and overhand throwing problems. In Grana WA, Kalenak A (eds): Athletic Injuries. WB Saunders, Philadelphia, 1991, with permission.

Figure 9-3 from Perry J: Biomechanics of the shoulder. p. 1. In Rowe CR (ed): The Shoulder. Churchill Livingstone, New York, 1988, with permission.

Figure 9-4 from Rockwood CA, Young DC: Disorders of the acromoclavicular joint. p. 413. In Rockwood CA, Matsen FA (eds): The Shoulder. WB Saunders, Philadelphia, 1990, with permission.

Figure 9-5 from Pappas AM, Goss TP, Kleinman PK: Symptomatic shoulder instability due to lesions of the glenoid labrum. Am J Sports Med 11:279, 1983, with permission.

Figures 9-6A from Ferner H, Staubesand J (eds.): Sobotta Atlas of Human Anatomy, Vol I: Head, Neck, Upper Extremities. p. 311. Urban & Schwarzenberg, Baltimore, 1983, with permission

Figures 9-6B from Prodromos CC, Ferry JA, Schiller AL et al: Histological studies of the glenoid labrum from fetal life to old age. JBJS 72A(9):1344, October 1990, with permission.

Figure 9-7 from Ferrari DA: Capsular ligaments of the shoulder: anatomical and functional study of the anterior superior capsule. Am J Sports Med 18:20, 1990, with permission.

Figures 9-11, 9-19, and 9-24 from Pappas AM, Zawacki RM, McCarthy CF: Rehabilitation of the pitching shoulder. Am J Sports Med 13:223, 1985, with permission.

Figures 9-16A, B, C from Pappas AM, Zawacki RM, Sullivan TJ: Biomechanics of baseball pitching: A preliminary report. Am J Sports Med 13:216, 1985, with permission.

Figures 9-16D from Pappas AM: Injuries of the shoulder complex and overhand throwing problems. In Grana WA, Kalenah A (eds): Athletic Injuries. WB Saunders, Philadelphia, 1991, with permission.

Figure 9-20 from Sports Illustrated.

Table 10-1 from Hawkins RJ, Bokor DJ: Clinical evaluation of shoulder problems. p. 149. In Rockwood CA, Matsen FA (eds): The Shoulder. WB Saunders, Philadelphia, 1993, with permission.

Appendix 10-1 from Kendall FP, McCreary EK, Provance PG: Lower extremity strength test. p. 177. In Muscles: Testing and Function. 4th Ed. Williams & Wilkins, Baltimore, 1993, with permission.

Figure 10-2 from U.S Public Health Service, Agency for Health Care Policy and Research, Dept. of Health and Human Services: Acute Pain Management: Operative or Medical Procedures and Trauma; Methods for Pain Assessment. p. 113, February 1992.

Figure 10-10 from Pappas AM, Zawacki RM, McCarthy CF: Rehabilitation of the pitching shoulder. Am J Sports Med 13:223, 1985, with permission.

Figures 11-12 and 11-15 from Neer CS: Dislocations. p. 273. In Neer CS (ed): Shoulder Reconstruction. WB Saunders, Philadelphia, 1990, with permission.

Figures 14-1 and 14-2 from Rockwood CA: Disorders of the Aurerioclavicular Joint. p. 413. In Rockwood CA, Young DC (eds): The Shoulder Vol. I. WB Saunders, Philadelphia, 1990, with permission.

Figure 14-4 from Rockwood CA: Disorders of the Aurerioclavicular Joint. p. 413. In Rockwood CA, Young DC (eds): The Shoulder Vol. I. WB Saunders, Philadelphia, 1990, with permission.

Figures 14-5, 14-14, 14-15, 14-16, and 14-17 from Goss TP: Double disruptions of the superior shoulder suspensory complex. J Orthop Trauma 7:99, 1993, with permission.

Figure 14-9 from Neer CS: Dislocations, p. 273. In Neer CS: Shoulder Reconstruction. WB Saunders, Philadelphia, 1990, with permission.

Figure 14-18 from Post M: Dislocations of the Shoulder, p. 518. In Post M (ed.): The Shoulder. Surgical and Nonsurgical Management. 2nd ed. Lea & Febiger, Philadelphia, 1988, with permission.

Figure 14-19 from Rockwood CA: Disorders of the Sternoclavicular Joint, p. 477. In Rockwood CA, Matsen FA (eds.): The Shoulder Vol. I. WB Saunders, Philadelphia, 1990, with permission.

Figure 15-12 from Goss TP: Fractures of the glenoid cavity (current concepts review). J Bone Joint Surg Am 74A:299, 1992, with permission.

Figures 15-4, 15-5, and 15-18 from Goss TP: Double disruptions of the superior shoulder suspensory complex. J Orthop Trauma 7:99, 1993, with permission.

Figures 15-10 and 15-11 from Goss TP: Fractures of the glenoid neck. J Shoulder Elbow Surg 3:42, 1994, with permission.

Figures 15-15 and 15-16 from Goss TP: Fractures of the glenoid cavity: operative principles and techniques. Techniques Orthop 8:199, 1994, with permission.

Figures 15-1, 15-3, 15-9, 15-20, 15-21, 15-22, 15-23 from Neer CS: Fractures, p. 363. In Neer CS: Shoulder Reconstruction, WB Saunders, Philadelphia, 1993, with permission.

Figure 15-24 from Rowe CR, Colville M: The glenohumeral joint. p. 331. In Rowe CR (ed): The Shoulder. Churchill Livingstone, New York, 1988, with permission.

Figures 17-1 and 17-3 from Henry AK: Extensile Exposure. 2nd Ed. Williams & Wilkins, Baltimore, 1966, with permission.

Figure 17-4 from Anson BJ, McVay CB: Surgical Anatomy Vol. 2, 5th Ed. WB Saunders, Philadelphia, 1971, with permission.

Figures 17-5, 17-6, 17-11, and 17-17 from Morrey BF (ed): The Elbow and Its Disorders. 2nd Ed. WB Saunders, Philadelphia, 1993, with permission.

Figures 17-7 from Anderson TE: Anatomy and Physical Examination of the Elbow, p. 273. In: Nicholas JA, Hershman EB (eds.): The Upper Extremity in Sports Medicine. CV Mosby, St. Louis, 1990, with permission.

Figure 17-8 from Anderson TE: Anatomy and Physical Examination of the Elbow, p. 273. In: Nicholas JA, Hershman EB (eds.): The Upper Extremity in Sports Medicine. CV Mosby, St. Louis, 1990, with permission.

Figures 17-9 and 17-18 from Langman J, Woerdeman MW: Atlas of Medical Anatomy. WB Saunders, Philadelphia, 1976, p. 265, with permission.

Figure 17-13 from Grant's Atlas of Anatomy 6th Ed. 1972 Fig. 78.1. Williams & Wilkins, Baltimore, with permission.

Figure 17-14 from Gray's Anatomy 37th Ed. 1989 Fig. 5.65, p. 617. Churchill Livingstone, Edinburgh, with permission.

Figure 17-15 Gray's Anatomy 37th Ed. 1989 Fig. 5.72, p. 623. Churchill Livingstone, Edinburgh, with permission.

Figure 17-16 from WH Hollinshead (ed.) Anatomy for Surgeons 2nd ed.: Vol. 3. E.H. Henderson. The Back and Limbs. Chapter 5: Arm, Elbow, Forearm: pp. 349–445. New York, Harper & Row, 1969, with permission.

Figure 17-20 from O'Driscoll SW, Horii E, Carmichael SW et al: The cubital tunnel and ulnar neuropathy. JBJS 73(B4): 613, 1991, with permission.

Figure 17-23 from Pappas AM, Zawacki RM, Sullivan TJ: Biomechanics of baseball pitching. Am J Sports Med 13:126, 1985, with permission.

Figure 18-1 from Acute Pain Management Guideline Panel 13 Acute Pain Management: Operative or Medical Procedures and Trauma. Clinical Practice Guideline. AHCPR Pub No 92-0032. Rockville, MD: Agency for Health Care Policy and Research, Public Health Service, U.S. Dept. of Health and Human Services. February 1992.

Figure 18-4 from Henry AK: Extensile Exposure. 2nd Ed. Williams & Wilkins, Baltimore, 1966, with permission.

Figure 18-5 from Gray's Anatomy 37th Ed. 1989 Fig. 5.72, p. 623. Churchill Livingstone, Edinburgh, with permission.

Figure 18-7 from Gray's Anatomy 37th Ed. 1989 Fig. 5.65, p. 617. Churchill Livingstone, Edinburgh, with permission.

Figures 20-2 and 20-5 from Green DP: Carpal dislocations and instabilities. p. 861. In Green DP (ed): Operative Hand Surgery. Vol. 1. 3rd Ed. Churchill Livingstone, New York, 1993, with permission.

Figure 20-9 from Bowers WH: The distal radioulnar joint. p. 973. In Green DP (ed): Operative Hand Surgery. Vol. 1. 3rd Ed. Churchill Livingstone, New York, 1993, with permission.

Figure 20-14 from Herbert TJ (ed): The Fractured Scaphoid. Quality Medical Publishing, St. Louis, 1990, p. 13, with permission.

Figure 20-16 from Whipple TL (ed): Wrist Arthroscopy. In: The Wrist. JB Lippincott, Philadelphia, 1992, p. 105, with permission.

Figure 20-17 from Taleisnik J: The Bones of the Wrist. p. 1. The Wrist. Churchill Livingstone, New York, 1985, with permission

Figures 23-2 from Gilula LA, Totty WG: Wrist trauma: roentgenographic analysis. p. 225. In Gilula LA (ed): The Traumatized Hand and Wrist. Radiographic and Anatomic Correlation. WB Saunders, Philadelphia, 1992, with permission.

Figures 24-1 from Amadio PC, Taleisnik J: Fractures of the carpal bones. p. 799. In Green DP (ed): Operative Hand Surgery. 3rd Ed. Churchill Livingstone, New York, 1993, with permission.

Figure 24-25 adapted from Eversmann WW Jr: Entrapment and compression neuropathies. In Green DP (ed): Operative Hand Surgery. 2nd Ed. Churchill Livingstone, New York, 1988, with permission.

Figures 25-3B, 25-4, 25-5, 25-6, 25-13, and 25-15 from Breen TF: Wrist and Hand Injuries (Including Upper Extremity Nerve Injuries). p. 91. In: Steinberg GG, Akins CM, Baran DT (eds): Ramamurti's Orthopaedics in Primary Care. 2nd Ed. Williams & Wilkins, Baltimore, 1992, with permission.

Figure 25-25 from Breen TF: Metacarpal rotational osteotomy for metacarpal and phalangeal fracture rotatory malunions. Techniques Orthop 6:19, 1991, with permission.

Index

Page numbers followed by *f* indicate figures; those followed by *t* indicate tables.